Frontiers in Anti-Infective Drug Discovery

(Volume 6)

Edited By

Atta-ur-Rahman, *FRS*

Kings College, University of Cambridge, Cambridge, UK

&

M. Iqbal Choudhary

H.E.J. Research Institute of Chemistry,International Center for Chemical and Biological Sciences, University of Karachi, Karachi, Pakistan

Frontiers in Anti-Infective Drug Discovery

Volume # 6

Editors: Atta-ur-Rahman and M. Iqbal Choudhary

ISSN (Online): 1879-663X

ISSN (Print): 2451-9162

ISBN (Online): 978-1-68108-479-4

ISBN (Print): 978-1-68108-480-0

First published in 2017.

General:

1. Any dispute or claim arising out of or in connection with this License Agreement or the Work (including non-contractual disputes or claims) will be governed by and construed in accordance with the laws of the U.A.E. as applied in the Emirate of Dubai. Each party agrees that the courts of the Emirate of Dubai shall have exclusive jurisdiction to settle any dispute or claim arising out of or in connection with this License Agreement or the Work (including non-contractual disputes or claims).
2. Your rights under this License Agreement will automatically terminate without notice and without the need for a court order if at any point you breach any terms of this License Agreement. In no event will any delay or failure by Bentham Science Publishers in enforcing your compliance with this License Agreement constitute a waiver of any of its rights.
3. You acknowledge that you have read this License Agreement, and agree to be bound by its terms and conditions. To the extent that any other terms and conditions presented on any website of Bentham Science Publishers conflict with, or are inconsistent with, the terms and conditions set out in this License Agreement, you acknowledge that the terms and conditions set out in this License Agreement shall prevail.

Bentham Science Publishers Ltd.
Executive Suite Y - 2
PO Box 7917, Saif Zone
Sharjah, U.A.E.
Email: subscriptions@benthamscience.org

BENTHAM
SCIENCE

CONTENTS

PREFACE

Infections kill more people than all other diseases combined. Despite the tremendous development in this field, infections are increasingly difficult to treat today because of the development of organisms resistant to antibiotics. Human sufferings because of bacterial, fungal, parasitic, and viral infections are therefore likely to increase many fold in the new future. Emerging antibiotic resistance in all infection-causing microorganisms is making many believe that the era of antibiotics is coming to an end. Recent reports establish that the chances of dying from hospital-acquired pneumonia or septicaemia are much higher from drug-resistant infections. In this context, extensive research, both in academia and in pharmaceutical industries, has begun, covering various aspects of this complex topic, such as infection biology, genomics of resistance, new drug target identification, and search for new antibiotics. It is often difficult, even for a prolific reader, to keep pace with these exciting developments. Thus, the need of a comprehensive book review series is greatly felt. The present series of volumes, partly addresses this need.

The last five volumes of the ebook series "*Frontiers in Anti-Infective Drug Discovery*" have attracted great scientific interest, as a welcome addition to the global literature in this active area of research. The present volume of this internationally recognized books series comprises of six carefully selected reviews on various aspects of infection, etiology, and treatment, contributed by leading experts in this field. Each review is focused on important aspects of anti-infection drug discovery and development, based on various innovative approaches, including relationship between infections and neurological disorders, identification of new molecular targets, outcomes of pre-clinical and clinical studies on new and novel classes of antimicrobial and antiviral drugs, combination therapies, and strategies to overcome emerging antibiotic resistance.

Pantazaki *et al.*, have reviewed some of the most striking recent reports on the relationship of infectious and inflammatory etiology with the on-set of Alzheimer's diseases (AD). Recent research has shown that many microorganisms, such as bacteria (*Helicobacter pylori*), viruses (*Herpes simplex virus*, *influenza*, CMV, *etc.*) and fungi can cause AD. It has been reported that these microorganisms and viruses can cross the blood brain membrane and cause mild to severe infections in the brain. Persistent or acute neuronal and peripheral inflammatory response against these infectious agents lead to accumulation of amyloid protein aggregates which are the major cause of AD. It has also been reported that an alternation in normal gut microbiota can cause the accumulation of functional amyloid proteins which are then transported to the Central Nervous System (CNS) causing neurologic and psychiatric disorders, such as schizophrenia, anxiety, and AD. The review provides an interesting description of the effects of chronic inflammatory responses against immune-reactive proteins as risk factors for nervous system disorders. The authors have also recommended the consumption of natural products and natural diets, such as Mediterranean and Asian diets, which are capable of preventing AD or reducing the risk of AD, and strengthening the body's ability to confront infections. In brief, this review is a comprehensive commentary based on recent literature on the possible relationship between the infection, microbiota and the on-set of Alzheimer's diseases. The authors thus support the use of chemotherapeutic and dietary approaches for the prevention of AD.

The review contributed by Dwivedi *et al.*, focuses on the conventional and current treatments of malaria comprising of natural substances and synthetic analogues. The choice of therapeutic agents against malaria depends on the species of parasite, the pattern of resistance, and the seriousness of the infection. Despite major developments in the understanding of the aetiology of malaria at the molecular level, and the introduction of new drugs, the disease is causing considerable morbidity and mortality in Asia, South America, and Sub-Saharan Africa. According the WHO, malaria kills more people world-wide than all other parasitic diseases taken together. The emergence and spread of multidrug resistant strains of malarial parasites have further limited the choice of antimalarial chemotherapeutics. This highlights the urgent need of efficient research for developing newer and broad spectrum antimalarial drugs. The development of an effective malaria vaccines has remained a major challenge for scientists, with only limited success achieved so far. This review highlights the importance of the development of new drug delivery systems which maximize the *on-site effect* and minimize the adverse effects of existing antimalarial drugs. Recent development of nanoparticles as careers for malaria chemotherapy which can minimize the side effects and improve bioavailability and selectivity of the drugs has also been discussed in this review. The authors have emphasized the need for continuous search for antimalarial drugs, giving the example of arteether (ART) and bulaquin. The review provides a comprehensive account of challenges and opportunities in malarial chemotherapy, and proposes several directions for future research in this important field.

Zehra Küçükbay and Hasan Küçükbay have contributed a chapter on recent developments in the field of novel antibiotics and antimicrobial agents. Their review presents merits and demerits of various classes of antibiotics, such as b-lactams, macrolides, fluoroquinolones, tetracyclines, and aminoglycosides, in the context of emerging resistance against them. The authors have focused on natural products as possible antimalarial agents which can circumvent the emerging resistance issues while having limited side-effects. By providing examples of fascinating natural products used against infections such as aspirin (willow plant), opioids (opium poppy), atropine (*Atropa belladonna*), and quinine (cinchona), the authors have advocated the need for searching natural chemical diversity as a source of new antimicrobial and resistance-reversal agents against increasingly resistant infections. This review thus provides an in-depth look at the most significant developments in antimalarial drug development and prospects of natural products as sources of new antimalarial drugs.

Tuberculosis or TB is among the most serious infectious diseases that can affect almost any tissue of the body, especially the lungs. Once considered to be a disease of the developing world, TB has recently emerged in the developed world as a co-infection along with HIV, since people with a compromised immune system develop TB very quickly. Many strains of *Mycobacterium* have now developed resistance against the arsenal of available drugs, making the treatment increasingly difficult. TB patients are now required to take several types of medications for long durations to eradicate the infection, prevent relapse, and avoid the development of antibiotic resistance. Recently two drugs, Bedaquiline and Delamanid, have received conditional approvals for the treatment of MDR-TB, for patients where other treatments fail. Jawed Ahsan has reviewed the recent developments in the TB chemotherapy, including new and repurposed antitubercular drugs in advanced phases of clinical trials. He has also commented on various vaccine candidates which are in clinical development. The review also discusses the need of new diagnostics, and anti-TB drugs as well as TB vaccines to control the spread of TB pandemic in the developing and the developed world.

Naseem Ahmed has contributed a review on widespread hepatitis viral infectious disease and its treatment. Hepatitis is wide spread, particularly in the poor regions of the world. Various forms of the hepatitis virus (hepatitis A- E) are wreaking havoc to many the health care systems of the developing world. Among the various forms, hepatitis A, B, C, D, and E are the most common. Over a billion people are estimated to be either patients or carrier of hepatitis. Cases of non-viral, and autoimmune hepatitis are widely reported due to alcohol consumption, use of medications against chronic disorders, and spread of autoimmune diseases. Current treatment options are often expensive, and beyond the reach of poor patients. However recent developments in this field have been very promising. Interferons alone or pegylated interferons have been used with 35-40% success, and numerous side effects. New medicines which target NS3/4A protease, NS5B polymerase, and NS5A enzymes have been developed with phenomenal success of 70-90%. Several other inhibitors of NS5B and NS5A polymerase targets are in various stages of development. The chapter provides an excellent review of the recent literature on new antiviral drug development, identification of new targets, investigational and novel therapies and most importantly merits and demerits of existing anti-hepatitis medicines.

Finally, the review by Shukla *et al.*, is focused on the discovery and development of various classes of natural and synthetic peptides and polypeptides as novel anti-infective agents as well as structure -function relationships. The emergence of resistance has led to the development of non-classical antibiotics, including peptide antibiotics, especially cationic peptides. Several thousands of such peptides have been isolated from natural sources (plants, animals, microbial, *etc*), and many more have been synthesized. However only a few have entered into clinical trials. As antimicrobial peptides (AMPs) kill bacteria quickly by the physical disruption of cell membranes, the emergence of resistance against them is less likely. The authors have also discussed various aspects of uses of AMPs, including their possible use as delivery vectors to transport the cell impermeable drugs to the cell interior. Their diverse and broad spectrum antimicrobial activity has been described in literature. These peptides offer a potentially rich source of novel antimicrobial agents. The authors have presented numerous examples of AMPs along with reports of modifications in the existing peptides, isolation of novel peptides from nature, the introduction of non-natural amino acids in their structures, and their mechanisms of action.

We are pleased to express our gratitude to all the authors of the above cited reviews for their excellent scholarly contributions to the 6th volume of this ebook series. We also appreciate the efforts of the brilliant publication team of Bentham Science Publishers for the efficient processing of the treatise. The skills and efforts of Ms. Fariya Zulfiqar (Assistant Manager Publications) & Mr. Shehzad Naqvi (Manager Publications), and excellent management of Mr. Mahmood Alam (Director Publications) are greatly appreciated. We also hope that like the previous volumes of this internationally recognized book series, the current volume will also receive a wide readership from scientists and research students.

Atta-ur-Rahman, *FRS*
Kings College
University of Cambridge
UK

&

M. Iqbal Choudhary
H.E.J. Research Institute of Chemistry
International Center for Chemical and Biological Sciences
University of Karachi Pakistan

List of Contributors

Anastasia A. Pantazaki	Laboratory of Biochemistry, Dept. of Chemistry, Aristotle University, "G. Papanikolaou" Hospital, Thessaloniki, Greece
Anil Kumar Dwivedi	Division of Pharmaceutics, CSIR-Central drug Research Institute, Lucknow, India Academy of Scientific and Innovative Research (AcSIR), Chennai-600113, India
Abhishek Arya	Division of Pharmaceutics, CSIR-Central drug Research Institute, Lucknow, India Academy of Scientific and Innovative Research (AcSIR), Chennai-600113, India
Dugeshwar Karley	Biofouling & Thermal Ecology Section, Water & Steam Chemistry Division, BARC Facilities, Kalpakkam, 603 102, India
Euphrosyni S. Koutsouraki	First Department of Neurology, Aristotle University, "G. Papanikolaou" Hospital, Thessaloniki, Greece
F. Zehra Küçükbay	Faculty of Pharmacy, Department of Basic Pharmaceutical Sciences, İnönü University, 44280 Malatya, Turkey
Georgios K. Katsipis	Laboratory of Biochemistry, Dept. of Chemistry, Aristotle University, "G. Papanikolaou" Hospital, Thessaloniki, Greece
Hafsa Ahmad	Division of Pharmaceutics, CSIR-Central drug Research Institute, Lucknow, India
Hasan Küçükbay	Faculty of Arts and Science, Department of Chemistry, İnönü University, 44280 Malatya, Turkey
Magda N. Tsolaki	Third Department of Neurology, Aristotle University, "G. Papanikolaou" Hospital, Thessaloniki, Greece
Marilia A. Chatzithoma	Third Department of Neurology, Aristotle University, "G. Papanikolaou" Hospital, Thessaloniki, Greece
Mohammed Jawed Ahsan	Department of Pharmaceutical Chemistry, Maharishi Arvind College of Pharmacy, Ambabari Circle, Jaipur, Rajasthan, India
Naseem Ahmed	Department of Chemistry, Indian Institute of Technology Roorkee, Roorkee-247 667, India
Pankaj Dwivedi	Division of Pharmaceutics, CSIR-Central drug Research Institute, Lucknow, India
Pavlos Gr. Myserlis	Third Department of Neurology, Aristotle University, "G. Papanikolaou" Hospital, Thessaloniki, Greece
Satish Agrawal	Division of Pharmaceutics, CSIR-Central drug Research Institute, Lucknow, India Academy of Scientific and Innovative Research (AcSIR), Chennai-600113, India
Sudhir K. Shukla	Biofouling & Thermal Ecology Section, Water & Steam Chemistry Division, BARC Facilities, Kalpakkam, 603 102, India Homi Bhabha National Institute, Mumbai 400094, India

T. Subba Rao Biofouling & Thermal Ecology Section, Water & Steam Chemistry Division,
BARC Facilities, Kalpakkam, 603 102, India
Homi Bhabha National Institute, Mumbai 400094, India

CHAPTER 1

Alternative Anti-Infective/Anti-Inflammatory Therapeutic Options for Fighting Alzheimer's Disease

Magda N. Tsolaki[1], **Euphrosyni S. Koutsouraki**[2], **Georgios K. Katsipis**[3], **Pavlos Gr. Myserlis**[1], **Marilia A. Chatzithoma**[1] and **Anastasia A. Pantazaki**[3,*]

[1] *Third Department of Neurology, Aristotle University, "G. Papanikolaou" Hospital, Thessaloniki, Greece*

[2] *First Department of Neurology, Aristotle University, "AHEPA" Hospital*

[3] *Laboratory of Biochemistry, Dept. of Chemistry, Aristotle University, 54124 Thessaloniki, Greece*

Abstract: Neurodegenerative diseases (NDs) have a serious impact on global health with no effective treatments yet available. Alzheimer's disease (AD) is an incurable, progressive neurodegenerative disorder, considered to be the most common cause of dementia. There is increasing evidence for the infectious/inflammatory etiology of AD. Although brain is assumed to be an immunologically isolated organ, many bacteria (*Helicobacter pylori*), viruses (*Herpes simplex virus*, *influenza*, CMV *etc.*), fungi, toxoplasma, are associated with AD. The presence of immune-related antigens around amyloid plaques, activated complement factors, cytokines and a wide range of related receptors in the brain of AD patients, led to the concept of "neuro-inflammation". Persistent or acute neuronal and peripheral inflammatory response to infectious agents is gradually gaining more attention, as a risk factor for someone to develop sporadic AD. The human microbiome (HM) has a pivotal role in nutrition, health and disease. About 100 trillion bacteria from up to 1000 bacterial species inhabit the gastrointestinal (GI) tract, contributing, at least in part, to what is known as the "human-biochemical" or "genetic-individuality" and resistance to disease. Several pathologies, including AD and inflammatory bowel disease, are associated with alterations in gut microbiome. Microbes of the gut microbiota or of extracorporeal origin possess the ability of producing functional amyloid proteins. These amyloids, *via* lymphatic and systemic transport to the Central Nervous System (CNS), seem to have an important role in the expression of neurologic and psychiatric disorders, such as schizophrenia, anxiety and AD. Cross-seeding of the neurodegenerative disorder proteins may be induced by these amyloids. Moreover, chronic inflammatory response to these immune-reactive proteins can also be an important risk factor for CNS well-being. Therapeutic/preventive options for halting CNS disorders' onset, could include: (a) Anti-inflammatory,

* **Corresponding author Anastasia A. Pantazaki:** Laboratory of Biochemistry, Dept. of Chemistry, Aristotle University, 54124 Thessaloniki, Greece; Tel: +30-2310-997838; Fax: +30-2310-997689; E-mail: natasa@chem.auth.gr

Atta-ur-Rahman & M. Iqbal Choudhary (Eds.)

anti-amyloid drugs (β-sheet breakers and other inhibitors of amyloid fibrillization), monoclonal antibodies, nanoparticles, which target pathological components of AD, or other medical interventions to remove infectious agents or to ameliorate their biochemical influence on GI-CNS tract, (b) Prebiotics to enhance the growth of desired organisms and reduce oxidative stress - a cause that has been implicated with AD, (c) Probiotics to provide both the desired bacteria, which increase the competitive effects with pathogens, and essential metabolic products, and to modulate the host immune system to resist in infection (d) The consumption of natural products, and the dedication to the Mediterranean (MeDi) and Asian (AsDi) Diets, abundant in bioactive compounds, are capable to prevent AD or reduce danger of AD, and strengthen the host's ability to confront infections. The significance of diet diversity leading to the microbiota diversity is a new clinically important concept. Finally, and (e) preventive medical and/or other therapies to alter the amyloids produced by bacteria, to decrease their production or stimulate their removal. This chapter is addressed to, and urges the excellent cooperation between experts of neurology/psychiatry, microbiology, biochemistry, dietary and nutritional sciences, in order to confront AD.

Keywords: Alzheimer's disease, Infection, Inflammation, Dietary interventions, Natural products, Mediterranean Diet (MeDi), Asian Diet (AsDi), Anti-amyloid treatment, Monoclonal antibodies, AD diagnosis, AD treatment.

1. ALZHEIMER'S DISEASE (AD)

1.1. Epidemiology

AD is a progressive neurodegenerative disorder affecting millions of people worldwide.

Due to an increasingly aging population, AD represents a crucial issue for the healthcare system because of its widespread prevalence and the burden of its care needs. It is one of the most devastating diseases for the older population, and has become a major healthcare burden in the increasingly aging society worldwide. Currently, there are still only symptomatic treatments available, just to manage the symptoms and slow down disease progression. It is a progressive brain disorder that minimizes memory ability and other cognitive functions associated with intellectual and social skills. It has become a colossal medical and socio-economic challenge in the growing elderly population. As the most common dementia known, AD affects 5.4 million Americans, 10 million Europeans and nearly 47 million people worldwide [1]. The number of dementia cases is anticipated to triple by 2050 [2]. Two forms of AD are known: sporadic and familial AD. Sporadic AD affects people mostly after age 60 and makes up about 97% of all cases. Familial AD occurs at an earlier age between 30-50 and results when one parent passes a mutated gene associated with this dementia to their offspring. Each child of an individual with familial AD has a 50% chance of inheriting the mutated gene and developing this dementia. There is an amyloid precursor protein (APP) mutation [alanine-673-->valine-673 (A673V)] that causes disease only in the homozygous state, whereas heterozygous carriers were unaffected, consistent with a recessive Mendelian trait of inheritance. The A673V mutation affected APP processing, resulting in enhanced beta-amyloid (Aβ) production and formation of amyloid fibrils *in vitro* [3].

It is a considerable and galloping public health anxiety, with significant augmentation reflected in the future, especially in low-to-middle income countries [4]. Moreover, there is at present unanimity that a considerable analogy of cases are potentially preventable [5]. Preventing or delaying the clinical onset of dementia would have a substantial effect on disease numbers [6]. It has been suggested that approximately a third of AD cases could be attributed to seven potentially modifiable risk factors: diabetes, midlife hypertension, obesity, smoking, depression, cognitive inactivity, and low educational attainment [7].

1.2. Pathogenesis

Several hypotheses have been proposed for the pathogenesis of AD, but none of them is satisfactory enough to elucidate its full spectrum. Most possibly this is why the current therapeutic strategies have shown limited – if any – effectiveness [8]. In the last two decades, more evidence has supported a role for neuro-inflammation and immune system dys-regulation in AD [9 - 11]. It remains unclear whether astrocytes, microglia and immune cells influence disease onset, progression or both. Aβ peptides that aggregate extra-cellularly in the typical neuritic plaques generate a constant inflammatory environment. This engenders a protracted activation of microglial and astroglial cells that excite neuronal injury and provoke the alteration of the blood brain barrier (BBB), damaging the permeability of blood vessels. Recent data support the role of the BBB as a link between neuro-inflammation, the immune system and AD [12 - 14]. Hence, a thorough investigation of the neuro-inflammatory and immune system routes that affect neurodegeneration and unusual enthralling findings like microglia-originated micro-vesicles, particulate as inflammasomes and signalosomes will ultimately contribute to the elucidation of the pathological process. Finally, we should advance with attention in order to define whether the role of neuro-inflammation in AD is "causal or sequential", but rather focalize on the identification of its precise pathological participation [15].

Two basic discoveries spurred research into inflammation as a driving force in the pathogenesis of AD. The first was the identification of activated microglia in association with the lesions [16]. The second was the discovery that patients with rheumatoid arthritis, who regularly consume anti-inflammatory agents, were relatively spared from the disease [17]. These findings led to the inflammatory pathways that were involved in AD pathogenesis. A pivotal advance was the discovery that Aβ activated the complement system [18]. This drew attention on the anti-inflammatory blockage of complement activation. More than 15 epidemiological studies indicated a sparing effect of non-steroidal anti-inflammatory drugs (NSAIDs) in AD; the longer the NSAIDs were used prior to clinical diagnosis, the greater the sparing effect. However clinical trials with NSAIDS in elderly people demonstrated many side effects [19].

It is accepted that the onset of AD initiates at least ten years before cognitive impairment allows clinical diagnosis, expunging the participation of NSAIDs, other anti-inflammatory drugs, or complement activation blockers, in the treatment of AD. The essential role of neuro-inflammation in AD has been indicated more than 30 years before. The inhibition of neuro-inflammation has become a key issue for AD and other chronic neurological disorders. Additionally, inflammation, as a reaction to amyloid deposition, is thought to accelcrate cognitive decline [20].

The discovery that certain early-start familial forms of AD seems to be originated by an increased precipitation of Aβ peptides directs towards the hypothesis that amyloidogenic Aβ is closely associated in the AD pathogenic process [21]. There is proof that the primordial pathology in AD is stimulated by oligomeric species and Aβ-sheet comprising amyloid fibrils, originating from full-length Aβ1-42 [22]. Numerous variants of Aβ1-42 oligomers have been discussed as pathological factors in AD [23]. Recently, it was pointed out that, due to their biophysical characteristics, Aβ1-42 oligomers tend to aggregate into inert amyloid plaques in contrast to N-truncated Aβ4-42 and pyroglutamate Aβ3-42 (Aβ pE3-42)-m-peptides, who remain soluble and maintain their toxic profile for a longer time period [24, 25]. Although Aβ4-42 is highly abundant in AD brains and was discovered as the first N-truncated peptide [26], it's possible role in AD pathology has been largely overlooked [9].

1.3. Diagnosis

Current studies address four main questions:

1. Are the current diagnostic criteria for dementia reliable?
2. Are the current diagnostic criteria able to establish a diagnosis for the widespread dementias in the aged people?
3. Do laboratory trials ameliorate the precision of the clinical diagnosis of dementia?
4. What co-morbidities should be evaluated in elderly patients undergoing an initial assessment for dementia?

Diagnostic criteria for dementia have improved since 1994, using more accurate clinical definitions and the new techniques of neuro-imaging, biomarkers, and genetic tests [27].

1.3.1. Monoclonal Antibodies in the Diagnosis of AD

Current diagnostic methods using sequence-specific antibodies against less toxic fibrillary and monomeric Aβ42 run the risk of false positive. Hence, conformation-specific antibodies against neurotoxic Aβ42 oligomers have garnered much attention for developing more accurate diagnostics. Antibody 24B3, highly specific for the toxic Aβ42 conformer that has a turn at Glu22 and Asp23, recognizes a putative Aβ42 dimer, which forms stable and neurotoxic oligomers more potently than the monomer. 24B3 significantly rescues Aβ42-induced neurotoxicity, whereas sequence-specific antibodies such as 4G8 and 82E1, which recognize the N-terminus, do not. The ratio of toxic to total Aβ42 in the cerebral spinal fluid (CSF) of AD patients is significantly higher than in control subjects as measured by sandwich ELISA using antibodies 24B3 and 82E1. Thus, 24B3 may be useful for AD diagnosis and therapy [25].

According to the recent 2011 guidelines of the National Institute on Aging and the Alzheimer's Association workgroup, CSF neurodegenerative biomarkers are now recommended in addition to patient's medical history, clinical examination, neuropsychological testing and laboratory assessment in order to enhance the certainty of the diagnosis of AD *in vivo* [28].

1.4. Treatment

The current treatment of AD is based on four acetylcholinesterase inhibitors (AChEI) – Tacrine and its successors Donepezil, Galantamine, Rivastigmine – affecting the cholinergic system and memantine – an N-methyl-D-aspartate receptor (NMDAR) antagonist, affecting the glutamatergic system (Table **1**).

Since 2003, no new drugs have been approved for treatment of AD. Despite recent debate regarding the so-called Aβ cascade hypothesis, new evidence supports the concept that an imbalance between production and clearance of Aβ42 and related Aβ peptides is a very early, often initiating event in AD. Confirmation that presenilin is the catalytic site of γ-secretase has provided a linchpin: all dominant mutations causing early-onset AD occur either in the substrate APP or the protease (presenilin) of the reaction that generates Aβ. Duplication of the wild-type APP gene in Down's syndrome leads to Aβ deposits in the teens, followed by microgliosis, astrocytosis, and neurofibrillary tangles typical of AD [29]. Apolipoprotein E ε4, which predisposes to AD in > 40% of cases, has been found to impair Aβ clearance from the brain [30]. Soluble oligomers of Aβ42 isolated from AD patients', can decrease synapse number, inhibit long-term potentiation, and enhance long-term synaptic depression in rodent hippocampus. Moreover, a cerebral injection of these isolated peptides in healthy rats, impair memory [31]. The human oligomers also induce hyper-phosphorylation of tau at AD-relevant epitopes and cause neuritic dystrophy in cultured neurons [32]. Crossing human APP with human tau transgenic mice enhances tau-positive neurotoxicity. In humans, new studies show that low CSF Aβ42 and amyloid-PET positivity precede other AD manifestations by many years. Most importantly, recent trials of three different Aβ antibodies (solanezumab, crenezumab, and aducanumab) have suggested a slowing of cognitive decline in post hoc analyses of mild AD subjects [33]. Although many factors contribute to AD pathogenesis, Aβ dys-homeostasis has emerged as the most extensively validated and compelling therapeutic target. To date, phase 3 immunotherapy trials with humanized monoclonal antibodies (mAb) targeting cerebral amyloid in patients with mild to moderate AD have not shown significant improvements in cognitive or functional outcomes [21, 34, 35]. Ongoing clinical trials with Aβ antibodies (solanezumab, gantenerumab, crenezumab) in early stages of the disease seem to be promising, while vaccines against the tau protein (AADvac1 and ACI-35) are now in early-stage trials [36].

Table 1. Chemical structure of FDA-approved current drugs for AD.

Drugs Formula Action		
Memantine	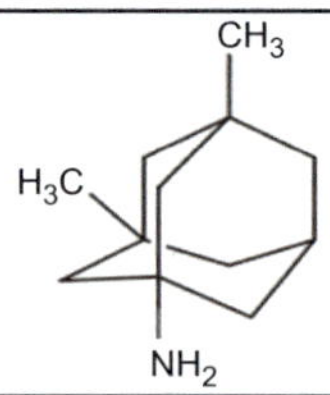	Glutamatergic system NMDA receptor antagonist
Donepezil	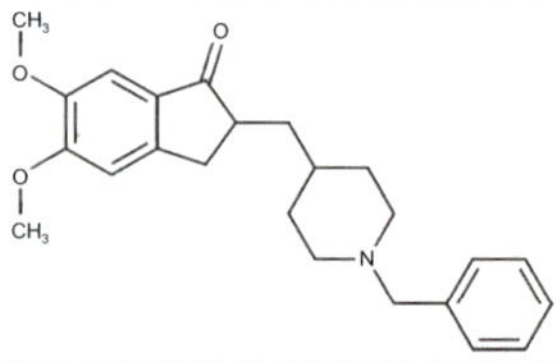	Cholinergic system AchEI
Galanthamine	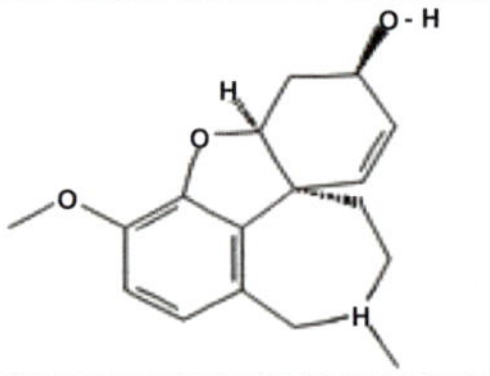	Cholinergic system AchEI

(Table 1) contd.....

Drugs Formula Action		
Rivastigmine	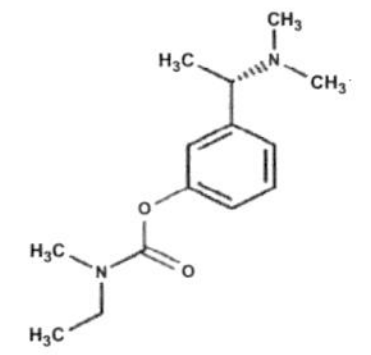	Cholinergic system AchEI
Tacrine	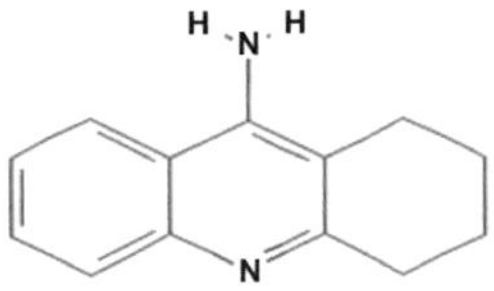	Cholinergic system AchEI

2. INFECTION AND INFLAMMATORY RESPONSE

Inflammation is the process by which the immune system defends the host from organisms or material perceived as foreign and potentially threatening. As far back as the first century AD, the Roman encyclopaedist Celsius identified inflammation as a constellation of four physical signs: Heat, pain, redness, and swelling, or in classical medical language, "Calor, dolour, rubor, and tumour." They reflect the actions of various cellular and chemical mediators that are part of the immune response [37]. Affected individuals frequently carry tell-tale signs of inflammation in their blood or in the organ system involved. These tell-tale signs, referred to as biomarkers or inflammatory markers, are found in all people, but are frequently at higher levels in people with chronic inflammatory diseases. The inflammatory markers include substances such as C-reactive protein, tumour necrosis factor (TNF), prostaglandin E2 (PGE2), and others. Inflammatory markers are signs of immune system activation, a process emerging as central to the aetiology of chronic diseases in the developed world.

It has become clear that inflammation contributes to chronic neuro-degeneration but its precise role is not clear yet and there are no effective treatments for slowing the progression of chronic conditions such as AD and Parkinson's Disease (PD). There is substantial epidemiological evidence that inflammatory co-morbidities are significant risk factors for dementia [38 - 40] and taking non-steroidal anti-inflammatory drugs protects against subsequent development of AD [41].

Consistent with a role of co-morbid inflammation, many researchers have shown that systemic inflammation can robustly alter brain inflammatory status, inducing a switching of microglial phenotype from 'primed' to activated, with the consequence of acutely elevated brain levels of IL-1b [42 - 44]. The pro-inflammatory cytokine IL-1b has been shown to contribute to impaired cognitive function and decreased neuronal viability [45 - 47]. In animal models of chronic neurodegeneration, such superimposed inflammatory activation can exacerbate the progression of neurodegenerative disease [48 - 50]. However, the mechanisms by which systemic inflammation exacerbate neurodegeneration remains unclear.

Another very interesting phenomenon is the aging of the immune system which is a continuous and dynamic process and it may be secondary to mechanisms activated by the response to the pathogens.

Innate immune response is partially affected by human aging. A decrease in the main functions of innate immunity cells, as a consequence of changes in the expression of a variety of innate immune cell receptors and altered signal transduction pathways have been reported. These defects may result in a reduced capacity to respond against bacterial and viral pathogens [51].

Adaptive immune responses also progressively decline with age [52]. Recent investigations focused on immune senescence suggested that the progressive decline of immune defense efficiency might be an adaptation mechanism to the microorganism exposure experienced by the aging organism over the life time [53 - 56]. Therefore, chronic sub-clinical infections represent important environmental factors, able to induce a reshaping of the immune system by antigen load during aging.

Several pathogens are able to induce a reshaping of adaptive immune responses and to impair the regulation of both peripheral and central immune defensive mechanisms. Defective immune defenses against some pathogens, both viruses and bacteria, may play a role in triggering chronic inflammatory responses and directly or indirectly activate neuro-inflammation [57]. In the individuals developing clinical AD, immune protective mechanisms appear to be defective. Therefore, persistent subclinical infections activate and amplify chronic neuro-inflammation and neurodegenerative mechanisms leading to progressive neuronal loss and cognitive impairment.

3. RELEVANCE OF INFECTION/INFLAMMATION TO AD PATHOGENESIS

3.1. The Role of the Innate Immune System in AD Brain

Immune responses in the CNS can be mediated by resident microglial cells and astrocytes, which are immune cells residing in the CNS and lack direct counterparts in the periphery. Furthermore, CNS immune reactions often take place in virtual isolation from the innate/adaptive immune interplay that characterizes peripheral immunity. However, microglias and astrocytes also engage in significant cross-communication with T-cells that have access to the CNS and other components of the innate immune system. It is known that chronic neuro-inflammation includes not only the long-term activation of microglial cells (and the resulting prolonged release of inflammatory facilitators), but also the resulting peak in oxidative stress. This pronounced release of inflammatory facilitator results in triggering the persistent inflammatory cascade, by recruiting additional microglial cells, effecting their proliferation, and resulting in the increased release of inflammatory factors. NDs, including AD, have been associated with chronic neuro-inflammation and elevated levels of a number of cytokines.

3.2. Inflammation in the Brain

Inflammation in the brain is largely regulated by the support cells of the CNS, the glial cells. This group of cells includes the astrocytes (which assist the metabolism in the neurons), the oligodendrocytes (which secrete the myelin insulating the neuronal axis and, thus, securing the efficient propagation of the nerve impulses) and the microglias (which serve as a local specialized immune system). Activation of the glial cells is a pivotal aspect of brain inflammation. When activated, microglias produce inflammatory facilitators, which activate other cells inducing the production of additional inflammatory facilitators. Thus, these molecules are able to complete positive feedback loops, thereby amplifying the resulting inflammation. Inflammation of the brain becomes more frequent with senescence and the process has been found to include the increased activation of microglia and astrocytes. Brain inflammation is also a key feature of AD. Even from the early stages of this ND, both oxidative damage and inflammation are usually present, and they are understood to be the result of amyloid plaques formation and the widespread apoptosis of nerve cells [58, 59].

It has been suggested that in AD, there is a period of equilibrium before the clinical outbreak of the disease; this equilibrium involves a competition between the restorative function of the immune system and the factors precipitating the disease. The symptomatic aspect of the disease is only revealed, when the immune system fails to cope with such locally-emerging threats [60]. This failure of the immune system could be the result of increasing levels of disease-causing factors, and that the immune system is no longer able to contain them, or a situation in which the immune function deteriorates or is suppressed, while the disease progresses, because of factors related (directly or indirectly) to the underlying cause of the disease. T-cell deficiency can be manifested at several levels: deficiency in memory T-cells specific for certain antigens, increased levels of regulatory T cells or of myeloid suppressor cells (MSCs) that suppress effectors' T-cell activity, or premature aging of the adaptive immune system [61].

Until recently a separating specialization was in place, with mostly neuroscientists studying the brain and mostly immunologists studying the immune system, and this specialized approach generated the tendency to consider these two systems as isolated entities. However, since more data has accumulated, strongly suggesting the importance of the immune system in regulating the aging processes in the brain, it became evident that these systems can no longer be considered independent and separate, and the need for a new interdisciplinary approach has solidified. A cardinal question that needs to be addressed is whether, with age, certain immune and inflammatory pathways become excessively activated and this, in turn, promotes degeneration, or if weak immune responses, which fail to cope with age-related stress, may contribute to disease [62].

3.3. Neuro-Inflammation in AD

There are many parallels between different NDs including atypical protein assemblies as well as induced cell death. Neurodegeneration can be found in many different levels of neuronal circuitry ranging from the molecular to systemic [63, 64]. Once viewed as a region where the immune system acts with restrictive access, because of the presence of the BBB, it is now clear that while the peripheral immune access is, indeed, restricted from and heavily regulated in the CNS, the last retains the ability to offer dynamic immune and inflammatory responses to a variety of attacks [65]. Infections, toxins, trauma, stroke and other hostile factors are capable of triggering an immediate yet transient activation of the innate immune system within the CNS [66, 67]. This acute neuro-inflammatory response includes the activation of the resident immune cells (microglia), which mature into phagocytes and the release of inflammatory mediators, such as cytokines and chemokines [68].

The sustained release of inflammatory mediators works to perpetuate the inflammatory cycle, activating additional microglia, promoting their proliferation, and resulting in further release of inflammatory factors. Due to the chronic and persistent nature of the inflammation, there is an often compromise of the BBB which increases the possibility of infiltration by peripheral macrophages into the brain parenchyma that result in further perpetuating the inflammation [65]. Under such condition, rather than assuming a protective role (as acute neuro-inflammation does), chronic neuro-inflammation has been shown to often have a detrimental and damaging effect on nervous tissue. Thus, whether neuro-inflammation results in either beneficial or harmful outcomes, in the brain may well depend on the very duration of the inflammatory response.

AD is associated with chronic neuro-inflammation as well as elevated levels of several cytokines [69 - 71]. Neuro-pathological and neuro-radiological studies have pointed towards these neuro-inflammatory responses, to initiate prior to any significant loss of neuronal populations in the progression of AD. While there is no clear evidence to support a pivotal role to any particular cytokine in the direct triggering of AD, cytokine-driven neuro-inflammation and neurotoxicity may well act as modifiers during the progression of the disease. Nevertheless, inflammatory challenges might act as triggers to uncover underlying genetic tendencies that contribute to neuronal dysfunction and death. Alternatively, viruses or bacteria might "prime" the immune system to respond aberrantly to subsequent environmental challenges. If the available evidence supports a role for neuro-inflammation in AD, it may be possible to alter the progression of disease, in affected individuals, with anti-inflammatory therapy [72].

3.4. The Role of Microglias

In the CNS, the resident tissue macrophages system consists of microglias, which are the principle mediators of inflammation. In their resting state, microglias have been observed that form a small cell soma and numerous branching processes (a ramified morphology). In healthy brain tissue, these processes are dynamic structures that are extended and retracted depending on the immediate microenvironment. During the resting state, several "key" surface receptors are expressed at low levels; these include the tyrosine phosphatase (CD 45 - also known as the leukocyte common antigen), CD14, and CD11b/CD18 (Mac-1). Moreover, cell surface receptor-ligand pairs, such as CD200R/CD200, are present to maintain neuron-glias' communication in the CNS [73].

In the presence of an activating stimulus, microglial cell-surface receptor expression is modified and the cells change from a monitoring role to protecting and repairing ones [74]. In addition to the up-regulation of the "key" surface receptors mentioned above, there is also up-regulation of proteins such as CD1, lymphocyte function-associated antigen 1 (LFA-1), intercellular adhesion molecule 1 (ICAM-1 or CD54), and of the vascular cell adhesion molecule (VCAM-1 or CD106). Activated microglias secrete a variety of inflammatory mediators including cytokines (TNF, and interleukins IL-1β and IL-6) and chemokines (macrophage inflammatory protein MIP-1α, monocyte chemo-attractant protein MCP-1 and interferon (IFN) inducible protein IP-10) that promote the inflammatory state. The morphology of the cells alters from ramified to amoeboid, as they assume their phagocytic role. These moderately active microglias are thought that perform beneficial functions, such as scavenging for neurotoxins, removing dying cells and cellular debris, and secreting trophic factors that promote neuronal survival. Persistent activation of brain-resident microglias may decrease the effectiveness of the BBB and promote quickened infiltration by peripheral macrophages, the phenotype of which is critically determined, by the microenvironment they encounter in the CNS [18].

Hypoxia and trauma reduce neuronal survival and, indirectly, trigger neuro-inflammation, as microglia becomes activated in response to the attack, in an attempt to limit further injury. Infectious agents activate microglias either through damage to infected cells or direct recognition of foreign (viral or bacterial) proteins. Following exposure to neurotoxins, such as the mitochondrial complex I inhibitor 1-methyl-4-phenyl-1,2,3,6-tetrahydropyridine (MPTP), the dopamine analogue 6-hydroxydopamine (6-OHDA), or the pesticide paraquat, microglias become activated and primed. Microglial responses to these toxins may contribute to neuronal dysfunction and eventually quicken neuro-degeneration [54]. In addition, genetic mutations that give rise to increased production of toxic oligomeric, aggregated/truncated, or oxidized protein species, promote sustained activation of microglias, and may prime the immune system for abnormal responses to subsequent attacks. Regardless of the initiating factor, all of these external or internal stimuli seem to retain the ability to precipitate a self-perpetuating inflammatory response, which, if is allowed to continue unhindered, may contributes to neuronal death.

3.5. Oxidative Stress in the Brain

Oxidative stress and inflammation are among several mechanisms, which interact through a number of pathways that contribute to neuronal loss. Other mechanisms include excessive stimulation of neurons (excitotoxicity), mis-folding and dysfunction of cardinal proteins, deregulation of gene expression, mitochondrial dysfunction, problematic calcium homeostasis, altered phosphorylation, cytoskeletal disorganization, increased extracellular matrix turnover, altered proteases/inhibitors, cell membrane malfunctions, reduced blood supply, and ineffective stress responses. These processes seem to be interconnected. Within the mitochondria, ROS are continuously produced by oxidases and the electron transport chain associated with oxidative phosphorylation. Other reactions pr-oducing ROS include the activities of cyclooxygenases, lipoxygenases, dehydrogenases and peroxidases. The subcellular sites, where these reactions take place include virtually all components of the cell, including the nucleus, the mitochondria, the lysosomes, the peroxisomes, the endoplasmic reticulum, the cytoplasm and the plasma membrane.

Oxidative damage to mitochondria has also been proposed to be a very important underlying finding in AD. This theory is supported by the observed reduction in brain metabolism, which occurs in AD patients, indicating reduced mitochondrial function. Reduced brain metabolism has been reported to precede the development of abnormalities in neuropsychological testing; suggesting that impeded brain metabolism plays a crucial role in the web of AD pathogenesis [55]. These findings are part of a growing body of evidence, suggesting that oxidative stress is indeed an important pathologic mechanism in NDs, and its onset can begin early in the diseases' process [56 - 60].

3.6. Oxidative Stress and Inflammation

Oxidative stress and inflammation may follow distinct biochemical cascades; nevertheless, both processes are closely interweaved and generally function in tandem, particularly in the brain, which is especially prone to oxidative stress. Whenever evidence of oxidative stress is found in brain specimens (*i.e.* ROS and the markers of their damage), evidence of inflammation (cytokines and other inflammatory mediators, activated immune cells, *etc.*) is also generally present. While much remains to be explored regarding oxidative stress and inflammation - and their interactions - at least two major points of convergence have been recognized and these explain their tendency to occur simultaneously and positively reinforce each other. The inflammatory response can trigger or increase oxidative stress and then the resulting activated microglias produce ROS, in their quiver of defences against pathogens and their markers. If the ROS overwhelm the cell's detoxification capacity, oxidative stress results in consequent damage to essential molecules and tissues [59].

Oxidative stress can trigger or increase inflammation through the activation of nuclear factor kappa B (NF-κB), which is known to be sensitive to oxidative stress. NF-κB is a transcription factor and, as such, it controls the expression of various genomic targets, including a variety of genes involved in the inflammatory response. NF-κB is generally associated with chronic inflammation and has also been linked to several forms of cancer with evidence suggesting that NF-κB is pivotal in the pervasive effects of oxidative stress [75].

At the same time, evidence is suggestive of Aβ, an important factor in AD, interacting in numerous ways with inflammation and oxidative stress. While there is evidence of complex interactions - with Aβ causing ROS/inflammation [76], and ROS/inflammation causing Aβ production [77, 78], an increasing body of evidence point towards this process to be initiated commonly by oxidative stress and inflammation [79 - 82].

3.7. Toll-like Receptors as Major Players in Neurodegeneration

Toll-like receptors (TLRs) are the main trans-membrane protein receptors on innate immunity cells; they bind typical, highly conserved structural motifs essential for pathogen survival, as lipopolysaccharides (LPSs) of gram-negative bacteria, peptide-glycans and lipo-peptides of gram-positive bacteria, fungal zymosan, viral double-stranded and single-stranded RNA [83, 84]. Nearly all cells within the human body express TLRs, including cells within brain tissue; both neurons, and glial cells. In cell injury and infection TLRs trigger innate immune response and modify adaptive immune response [85] and also participate in several non-immune processes: are engaged in brain development, neurogenesis, and release neurotrophic, neuro-protective factors [84].

TLRs could be activated not only by invading pathogens, but also by various mediators released from stressed or injured cells, in the absence of microbial infection [83]. In aging human brain, up-regulated transcription of pro-inflammatory cytokine genes is accompanied by markedly changed transcription of TLR receptor proteins; expression of TLR1, TLR2, TLR4, TLR5 TLR7 is elevated, whereas that of TLR9 is down-regulated. The cellular source of over-expressed TLRs in aging human brains was identified to be the mononuclear phagocytes – microglia [86]. Altered expression of TLRs in normal aging brain could be associated with greater susceptibility to AD in aged people.

3.8. TLRs in AD

Aβ is able to activate TLRs and, hence, elicits the production of pro-inflammatory cytokines, reactive oxygen and nitrogen radicals in activated microglial cells [87, 88]. The recognition of fibrillary Aβ by microglial cells occurs through its interaction with a cell surface receptor complex for fibrillary proteins, including CD36, CD47, integrin α6β1, and scavenger receptor A [89]; however, activation of TLR2, TLR4 and their co-receptor CD14 is required for linking the recognition event to mechanisms of Aβ phagocytosis and reactive oxygen production by microglia [88].

Recently, it has been demonstrated that TLR4, which is mainly expressed on microglias within the brain tissue, can mediate extensive neuronal and oligodendrocyte death, when activated with LPSs in mixed cell cultures and *in vivo* in mice. In primary cultures of mouse parietal cortex neurons Aβ42 and lipid peroxidation product 4-hydroxynonenal (HNE) increased expression of TLR4 which lead to neuronal apoptosis, whereas neurons from TLR4 mutant mice were protected against apoptosis induced by Aβ42 and HNE [90]. The loss of function mutation of *tlr4* gene strongly inhibits microglial activation by fibrillary Aβ, resulting in significantly lower release of IL-6, TNF-α and nitric oxide [76].

These results strongly suggest an important role played by TLR4 in neuro-inflammation and neurotoxicity in AD [76]. Humans bearing functional *tlr4* gene polymorphism (Asp299Gly) exhibited reduced inflammatory reactions and lower susceptibility to late-onset AD [91]. It should be emphasized, that an activation of microglial TLRs in early stage of AD elicits desired effect by reducing the Aβ burden; however, in more advanced stages of the disease, TLRs activation encourages neuro-inflammation and participates in neurodegeneration. Therefore, any potential treatment approach directed on TLRs should be modified to reflect the corresponding stage of the disease.

3.9. Conclusions

A growing body of research findings highlights the role of "immune molecules" (such as the microglias, the complement, the class-I major histo-compatibility complex and the TLR system of innate immunity) in CNS development and plasticity as well as in the general pathogenesis mechanism of neurodegeneration [83, 84, 92, 93].

Even in the absence of clear evidence to attribute a clear role for the classical inflammatory cytokines (such as TNF-α and IL-6) in neurodegeneration, and a gain of neurotoxic function by microglias, albeit, there are also promising experimental results, which describe deficits of immune activation in degenerating brain tissue, that leave room for loss-of-function paradigms. Apart from vaccines, however, medicine appears to be more successful in inhibiting the immune system rather than stimulating it. A strategy for blunting inflammatory reactions within the brain tissue should be focused on TLRs on microglias or macrophages during clinical course of neuro-degeneration. In the meantime, we need to further explore and understand the molecular events in immune cell function that occur in healthy people [63, 72].

4. INFECTIVE CAUSES

Many authors speculate that mental illnesses could be epidemic [94, 95]. Although the aetiology of the many neuropsychiatric diseases remains elusive, it is thought to entail genetic and environmental causes, and microbial pathogens have also been envisioned as contributors to the phenotype. The inability to establish unique and consistent relationships between specific environmental factors and individual neuropsychiatric conditions, has recently led to reflection upon host responses to these agents. These conditions have been attributed to various imbalances triggered either by infection, xenobiotics, diet and other environmental agents [96]. Recently, the vigorous search for microbes, their metabolites and other indications of a common mechanism, which leads to a neuropsychiatric illness, involves also the auto-immunity.

This opinion was empowered, as evidence accumulated, to support the theory that errors, in the bidirectional communication between the brain and the immune system, are substantial contributors to the aetiopathology of a big spectrum of conditions [97, 98]. New evidence supports the possibility that, except the microbes associated with infections, bacteria of the gut microbiome, also known as microbiota, can produce auto-antibodies, which target the brain, and they could provide the critical correlation between neuropsychiatric disorders and infection.

Trillions of microorganisms, collectively designated as the gut microbiota, reside throughout the GI tract, broadening host metabolic [99], digestive [100], immune [101], and neural function [102]. These microbes modulate the distant and complex center of the nervous system, the brain. Sequentially, the CNS deploys top-down regulation, forming gut microbial composition and physiology *via* inflammatory responses [103] and hypothalamus-pituitary axis (HPA). This bi-directional communication takes place through varied and mostly unexplored mechanisms, involving immune, endocrine, and neural pathways [104]. The acknowledgment of the human microbiome (HM) as a crucial contributor to health, proper nutrition, and disease aetiopathology is relatively new, and only a few peer-reviewed studies correlate the alterations in microbiota with the aetiology of human disease. Indisputable clinical evidence supports the view that it is important for the preservation of optimal health to maintain a stable and diverse gut microbial configuration. In fact, altered microbiota compositions have been correlated with various human illnesses, such as cardiovascular disease [105 - 108]. On one hand, changes in the microbial community affect behavior and vise-versa [109]. However, the microbiota is affected by countless environmental and host-related factors. Microbial metabolites regulating the axis could be one of the most important mediators [104]. The blood circulation is a sealed system and blood in healthy persons was initially considered a sterile environment [110, 111]. This definition applies mostly as the absence of microbes that can be cultivated, since blood can be an environment suitable for microbial growth [112 - 115], and bacteremia or sepsis, even at 1– 10 cells per mL [116], is potentially life-threatening [117 - 120]. Nevertheless, the idea that only truly sterile blood is found in healthy humans has been called into question, as it does not mean that non-cultivable forms of organisms or dormant microbes are absent.

Recently, thanks to the NIH's Human Microbiome project (HMP) and the European MetaHIT project, the gut metagenomics have been systematized in order to decipher the function and structure of the gut microbiota [121 - 123]. This information can be used to correlate diseases with changes in the microbiome. The Integrative HMP, the second phase of the NIH HMP, studies the interactions by analyzing host activities and microbiome in longitudinal studies of disease-specific cohorts and by developing integrated data sets of microbiome and host functional properties (The Integrative HMP (iHMP) Research Network Consortium 2014), giving us the ability to analyze microbial and host DNA (genome) and RNA (transcriptome) sequences [123]. However, the main anatomic sites, in the HMP study, where samples are collected from mouth, nose, skin, colon and vagina [124]. This means that the blood microbiome remains out of focus in spite of the blood sterility, being a subject of controversial discussion.

Other sources have recently associated the oral microbiome with AD, because it produces a chronic inflammatory response, particularly when the human immune system grows old, meaning that the cells-mediated and humoral responses are reduced. Immuno-senescence entails that the innate immune system prevails, and therefore the levels of pro-inflammatory cytokines, such as TNFa, increase. Thereafter the BBB is exposed in those cytokines' levels, and as result its coherence is jeopardized.

In addition to the rise in the bacterial load and the sterility of areas, such as blood and CSF, both of which lately have been questioned by numerous sources, they could contain immunologically-tolerated bacteria capable to be multiplied silently, escaping the detection, and to generate during the time a chronic inflammatory response. Such mechanisms are considered to play a role in the aetiopathology of back pain and atherosclerosis. AD has been correlated with inflammatory processes, but it yet remains unclear, whether this association could be essential for prevention or even therapy of the disease [125].

4.1. Bacteria

"Normal microbial flora" or as it's called lately "microbiota" is the term that describes the population of micro-organisms that inhabit the skin as well as mucous membranes of healthy individuals. This normal microbiota provides the first line of defense against microbial pathogens, assists in digestion, plays a role in toxin-degradation, and contributes to the maturation of the immune system. Changes in the normal microbiota or inflammatory stimuli can result in diseases such as inflammatory bowel disease. An attempt to understand the role played by resident microbial ecosystems in human health and disease, the HMP was launched. Many observations have already been made. For instance, it has been clarified that there are quite notable differences between individuals as far as numbers and types of species of microorganisms colonizing the colon. This field is evolving with a quick pace and our understanding of the microbiota will soon change as more information about microbial communities becomes accessible through the HMP.

4.1.1. Bacteria and CNS Assosiation

The microorganisms can be considered culpable, among the most important contributors in the generation of the amyloid plaques in AD, as already proposed a century ago by Alois Alzheimer and colleagues. These microbes originated primarily from the gut microbiota and secondly from the oral cavity that lives in co-habitation in humans, are able to arrange the nutrition and metabolism of the host organism affecting crucially the evolvement and functionality of the immune system. A number of recent evidence turns in the perception of the infectious hypothesis for AD [57, 126 - 128].

4.1.1.1. Mouth Microbiota

At birth, the mucous membranes of the pharynx and the mouth are usually characterized by sterility but can be contaminated during birth. Within 4-12 hours, the most prominent members of the local flora are viridian *streptococci* and remain so until death. They most likely come from the respiratory tracts of the mother and other individuals in the same environment. Early in life, anaerobic and aerobic *Staphylococci*, as well as gram-negative diplococci (*Moraxella catarrhalis, neisseriae*), some diphtheroids and sporadic *Lactobacilli* compose the microbiota. When teeth start to erupt, the anaerobic spirochetes, *Capnocytophaga* species, *Rothia* species, *Fusobacterium* species, and *Prevotella* species establish themselves, accompanied by some anaerobic vibrios and lactobacilli. *Actinomyces* species are normally present in tonsillar tissue and on the gingivae in adults, and a variety of protozoa may be present too. Recent studies support the association of periodontal infection and its putative links with AD [129 - 131].

4.1.1.2. Microbiota of the Intestine

At birth, the intestinal tract is sterile, but that changes when nutrition begins. In breastfed children, in the intestine environment, multiple species of lactic acid streptococci and lactobacilli are involved. They are aerobic and anaerobic, Gram-positive, non-motile organisms that produce acid from carbohydrates and thrive in pH 5.0. We encounter a slightly different environment in bottle-fed children, which is a more mixed flora, where lactobacilli are less dominant. The intestine flora alters as food habits mature towards that of an adult. Diet plays the significant part on the relative composition of the fecal and intestinal microbiome. In the adult esophagus, microorganisms arrive with food and saliva. The acidity of the stomach maintains the number of micro-organisms at a minimum. The normal acid pH of the stomach acts protectively against many pathogens and subsequently its decrease can cause extensive changes in the microbiota of all the GI, something that occurs in a degree with aging.

As the intestine pH becomes alkaline, flora gradually increases. In the duodenum, there are approximately 103-106 bacteria per gram, in the jejunum and ileum about 105-108 bacteria per gram, and in the cecum and transverse colon, 108-1010 bacteria per gram of contents. *Lactobacilli* and *Enterococci* are dominant in the upper intestine, but in the lower ileum and cecum, the microbiota is fecal. In the sigmoid colon and rectum, are found approximately 1011 bacteria per gram, composing 60% of the fecal mass. In the adult colon, 96-99% of the bacterial flora consists of anaerobes which are *Bacteroides* species and anaerobic gram-positive cocci. From it, 1-4% is facultative aerobes. Most likely there are more than 500 species of bacteria in the large intestine in an unknown percentage undesignated [132]. Many recent reports support the association of intestinal microbiota with AD [133 - 139].

An obstacle in defining the correlation between a particular pathogen and a particular CNS disorder is that even if the link is existent, it may, however, be nonspecific, as far as both the type of infectious factor which induces brain dysfunction, as well as the neurobehavioral changes that arise, are concerned. A variety of studies on animals demonstrates a clear effect on offspring brain development and behavior short after prenatal or in early postnatal exposure to non-infectious factors that mimic an actual influenza infection [140 - 146] Therefore, illustrating how maternal immune responses may modify post-infectious aftermaths in the offspring [147 - 149]. So, it becomes clear that neurobehavioral damage demands molecules that derange brain development and stem from the innate immune and inflammatory system and their cognate receptors a characteristic example being TLR3 and TLR4 [150, 151]. Pathogen-associated molecular patterns (PAMPs) are sequence motifs on infectious factors that can be recognized by pattern recognition receptors (PRRs) on dendritic cells, macrophages, microglias and other cells of the immune system [98]. Maternal activation of the immune system is also correlated with alterations in offspring immune responses in the peripheral blood [152] and the brain [140]. Such changes include reductions in T regulatory cells (Treg) and shifts toward a T helper type 2 cytokine phenotype (Th2, associated with allergic or autoimmune disorders) in studies on mice. An interesting development was that through bone marrow transplantation except for the immune disturbances in these mice, the autism-like behavior was also abolished [152]. Thus, accumulating evidence suggests that it may be the innate immune system and its metabolites dysfunction, triggered by a possible infection of neurons and glial cells. Recently, the presence of particular commensal microbes in the GI proves to be essential for brain development and health [104, 153, 154]. Some probiotics have been used in order to modify behavioral abnormalities [155 - 159]. A mechanism by which microbiota could affect the CNS is the production of bacterial metabolites that endanger the barrier integrity of the GI epithelium, allowing bacterial products with neuro-active properties to enter into the circulation. Some children with Autism Spectrum Disorder (ASD) were found to have the levels of p-cresol (4-methylphenol) elevated in their urine. P-cresol is an organic compound originating by the GI microbiota that contains the enzymes for its synthesis, but that can also stem from the environment as a contaminant [160]. Another study identified a microbe called *Sutterella*, which is rarely mentioned, in the intestine microbiome of the cecum and ileum of ASD children with GI irritations and a high ratio of behavioral recrudescence, but not in age and sex-matched control children [161]. Furthermore, deficiencies were found in the expression of glucose transporter genes and disaccharidase in the GI, parallel with the atypical representation of bacteria in their GI microbiome [162]. Although the correlation of these agents to CNS dysfunction is unknown, atypical patterns of GI microbiota are also found in some autoimmune diseases such as Type 1 diabetes [163, 164].

4.1.1.3. Appetite Regulation

Bacteria which produce short-chain fatty acids are undoubtedly regulators of appetite. On top of that, the neural function is also regulated by microbiota-mediated tryptophan metabolism [165]. The gut bacteria *Clostridium* sporogenes and *Ruminococcus gnavus* can decarboxylate tryptophan to tryptamine [166], which induces the release of serotonin by enterochromaffin cells [167]. The availability of serotonin in the colon increases under the influence of stress [168, 169]. A recent study indicates that spore-forming bacteria from gut microbiota boost the serotonin biosynthesis in the colon, thus controlling GI motility as well as platelet function [165]. This could be a mechanism in which gut microbiota affects the CNS [170].

4.1.1.4. Common Factor in Various Neurologic Conditions

There is a theory, which suggests that mis-folded proteins play an important role in the aetiopathology of some brain disorders [171]. A cause for protein mis-folding could be brain inflammation, which in turn results from inflammation in the gut microbiota since these two systems share a bi-directional connection [172, 173]. The same hypothesis applies to numerous autoimmune diseases like Multiple Sclerosis (MS), considering that dysfunctional gut microbiota promotes a pro-inflammatory state [174]. MS is frequent in Western countries [175], where diet habits considered less healthy due to disrupting GI microbiota and promoting pro-inflammatory state [176]. Interestingly, LPSs and specific antibodies have been found in patients with PD and MS with both markers indicating increased intestinal permeability [177, 178]. Studies in animals have shown that age-related changes in the brain that are found in ND, such as AD and MCI, along with immune dysfunction and extensive oxidative stress, are related with diet disrupted gut microbiota [179, 180]. Another issue, where gut microbiota seems to play an important role, is referring to the levels of the brain-derived neurotrophic factor (BDNF) that participates in the survival of neurons, and are decreased in people suffering from AD [181]. Therefore, an age-related shift in the microbiota environment might be linked to age-related neurodegeneration [182]. Notably, unhealthy dietary habits that influence the GI microbiome negatively are also risk factors for older adults with depression to demonstrate cognitive decline [183, 184].

4.1.2. Microbial-Generated Amyloids

Amyloid is a term for any insoluble, aggregated, lipoprotein-rich deposit exhibiting β-pleated sheet structures, which are oriented perpendicular to the fibrillary axis [185 - 188]. Amyloid fibrillation initiates as protein monomers that self-aggregate into dimers, oligomers, fibrils, and accumulate over time; a process resulted from the hydrophobic tendency of the aromatic amino acid peptides, which comprise the primary sequence of the amyloid [189, 190]. Amyloidogenic proteins polymerize in a cooperative way, thus can be expanded as amyloid aggregates, stemming from the already-accumulated protein, in a similar to a seeding procedure way. "Amylome" is a term used to classify amino acid sequences in proteins with inner, self-complementary interfaces and high fiber-forming ability. Its description improved our comprehension of the characteristic to form amyloids consisting of different proteins that play part in diseases [189 - 191]. The aetiopathology of amyloid-accumulating diseases, including AD, involves a prominent local response of the inflammatory system, where amyloid deposition takes place, mediated by microglial cells acting like the macrophages of the CNS. Microglias have molecular receptors on their exterior, with TLR2 being a crucial representative, in order to detect abnormal amyloid forms and begin a phagocytic response [192 - 194].

The microbiome of the GI tract has the largest population and variety of microbes in the human organism, composed from about 1014 microbes. More than 99% of the intestine microbiota constitute anaerobic bacteria with fungi, archae-bacteria, protozoa, and other micro-organisms, which consist of the rest 1% [195 - 197]. Human eukaryotic cells are largely outnumbered by about 100 to 1 from the prokaryotic cells of the microbiota, and in total, the genetic material of the microbiota outnumbers human genes by 150 to 1 [196, 197]. A recent analysis of the microbiome showed that 98% of the GI tract microbiota species fit in only 4 bacterial categories: the gram-positive *Firmicutes* (64%), gram-negative *Bacteroidetes* (23%), *Proteobacteria* (8%) and *Actinobacteria* (3%). The remaining 2% is composed of minor and quite diverse divisions [196, 198, 199]. Amyloid is also secreted by other microbiome fungi and bacteria included [196, 200]. *Escherichia coli* are equipped with extra-cellular amyloids called curli fibers, which are composed by several types of curlins, such as CsgA, CsgB, CsgC, CsgD, CsgE, CsgF, and CsgG, but the majority of the structure is composed by CsgA subunits.

These amyloids are a common secretory component that assists surface attachment, adhesion, development of biofilm and thus protection against host immune responses [199, 201]. Biofilms are roughly composed of a matrix of polymeric amyloids and lipoproteins, built in multiple forms in the extracellular environment. Intriguingly, CsgA as a decisive amyloid component, contains a PAMP, which is identified by TLR2 [202]. The list of amyloid systems that the gut microbiota employ, gradually expands including those correlating with gram-negative species of *Bacillus, Streptomyces, Staphylococcus, Pseudomonas* and others, suggesting that amyloids are a broad phenomenon exploited by a diversity of bacteria in the gut [196, 199, 201]. Consequently, considering the immense number and plethora of bacteria in the GI microbiota and their ability to construct large quantities of amyloids suggests that the human organism may be exposed to a potentially hazardous amyloid burden, particularly during senescence when the GI epithelial barrier and the BBB grow significantly permeable [195, 203, 204]

4.1.3. The Amyloid Peptides of AD and Endotoxin-mediated Inflammation

An amino acid type 3 transmembrane βAPP, *via* synergy with membrane proteins and secretase cleavage, yields Aβ peptide monomers, with Aβ40 and Aβ42 being most abundant [189, 205, 206]. Lesions in AD are associated with Aβ40 peptides, which relate with the cerebral vascular endothelium, and Aβ42 peptides which are less abundant, albeit more neurotoxic and hydrophobic. Specifically, they comprise the nuclei of the senile plaque (SP) [189, 207]. Numerous toxic biophysical qualities, as well as self-aggregation, seem to be attributed to the two hydrophobic amino acids that are found in Aβ42 and form this slightly larger molecule than Aβ40 [202, 206, 208]. The identification of Aβ42 peptides and their mis-folded clusters by microglial recognition systems, and the inefficacy of microglial cells to cope with these toxic, pro-inflammatory insertions are considered to build the molecular base for the increased oxidative stress, atypical activation of the inflammatory system and chronic inflammation indicative of a brain suffering from AD [193, 205, 209 - 214]. Thought-provoking are the facts, firstly that βAPP-originated Aβ42 peptides provoke a motif of expression of inflammatory genes characteristic of the typical immune response and inflammatory process induced by infectious factors such as LPSs, a widespread endotoxin stemming from the exterior of gram-negative bacteria [193, 215] and secondly that the existence of bacteria, LPSs or inflammation is strongly conducive to neurotoxicity caused by amyloids [187, 213, 216 - 219].

4.1.4. Molecular Mimicry

Molecular mimicry (MM) is a theoretical explanation for the aetiopathology of autoimmunity and for the survival of micro-organisms in hostile environments.

MM is based on the fact that there are various molecular similarities, both in structure and in sequence, between microbes and the host, including amyloids. This similarity is proposed that is sufficient to result in the activation of the immune system, since host molecules are now considered hostile, causing autoimmunity. MM may also be a powerful strategy that microorganisms utilize to thrive, despite the defensive host cell functions [196, 220, 221]. For instance, mitochondria are now considered to have originated from archaebacteria, which formed early in the evolutionary history through endo-symbiotic processes. Sequentially, cross-reactivity to bacterial products may exert destructive effects on mitochondria. With aging, while GI tract epithelium and BBB become more permeable, these autoimmune responses may exacerbate [195, 203, 204, 221]. This theory is partially confirmed by extragastric diseases such as rheumatic fever, basal ganglia disorder, Sydenham's chorea, low-grade systemic inflammation and their connection to the *Firmicute Streptococcus* and the gram-negative *Proteobacteria Helicobacter pylori* [95, 154, 196, 220, 222, 223]. Accordingly, a response to bacterial infection or symbiosis may result in the formation of antibodies that react with CNS mitochondria or amyloids and up-regulate CNS inflammation [221, 224]

The immense surface of the oral and nasal cavities as well as of the gut epithelium is the paramount interface for intercommunication between bacteria and human cells. It is fundamental to the immune system and the preservation of its homeostasis that it remains alert of the GI microbiota. With the gut being the bigger immune organ in the human body and the enormous microbial load contained within, it would be hazardous if it was not subject to unceasing surveillance [225]. On the other hand, this communication is bi-directional; a recent example is that anti-inflammatory Treg cell production may be amplified by a rationally selected mixture of *Clostridia* strains [226]. Moreover, it has been suggested that the immune system undergoes a sort of education by the intestinal microbiota, as it has been found that germ-free mice have weak immunity [227]. Immune cells like monocytes, macrophages, and dendritic cells are capable of recognizing pathogen-associated molecular patterns (PAMPS), enhancing antigen surveillance [228]. As it was previously mentioned bacterial amyloid is identified as a PAMP and activates TLR2 and other significant mediators of inflammation such as NFκB, TLR1, and CD14 [229, 230]. TLRs are presented on immune and neuronal cells and affect the production of a large group of inflammatory molecules such as cytokines and chemokines [231]. TLR2s are activated by a relatively wide faction of molecules, including lipoteichoic acid, peptidoglycan as well as amyloid [228].

Large quantities of T cells are located in the GI wall. They circulate extensively and may go in the brain as well [232]. The nervous system of the gut is quite extensive, including fibers supplying the epithelium, smooth muscle, blood vessels, as well as Peyer's patches. Accordingly, molecules of the immune system in the blood can reach the brain employing a handful of mechanisms. These may be active transportation through the BBB, signaling in the GI tract and proliferation of secondary agents into the brain, through the circum-ventricular organs, or signaling over nerves like the vagus [231 - 233]. Consequently, inflammation in the brain may be associated with cerebral amyloid which mimics viral or bacterial infection, activating glial cells *via* TLRs [234]. Furthermore, Notch1 up-regulation has been reported following TLR2 activation, which may intensify processes inducing AD [235].

It is now confirmed that ND associate with sterile inflammation in the brain [236, 237]. For instance, neuro-inflammation has also been reported in PD, with activation of TLR2 and stimulation of microglia [238]. In transgenic mice TLR2 assists in purging the brain from Aβ [239]. In AD, mononuclear cells found in peripheral blood, showed elevated expression of TLR2 and TLR4 [233]. Moreover, TLR2 has been demonstrated to be essential for maintaining the integrity of the GI barrier [234]. Another field where innate immunity plays an important role is goblet cell activation which influences mucus secretion and by that the gut-blood barrier [240].

CD14 is another crucial molecule of the innate immune response, which contributes to the activation of the TLR1/TLR2 complex when it is triggered by LPSs, bacterial amyloid, or by the immune reply to pathogens [241, 242]. Several processes in the peripheral inflammatory system were found to influence considerable types of neurodegeneration [231, 243]. In mice, it was reported that inflammation induced in the peripheral system, puts into action the complement pathway of the microglia, thus damaging dopaminergic neurons [244].

Inflammation and oxidative toxicity may result from TLR1/TLR2 complex activation which triggers a series of events; up-regulation of CD14 and sequentially NFκB expression and therefore activation of nitric oxide synthase (NOS) [230]. All neurodegenerative disorders are strongly linked with oxidative toxicity stemming from the production of free nitrogen and oxygen radicals [80]. It has been proposed that oxidative toxicity is considered an essential process in AD, with free radical construction leading to Aβ deposition [245].

Recent findings of rare genetic risk agents (TREM2 and clusterin) for AD, frontotemporal dementia (FTD), and PD support the crucial role of inflammation in ND [246, 247] TREM2 (Triggering Receptor Expressed on Myeloid cells 2) is expressed on a wide range of cells, including microglia, circulating and myeloid cells. TREM2 has several functions; it stimulates phagocytosis, reduces cytokine production and suppresses inflammation and it also suspends TLR activation in dendritic cells and macrophages. Clusterin is also a member of the innate immune system, which was found to be genetically associated with AD. Clusterin is mostly expressed on the microfold cells and dendritic cells of Peyer's patches in the human GI tract [248].

Therefore, following the same pattern as ankylosing spondylitis, oxidative toxicity, as well as inflammation in AD and PD, may be influenced by the exposure to bacterial products. As it was previously mentioned, bacterial amyloids and the Aβ amyloid are identified as PAMPs by a TLR2 pathway, causing oxidative toxicity and inflammation. As a result, cells of the immune system previously exposed to bacterial amyloid may react aggressively to the Aβ amyloid in the brain. These exposed cells include circulating macrophages as well as brain microglia [232]. Stimulation of the immune system by the gut microbiota may also withhold destruction of crucial brain proteins like Aβ, which normally are wiped by perivascular pathways [249, 250].

A handful of research groups observed that Aβ deposits are not necessarily connected to dementia [251]. They found that people with Aβ deposits without dementia show signs of minor inflammation compared to people with dementia and Aβ deposits [237]. Thus, bacterial amyloid may be responsible for the development of dementia, *via* priming immune cells and enhancing immune responses to overreact when they contact Aβ and other types of amyloid [243, 252].

Neurodegeneration and its connection to inflammation have yet to be fully clarified. For instance, in ND inflammation involves activation of the microglia, astroglia and the complement, as well as up-regulation of cytokine expression inducing oxidative stress without the participation of lymphocytes or macrophages [253]. The response of the immune system to bacterial amyloid may vary from pathogenic to protective, which means they can either provoke oxidative stress and up-regulate harmful cytokines, or increase clearance of hazardous oligomers. A mouse model showed that a deficiency in complement C3 obstructs priming in the microglia and increases the deposition of the plaque, thus suggesting a beneficial role of the complement component [254].

On the other hand, chaperones, which are cellular proteins that assist in folding or unfolding of other macromolecular structures, may be occupied with the non-endogenous amyloids, leading to the increased possibility of endogenous mis-folding peptides. It is also possible that by inhibiting the fibrillization of the peptides, more oligomers may be available for seeding [255, 256]. Taking all these into consideration, it seems over simplified to conclude .whether immune responses in ND are entirely protective or pathogenic.

Homology in nucleotide and peptide sequence either in primary, secondary, or tertiary structure may affect the immune system through numerous mechanisms. Molecular mimicry may enhance salutogenic developments or inhibit multiple disease progressions. Conservation of protein sequences and forms that occurred during evolution must be taken into consideration, as well as the countless opportunities for the human immune system to be altered by interactions with various forms of life like plants, viruses, and bacteria. The gut microbiota is a considerable source of such interactions, therefore MM originating in the GI tract is a strong prospect. Amyloid structured proteins are quite common due to their adaptive nature. There is speculation upon the possibility that amyloid proteins, from non-mammalian sources, could work as prions in humans. Recent studies on iatrogenic Creutzfeldt-Jakob disease (CJD), supports the concept that NDs have common features concerning propagation of disease-associated proteins as seeds. They raised concerns that Aβ, one of the hallmark injuries of AD, may be transmitted from human-to-human. Nevertheless, until further evidence emerges, prions of transmissible spongiform encephalopathies are the only NDs-associated proteins proven to disseminate clinic-pathological phenotypes [257].

Computer modeling could be used in the near future as technology advances, for predicting cross-seeding between specific proteins or peptides. Unfortunately, we don't have the means yet nor the exact knowledge of protein forms and cross-seeding mechanisms to materialize a research of that scale. In addition, researching homologous sequences is not enough anymore, since secondary and tertiary structures have to be studied as well when searching for MM mechanisms.

4.2. Viruses

Another group of researchers focusing on the potentially infectious side of AD studied the possible viral involvement instead of the prokaryotic. Elderly people have viruses and other micro-organisms present in the brain, but they are mostly dormant [258 - 260]. Nonetheless, reactivation may occur in conditions of stress and suppression of the immune system; for instance, the DNA of *herpes simplex virus* type 1 (HSV1) is amplified in the brain of patients with suppressed immune system [261]. Evidence that viruses could play a part in the aetiopathology or progression of AD has been accumulated;

i. Herpes simplex encephalitis (HSE) damages regions of the CNS associated with the limbic system, linked with memory, affective and cognitive processes and personality, the same as AD-related deficiencies [262].
ii. AD pathology in the brain of AD patients co-localizes with pathogen marks such as HSV1 DNA [260, 263, 264].

iii. The development of AD is greatly correlated with HSV infection [265 - 268].
iv. Except from the prominent inflammatory character of AD that has been already analyzed and indicates an infectious disease model [269, 270], polymorphisms of the apolipoprotein E gene (APOE), which regulates the function and efficacy of the immune system against infections [271], also affect AD risk [272, 273].
v. Studies focusing on the genome indicate that further components of the immune system, such as mutated cellular receptors used by viruses for cellular entry and intracellular transport, are AD risk factors as well [274 - 279].
vi. Intra-cerebral infusion of AD brain extracts into primates [280] and mice [281, 282] showed that some traits of AD are transmissible, probably by an amyloid seeding process.

Additionally, facts that may connect the viral infection with the aetio-pathology have also been discovered;

i. In humans, in some occasions, brain infection (*e.g.* by HIV, HSV, or measles) has symptoms similar to the ones associated with AD pathology [283 - 288]. Syphilitic dementia, generally it is recognized, that caused by the invasion, the persistence and the accumulation of *T. pallidum* in the brain. *T. pallidum,* the causative agent of syphilitic dementia, also reproduces the pathological hallmarks of AD. Moreover, several types of spirochetes, in a similar way to *T. pallidum*, can cause dementia and reproduce the characteristic hallmarks of AD [128].
ii. In cell cultures and in mice, hallmarks of AD-like Aβ deposition and tau abnormalities are recognized after infection with HSV1 [200 - 209] or bacteria [263, 289 - 291]. Antiviral medication, such as acyclovir, blocks *in vitro* HSV1-caused Aβ and tau pathology [292]. An early symptom of AD is olfactory deterioration [293]. The lateral entorhinal cortex, where the olfactory nerve leads, is the site where AD pathology subsequently advances *via* the brain [294, 295]. Therefore, it is a potential entrance to the brain for viruses [296], HSV1 included [297], together with *Chlamydia pneumonia* [298]. Furthermore, brain stem areas that shelter dormant HSV irrigate these regions directly. Thus, virus reactivation in the brainstem would disrupt tissues as those affected by AD [299].
iii. A viral infection up-regulates the gene encoding cholesterol 25-hydroxylase (CH25H) and its product (25-hydroxycholesterol, 25OHC) enhancing the innate antiviral response [300, 301].
iv. Polymorphisms in the CH25H gene dictate susceptibility to AD and deposition of Aβ [302], indicating that 25OHC may induce Aβ deposition, suggesting a link between viral infection and Aβ production [303].
v. Aβ is a peptide with antimicrobial features against numerous bacteria and yeast

[304], as well as antiviral features [305 - 307]. Another peptide with similar activity is β-defensin 1 and it also undergoes up-regulation in AD patients [308].

As far as HSV1 is concerned, there are numerous publications by various research groups, which show that this virus plays a great part either directly or indirectly in the disease's appearance and evolution. Some studies suggest that the virus endorses the risk of the disease, when it coexists in the brain of people with the ε4 allele of *APOE* [309], with that allele being a confirmed susceptibility agent for AD as well as for other infectious diseases [310], such as *herpes labialis*. Of course, there are reports that oppose that view dating over a decade ago [311 - 313], making the topic a controversial one, despite the recent supportive findings. It is not hard to recall the opposition that initially existed, against theories and data supporting that cancer in some cases could be of viral infection, or that ulcer could be caused by bacteria. Therefore, infectious agents, such as HSV1, *Chlamydia pneumonia*, and spirochetes, may reach the CNS and inhabit there in dormant form. In the passage of time, either because of senescence, stress, or other conditions that lead to immunosuspension, these agents may be reactivated. Consequently, the damage to the neurons (either caused directly by viruses, or by virus enhanced inflammation) leads to gradual synaptic malfunction, neuronal degeneration, and finally to AD. This damage involves the induction of Aβ, which may initially have a defensive role, but its accumulation later through "the seeding process" leads to further damage.

4.3. Fungi

New perspectives opened, when it has been considered the possibility that fungal infection could be a risk factor for AD or even that AD could be a fungal disease. Recent findings show that fungi can be found in brain tissue from various regions of the CNS in AD patients. In a small study, all eighteen samples out of AD patients showed clear evidence of fungal cells inside neurons or extra-cellularly [314]. Thus, 100% of the AD patients who were analyzed this far by that laboratory, display fungal cells and material in the CNS. Moreover, fungal macromolecules, such as polysaccharides, proteins and DNA have been found in the blood serum from AD patients [315]. Additionally, from the frozen tissue of AD brains, fungal proteins and DNA were identified by proteomic analyses and PCR [316]. Findings from other laboratories reinforce the possibility of fungal infection in AD. For instance, in AD brains have been also found chitin bodies [317, 318]. One explanation for their presence, is that they are abnormally produced by neuronal cells and participate in the amyloidogenic process [319]. However, chitin is also a component of the fungal cell wall, therefore these chitin polysaccharides may stem from fungi. In AD patients increased chitinase levels, which are detected in blood serum and cerebrospinal fluid, support this theory [320 - 323]. Supposedly, the substrate, in this case, fungal chitin, enhances the production of chitinases. Additionally, in two patients diagnosed with AD, antifungal treatment has reduced clinical symptoms [324, 325]. Although a possible interpretation, in that case, is that these patients were misdiagnosed, it offers an alternative perspective as to a potential connection. Intriguingly, Aβ peptide has strong antimicrobial activity, especially against *Candida albicans*. Consequently, a chronic fungal infection in CNS could be a potential trigger agent for the production of Aβ deposits and thereafter of AD.

Hypothetically accepting that fungi are the etiological factor of AD, all of the symptoms detected in AD patients can be promptly explained. For instance, the gradual progression of the disease agrees with the chronic nature of fungal infections when they remain untreated. Furthermore, activation of the immune system may be caused by an infectious fungal factor. Spread fungal infections can enhance the production of cytokines [326 - 328], which may occur years before the outbreak of the cognitive decline observed in AD patients. Sequentially, this disseminated infection may gradually extend to the CNS, with synaptic dysfunction and neuronal loss following, when the microbial burden in the CNS increases. The presence of one fungal infection can promote the settlement of other fungal species that may affect more areas of the CNS, concluding to mixed fungal infections. The differences observed in AD patients, as it concerns both severity and evolution of the related symptoms, could possibly be mirrored in the diversity or the combination of fungal species that may infect the CNS. Moreover, the pathologic physiology of the blood vessels found in AD can be interpreted as fungal infections, particularly in arteries, where the oxygen distribution is higher [329 - 331]. Finally, the symptoms characterizing AD pathology do not seem incompatible with the possibility that AD may be of fungal origin. The presence of fungal infection in AD may be due to its participation in the aetiopathology of the disease, but on the other hand, it could also mean that AD patients are prone to this type of infection [332, 333]. Immune senescence, diet changes that come with age and hygiene habits, may contribute in ways not yet clarified to that particular microbial profile. Therefore, further research on the subject must take place, in order for safer conclusions to be extracted, as in what measure fungal infection participates in AD aetiopathology.

5. INFLAMMATORY FACTORS

5.1. LPSs-Induced Neuro-Inflammation

5.1.1. LPSs: Structure, Role, Biological Effects

LPSs are antigenic constituents of the outer membrane (OM) of Gram-negative bacteria, which surrounds peptidoglycans layer. Up to $3.5x10^6$ LPSs molecules, can be present on the bacterial cell surface [334, 335]. Alongside phospholipids and OM lipoproteins (OMPs), LPSs are part of a mosaic-type membrane from which they project towards their outer environment, as proved by their functions as recognition patterns for bacteriophages and innate immune system receptors [336, 337]. LPSs are amphipathic molecules and are comprised of three main domains – a hydrophobic lipid anchor, the core oligosaccharide and the hydrophilic O-antigen.

The lipid anchor (termed lipid A) consists of a disaccharide bound to variable numbers (usually six) of fatty acids and is the most highly conserved part of the molecule, whereas variations still exist and studied for plenty of bacteria. Lipid A is the most prominent biological effector of the molecule, and its chemical identity and integrity are essential for the antigenic reaction. Altered or prodromal forms of Lipid A are not partially or at all able to induce the release of inflammatory markers, as has been extensively studied and referenced before [338, 339]. The core oligosaccharide – constructed mainly by hexoses – is much more variable, even at the same-organism. Finally, the O-antigen is built by repeating units of mono- or oligosaccharides and is highly variable in structure [334].

LPSs are considered to be indispensable for the viability of Gram-negative bacteria in their hosts. The low fluidity of the highly ordered structure of the LPSs monolayer helps bacteria to resist both hydrophobic and hydrophilic antimicrobial compounds [340]. Also, LPSs layer is stabilized by associated divalent cations and represents an effective barrier of the bacterial cell towards external stress factors. Many compounds with antibiotic properties, such as the group of poly-myxin, cationic proteins, and peptides or polyamines, and also chelators like ethylene di-amino-tri-acetic acid (EDTA) or nitrile-tri-acetic acid (NTA), take advantage of that property, by destabilizing the tight interactions of the LPS-cation-network on the bacterial surface and increasing the permeability of the outer membrane [341].

LPSs immuno-stimulatory ability is extremely weak when it is incorporated into the bacterial OM [342], but after release from the bacterial wall, its toxic constituent - lipid A - is recognized by immune cells, causing inflammatory responses. LPSs and other cell wall constituents are shed from the bacterial cells when they multiply but also when bacteria die or lyse [343]. In addition, several antibiotics are known to cause the release of LPS from bacteria, due to filamentation, cell-wall breakage and cell lysis [344 - 346].

Recognition of PAMPs by the human innate immune system is a core process for harnessing bacteria outgrowth and viral replication and spread. Several microbial components are recognized as PAMPs, including glycolipids, cell-wall acids and nucleic acids. Lipid A is one the most well-studied PAMPs [347]. Minute amounts of LPSs at bloodstream are an early sign of infection and prepare the immune system to confront invading bacteria. They can also lead to fatal septic shock syndrome, if the inflammatory response is amplified and uncontrolled. Luckily, commensal bacteria continually produce and release a steady, non-toxic amount of LPSs at body fluids and tissues, thus helping immune system to adapt to it. However, when more generalized septic phenomena are in progress, greater quantities of these bacterial antigens are released and subsequently cause a larger scale immune reaction. This widespread activation of cells responsive to bacteria or bacterial components results in the release of various inflammatory mediators [343].

5.1.2. LPSs Signal Transduction via Toll-Like Receptor 4 (TLR4)

Given their conserved architecture, it is mostly anticipated that most types of lipid A molecules would be detected at an extremely sensitive fashion. Indeed, very low quantities as less as pico-molar levels, can stimulate an ancient receptor of the innate immune system present on macrophages and endothelial cells of animals – the TLR4 [348, 349]. TLR4 is a membrane spanning protein that is distantly related to the IL-1 receptor and is a member of TLRs family. Mice strain that are resistant to LPSs toxic effects, as demonstrated by Beutler's group, have a missense mutation in the third exon of TLR4, thus proving that signaling *via* this receptor is an important event for sensing LPSs [350].

In order for the innate immune system cells to respond to LPSs presence, various proteins are recruited [347]. LPSs binding protein (LBP) is possibly the very first of those. LBP is a 60 kDa serum glycoprotein that binds to the lipid A moiety of LPSs with a dissociation constant of 3.5 nM [351]. LPB acts as a lipid transferase, thus exchanging LPSs with CD14, a myeloid cell-surface receptor and soluble plasma protein. Both of them are also needed for transferring LPSs from bloodstream and bacteria cell-wall to high-density lipoprotein (HDL) particles, leading to its neutralization [352]. CD14 then transfers LPSs to TLR4, employing MD2 protein – a soluble protein than non-covalently associates with TLR4 and is essential for both TLR4 targeting and LPS binding [353, 354]. LPSs interact with a large hydrophobic pocket in MD-2 and directly bridges the two components of a multimeric complex resulting from the association of at least two TLR4 complexes [354].

A plethora of adaptor proteins operate downstream of TLR4, facilitating the signaling cascade events that lead to the activation of transcription factors like nuclear factor-κB (NFκB), activator protein-1 (AP-1) and interferon regulatory factor (IRF).

Two major pathways (depicted in Fig. (**1**)) are now recognized: myeloid differentiation primary response gene 88 (MyD88)-dependent pathway and a MyD88-independent pathway [347, 355]. MyD88-dependent pathway employs the adaptor proteins MyD88 and toll-interleukin-1 receptor (TIR)-domain containing adaptor protein (TIRAP). TIRAP contains a phosphatidyl inositol 4,5-biphosphate binding domain, which recruits TIRAP to the plasma membrane. TIRAP then facilitates the association between MyD88 and TLR4 to initiate MyD88-dependent signaling [356]. MyD88-independend pathway is fueled from the interactions of TLR4 with TIR-domain containing adaptor inducing IFN-β (TRIF) and TRIF-related adaptor molecule (TRAM). TRAM is employed to the plasma membrane *via* myristoylation and then recruits TRIF [357].

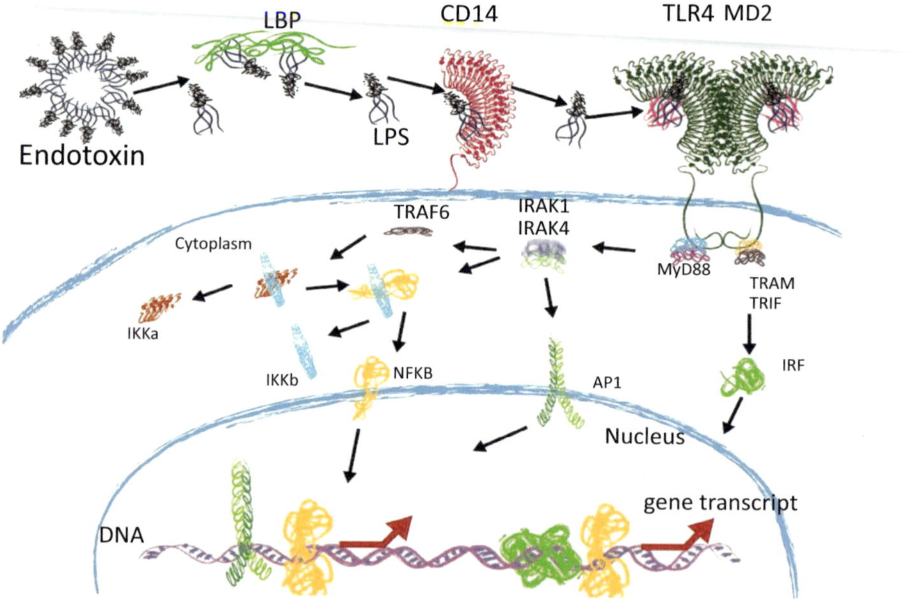

Fig. (1). LPSs–related signaling *via* TLR4. Two main pathways are now recognized, namely MyD88-dependent and MyD88-independent. MyD88-dependent pathway leads to the expression of cytokines, chemokines and inflammatory-promoter enzymes. MyD88-independent pathway is mostly responsible for the production of interferons of type I. Scheme kindly granted from Nijland *et al.*, 2014 [355].

Both of these pathways lead to the activation of specialized protein kinases, like mitogen-activated protein kinase (MAPK), phosphorylate transcription factors and lead to their translocation to the cell nucleus. Especially, MyD88-dependent pathway is responsible for the major activation of NFκB and AP1, although MyD88-deficient macrophages display a delayed activation of NFκB as well [358]. This pathway leads to the expression of pro-inflammatory cytokines, like TNFα, IL-1β, IL-6, chemokines like MCP-1, MIP-3α and IL-8 and inflammation-promoting enzymes, like inducible NO synthases (iNOS) and cyclooxygenase-2 (COX-2) [348, 359]. MyD88-independent pathway employs mainly IRF activation that, alongside NFκB, lead to the expression of Type I interferons and interferon-inducible genes [360].

5.1.3. LPS's Effect on the Permeability of the BBB

BBB is a formation established through the neurovascular system, controlling the interchange of chemicals between the CNS and the bloodstream, retaining its homeostasis and rejecting any neurotoxic substances. BBB's integrity is shielded by three modifications of the capillary bed: an induction of tight junctions that prevents intercellular (paracellular) leakage, a decrease in micropinocytosis, and a loss of intracellular pores and fenestrae [361]. Despite the austerity of BBB regarding molecular trafficking through it, peripheral injections of LPS, systemic inflammation and infections, have been proven to be able to induce neuro-inflammation, while BBB integrity is still intact and LPS is excluded from most of the cerebrum [65]. Brain dysfunction and alterations in brain metabolism and function are observed in almost 70% of septic patients. Previous studies indicate significant and occasionally long-lasting cognitive impairment, apoptotic events and neurodegeneration in animals subjected to mild systemic inflammation or septic shock [362]. How do the peripheral signals pass on through to CNS?

First of all, brain is not an absolutely isolated organ. The circumventricular organs (CVO) (*e.g.* organum vasculosum of the lamina terminalis, subfornical organ, median eminence and the area postrema) are able to detect PAMPs in the blood. These regions of the brain are characterized by a rich vascular plexus, specifically packaged blood vessels and non-tight junctions between endothelial cells, allowing large molecules from the capillaries to pass through and into the CNS. The choroid plexus and leptomeninges are also highly vascularized and local immune cells like microglia are rapidly activated by circulating pathogens [65]. Activated microglia is able to respond and spread on the message, leading to a more generalized reaction of the brain parenchyma to the infectious cause and/or its products, as will be discussed below.

Secondly, infection by bacteria, fungi or viruses (HIV, rabies virus, west Nile virus) has been proven to be able to alter the permeability of the BBB. Sometimes, this disturbance is so intense, that leads to bacteria relocation from blood to CNS and subsequently to neuro-inflammatory reactions and central diseases like meningitis and encephalitis [363 - 365]. On the one side, this mechanism is probably a rather sophisticated action of the innate defense, in order for immune cells to infiltrate CNS and confront the infectious agents. Rabies virus infection caused by the bite of silver-haired bats is a leading cause of rabies death in USA and Canada, due to ineffective inflammatory reaction in the CNS. It is proposed that an induction of BBB's permeability in these cases is not manifested, leading to an asymptomatic, mostly lethal disease [366]. On the other side, infective agents infiltration to the brain manifested by both the neuro-inflammatory stress and BBB's leakage, is the cause of encephalitis [363, 367].

BBB disruption is an effect of endotoxin administration been noted extensively. Peripheral injection of 3 mg/kg LPSs at rats induced increased takeover of insulin [368], albumin and sucrose [361, 368, 369] to all brain compartments after 24 hours, indicating increased leakage of peripheral capillary beds. Especially thalamus, frontal cortex, cerebellum, and pons-medulla had increased glucose *versus* control of over 50%. Lower doses of 0.3 mg/kg or even less, were not able to disrupt BBB's integrity, but led to weight loss, thus proving that LPS can impose its pyrogenic effects independently of BBB's disruption [361]. *In vivo* as well as *in vitro* studies investigating unbalanced sucrose and albumin ratios between central and peripheral circulation, elaborate that BBB's disruption is manifested in both para-cellular and transcellular manner [361, 370].

The mechanism, by which the BBB is disrupted during sepsis and LPSs exposure, is not yet clear, but there is a lot of research around pharmacological interventions against it. TNFα most possibly possesses central role at this matter, as a peripheral shot alone is enough to induce BBB opening [371]. Moreover, LPSs-activated pro-inflammatory mediators are known to modulate the activity and expression of P-glycoprotein (P-gp), a main transporter at the BBB, which also limits brain penetration by neurotoxins. Neuro-inflammatory factors modulate both the activity and expression of P-gp. Short-term treatment of brain endothelial cells with TNFα and NO, reduced P-gp activity [372, 373], while long-term treatment increased both its activity and total levels [373]. Microglial ROS produced by NADPH oxidase are possibly important at this route, as shown by a study employing a NADPH-oxidase inhibitor [374, 375]. LPSs are not able to cross the vasculo-endothelial barriers. Instead, it interacts with the endothelial cells, disrupting the tight junctions and possibly leading to their death. Some of the immediate noticed effects are increased NO release, architecture disruption of the tight junction proteins, high inflammatory activity of the abluminal neurons characterized by a sequential increase in TNFα, IL-1 and apoptotic factors including IL-10 and caspase-8, which resolve inflammation and induce apoptosis [369]. Inhibiting microglial activation by blocking iNOS and other generators of NO or blocking ROS prevented injury in microglial/endothelial co-cultures. Inhibition of downstream effectors of TLR4, also decreased microglial activation and BBB injury [376].

5.1.4. Neuro-Inflammation and Apoptosis Due to LPSs

Microglia is considered the main cell of the innate immune system of the CNS. Peripheral macrophages and lymphocytes are restricted, until infection or injury at the CNS generates signals leading to their recruitment. Thus, CNS-resident cells such as microglia and possibly astrocytes, represent the first line of defense against invading pathogens and potentially provide innate immune signals leading to subsequent adaptive immune responses [65]. In mice, microglia numbers in several brain regions (including hippocampus and frontal cortex) are increased as a response to an LPSs systemic shot [377]. Human brain microglia [378], astrocytes [379] and pericytes [380], have all been recognized to express TLR4 and possibly be sensitive to LPSs at cell cultures [381]. However, Tarassishin's team have argued that human astrocytes (in contrast to murine ones) are not immediately responsive to LPSs, providing evidence for the absence of CD14 expression from these cells [379]. LPSs also bind to soluble CD14 molecules in plasma, that can signal downstream to TLR4 of brain endothelial cells, in a manner needless of endocytosis and crossing of BBB, as seen by a MALDI-TOF mass spectroscopy of the hypothalamic paraventricular nucleus [382].

It is well established that the prime reaction to LPSs is TNFα production, followed by other cytokines and chemokines expression. After both systemic/intraperitoneal [178, 383] or intracerebroventricular [384] injection of *E. coli* LPSs, a dramatic increase in cerebral TNFα mRNA levels and expression has been verified. Most probably, TNFα expression is enhanced firstly at the liver, followed by peak plasma levels 1 hour after the injection. Brain showed an increase in TNFα mRNA (7,336%) and protein levels (653%) that both peaked at 1 hour. Brain TNFα mRNA synthesis occurred shortly after liver TNFα mRNA synthesis, very likely after the TNFα protein was able to enter the brain. TNF receptors (TNFR) 1 and 2 are indispensable for brain sensitization and relocation of systemic TNFα, as proven by TNFR-knock-out mice [178]. Even when LPSs are shot in the cerebroventricular system, plasma levels reach a plateau after 2 hours in parallel with TNFα peak plasma levels, indicating that the main site of immune-response to LPSs is the periphery [384]. These results support that liver-derived TNFα induced the synthesis of TNFα in the brain and that TNFα receptors in brain are essential for LPSs induced elevations of brain TNFα.

Most interesting is that, although plasma and liver levels of TNFα decline and returned to basal levels after 9 hours and 1 week respectively, levels at the brain remain high for at least 10 months. At the same time, extensive induction of microglia of substantia nigra, hippocampus and cerebral cortex is identified, amplifying TNFα expression and further increasing the expression of brain pro-inflammatory factors. This persistent neuro-inflammation should not attributed to LPSs toxicity, as a peripheral shot of TNFα induces similar effects on the brain [178]. Repeated central shots can also lead to impaired spatial memory and extensive inflammatory reaction of microglial cells within the ventral temporal lobe structures, mainly hippocampus. Also activated, hypertrophic astrocytes were spotted throughout the brains of LPSs-treated rats, increased levels of IL-1β and TNFα, and also APP, as is often found in AD patients [9]. These results demonstrate that both acute and chronic LPSs challenge, are able to induce extensive neuro-inflammatory reactions, with detrimental effects for the psychopathological status of the brain.

Apoptosis of neurons due to LPSs administration, especially those of the substantia nigra (SN), has been studied and reported. Dopaminergic (DA) neurons of the SN are shown to be the most susceptible at LPSs-induced neuro-inflammation, possibly due to the extensive number of microglia residing in it. A single systemic administration of LPSs in mice modes, results in significant loss of DA neurons beginning at 7-months post-treatment (23% loss) and reaching as high as 47% loss after 10 months [178]. An apoptotic/necrotic profile in hippocampal cells has also been established after LPS systemic challenge, with increased expression of genes encoding iNOS, COX-2 and TNFα after 3 hours, followed by sub-structural and morphological alterations, high caspase-3 activity and apoptosis-inducing factor immuno-reactivity after 24 and 48 hours. Swollen synapses and reactive, hypertrophic glial cells have also been visualized, revealing the sensitivity of hippocampus to systemic LPSs [385].

Activation of iNOS by TNFα and Interferon γ (IFN-γ) and its subsequent release in SN is a possible cause for these apoptotic events. IFN-γ is released by lymphocytes reaching site of inflammation after their co-activation by killer cells' IL-12 and IL-18 and it is imperative for the rapid expression and cytotoxic effect of iNOS [386, 387]. Whereas calcium-dependent NO synthases produce acutely low quantities of NO to serve as a neurotransmitter and signaling transducer, iNOS, when activated, produce NO over prolonged periods. High quantities of NO react with superoxide to produce peroxy-nitrite, establishing a highly-oxidizing cytotoxic environment able to cope contaminants and tumor cells. Activated microglia also produces abundant superoxide through the membrane-associated NADPH oxidase [388]. Intracranial injection directly to SN of mice lead to time- and dose-dependent activation of iNOS in microglia, with a peak at about 24 hours and return to basal levels after 7 days. Increased amounts of total nitrates plus nitrites – the end-products of NO – were also measured and increased in parallel to iNOS levels [389].

In co-cultures containing both microglia treated with LPS and cortical neurons, LPSs-activated microglia caused the death of 78±3% neurons at 48 hours. Indirect measurement of NO revealed a peak at 14 hours and a gradual decline until 48 hours. Similarly, the superoxide and/or peroxy-nitrite generated by microglia cells peaked at 12 hours. Inhibiting NOS action was enough to spare 97% of the neurons from apoptosis, whereas blocking TNFα expression did not bring up the same effects [388]. In another study, employing mixed glia and neurons, a loss of neuronal mitochondrial trans-membrane potential occurs by 12 h after LPSs and IFN-γ treatment, attributed to the activation of glial cells and up-regulation of iNOS and IL-1β [387]. Loss of the mitochondrial inner trans-membrane potential is often associated with the early stages of apoptosis [390].

5.1.5. Concluding Remarks - Probable Link to AD

LPSs are an essential component of Gram negative bacteria OM, helping them to adapt to the most unfavorable environment of their hosts. Some of these microorganisms symbiotically inhabit most of the tissues of the human body, especially the gastrointestinal gland. So, our innate immune system is constantly exposed to some quantities of LPSs shedding from these bacteria during physiological metabolic processes, or after their lysis. This exposure is probably minimal, way lower than the LPSs neuro-inflammatory levels used at the experimental models referenced above. However, when chronic bacterial infections like periodontitis, inflammatory bowel disease and *Helicobacter pylori*-mediated gastric ulcers are in progress, a larger and chronic exposure to LPS is expected. Indeed, TLR4 is overexpressed and especially TLR2 and TLR5 are stimulated after infection of gastric epithelial cells, leading to cytokines production [391 - 393]. A constant increment of gingival LPSs (354% after 2 weeks to 373% after 6 weeks) and cytokines has been documented in periodontitis rat models [394] and four- to five-fold higher level of circulating endotoxin levels and higher values in a large panel of inflammatory markers in aggressive, early-onset periodontitis [395]. Finally, in Crown's Disease, patients at the active phase of the disease have significantly higher serum levels of LPSs than quiescent-phase patients and healthy donors [396].

All of the aforementioned and other bacterial diseases, especially periodontitis [397 - 400] and *H. pylori* infection [401, 402] are linked with an increased probability for someone to develop dementia and AD. Although the link cannot be easily established, as both bacterial infections and AD are very complicated and multifactorial diseases, LPSs neuro-inflammation should be examined carefully. A single study on the circulating levels of LPSs in patients suffering from NDs like amyotrophic lateral sclerosis (ALS) and AD, identified a statistically higher titer of endotoxin compared to healthy controls, as well as a positive correlation with the levels of activated monocytes [403]. More research on the matter must be pursued, in order to elucidate the biochemical pathway to this disturbance.

It has been already noted that the main pathway for LPSs inflammation initiates by mainly peripheral and to a lesser extent, central recognition of its PAMP – lipid A, by TLR4 and possibly other TLRs. This recognition leads to intracellular signaling cascades at both infected tissues and immune cells and thus to the production of cytokines and chemokines, like TNFα, ILs and IFNs. These molecules, even if they are not produced at the brain, they can reach it and stimulate their receptors near BBB, inducing brain microglia, astroglia and even pericytes to transduce the signal and evoke an inflammatory reaction. At the same time, BBB's isolative nature is disrupted, letting more molecules to cross into the brain *e.g.* cytokines, chemokines, toxins and immune cells like macrophages and affect the neuronal environment during inflammatory process.

Constantly high values of LPSs and inflammatory factors, like the ones documented at chronic infections, most probably are able to induce a vicious cycle, constantly enlarging the inflammatory reactions in progress, while the immune system tries to cope up with the infective agents. Normally these inflammatory reactions should ameliorate over time, but when the pathogens are extremely resistant, the inflammatory challenge persists. Then, extensive inflammation can lead to prolonged cytotoxic conditions in the CNS, that are at least able to result in neuronal death and higher susceptibility of brain integrity, as demonstrated by BBB's leakage.

A lot of research brought up a possible role between A*β* clearance, tau hyper-phosphorylation and LPSs signaling. A*β*, one of the main constituents of proteinaceous aggregates in AD patients, can be cleared by microglia in the brain in TLR-pattern, but this route seems to be defective in AD [404]. Tau, a phosphoprotein that stabilizes neuronal microtubules, is maybe the most prevalent defective protein in AD brains. Tau hyper-phosphorylation mediated by various kinases *e.g.* apoptotic cyclin-dependent kinase 5 (cdk-5), glycogen synthase kinase-3β (GSK-3β), p38–MAPK and c-Jun N-terminal kinases (JNK), destabilizes the cytoskeleton of neurons and is one of the mechanisms leading to neurodegeneration in AD [405].

Activating TLRs and their co-activator CD14 were shown to stimulate the phagocytosis of fibrillary A*β* [404]. Neuro-inflammation induced by central or peripheral LPS treatment in AD mice models, lead to increased deposition of Aβ plaques [10, 48], whereas a moderate LPS-induction in the hippocampus lead to a moderate clearance of plaques [406]. Disturbance at the processes of Aβ transport through the BBB have also been studied. Lipoprotein receptor-related protein-1 (LRP-1) and P-gp, are the main proteins that mediate soluble Aβ clearance from the brain. LPSs administration can indirectly decrease the redistribution of Aβ from brain parenchyma to brain vasculature and decrease entry into blood, impair peripheral clearance of injected Aβ, increase influx through BBB, downregulate LRP-1 levels and cause its mis-localization in cultured brain endothelial cells [407, 408]. Repeated systemic administration of LPSs to 3xTg-AD mice, led to extensive microglia activation, two-fold higher levels of AT8 antibody immunoreactivity, which recognizes tau phosphorylated at Ser202 and Thr205 and AT180 antibody which recognizes tau phosphorylated at residues Thr231 and Ser235. Also, cdk5 activity was nearly twofold higher in the LPSs-treated 3xTg-AD brains studied, attributed to the higher levels of its effector p-25 protein. Amyloid metabolism did not appear to be affected at this study [405]. On the other side, both amyloid and tau metabolism is affected after LPSs treatment and after infection with *Borrelia burgdorferi, in vitro* [290]. An enhanced tau aberrant phosphorylation is referenced in rTg4510 mice, after LPSs central injection, but not of argyrophilic inclusions or total tau [409].

6. DIETARY INTERVENTIONS

Hippocrates of Kos (460 - 377 BC), the father of Medicine, was a great believer in dietary measures, in the treatment of disease. He is often quoted "Preventing is better than treating" and "let food be thy medicine and medicine be thy food".

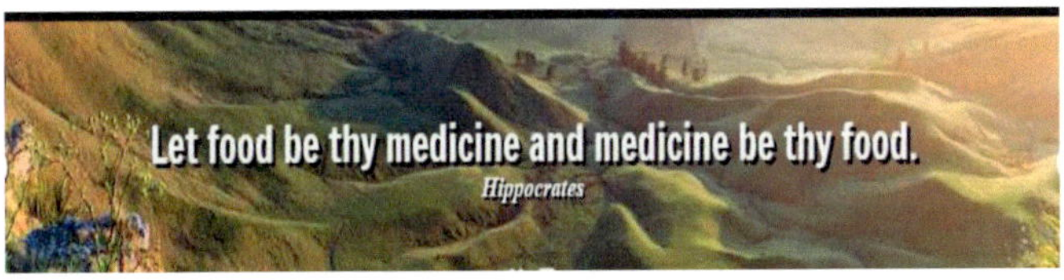

http://www.brainyquote.com/quotes/authors/h/hippocrates.html

6.1. Nutrition (Overview)

Drugs currently utilized in the cure of cognitive impairment and dementia, exhibit a very restricted therapeutic value, indicating the need to create potentially new individualized tactics (and practices), capable to impede and to delay the progression of the preliminary stages of dementia syndromes. Diet is an essential factor, which affects the risk of modern-day metabolic diseases, including cardiovascular diseases, obesity, diabetes mellitus as well as AD. The potential ability of certain foods, as well as their bioactive compounds, to reverse or prevent the advancement of the pathogenic operations, which affect these diseases, has concentrated much research interest. Plethora of nutritional constituents like antioxidants, vitamins, trace minerals, flavonoids, metabolic substrates and modulators, as well as omega-3 fatty acids among others, were collectively reported as candidate to positively multiply influences on various cellular pathways and metabolic processes, including these implicated to neurodegeneration in AD.

Many interventions were proposed to prevent or ameliorate AD. Numerous experimental studies investigated the eventual relationship between dedication to the MeDi and cognitive decrease. Specifically, it has been demonstrated that all these agents down-regulated several of the various processes involved in development of AD pathology comprising aging, amyloid deposition, neurofibrillary degeneration, synapse loss, inflammation, metabolic compromise, loss of vascular integrity, and neuronal injury and loss.

6.1.1. Prebiotics

In 1995, Gibson and Roberfroid introduced the concept of prebiotics as "a non-digestible food ingredient that beneficially affects the host by selectively stimulating the growth and/or activity of one or a limited number of bacteria in the colon, and thus improves host health" [410]. Since then, the definition has been revised many times [411 - 415], with the latest update given in the 6th Meeting of the International Scientific Association of Probiotics and Prebiotics (ISAPP) where scientists defined a prebiotic as "a selectively fermented ingredient that results in specific changes in the composition and/or activity of the gastrointestinal microbiota, thus conferring benefit(s) upon host health" [415]. Until now, there is ongoing debate on several aspects of prebiotics, with regards to specificity (stimulation of certain genera of microflora) and mechanism of action [416, 417].

Bacteria can be categorized as either beneficial or potentially harmful, based on their fermentation end products and metabolic processes. In general, colonic bacteria having an almost exclusive saccharolytic metabolism are considered beneficial. This is because the end products from a saccharolytic gut fermentation, short chain fatty acids (SCFA) namely lactate, acetate, propionate and butyrate, are considered to confer multiple beneficial physiological, metabolic and immunologic effects [410, 418 - 422]. On the other hand, substances from protein and amino acid fermentation, such as amines, ammonia and phenolic compounds can be harmful towards host health [423, 424]. Thus, genera with a peptolytic or mixed saccharolytic/peptolytic metabolic profile are considered detrimental, especially when they have the ability to form toxins or have pathogenic or opportunistic pathogenic activity [415]. Typically, *Bifidobacteria* and *Lactobacilli* (and sometimes *Eubacterium* and *Roseburia*) are generally considered beneficial [410, 415, 418], while *Bacteroides* and *Clostridia* are considered harmful [410, 415, 425].

Any ingredient that (a) is non-digestible and (b) enters the large bowel can be a candidate prebiotic. These include polysaccharide carbohydrates, proteins and lipids; however, most prebiotics are non-digestible oligosaccharides, which exert certain fermentation selectivity towards beneficial bacteria. The criteria for prebiotic classification are: i) resistance to gastric acidity, to hydrolysis by mammalian enzymes, and to gastrointestinal absorption; ii) fermentation by intestinal microflora; and iii) selective stimulation of the growth and/or activity of those intestinal bacteria that contribute to health and well-being [412].

Based on the above criteria, the majority of studies (both experimental and human) have been focused on two chemical groups: inulin-type fructans (inulin, fructo-oligosaccharides) and galacto-oligosaccharides (GOS) [426]. Strong evidence exists also for lactulose [427]. These have consistently demonstrated the ability to selectively stimulate the growth of *Bifidobacteria* and Lactic acid bacteria. However, other substances have also been studied, including manno-oligosaccharides [428], pectic-oligosaccharides [429], soybean oligosaccharides [430], isomalto-oligosaccharides [431], xylo-oligosaccharides [432] and others, but they are currently listed as candidate prebiotics, since further research is needed.

In this section, we will discuss some the above substances in association with their effect on cognitive function and AD, where applicable.

6.1.1.1. Inulin-Type Fructans

Inulin-type fructans (ITF) are linear carbohydrates consisting mainly of β-(2→1) fructosyl-fructose linkages [433]. A starting α-D-glucose moiety can also be present. ITF contain both GpyFn (α-D-glucopyranosyl-[β-D-fructofuranosyl]$_{n-1}$-D-fructofuranoside) and FpyFn (β-D-fructopyranosyl-[β-D-fructofuranosyl]$_{n-1}$- D-fructofuranoside) with fructose units ranging from 2 to 70.

Inulin is a natural occurring polysaccharide found in many plants that are part of the human diet, including leeks, asparagus, onions, wheat, garlic, chicory, bananas and artichokes [433]. It is a polymer composed mainly of fructose units, with a terminal glucose. Its degree of polymerization (DP) ranges from 2 to 60. It has been shown to be a prebiotic [433, 434], but it is probable that other characteristics may be attributable for the changes in behavior after its consumption. Studies have shown that, *in vitro*, inulin selectively stimulates the growth of *Bifidobacteria* and *Lactobacilli* [435]. It is commonly extracted from the chicory root for commercial purposes and is added to many foods, mainly to increase dietary fiber and to replace fats or carbohydrates.

Hydrolysis of inulin gives rise to a subgroup of ITF, fructo-oligosaccharides (FOS), which are defined as a fraction of oligosaccharides with a DP of less than 10 [433]. FOS can also be produced with the action of the enzyme β-fructosidase of *Aspergillus niger* on sucrose [436]. Hydrolysis of inulin also occurs in nature, owning to the high concentrations of FOS in a large number of plants, particularly Jerusalem artichoke, chicory and the Blue Agave plant [437]. Shorter FOS includes short chain FOS (scFOS), with a maximum of 5 fructose units. Inulin is usually combined with oligo-fructose and most of the published research findings have been based on the combination of the two substances.

In a 2005 animal study by Messaoudi *et al.*, researchers found that inulin ingestion may lead to improved cognitive function [438]. The study examined the behavioral and cognitive effects of oligo-fructose-enriched inulin at doses 5% and 10% in the diet, orally ingested daily during two weeks, utilizing a functional observational battery (FOB) and the light extinction test in male Wister rats. The control group received a standard diet and was tested in the same test situations. The behavioral effects were evaluated two days before and 14 days after the beginning of the intervention period and the cognitive effects were assessed after the administration period by lever-pressing activity and learning discrimination using the light extinction test paradigm. The study showed that oligo-fructose-enriched inulin at 5% in the diet, and especially at 10% in the diet, increased relaxation and stimulated and increased the general activity and interest of the rats to the test environment, compared to the control group. Both doses were associated with significant effects on learning discrimination in male rats. These findings suggested that oligo-fructose-enriched inulin, particularly at the dose of 10%, improved cognitive function and the general well-being of the male rats. However, high doses of this regimen are associated with gastrointestinal symptoms in humans and most research has used doses of less than 15 g. In a more recent study, Rozan *et al.* aimed to investigate the effects of long-term intervention with oligo-fructose-enriched inulin on behavioral, cognitive and visuomotor coordination in rats [439]. The two groups of rats were receiving either a diet with 10% oligo-fructose-enriched inulin or a standard diet tested at 12, 18 and 24 months of age. Supplementation of diet with oligo-fructose-enriched inulin was associated with age- and sex-related improvements in spatial learning abilities, depression, anxiety and vasomotor speed, indicating that long-term intervention with this substance may improve cognitive and emotional aspects of aging.

Concerning human studies, Smith *et al.* were the first to investigate the effects of regular consumption of oligo-fructose-enriched inulin on well-being, mood and cognitive performance [440]. They found that oligo-fructose-enriched inulin had no negative effects but did not improve well-being, mood or performance (both subjective reports and objective measures). In a successive study in 2015, the same authors attempted to assess the acute effects of oligo-fructose-enriched inulin over a 4-hour period, during which the participants remained in the laboratory [441]. In a double-blind, placebo-controlled trial of 47 subjects, they evaluated mood and cognitive performance at baseline and then following inulin or placebo, at two sessions, one week apart. Volunteers consumed one sachet of 5 g inulin or placebo in powder form, in decaffeinated tea or coffee with breakfast. With regards to cognitive function, the authors found that the most consistent effects were on episodic memory, where consumption of inulin was associated with great accuracy on a recognition memory task and improved immediate and delayed recall performance. There were no significant effects of inulin on mood, psychomotor performance and selective and sustained attention. However, these immediate effects of inulin (two hours after ingestion) essentially rule out a prebiotic effect and authors concluded that further research is needed in order to identify the mechanisms that underlie the acute effects of inulin.

In a small number of animal studies, FOS has been linked to improvement in oxidative stress states, similar to that seen in AD. In a 2011 study by Hsia *et al.*, the researchers aimed to determine the effects of FOS (including fructosyl-nystose, nystose and kestose) on the D-galactose (DG)-induced oxidative damage of lipids, proteins and mitochondrial DNA [442]. Subcutaneous (s.c.) DG treatment of C57BL/6J mice has been shown to be associated with enhancement of parameters of AD [443] and neurological impairment [444, 445]. The study found that, among others, FOS systematically normalized DG-induced elevations in the levels of malonaldehyde dimethyl acetal (MDA) in the cerebral cortex and protein carbonyls in the hippocampus, suggesting that this treatment could reduce oxidative damage in the brain, which is associated with age-related neurodegeneration and AD [446]. Similarly, a more recent study by Yen *et al.* sought to assess the effects of dietary FOS on the brain Aβ, amyloid-associated enzymes, cognitive performance and plasma antioxidant levels of DG-treated BALB/cJ mice [447]. They found that FOS supplementation (1) reduced the DG-induced Aβ density in the cortex and hippocampus and (2) attenuated the DG-induced protein expression of Aβ and beta-site amyloid precursor cleaving enzyme of the whole brain in a dose-response manner, suggesting that FOS' effects could be dependent on the anti-oxidant pathway. Of note, FOS was also associated with improvements in spatial learning/memory function after one day of training.

In conclusion, despite the early, promising results on the beneficial effects of an oligo-fructose-enriched inulin diet on cognitive function, mood and general well-being of animal subjects, the recent human studies have raised considerable concerns as to the real benefits of the above diet. It may be possible that inulin does confer some benefit on cognitive and behavioral performance; however, it is not sure whether this effect can be attributed to a prebiotic effect or some other effect of inulin. Similarly, FOS supplementation seems to be associated with improvements in many parameters of AD, systemic inflammation and neurodegeneration. However, how a soluble fiber diminishes the DG-induced oxidative stress and AD parameters remains to be determined. Although these preliminary studies seem promising, with regards to the effects of ITF on cognitive function, conclusions should not be drawn regarding their effect on human cognition, until properly designed clinical trials are executed and evaluated. Additionally, multiple research efforts are of vital importance, since reproducibility of the results is needed in order to reach a certain conclusion, either positive or negative.

6.1.1.2. Galacto-Oligosaccharides

Galacto-oligosaccharides (GOS) are typically formed by enzymatic treatment of lactose by β-galactosidase to produce oligomers of variable chain lengths [39]. Typically, they have a degree of polymerization ranging from 2 to 10 with a terminal glucose. The trans-galactosylation activity of β-galactosidase on lactose results in the formation of 4′- or 6′- galactosylactose, longer oligosaccharides, trans-galactosylated disaccharides and non-reducing oligosaccharides [448]. GOS are mainly produced from whey-derived lactose, but the raw material can also be lactose in cow's milk [449]. GOS are utilized in several commercial products, such as infant formulas, dairy products, sauces, soups, cereals, beverages, snack bars, ice creams, bakery products, animal feeds and as sugar replacements [450].

Only a small number of studies have investigated the potential effects of GOS on cognitive function. Namely, Waworuntu *et al.* have recently reported on the impact of dietary prebiotics poly-dextrose (PDX) and GOS, during normal early postnatal development on cognition, social- and anxiety-related behaviors in C57BL/6J mice, Sprague Dawley (SD) and Long Evans (LE) rats [451]. They found that mice fed with prebiotic diet performed better at anxiety tests, SD-prebiotic fed rats showed more positive social interactions than the controls and LE-prebiotic fed rats had higher recognition index in the novel object recognition test than the control group, indicating better memory performance. Consecutively, they performed a second group of experiments, assessing whether alterations in the gut microbiota were associated with the improved cognitive performance, observed in these animals [452]. They found a significant shift in the gut microbiota in prebiotic fed rats, in comparison to controls. Prebiotic diet resulted in significantly higher proportion of the short-chain fatty acid producing bacteria *Allobacculum*, and lower proportion of *Clostridium*.

The above results suggest that there may be an association between GOS diet and improvement in cognitive function, mediated through alterations in gut microbiota. Further research need to be done, both in animals and in humans, in order to assess the potential effects of GOS-enhanced diet on cognition.

6.1.1.3. Lactulose

Lactulose is a non-absorbable disaccharide comprised of one molecule of each galactose and fructose, linked by a β (1-4) bond [453]. It is produced commercially by isomerization of lactose. It has commonly been used for constipation and hepatic encephalopathy [454]. Limited evidence suggests its use for the treatment or prevention of neurodegenerative processes. Namely, a recent study by Lee *et al.*, evaluated the efficacy of lactulose and melibiose in treating aggregation-mediated neurodegenerative diseases, such as Alzheimer's, Parkinson's and polyglutamine (polyQ)-mediated diseases [455]. Using polyQ-mediated spinocerebellar ataxia type 17 (SCA17) cell and slice cultures, they found that lactulose effectively inhibited the aggregation in neuronal and Purkinje cells. They speculate that this was mediated through the up-regulation of autophagy of aggregated cytosolic proteins. Although the aggregates found in AD (tau and β-amyloid) differ in structure and composition from the intranuclear, perinuclear and neuritic inclusions found in polyQ SCAs, fundamental findings can shed light on the pathogenesis and potential treatment of other neurodegenerative diseases.

6.1.1.4. Candidate Prebiotics and Other Substances

Several of the ingredients below are being assessed for prebiotic activity. However, evidence is not sufficiently strong in order to classify them as prebiotics, according to the criteria presented above [412], compared to fructans or galactans.

Soybean Oligosaccharides (Glycine max L.) are a source of a wide variety of nutrients [456]. It contains oligosaccharides, vegetable protein, dietary fiber, vitamins and minerals. It can be found in many forms, including soybean flour, tofu and temphe [457]. The most important oligosaccharides found in soybean are the trisaccharide raffinose and the tetrasaccharide stachyose, which were found to have bifidogenic activity [458]. They have revealed prebiotic potential in a number of studies [430, 459, 460].

Although soy isoflavones has been the ingredient of soybeans most widely studied with regards to cognitive function and oxidative damage [461 - 466], the underlying mechanism is still not fully understood. Recent studies investigating the effect of soybean supplementation, and not isoflavones in particular, on cognitive function have also reported positive outcomes [467 - 469]. These include reversal of alprazolam- and scopolamine-induced memory deficits in experimental animals as well as suppression of cognitive dysfunctions in mice fed with green soybean through reduced Aβ accumulation, increased in Ptgds (an Aβ-chaperone) and decreased Aplp1 (a homologue of amyloid precursor protein) expression. Of note, Unno *et al.*, speculate that it may not be solely the high content of isoflavones in soybeans that is responsible for the reductions in Aβ aggregation [466]. The high levels of oligosaccharides, which stimulate Bifidobacterium growth, may increase the production of aglycones (genistein from genistin and daidzein from daidzin, required for their effective absorption) by intestinal microflora. Thus, the combination of these components may have synergistic effect on therapeutic potential.

Resistant Starch (RS) is a fiber that has many beneficial effects. There is some evidence that RS and its derivatives may act as prebiotics [470, 471]. Concerning its effects on cognition and behavior, a study by Zhou *et al.* found that RS-fed aged mice exhibited better glucose sensing and motor coordination [472]. However, Lyte *et al.* recently found that RS diet was associated with undesirable effects, such as increased anxiety-like behavior [473].

Mannan-oligosaccharides, derived from yeasts have also shown prebiotic potential [474]. Jiang *et al.* have demonstrated that the synthetic β-(1,4)-D-mannosyl oligosaccharides 6, 9, 12, 15 and 17, derived from the heterogeneous β-(1,4)-D-oligomannurate 971, have neuroprotective potency against Aβ toxicity, *in vitro*, with compounds 6 and 9 showing even more activity than 971, indicating a probable intervention against AD [475].

Glucans, consisting mainly of oligosaccharides and polysaccharides, referred to as glucooligosaccharides (GIOS) are another substance studied for their prebiotic effect [476]. Limited evidence suggests that these substances, derived from L. japonica, can directly inhibit $A\beta_{42}$ aggregation and reduce neurotoxicity induced by $A\beta_{42}$ in a dose-dependent manner, *in vitro*, presenting another potential treatment for AD [477].

Pectic Oligosaccharides have also been reported to exert selective fermentation by *Bifidobacteria*, eubacteria and *lactobacilli* [478 - 480]. In a recent report, pectin supplementation did not affect cognitive function but increased cecal short-chain fatty acids in mice [481].

Non-starch Polysaccharides (NSP) have also shown prebiotic activity [482]. Multiple clinical studies have elucidated the potential cognitive benefits of NSP supplements, in terms of improved attention, concentration and memory performance both in acute and chronic intake [483 - 487], although the exact mechanisms underlying these effects remain to be investigated.

6.1.2. Probiotics

According to an expert consultation of international scientists on behalf of the Food and Agriculture Organization of the United Nations (FAO) and the World Health Organization (WHO) in 2002 and a consensus statement provided by the International Scientific Association for Probiotics and Prebiotics (ISAPP) in 2013, a probiotic is "a live microorganism that, when administered in adequate amounts, confers a health benefit on the host" [488, 489]. The concept of probiotics was introduced by Metchnikoff who hypothesized that the normal gut microflora could have adverse effects on the host and that consumption of specific bacteria could reverse this effect [490].

One of the core elements of probiotics, as highlighted by the definition, is that the microorganism has to be alive when administered [491 - 493]. It is of vital importance that probiotics have undergone controlled evaluation to document the health benefits on the host. In fact, only products that contain live organisms that provide health benefits shown in reproducible research on human subjects can actually be claimed as probiotics [494 - 496]. A probiotic must be a taxonomically defined microbe or combination of microbes. A precise identification of the strain is (genotypic and phenotypic characterization of the tested microorganism) is an absolute necessity, since most effects of probiotics are considered to be strain-specific and cannot be extended to other probiotics of the same genus or species [493, 497]. Finally, probiotics must be administered in adequate numbers, defined as the number that is able to trigger the targeted effect on the host. This depends on strain specificity, process and matrix and targeted effect.

With regards to safety of use, according to the 2002 FAO/WHO guidelines, even for bacteria that are Generally Recognized as Safe (GRAS), the safety of the potential probiotic should be assessed by the minimum required tests:

- Determination of antibiotic resistance patterns
- Assessment of certain metabolic activities (*e.g.* D-lactate production, bile salt de-conjugation)
- Assessment of side-effects during human studies
- Epidemiological surveillance of adverse incidents in consumers (post-market)
- If the strain under evaluation belongs to a species that is a known mammalian toxin producer, it must be tested for toxin production

- If the strain under evaluation belongs to a species with known hemolytic potential, determination of hemolytic activity is required

Most of research has focused on the use of intestinal isolates of bacteria as probiotics [415]. These include lactic-acid producing bacteria, such as *lactobacilli, streptococci, enterococci, lactococci* and *bifidobacteria*, but also *Bacillus* spp. and fungi/yeasts (*Saccharomyces* spp. and *Aspergillus* spp.). According to Health Canada, the following species can be classified as probiotics, when delivered in food at a level of $1x10^9$ colony forming units (CFU) per serving: *Bifidobacteria* (*adolescentis, animalis, bifidum, breve* and *longum*) and *Lactobacilli* (*acidophilus, casei, fermentum, gasseri, johnsonii, paracasei, plantarum, rhamnosus* and *salivarius*) [498]. We will focus on the above species, classified as probiotics, and their association with cognitive function and Alzheimer's disease (AD).

6.1.2.1. Lactobacilli

A significant amount of studies has indicated that probiotic supplements can effectively improve several aspects of cognitive function, based on a variety of animal models [104, 499 - 505]. However, most evidence exists on *lactobacilli*.

Gareau *et al.* recently sought to determine the behavioral effects of acute enteric infection with *Citrobacter rodentium* on C57BL/6 mice or germ-free Swiss-Webster mice [506]. They found that memory impairment, induced by acute stress on the above groups, was prevented by treatment with a combination of probiotics including *Lactobacillus (L.) rhamnosus* R0011 and *L. helveticus* R0052. *L. helveticus* R0052 administration has also shown to prevent the negative effects of a Western-style diet and inflammatory state on anxiety-like behavior and memory [507]. Similarly, in a 2014 study aiming to determine the effects of the adaptive immune system and psychological stress on behavior in Rag^{-1-} mice, Smith *et al.* found that probiotics (*L. rhamnosus* R0011 and *L. helveticus* R0052) successfully ameliorated the immune-mediated deficits on learning, memory and anxiety-like behavior [508]. The role of *L. helveticus* NS8 on cognition was also assessed in a study by Liang *et al.* [509]. They found that supplementation with this probiotic improved chronic restraint stress-induced behavioral and cognitive dysfunction in Sprague-Dawley rats, an effect similar to and even better than that of citalopram. A *L. helveticus*-fermented milk product (Calpis sour milk whey) has also demonstrated beneficial effects on cognitive performance [510]. In particular, it was observed that the powder of this product, when administered orally, could improve scopolamine-induced cognitive impairment and memory. Another recent study evaluated anxiety-like behavior and recognition memory in a dextran sodium sulfate (DSS) mouse model of acute colitis and how probiotics could ameliorate potential cognitive disturbances seen in this state [511]. Researchers found that the mixture of *L. rhamnosus* R0011 and *L. helveticus* R0052 could effectively prevent the impaired recognition memory and anxiety-like behavior seen in this murine model of inflammatory bowel disease. It is evident that, as previously discussed, the effects of the probiotics are strain-specific.

With regards particularly to AD pathogenesis, one study evaluated fermented milks cultured with probiotic strains that improved amyloid precursor protein (APP) metabolism [512]. Initially, ethanol precipitates of the fermented milk cultured with multiple strains and isolates, including *Bifidobacterium* (B.) *bifidum, B. lactis, B. longum, L. acidophilus, L. gasseri, L. helveticus, L. johnsonii and L. rhamnosus*, were evaluated in a cell-based assay measuring APPβ level using APP and β-secretase over-expressing BA-3cells. Many precipitates decreased βAPP level, demonstrating a strain-specific effect, with *L. johnsonii, B. longum, L. gasseri* and *L. helveticus* strains showing the strongest inhibitory activities. In particular, ethanol precipitate 1:2 from *L. helveticus* IDCC3801 (EPH 1:2) demonstrated the highest decrease of sAPPβ. Further analysis showed that EPH 1:2 led to the increase of total APPα level. This is consistent with observations of APP processing, where decrease of APPβ inversely leads to increase in total APPα. Therefore, EPH 1:2 effectively blocked amyloidogenic pathway *via* the simultaneous stimulation of non-amyloidogenic pathway in APP processing. The *in-vivo* effects of EPH 1:2 were also evaluated, especially the Aβ-lowering activity in rat models. When administered orally, EPH 1:2 led to a decrease of serum Aβ40 level to more than 50%. Consequently, using the Morris water maze task, it was found that EPH 1:2 significantly improved scopolamine-induced memory impairments. Overall, the above results indicate that this strain of *L. helveticus* improved APP processing and amnesia, suggesting a potential therapeutic agent for AD.

Another probiotic agent that has been examined for its effects on several cognitive functions is the *Lactobacillus*, strain C29 (*Lactobacillus pentosus var. plantarum* C29), derived from fermentation of kimchi, a traditional Korean food. In 2012, Jung et al. were the first to report that *Lactobacillus pentosus var. plantarum* C29 protects against scopolamine-induced memory impairment in mice, as demonstrated in passive avoidance, Y-maze and Morris water maze tests [513]. Additionally, they found that C29 protects brain derived neurotrophic factor (BDNF) and cAMP response element-binding protein (CREB) expression in the hippocampus, which were reduced by scopolamine, indicating potential benefits for AD treatment, where BDNF is decreased [514]. Shortly after that, Woo *et al.* validated these results in D-galactose-induced accelerated aging mouse model [515]. They found that supplementation with C29 reduced D-galactose-induced memory deficits in the same tests (passive avoidance, Y-maze and Morris water maze tests) and that it also reversed the suppression of BDNF and CREB activation. Similarly, Jeong *et al.* recently found that C29 ameliorates memory impairment in Fischer 344 rat models by restoring doublecortin (DCX) and BDNF expression and CREB activation [516]. Other mechanisms implicated and suggested to contribute to memory improvement following C29 treatment, include suppression of p16, p-p65, p-FOXO3a, COX-2 and iNOS activation as well as activation of Akt, mTOR and NF-κB in the hippocampus [515, 516].

Other *lactobacilli* strains that have shown memory-enhancing potential include *Lactobacillus curvatus* HY7601 and *Lactobacillus plantarum* KY1032. The mixture of the above strains has been shown to attenuate age-dependent memory deficits in Fischer 344 rats (seen in Y-maze task), restore DCX and BDNF expression and reduce p16, p53, COX-2 expression, phosphorylation of Akt and mTOR and activation of NF-κB in the hippocampus [517]. *Lactobacillus plantarum* strain TWK10-fermented soymilk has also been shown to improve learning and memory in animal models of vascular dementia (H_2O_2-, oxygen-glucose deprivation (OGD) - and deoxycorticosterone acetate (DOCA)-salt-induced rat models), indicating a potential intervention for oxidative stress observed in neurodegeneration and AD [518].

Although the effect of *lactobacilli*, used as prebiotic supplements, on cognitive function has been investigated in numerous experimental studies, less results have been drawn from human clinical trials. In 2007, Benton *et al.* were the first to report in a double-blind placebo-controlled trial that a yoghurt product containing *L. casei*, Shirota strain, improved the mood of those most depressed at baseline [519]. Since poor mood is associated with poor memory, this finding had many implications on this area of research [520]. However, they also found that, with regards to any direct association of probiotics with cognition, the consumption of probiotics negatively affected memory performance, as measured by the Wechsler Memory Scale, while the placebo group performed significantly better at the memory evaluations. In a randomized, double-blind, placebo-controlled trial, Rao *et al.* showed that subjects with chronic fatigue syndrome (CFS) receiving a mixed probiotic supplement, containing *L. casei* Shirota had less anxiety symptoms than those receiving a placebo supplement [521]. Since CSF is associated with neuropsychological impairments, this trial further strengthened the evidence supporting *L. casei's* use for cognitive decline and depressive symptoms. Furthermore, based on previous findings as discussed, Chung *et al.* sought to determine any possible effects of *L. helveticus* IDCC3801 – fermented milk powder (LHFM) on the cognitive performance of a healthy aged population [522]. They designed a 12-week, double-blind, randomized controlled trial assessing the cognitive function of 36 older adults using a neuropsychological test battery containing the digit-span, story recall, and verbal-learning tests in order to investigate attention, working memory, and short- and long-term memory. They also administered a cognitive fatigue test battery including a rapid visual information-processing (RVIP) task and Stroop color-word test evaluating sustained attention, working memory and selective attention/freedom from interference. Additionally, the evaluated the perceived stress scale (PSS), the geriatric depression scale-short form (GDS-SF), BDNF and whole blood viscosity (WBV). Of note, probiotic supplementation was associated with better performance in RVIP and Stroop color-word tests, indicating that LHFM may have a beneficial effect especially during cognitively demanding tasks. No changes in PSS, GDS-SF, BDNF and WBV were observed with administration of the probiotic, indicating that the improvements in the cognitive fatigue battery are not implicated by improvements in stress, depression or other biologic markers.

6.1.2.2. Bifidobacteria

Evidence concerning *Bifidobacteria* is not as abundant compared to *lactobacilli*, with regards to neurodegeneration and prevention of cognitive decline. The effects of *bifidobacteria* on cognition and memory are mainly strain-specific. A recent study found that supplementation with B. Breve NCIMB 702258, combined with α-linolenic acid, resulted in high levels of docosahexaenoic acid (DHA) in the brain of BALB/c mice [523]. It is known that elevation of DHA results in reduction in synthesis of inflammatory eicosanoids from arachidonic acids, leading to an anti-inflammatory profile beneficial to many conditions, including AD, where excessive production of eicosanoids is observed [524]. The same researchers had similar results (elevation of DHA levels by administration of *B. breve* NCIMB 702258) when they used another model, wild-type C57BL/6 male mice, strengthening their previous results [525]. Additionally, following another neurodegeneration and AD pathway, O'Sullivan *et al.* found that treatment of maternally separated (MS) and non-separated (NS) Sprague Dawley rats with *B. breve* 6330 significantly reduced BDNF exon IV mRNA in NS rats [526]. However, *B. breve* 6330 did not affect BDNF total mRNA or BDNF exon IV in MS rats. Savignac *et al.* have also recently shown that both *B. longum* 1714 and *B. breve* 1205 had a positive effect on memory and cognitive tasks in stressed BALB/c mice [527].

Some evidence exists also for the modulation of behavior (especially anxiety-like behavior) through *Bifidobacteria* supplementation. Several studies have reported that certain *Bifidobacteria* strains, including *B. longum* and *B. breve,* can have a beneficial effect on stress, anxiety and general anxiety-like behaviors [528 - 534]. This is particularly important since stress and anxiety can be associated with impaired cognition, and modulation of these behavioral characteristics through probiotic supplements can possibly have an indirect effect on cognitive function [535, 536].

6.1.2.3. Other Bacilli and Mixed Supplements

There are a number of other probiotic substances that have proven to be effective against cognitive decline, in animal models. Notably, it has been previously described that *Bacillus subtilis*-fermented soymilk (PFSM) can be protective against AD [537]. In particular, Kim *et al.* found that PFSM effectively reduced nitric oxide (NO) formation and lipid peroxidation in the brain of ICR mice injected with Aβ, indicating strong anti-oxidative activities of *Bacillus subtilis*. Furthermore, they found that PFSM improved learning and memory abilities, evaluated by T-maze, novel object recognition and Morris water-maze tests. The exact strains of *Bacillus subtilis* were *Bacillus subtilis* 2829 PNU-15 and it was extracted from cheonggukjang, a traditional fermented Korean food. Fermentation of another traditional product, chungkookjang, with *Bacillus licheniformis* has also shown anti-Aβ activities [538]. It was found that standardized chungkookjang fermented with this probiotic strain can ameliorate cognitive decline, measured by the water maze test, and decrease Aβ levels in β-amyloid-induced diabetic rats. Supplementation of mixed probiotic strains has also proven to be beneficial for cognitive impairment. In a 2013 study by Davari *et al.*, it was observed that a mixture of *L. acidophilus, B. lactis* and *L. fermentum* strains (ATCC 4356, DSM 10140 and ATCC 9338 respectively) was beneficial in a number of behavioral, electrophysiological and biochemical tests [539]. Namely, this probiotic intervention improved spatial learning in Morris water maze task and positively affected the basic synaptic activity and synaptic plasticity in a diabetes mellitus rat model.

Several mixed probiotic supplements have been investigated for their efficacy in clinical settings, concerning potential benefits on human cognition. In a mixed animal-clinical study Messaoudi *et al.* found that administration of a *L. helveticus* R0052 and *B. longum* R0175 resulted in reduction in psychological distress in human volunteers, as evaluated by the Hopkins Symptom Checklist (HSCL-90) and the Hospital Anxiety and Depression Scale (HADS) [540]. They found that this mixed probiotic supplement was associated with improvements in global severity index, somatization, depression and anger-hostility. In a randomized clinical trial, Steenbergen *et al.* found that a multispecies probiotic containing *B. bifidum* W23, *B. lactis* W52, *L. acidophilus* W37, *L. brevis* W63, *L. casei* W56, *L. salivarious* W24 and *L. lactis* W19 and W58 was associated with less cognitive reactivity to sad mood [541]. Since cognitive reactivity is a vital component of depression pathogenesis, interventions aiming to ameliorate this characteristic may have an important impact on cognitive function [494, 542 - 549]. Lastly, Tillisch *et al.* reported that administration of a fermented milk product containing

B. animalis subsp lactis I-2494, *Streptococcus thermophilus* I-1630, *L. bulgaricus* I-1632 and I-1519 and *L. lactis subsp lactis* I-1631 had a substantial effect on the activity of many brain regions and networks that control emotion and central processing in healthy women, suggesting potential implications on improvements in cognitive functions [548].

6.1.2.4. Conclusion

Overall, it seems that the evidence concerning the effect of probiotic supplements on cognition is preliminary and few assumptions can be drawn with regards to their use in clinical practice. As demonstrated by a recent systematic review of randomized controlled trials, probiotics may be associated with some improvements in behavioral and cognitive outcomes – anxiety, depression, autism spectrum disorder, obsessive-compulsive disorder and certain aspects of memory [549]. Since many experts have expressed their concern on the efficacy of many probiotic strains, it would be advisable that they are used only as supplementary products to a main intervention protocol for a possible cognitive decline in human subjects [494].

Of note, most of the animal studies that evaluated the efficacy of pre- and probiotics are based on dementia, learning, memory and attention of various mice/rat models, such as Wister, Sprague-Dawley, Long Evans and Fischer 344 rats, and C57BL/6, BALB/c, Swiss-Webster, Rag-1-, Dextran Sodium Sulfate (DSS) and ICR mice. No study exists on specialized transgenic AD mouse models, such as PDAPP, Tg2576, APP23, TgCRND8, APP-Dutch, PS1M1146V, PSAPP or 3xTg. The researchers, however, frequently administered substances in control mice/rats in order to induce alterations similar to that observed in AD and assessed the effectiveness of pre- and probiotics on these models. Table **2** summarizes the characteristics of these models and the effect of the pre- and probiotics that were given in the respective studies.

6.2. Natural Products

A fascinating and still widely unexplored avenue seems to be provided by natural products or nutraceutical intervention for treating AD. The following is a list of phytochemicals present in commonly consumed foods that is yet endless. (https://en.wikipedia.org/wiki/List_of_phytochemicals_in_food#Stilbenoids)

6.2.1. Phenolic Compounds

6.2.1.1. Crocus Sativus L. (saffron)

Crocus sativus L. (saffron) is a flowering plant, member of the *Iridaceae* family

[550]. Saffron's essential oil, obtained from the extract of its stigmas, consists of approximately 150 compounds (volatile and aromatic compounds) belonging to terpenoids and flavonoids, but only about one-third of those constituents have been isolated and characterized [551]. Principal components of the stigma of this plant comprise crocins, safranal, picrocrocin, ketoisophorone, isophorone, and glycosidic terpenoids [552]. Among the numerous non-volatile active components are zeaxanthin, lycopene, and various α- and β-carotenes derived from anthocyanins carotenoids.

Pharmacological studies have demonstrated several beneficial effects of saffron and its constituents, which possess a wide range of activities including anti-oxidant capacity [553 - 555], anti-inflammatory potential [556] and neuroprotective activities in memory impairment and learning amelioration [557 - 561].

Table 2. Characteristics of AD animal models used.

Substance Administered	Mouse/Rat Model	AD-specific Alterations	Pre-/Probiotic Used	Pre-/Probiotic Effect	Refs.
D-galactose	BALB/cJ mice	↑ oxidative stress levels and MDA levels in cerebral cortex; ↑ protein carbonyls in the hippocampus	FOS	↓ MDA levels in cerebral cortex; ↓ protein carbonyls in the hippocampus	[427]
	BALB/cJ mice	↑ Aβ density in the cortex and hippocampus; ↑ protein expression of Aβ and beta-site amyloid precursor cleaving enzyme of the whole brain	FOS	↓ Aβ density in the cortex and hippocampus; ↓ protein expression of Aβ and beta-site amyloid precursor cleaving enzyme of the whole brain	[432]
	C57BL/6J mice	↓ BDNF and CREB expression in the hippocampus	*Lactobacillus pentosus var. plantarum* C29	↑ BDNF and CREB expression in the hippocampus	[500]
Scopolamine	Sprague-Dawley rats	↓ Ach and ↑ AchE activity in brain; ↑ COX-1 and COX-2 activity, ↑ IL-1β and ↓ IL-10 (enhanced neuro-inflammation)	Total isoflavones	↑ Ach and ↓ AchE activity in brain; ↓ COX-1 and COX-2 activity, ↓ IL-1β and ↑ IL-10 (suppressed neuro-inflammation)	[446]
	ICR mice	↓ BDNF and CREB expression in the hippocampus	*Lactobacillus pentosus var. plantarum* C29	↑ BDNF and CREB expression in the hippocampus	[498]

(Table 2) contd.....

Substance Administered	Mouse/Rat Model	AD-specific Alterations	Pre-/Probiotic Used	Pre-/Probiotic Effect	Refs.
Aβ-peptide	Wistar rats	↑ ROS in neurons (oxidative stress); Aβ deposition on mitochondrial membrane (destruction)	SIF	↓ ROS in neurons (oxidative stress); ↓ Aβ deposition on mitochondrial membrane	[447]
	ICR mice	↑ NO formation and lipid peroxidation in the brain (enhanced neuro-inflammation)	*Bacillus subtilis*	↓ NO formation and lipid peroxidation in the brain (suppressed neuro-inflammation)	[522]
-	Fischer 344 rats	↓ BDNF expression and CREB phosphorylation	*Lactobacillus pentosus var. plantarum* C29, *Lactobacillus* mixture	↑ BDNF expression and CREB phosphorylation	[501, 502]

Ach: acetylcholine; AchE: acetylcholinesterase; BDNF: brain derived neurotrophic factor; COX: cyclooxygenase; CREB: cAMP response element-binding protein; FOS: fructo-oligosaccharides; MDA: malonaldehyde dimethyl acetal; NO: nitric oxide; SIF: soybean isoflavones

Oxidative stress has been proved to be a contributor, which is implicated to promote AD pathological features. *C. sativus* stigma's constituents, thanks to their anti-oxidant and anti-amyloidogenic activities could be useful for inhibiting aggregation and deposition of Aβ in the human brain, reflecting also in a positive effect on cognitive function. It has been proposed that saffron could be used for the development of new therapeuticals for the prevention or delay of AD [555].

Crocin displays strong affinity for NMDAR [562], exhibits an inhibiting effect on tracheal muscles *β*2-adrenoceptors, and possibly on histamine (H1) receptors [563]. Trans-crocin displays channel opening activity justifying the use of saffron for CNS disorders, in accordance with pharmacokinetics and pharmaco-dynamics data [564, 565]. Bioavailability of crocin, after oral administration, is almost negligible in the systemic network, as pointed out by *in vitro* studies. However, crocin is subjected to hydrolysis/de-glycosylation in the GI route to de-glycosylated trans-crocetin, which afterward is converted to absorbable by passive diffusion. In this form, it is able to be transported rapidly and extensively through cells, and finally to penetrate through the intestinal barrier [564, 566, 567], while crocetin is capable to pierce slowly BBB in order to become disposable to CNS [564].

Basic and clinical studies showed that the cognitive functions in saffron-treated individuals with AD, were significantly better than placebo [568]. Amazing evidence demonstrates that *C. sativus* and its main component crocin are importantly implicated in cognition. It is noteworthy that the saffron's potency does not differ than that of the drug for AD, donepezil, an inhibitor of acetylcholinesterase (AchE), whereas the patients subjected to saffron-treatment did not present side effects compared to these subjected to the drug-treatment [569]. Various *in vitro* enzymatic and molecular docking studies, for the *C. sativus* and crocetin, demonstrated their binding in the catalytic center and in other peripheral sites that result in inhibition of the enzyme AchE. The importance of this inhibition reflects in the augmentation of the amounts of synaptic acetylcholine, a neuro-transmittant compound, which actively participates in cognitive operation [570].

Recent preclinical trials in mouse and rat models, and clinical trials performed on the effects on cognition of *C. sativus* and its constituents, have been cumulatively recorded in details as well as the doses used. Outcomes from clinical investigations evaluating the effectiveness of saffron (but not crocin) in cognitive operation, pointed out that despite the moderate effects, which have been evidenced, they were not far from these of the drugs for AD donepezil and memantine. Despite the noteworthy safety evidence of saffron, which was displayed in all clinical studies, the research did not includes other cases of memory disorders that occur in other pathologies such as brain ischemia, traumatic brain injury, and cognitive impairments related to schizophrenia [569]. Several clinical trials of saffron and its constituents have been carried out to fight a wide spectrum of diseases recorded collectively, including AD, cardiovascular, and gynecology disorders *etc.* [565]. Recently, the efficacy of crocus in the management of amnesia and multi-domain MCI (aMCImd) was proved satisfactory by improving Mini-Mental State Examination scores ($p=0.015$), compared to that of the control subjects that deteriorated [561].

Significantly increased levels of acrolein, an unsaturated aldehyde, provoke toxicity mediated by induction of oxidative stress resulting in enhanced levels of tau phosphorylation and Aβ deposition in the brain, effects which are correlated with pathogenicity of NDs as AD [571]. Although acrolein causes activation of MAPKs signaling pathway, the co-supplementation with crocin weakened the pre-mentioned effects by affecting this pathway, and enabling crocin a promising approach for the AD treatment [572]. Crocin also displays neuroprotective capacity against acrylamide-induced cytotoxicity in PC12 cells [573].

Thanks to the anti-inflammatory activity and anti-Alzheimer properties among other beneficial activities of the extracts of *C. sativus,* due to its particular constituents (crocetin, crocin, safranal), it has been proposed as potential therapeutic for various nervous system disorders such as AD and PD. Their beneficial effects has been mainly attributed to their interactions with cholinergic, dopaminergic and glutamatergic systems [574].

Various studies regarding *C. sativus* toxicity have demonstrated its safety. Various biochemical and hematological parameters in mice ranged in physiological values. A later report, which focused on both acute oral or intra-peritoneal administration of a high dose (up to 3 g oral) and sub-acute (15-180 mg/kg intra-peritoneal), did not demonstrate appreciable toxicity of crocin [575]. Recently, also, the safety and toxicity of saffron was extensively discussed. In some clinical applications for the effectiveness of saffron for AD and depression, several minor adverse effects (including nausea, vomiting, dizziness, dry mouth *etc.*) were reported, after administering 15-30 mg/day [565].

Finally, extracts of the whole plant *C. sativus* or of its parts (stigma, stamen, leaves and colora), has been proposed to constitute an important source of antimicrobial agents against different bacteria (*Micrococcus luteus, Staphylococcus epidermitis, Staphylococcus aureus* and *E. coli*) and fungi *Candida albicans, Aspergillus niger* and *Cladospourium sp* [576].

6.2.1.2. Natural Mono-Phenols

6.2.1.2.1. Rosmarinic Acid (RA)

RA is a plant-originated polyphenolic carboxylate compound, isolated and characterized in 1958 from rosemary (*Rosmarinus officinalis*), a perennial herb. RA is an ester of caffeic acid and 3,4-dihydroxyphenyllactic acid but biologically is formed from 4-coumaroyl-4'-hydroxyphenyllactate. RA is mainly found in a variety of *Lamiaceae* species used commonly as culinary herbs but rather it is well known for being the active ingredient of rosemary and perilla oil, recorded among the natural products as promising drug candidates for the treatment of AD [577].

Oxidative stress has been recently considered as one of the preclinical neuropathological incidents of AD, resulting from the significant imbalance that occurs between the production of ROS by tissues and their subsequent removal by the antioxidant system [578, 579]. RA at concentrations ranging from 1 to10 μM) restrain the ROS generation and thus inhibited the apoptotic pathways, DNA breakage, and caspase-3 activation. Moreover, RA was found to reduce the tau protein hyper-phosphorylation [580], whereas RA supplementation (0.25-4 mg/kg, i.p.), impedes importantly the memory impairment caused by Aβ deposit, mostly by attacking NF-κB and TNF-α [581, 582].

RA and *Perilla frutescens* var. japonica extract (PFE) supplementation improved remarkably cognition function and object distinctions that were declined by A$\beta_{25\text{-}35}$ peptide, in the T-maze and object identification tests, respectively. Moreover, PFE diminished importantly the oxidative stress as reflected by the inhibition of NO and MDA formation in mouse brain after amyloid peptide A$\beta_{25\text{-}35}$-injection. Therefore RA can contribute to cognitive amelioration and to impedes AD, stimulated by Aβ [583].

6.2.1.2. Polyphenolic Compounds

Polyphenols nowadays have attracted a distinctive interest from the scientific society due to their anti-oxidant capacity and their ability to scavenge the free radicals generated during various pathological process including neurodegenerative disorders, cancer and cardiovascular diseases. Among the various polyphenolic compounds found in foods, a number of the most known and widely-consumed were recorded here, due to their involvement in the beneficial effect in AD disease. The largest and best-studied natural polyphenols are the flavonoids, which include several thousand compounds, among them the flavonols, flavons, flavan-3-ol (catechins), flavanones, anthocyanidins and isoflavonoids. The phenolic unit can be found dimerized or further polymerized, creating a new class of polyphenol.

6.2.1.2.1. Flavonoids

Flavonoids (or bioflavonoids) constitute a family of various plant-derived secondary metabolites, which are the most significant plant pigments responsible for flower coloration. Flavonoids are secreted by the root of their host plant and assist the *Rhizobia* during the infection stage, that live in a symbiotic condition with various legumes, like peas, beans, clover, and soy.

6.2.1.2.2. Flavonols

Flavonols that comprise among others quercetin are found in red and yellow onions, tea, wine, apples, cranberries, buckwheat, beans, lovage.

Quercetin (QCT)

Quercetin (QCT) is found in a broad diversity of foods including red and yellow onions, tea, wine, apples, cranberries, buckwheat, beans and lovage. Bioavailability of quercetin-rich food is very slow, exhibiting long half-lives of elimination from plasma, signifying that daily consumption of quercetin-containing foods reflects in increased quercetin levels in blood, whereas its conjugation with glucose ends in enhanced absorption from the small gut [584]. However, in various studies in humans, QCT at daily dose higher than 1,000 mg had not exerts hurtful effects neither in hematology and in serum electrolytes, nor in the various blood parameters, which reflect the physiological liver and kidney operation [585]. A number of biological activities were ascribed to quercetin including firstly its anti-oxidant ability acting as scavenger of ROS, one of its multiple faces in neuroprotection [586].

Among the various QCT's actions like anti-inflammatory, anti-cancer and antiviral ones, and focusing on QCT's pharmacological actions on AD disease, it should emphasize its anti-amyloidogenic activity [587, 588]. This anti-amyloidogenic action is exerted by inhibition of Aβ fibrils generation that might be occurred at concentration of 10 μM [589]. Doses of QCT (in the range 5-20 μM) exert a protective role and enfeeble the $A\beta_{1-42}$-triggered oxidative cell toxicity in hippocampal neurons cultures, in terms of protein oxidation, lipid peroxidation and apoptosis, while dose as high as 40 μM triggers cytotoxicity [590].

QCT and bilobalide (BB) stimulated neurogenesis and synaptogenesis in hippocampal neurons, when were administered in combination, acting with a common mechanism. Moreover, this combination causes important enhancement of phosphorylation of cAMP response element binding (CREB) protein and BDNF in brain mice [591]. QCT exerts ameliorative effect on several animal *in vivo* models of neural disorders attributed to an augmented permeability of BBB. Behavioral studies conducted to assure QCT intrusion in BBB and improved brain delivery certify its protective ability when administered encapsulated inside solid lipid nanoparticles (SLN) [592].

Despite the lack of QCT's toxicity in several animal studies, a danger for neurotoxicity cannot be excluded, due to the limited range of therapeutic doses used *in vitro,* and especially in the case that brain accessibility from QCT is increased as result from pathological or artificial causes like as delivery from liposomes, nanoparticles *etc.* [586].

QCT reduces the expression of activating transcription factor 4 (ATF4), which is upregulated in both AD brain and AD mouse model, indicating its latent roles in the pathogenesis of this disease and it might constitute a novel potential curative target for AD [593].

QCT might recall importantly memory in early-stage AD patients, as seen after the consumption for 4 weeks of a QCT-rich onion (Quergold) powder in respect of that of control onion ('Mashiro' white onion) powder [594].

6.2.1.2.3. Isoflavonoids

Isoflavones are a type of natural isoflavonoids, some of which act as phytoestrogens in mammals and are produced by the members of the *Fabaceae* (*i.e.*, *Leguminosae*, or bean) family.

Soybean Isoflavone

Soybean isoflavone (SIF) administered to rats at a dose 80 mg/kg/day before and after an injection of peptide 1-42 ($A\beta_{1-42}$). Then, the effects on the learning, on memory ability, on the integrity of ultra-micro structure of hippocampal synapses, and the expression of synaptic associated proteins, were examined. The pre-administration of SIF leads to amelioration of the learning decline and memory capability, in rats induced by $A\beta_{1-42}$ injection. Additionally, SIF pretreatment resulted to relieve the synaptic structural injury and compete to reset the down-regulated expressions of a range of proteins including synaptophysin and postsynaptic density protein 95 (PSD-95), calmodulin (CaM), Ca^{2+}/calmodulin-dependent protein kinase II (CaMK II), cAMP response element binding protein (CREB), as well as the levels of CaMK II and CREB phosphorylation (pCAMK II, pCREB) that all are induced by $A\beta_{1-42}$ injection. The suggested mechanism of action might be associated with the safeguard of synaptic plasticity by ameliorating the synaptic structure and arranging the proteins associated to synapses of rats [595].

A similar experiment, which was conducted that examined the influence of SIF on the structural synaptic injury induced by $A\beta_{1-42}$ in rats, since injuries of synapses constitute a crucial parameter of cognitive decline. More findings demonstrated that whereas $A\beta_{1-42}$ exerted a down-regulation effect on the levels of both mRNA and protein expression of the two subunits of NMDAR, as well as the levels of the mRNA expression of a number of protein including CaM, CaMKII, CREB, and BDNF, pre-administration with SIF abolished these events. The proposed mechanism of the SIF involvement is to interact with NMDAR and to interfere in the cascade of signaling pathway CaM/CaMKII/CREB/BDNF that affects synaptic plasticity [596].

Resveratrol (3, 5, 4'-Trihydroxy-Trans-Stilbene; RSV)

RSV is a plant flavonoid that belongs in the family of stilbenoids and it was found in grape (peels and seeds, grape wine), nuts, peanuts Japanese knotweed root. Plethora of activities was ascribed in RSV listed below. The pleoitropic potential of RSV was praised recording a list of activities and mechanisms that affects, including modulation of the transcription factor NF-κB, inhibition of the cytochrome P450 isoenzyme CYP1 A1, suppression of the expression and activity of inflammation-related COX enzymes, moderation of Fas/Fas-ligand-intervened apoptosis, p53, mammalian target of rapamycin, cyclins and diverse phosphodiesterases. This elevated cytosolic cAMP levels resulted in activation of the Epac1/CaMKKβ/AMPK/SIRT1/PGC-1α pathway that reflects in facilitation of many cellular functions, like augmented fatty acids oxidation, mitochondrial biogenesis and respiration, as well as gluconeogenesis process. A valuable addition in the list is the benefit in autoimmune diseases, since RSV enhances apoptosis of activated T cells and suppresses the expression of pro-inflammatory molecules including TNF-α, interleukin-17 (IL-17) *etc*. Furthermore, RSV efficacious involvement towards cancer might be explained with its capacity to inhibit the expression of both the hypoxia-inducible factor-1α and vascular endothelial growth factor. RSV affect and increase the synthesis and action of BDNF participating indirectly in prevention of bisphenol A-induced autism, type 2 diabetes mellitus, and metabolic syndrome, since BDNF is involved in the pathogenesis of the pre-mentioned diseases and is also altered in depression, schizophrenia, bipolar disorder, and autism. RSV also augments the levels of the anti-inflammatory lipid, lipoxin A4 *via* augmentation of the BDNF levels, since the levels of both BDNF and lipoxin A4 are low in diabetes mellitus. An extension in the list, merits adding the capacity of RSV to modify the composition of the gut microbiota, a crucial to AD-contributing factor recently reported, and to affect stem cell proliferation and differentiation. All the recorded RSV pleiotropic activities may explicate the amassing beneficial effects [597].

Despite rampant information including *in vitro* and *in vivo* epidemiological studies for evidences that emphasize the probable role of two polyphenols in contravening effectively in neurodegeneration, the outcomes of published trials (collectively five for curcumin, six for RSV) are discouraging, since do not allow to deduce upshot in respect their curative or neuroprotective capacity. These substances are attractive, thanks to their capability to interfere with diverse processes involved in the primary stages of dementia, and because of usefulness in prolepsis of the AD pathology. Conclusively it was suggested a more long-term treatment of clinical trials with these compounds and with increased bioavailability to benefit of the potential preventive properties of curcumin and RSV [598].

An important cellular degradative pathway of damaged proteins and organelles for removing "cell wastes or debris" is autophagy, dysfunction of which reflects in their accumulation and emergence of pathology. One of the most significant properties ascribed to RSV is its involvement in the autophagy regulation and clearance of vulnerable proteins' aggregation and of disintegrated organelles, by impeding the accumulation of pathological proteins, a hallmark of different neurodegenerative diseases, including AD, PD and Huntington's disease (HD) [599].

Plethora recent studies highlight the contribution of oxidative stress in induction of neuronal injuries, modulation of diverse intracellular signaling pathways that ends to apoptosis or necrosis of neuronal cells. Accumulated data were reviewed that confirm the anti-oxidative efficiency of polyphenols in diminishing the oxidative stress-derived consequences, in reducing neurotoxicity and neuronal death, and emphasize the neuroprotective role of phytochemicals against neurodegenerative diseases as PD or AD [600].

Despite the efforts to discover drugs that exert improvement, prolepsis or reversion of development of AD pathology, none of them have adequate effectiveness to perform that. RSV, notorious for its therapeutic outcomes on a wide range of age-related diseases and inflammation, was used also to confront and ameliorate the poisonous effects of an agonist of glutamate Ibotenic acid (IBO) in male Wistar rats by altering the respective receptors like NMDA receptor. RSV supplementation (20 mg/kg body weight, i.p.), was attenuated significantly the alterations of glutamatergic and cholinergic receptor, which are also associated with significant changes in the behavioral parameters in IBO-stimulated rats. In addition RSV reduced oxidative stress, ameliorated spatial learning execution, weakened immobility, and extemporary open field potency in IBO-exhorted rats [601].

RSV in combined administration with vitamin D acts synergistically, and it is able to reverse cytotoxicity exerted by tunicamycin and $A\beta_{25\text{-}35}$ peptide in SH-SY5Y cells, that reflected in increased levels of endoplasmic reticulum stress markers, a crucial factor contributing in the AD pathogenesis. However, supplementary studies are necessary for an *in vivo* application of similar therapy in human AD patients [602].

The dual factor of neuro-inflammation and oxidative stress ultimately have been implicated to contribute in neurotoxicity and as result many antioxidant practices were developed to fight and treat neurodegenerative diseases and dementia. A spectrum of herbal ingredients enriched in polyphenols including green tea polyphenol (-)- epigallocatechin-3-gallate, RSV, curcumin, quercetin and extract derived from elderberry, *Sambucus nigra* and others) have been proposed as powerful neuro-protectives possessing antioxidant ability for protection of neuronal cells against oxidative exposure [603]

Various dietary ingredients including (L-ascorbic acid, caffeic acid, caffeine, curcumin, (-)-epigallocatechin gallate (EGCG), gallic acid, propyl gallate, RSV, and α-tocopherol) are regarded as beneficial factors in AD pathogenesis due to their metal (iron, copper and zinc) chelating capacity, radical scavenging ability and the suppression properties of the Aβ fibrillation. Although the substances EGCG, gallic acid, and curcumin are regarded as multi-liturgical compounds;

nevertheless, their low brain intake might restrict their therapeutic impacts. Whereas the antioxidants L-ascorbic acid and α-tocopherol, although display a higher brain uptake, however, they need further study to fight oxidative stress within the AD brain [604].

A principal provenance of neurotoxicity has been regarded as the glyceraldehyde-originated Advanced Glycation End Products (AGEs) and it was demonstrated that the glyceraldehyde-AGEs increase the levels of Amyloid precursor protein (APP) and Aβ *via* ROS, leading to augmented neurotoxicity. In addition, AGEs provoke an up-regulation of APP hydrolytic processing (by enzymes BACE and PS1) and of the Sirt1 expression by means of ROS, whereas do not influence the expression of down-stream antioxidant genes HO-1 and NQO-1. Moreover, it was found that AGEs increase the glucose regulated protein-78 (GRP78) expression, which serves as the monitor to detect accumulation of misfolded/unfolded proteins, and enhance the cell death-related pathway p53, bcl-2/bax ratio, caspase 3. AGEs worsen the neuroprotective outcomes of Sirt1 and drive to neuronal cell death through ER stress. Finally, AGEs augment ROS generation, which excites the down-stream pathways associated to APP processing, Aβ formation, Sirt1, and GRP78, leading in the over-regulation of pathway related to cell death. This in-turn enhances neuronal cell death, which leads to the development of AD [605].

Modern cures, first and foremost, focalized on the improvement of cholinergic transmission to fight AD. Nevertheless, all these cures seem to be only coincidental, and for the moment there is still not a disposable drug for the administration in AD patients capable to confront AD. A complete conspectus focalized on the spectrum of beneficial outcomes including the anti-oxidant, anti-inflammatory, cognition-amplifying, anti-amyloidogenic, and neuroprotective ones, that exert a group of diverse nutraceuticals including curcumin, apigenin, docosahexaenoic acid, epigallocatechin gallate, α-lipoic acid and RSV, in respect of their potential for AD prolepsis and therapy [606].

The consequences of RSV administration on hippocampal astrocytes and the expression of TNF-α in AD rat models, were investigated. It was demonstrated that both the activation of astrocytes and the secretion of TNF-α can be inhibited by RSV in AD rat models. Specifically, the expression of GFAP in rats exposed in RSV and estradiol valerate reduced gradually with increasing RSV concentration (40, 80 mg/kg) compared to the reference group. Whereas the levels of TNF-α diminished significantly in RSV 20, 40, 80 mg/kg and estradiol valerate group compared with the model group ($P < 0.01$) [607].

The potential of RSV to confront inflammation stimulated by $A\beta_{1\text{-}42}$ and to protect the structural integrity of BBB was investigated in AD rats. The outcomes showed that RSV is advantageous at one hand since decreases the levels of insoluble $A\beta_{1-42}$ responsible for stimulation of neuro-inflammation and at the other hand protects the integrity of BBB, reflecting respectively in decreased expression of NF-κB a, and secondly in increase of Claudin-5 and decrease of advanced glycation end products (RAGE) and matrix metalloprotein-9 (MMP-9) [608].

RSV was safe and enough tolerate, and it and its metabolites permeate the BBB, able to exert diverse effects to CNS, as it was proved in a phase 2 trial in subjects with mild to moderate AD. The outcomes notably showed that the levels of Aβ40 peptide in CSF and plasma diminished more in the placebo subjects than these of RSV remedy, whereas brain volume loss was augmented by RSV therapy in comparison to placebo. Supplementary studies are necessary to explain alteration of some biomarkers [609].

RSV has been demonstrated to constitute an omnipresent panacea attributed to its inherent features associated to its stilbene structure, specifically for a broad spectrum of NDs. The diverse molecular targets of RSV were assessed *in vivo* and *in vitro* in respect its capability to confront drastically a number of NDs including AD, PD, HD and ALS. Despite the profound heterogeneity of the pathologies investigated, appeared that RSV, acting on relatively convergent protein targets, produces therapeutic outcomes in neuronal cells widely variable in morphological structure and particularly in their operation executed in the different anatomical areas to which is destined [610].

Aβ has been reported that induces production of ROS and oxidative stress in neuronal cells, which in turn up-regulates the β-secretase 1 (BACE-1) expression and the Aβ levels, thereby propagating oxidative stress and increasing neuronal injury. The biological behavior of a group of RSV derivatives, considered as inhibitors of neuronal cells death that is oxidative stress-stimulated (named oxytosis), was assessed against BACE-1, by means of homogeneous time-resolved fluorescence (TRF) assay. RSV and its derivatives exert an inhibitory activity on both oxytosis and BACE-1 suggesting the critical BACE1 mediation in oxytosis. Noteworthy that four of the assessed RSV analogues exhibited higher activity than that of RSV [611].

RSV at a concentration of 100 μM caused a 40% decrease in paralysis, in the transgenic *Caenorhabditis elegans* strain CL2006, expressing $A\beta_{1-42}$ under control of a muscle-specific promoter and responding to Aβ-toxicity with paralysis, used as a model. RSV reduces the Aβ-induced toxicity in a *C. elegans* model of AD by targeting specific proteins involved in proteostasis and thereby reduces the amount of aggregated Aβ [612].

One of the strategies that impede AD pathogenesis has been focus on inhibition of β- and γ-secretases, which create Aβ deposition from Aβ precursor protein (APP) through successive cleavages. A RSV trimer named miyabenol C, which was isolated from stems and leaves of the small-leaf grape (*Vitisthunbergii var. taiwaniana*), when either was added in cell cultures or administered in the brain of AD model mice resulted in decrease of the amounts of both Aβ and sAPPβ. Thus, miyabenol C might be considered as a distinguished β-secretase inhibitor, and must to be proposed as a substance candidate for drug development suitable for AD therapy [613].

A conspectus collecting the recent investigations of RSV neuroprotective outcomes, in both cell cultures and animal models, confers data about the molecular mechanisms of its neuroprotection and explores its therapeutic prospects in AD [614]. RSV exhibited the capacity to invert the debility of memory in mice induced as result of their exposure in LPS. Furthermore, it was confirmed that RSV enhanced markedly both the estradiol and neprilysin (NEP) levels associated to reduction of Aβ deposition. NEP is one of the most meaningful amyloid degrading enzymes, which is principally affected by estrogen. Thus, a correlation exist between the up-regulation of estradiol levels, which drives to augmentation of NEP levels, especially in brain, consequently resulting in increased degradation ending in diminished Aβ deposition [615].

A conspectus collectively records studies supporting the protective role of polyphenols especially RSV, its bioavailability in brain, as well as novel strategies and their impact in AD prolepsis even before the emergence of clinical symptoms. This review constitute part of a Special Issue entitled: RSV: Challenges in translating pre-clinical findings to improved patient outcomes [616]. Nutritional consumption of polyphenols is accepted that provides important potentiality to diminish the hazard of AD development and to counteract the changes occurred in AD. Several endeavors have been performed to unfold the molecular mechanisms of various biological pathways aiming to discover the specific interactions of polyphenols with their concrete targets [617]. The neuroprotective and anti-oxidant consequences of RSV on AD and its multi-potential mechanisms of action, as well as the alternative use of analogues to increase its bioavailability in plasma was summarized [618].

Many external or dietary factors influence epigenetic mechanisms causing reversible alterations, and some others associated with pathogenesis of AD. A spectrum of dietary nutrients was considered capable to trigger epigenetic alterations demonstrating a critical role in health and in prolepsis of some diseases specifically NDs. A collective overview provides information for epigenetic alterations connected to AD pathogenesis and the bio-dynamic nutrients capable to affect epigenetic mechanisms [619].

Stilbene including RSV exhibits neuroprotective activity in various models for toxicity studies. A broad spectrum of properties including the anti-inflammatory, the enhancer of the clearance of Aβ, the free radical scavenging, the modulatory of intracellular effectors correlated with oxidative stress (*e.g.* heme oxygenase), neuronal energy homeostasis (*e.g.* AMP kinase), program cell death (*i.e.* AIF) and longevity (*i.e.* sirtuins) have been ascribed to RSV, thanks to which intervene in several crucial mechanisms. RSV multi-target protective consequences and its eventual prophylactic role in NDs was reviewed [620].

Oral administration of RSV in AβPP/PS1 mouse model of AD exerts beneficial consequences, reflected in decrease of the amyloid encumbrance and increase of mitochondrial complex IV protein levels, in mouse brain. These protective outcomes executed by inducing activation of several neuroprotective routes involving Sirtuin 1 and AMPK pathways in mice. More RSV promotes alterations of the inflammatory situation, as deduced from increased IL1β and TNF gene expression. Conclusively RSV diminishes the detrimental events occurring in AβPP/PS1 mouse hippocampus, reflected in prolepsis of memory loss [621].

Lately, natural constituents and supplemental substances attract galloping interest as an alternative choice to cure AD due to extended information for their curative potentiality either preventative, protective or restorative to confront various NDs. Experimental and clinical outcomes relative to ingredients of nutritional supplements (*i.e.*, Cur, RA, RSV, acetyl-L-carnitine, and ω-3 (n-3) pol-yunsaturated fatty acids (PUFAs) that already showed auspicious remedial consequences on long-standing diseases including AD and other NDs derived from acute unpropitious episodes or traumatic brain injury, were reviewed [622].

Numerous efforts were executed to discover drugs to treat AD, while it has been designed and synthesized a series of new compounds, by combination of two pharmacophores RSV and clioquinol, taken into account the 'multi-target-directed ligands' (MTDLs) practice. Among them the compound (E)-5-(4-hydroxystyryl) quinoline-8-ol (10c) inhibited the Aβ aggregation both self-induced and copper(II)-induced, and exhibited potential anti-oxidant behavior and bio-metal chelation ability, whereas it did not show acute toxicity in mice at high doses of up to 2000 mg kg^{-1}. In addition, it was able to penetrate the BBB, as shown by a parallel artificial membrane permeation assay. It is noteworthy that compound 10c was suggested as an encouraging multifunctional compound for the development of novel drugs for AD [623].

RSV is a well-acknowledged for its antioxidant activities thanks to which modify the metal ion deregulation and the principal feature of AD brain. The capability of RSV to act as neuroprotective agent against dementia, and to oppose to the oxidative stress generated by amyloid and by metals metabolic dysfunction, was reviewed [624].

Because a critical hallmark of AD was considered the Aβ accumulation in brain, numerous curative practices appeared to target against Aβ deposition. A summarized study aimed to record collective evidence that concern especially pharmaceutical agents, which focused on the treatment of Aβ deposition, that were used at various stages of clinical trials. Moreover, because of the growing development of computational studies that provided a significant positive impact in the drug design area, natural products were investigated using *in silico* studies, as candidate therapeutic compounds in prolepsis of Aβ plaque creation [625].

Curcuminoids

Curcumin (Cur; or diferuloylmethane that oxidizes to vanillin), is a yellow polyphenolic phytochemical compound that is the basic curcuminoid found in turmeric (*Curcuma longa),* a rhizomatous herbaceous perennial plant, member of the ginger (*Zingiberaceae*) family. It is used as additive for food flavoring and coloring.

Plethora of activities was ascribed to Cur and its involvement in several cellular processes, providing a list that could be considered endless and emphasizing the most important. The neuroprotective potential of Cur as well as its limitations have been reported with emphasis on AD and are attributed to the anti-amyloidogenic, anti-inflammatory, anti-oxidative, and metal-chelating properties [626]. There is plentiful evidence that Cur is able to reduce soluble Aβ, relieve plaque burden, as well as attenuate neurotoxic effects caused by Aβ *in vitro* [627 - 629] and *in vivo* in animal models [630, 631]. However, there are contradictory reports for Cur effects found in cell culture studies, due to its instability in aqueous solution under physiological conditions (pH 7.2 and 37 °C), where degradation of up to 90% of Cur in solution can occur within 30 mins [632]. Cur inhibits with a dose-dependent manner the formation of Aβ fibril from Aβ monomers, and is capable to destabilize preformed Aβ fibrils using efficacious concentrations at levels of μM, (EC_{50}) of 0.1 – 1 μM [627], and (0.5 – 8 μM Cur) *in vitro* [597] as shown by electron microscopy analysis, while at 4 – 64 μM, Cur can also reduce the formation of Aβ oligomers [629]. Moreover, Cur, at concentrations ranging from 0.1 – 5 μM, potentially weakens cytotoxicity of SH-SY5Y human neuroblastoma cells, induced by oligomeric Aβ [629]. Similarly, it was demonstrated that Cur inhibits Aβ aggregation dose-dependently using thioflavin T cell-free assay [628].

It has been proposed that the mechanism through which Cur disorganizes Aβ assemblage and plaque formation takes place in two steps: firstly, the phenolic group of Cur may interact with the aromatic residues in Aβ fibrils, thereby disrupting peptide stacking; and secondly, the hydroxyl groups and -diketone unit of Cur may act as -sheet breakers *via* competitive hydrogen bonding [633].

It is interesting that nano-liposomal formulations of Cur were able to increase the ability of Cur in inhibiting the genesis of fibrillary and oligomeric Aβ *in vitro*, reflecting in increased affinity of Cur towards Aβ to nano-molar concentrations [634].

Cur, at concentrations 1, 10, and 20 μM, attenuated cytotoxicity on primary rat prefrontal cortical neurons [635], and at concentrations between 1 and 50 μM, rescues primary rat hippocampal neurons toxicity, caused from the intracellular Aβ [636], which it has been observed in early stage AD and correlates rather to cognitive impairment than extracellular Aβ deposition [637]. The protective action of Cur, against the intracellular Aβ-induced toxicity, is executed *via* inhibition of caspase 3, of phospho-AKT (Protein kinase B (PKB) [635], and *via* diminution of intracellular ROS levels [636]. The Aβ-caused cytotoxicity in SK-N-SH cells *in vitro* is reflected by morphological alterations, like short and reduced number of neurites, and Cur is able to attenuate this cytotoxicity that is concurred with recuperation in MAP2 protein levels [638].

Outcomes from a number of preclinical studies demonstrated that Cur may be helpful for the prolepsis and/or treatment of a spectrum of diseases including AD, cancer, cystic fibrosis and inflammatory diseases [639]. However, it should be noted that in phase I clinical studies, administration of Cur (up to 8,000 mg/day, p.o.) did not result in important side effects except mild nausea and diarrhea [640]. In contrast, excessive administration of Cur can result in alteration of the gut microbiota, intervening in the physiological homeostasis and the immune response [641]. Cur at concentrations ranging from 5-10 μM exerted protection of PC12 cells against neurotoxicity induced by Aβ, causing inhibition of oxidative damage, intracellular calcium influx, and tau hyper-phosphorylation, while concentrations as high as 50 μM provoke cellular cytotoxicity [642].

Cur at as low as concentration of 1 μM improved cognitive deficit *via* stimulation of brain derived neurotrophic factor (BDNF) and increase of GSH levels in hippocampi and modulation of NMDA receptor levels [643].

Accumulating evidence has suggested that the reactivation of *herpes simplex virus* type 1 (HSV-1) in the brain is a potent risk factor of AD. Cur diminishes HSV-1 infectivity and also slows HSV-1 replication. Orally administered Cur is absorbed by the GI system, enters the bloodstream, crosses the BBB, and then accumulates in the vicinity of the senile plaques. Of note, oral administration of low dosages of curcumin (160 ppm) for 6 months significantly reduced the Aβ plaque burden in the brain of APPSw mice [643]. The long-term oral consumption of Cur or some of its derivatives displays preventive effects, by attenuating the progression of AD thanks to its anti-inflammatory and antioxidant activity, and through its antiviral activity targeting against HSV-1 [644].

Recently its use was proposed to occur by means of a novel technique of a Cur derivative aerolization, FMeC1, to expedite its improved and safe distribution to the brain. It is noteworthy that currently Cur was administered in animal models and not in humans as unsuitable for use [645].

In the frame of discovering new therapies and of development of new drugs for fighting AD, a series of curcumin derivatives were designed, synthesized and assessed for their inhibitory capability for both tau protein and Aβ aggregation. Among others the compound 3-[(1E)-2-(1H-indol-6-yl)ethenyl]-5--(1E)-2-[2-methoxy-4-(2-pyridyl methoxy) phenyl] ethenyl]-1H-pyrazole (compound 4, PE859) was proposed as the more powerful inhibitor than Cur due to its pharmacokinetic properties and pharmacological efficiency *in vivo* providing the appropriateness as a drug for AD [646].

The affinity of three (nat/68) Ga-labelled Cur analogues for synthetic β-amyloid fibrils and for amyloid plaques was evaluated to be used as novel metallic radiotracers Cur-based, but further structural changes are required to ameliorate them for their utilization as radiotracers *in vivo* [647].

Cur is also a powerful agonist of Peroxisome Proliferator-Activated Receptor-Gamma (PPARγ), a probable target in which bound, exerting reduction of neuro-inflammation and amelioration of neuronal operation in AD [616]. Using both APP/PS1 transgenic mice and Aβ-induced neuro-inflammation in mixed primary hippocampus of neuronal/glial cultures, it was demonstrated that Cur injected intraperitoneally at 150 mg/kg and 4 mg/kg PPARγ inhibitor GW9662, daily per 4 successive weeks, decreased microglia and astrocytes activation and cytokine generation and thus suppressed neuro-inflammation, a critical cause of AD pathogenesis *via* inhibition of the NF-κB signaling pathway. Aβ can activate both microglia and astrocytes and the inflammatory response in the hippocampi of APP/PS1 mice was manifested by overproduction of multiple inflammatory mediators, *i.e.* TNF-a, IL- 1b, COX-2, and NO. Treatment of mice with Cur markedly suppressed the production of these toxic mediators [648]. Cur at 10 μM protected cholinergic neurons in mixed primary hippocampus of neuron/glia cultures and Cur alleviates spatial learning and memory deficits in APP/PS1 mice and promoted cholinergic neuronal function *in vivo* and *in vitro* at the same concentrations [648].

Using human neuroblastoma (SHSY5Y) cells, it was demonstrated that while Aβ was found to affect negatively mitochondrial dynamics, to restrict the biogenesis and operation of mitochondria, and to diminish synaptic activity, in contrast Cur augmented mitochondrial function and cell viability, and exerts protective effects against the mitochondrial and synaptic toxicity caused by Aβ. Cur is an auspicious molecule to be used as drug to treat AD patients [649].

A broad gamma of studies has been carried out concerning the physicochemical features and pharmacological outcomes of Cur on different diseases like AD, cardiovascular diseases, cancer, rheumatoid arthritis, diabetes, inflammatory bowel disease (IBD), and it comprises even wound healing. Formulations of nano-Cur displayed improved effectiveness and bioavailability under *in vivo* conditions and strong ability to regulate the cascade of signaling pathways of proliferation, inflammation, invasion, and apoptosis of various cancerous cells [650]. Cur may regulate the crucial biomolecules participating in the brain insulin signaling pathways and could be constituted one prospective theranostic component for the AD cures, to ameliorate the memory and learning capability of patients [651].

Cur and its analogues centralize considerable attention for the obstruction and cure of AD, both because of their ability to impede the creation of Aβ assemblage and its capacity to bind Cu (II) ion. Curcuminoids, the Cur's derivatives of K2T series, display the capability to inhibit the assemblage of the amyloid Aβ1-40 fibrils with a half maximal inhibitory concentration (IC_{50}) close to that of curcumin [652].

Hydroxycinnamic Acids

Caffeic acid found (CA) in artichoke, pear, apple, basil, thyme, oregano, olive oil *etc*. is an active phenolic compound that has a variety of pharmacological actions. Due to the inconclusive results from many epidemiologic studies, a meta-analysis of prospective cohort studies was conducted, which includes eleven prospective studies, and 29,155 participants for assessment of the relation between the daily coffee intake and the danger for cognitive impairment and dementia. It was concluded that higher coffee consumption is correlated with decreased hazard for AD but more controlled trials or well-designed cohort studies are required [653].

The protective activity of CA, which was fed orally at a daily dose of 10 or 50 mg/kg for duration of 2 weeks, in AD mouse model induced by $A\beta_{25-35}$ peptide injection, was assessed. Mouse cognitive capabilities were recorded by means of various behavioral tests, whereas the defense ability of CA against oxidative stress was determined, by measuring lipid peroxidation and nitric oxide (NO) generation. CA supplementation at a high dose of 50 mg/kg/day displayed the most powerful protective role by inhibiting lipid peroxidation and NO production in some tissues including brain, in comparison to the reference group (that was $A\beta_{25-35}$ peptide) and ameliorated spatial cognitive and memory functions [654].

Cinnamic Acid

Cinnamic acid is found in cinnamon and aloe. The consumption of the natural flavor-providing spice cinnamon as well as its metabolite sodium benzoate (NaB) was underlined to attenuate oxidative stress and to protect memory and learning, in experiments with transgenic mice models of AD. In addition NaB inhibited the generation of ROS in mouse microglial cells induced by bacterial LPS, by fibrillary Aβ and also by the compound 1-methyl-4-phenylpyridinium (+) [655].

It is known that $A\beta_{42}$ originated from βAPP hydrolysis, triggers the expression of a number of inflammatory genes, characteristic of the common immune-and inflammatory-response, which is promoted by infectious components such as bacterial LPS, a common toxic constituent located on the OM of Gram-negative bacteria. Amyloid neurotoxicity is due to the strong contribution of the presence of bacterial LPS or endotoxin-mediated inflammation [656].

Oral administration of cinnamon (*Cinnamonum verum*) powder in transgenic mice was followed by various ameliorative outcomes comprising repression of the neuronal apoptotic process, abolishment of glial activation, diminution of Aβ encumbrance in the hippocampus and safeguard of memory and learning. Consequently, cinnamon powder may be recorded in the list of the hopeful natural dietary supplements in pausing or retarding the evolution of AD [657].

6.2.1.2.4. Hydrolyzables Tannins

A novel search aimed to attenuate one of the AD features, the microgliosis, by a dietary intervention, which included pomegranate juice. This juice contains plentiful phyto-chemicals comprising a family of hydrolyzable tannins, (named ellagitannins), created from the binding of a carbohydrate with ellagic acid and/or gallic acid to compose pomegranate ellagitannins, also familiar with the name punicalagins [658]. It contains also a wide spectrum of vitamins like B1, B2, B3, B5, B6, B9, C, E and K, many microelements, and a number of other compounds responsible for the red color being ascribed to the family of anthocyanins, like delphinidin, cyanidin, and pelargonidin glycosides [659].

Mice 12-months-old, pomegranate-treated, have reduced microgliosis and Aβ plaque accumulation compared to the control, as it was shown by immunocytochemistry. Examination of brains from pomegranate-treated mouse during 3 months demonstrated reduced levels of TNF-α and of nuclear factor of activated T-cell (NFAT) transcriptional activity compared to controls. Two polyphenolic constituents of pomegranate juice, punicalagin and ellagic acid, were considered capable to diminish NFAT activity in a reporter cell line ($P < 0.05$) and secretion of Aβ-triggered TNF-α by microglia, exerting anti-inflammatory outcomes in brain and preventing AD progression [660].

Red Raspberries

Red raspberries (*Rubus idaeus* L.) are unique berries with a rich history and nutrient and bioactive composition. The putative health benefits of raspberries and raspberry-based products is potentially attributed to the presence of several essential micronutrients, dietary fibers, and polyphenolic components, especially ellagitannins, flavanols, flavonols and anthocyanins, the latter of which give them their distinctive red coloring. Red raspberry extracts (or the entire fruit) could reduce/or reverse the risk of metabolically-associated patho-physiologies due to their constituents' anthocyanins and ellagitannins (and probably *via* their metabolites ellagic acid or urolithin), acting through various mechanisms, as has been revealed in *in vitro* and *in vivo* studies. The ameliorative effects of red raspberries and selected components, in modulating the risk of metabolic diseases, especially cardiovascular disease, diabetes mellitus, obesity, and AD, all of which share critical metabolic, oxidative, and inflammatory links, were assessed. The body of research is growing and supports an eventual participation of red raspberries in decrease the hazard of metabolically-dependent long-standing diseases [661].

<u>6.2.1.2.5. Phenylethanoid</u>

Olive Oil

Olive oil contains a type of phenolic compounds characterized by a phenethyl alcohol structure like tyrosol and hydroxyl-tyrosol named phenylethanoids.

Oleocanthal is also a phenylethanoid, (also known as (-) - decarboxymethyl ligstroside aglycone and p-HPEA-EDA), which belongs to the secoiridoid phenolic group and is found in quantities ranging from 0.2 to 498 mg/kg in extra-virgin olive oil (EVOO) and from 55 to 144 mg/kg in oil industry wastes [662].

Oleocanthal possesses anti-inflammatory and anti-oxidant properties *in vitro,* it is considered as a potent non-specific inhibitor of the inflammation-responsible enzyme COX, since it acts similarly to the family of the non-steroidal anti-inflammatory drugs [662]. It is noteworthy that the therapeutic effect of oleocanthal was assessed to mimic drug *ibuprofen-like activity* as follows: An amount of 50 g (4 tablespoons) of a typical EVOO per day comprises a quantity of oleocanthal with an *in vitro* anti-inflammatory upshot, equivalent to 1/10 of the suggested dose of ibuprofen for adult pain relief [663].

Long-term intake of small oleocanthal quantities was proposed that may contribute partially for the preservation of low occurrence of heart diseases and AD, connected with MeDi [663, 664]. Oleocanthal has recently earned the interest of the scientific community, after it has been demonstrated that it can disturb Aβ and tau aggregation *in vitro* [665] and enhance Aβ clearance from mice brains [666].

Oleocanthal enhanced the effect of estradiol on the regulation of gene expression, involving estrogen receptor α, a process believed to be regulated through heterodimeric estrogen receptors. Oleocanthal binds to both estrogen receptors inducing estradiol-agonistic or anti-agonistic effects [667]. It has been suggested that AD is most prevalent in females than males, a fact that may be attributed partly in estrogen signaling impairment. Estrogens also play critical roles in neurogenesis and it is known to have a protective effect on the brain. Loss of estrogen during menopause could, in part, lead to the deficits seen in brain metabolism (mitochondrial impairment) in AD. Estrogens play a multi-functional role like both in reduction of Aβ generation, exerting favor in the non-amyloidogenic pathway *via* MARK/ERK activation and in the BACE1 levels, and promoting Aβ clearance by both modulating the levels of Aβ degradative enzymes or/and activating the microglial phagocytotic process [668].

Olive oil was also suggested as a principal and powerful dietary agent for its therapeutic effect against cognitive impairment, and evaluated by behavioral performance and neuropathology, due to its high content in sanitary constituents like oleuropein aglycone (OLE) and polyphenols [669].

OLE is also a phenylethanoid, a type of phenolic compound found in olive leaf together with other closely related compounds, which are tyrosol esters of elenolic acid with substitution of hydroxylation or glycosylation like 10-hydroxyoleuropein, ligstroside, and 10-hydroxyligstroside. It is also one of the main natural phenols found in argan oil.

OLE, a natural phenol plentiful in the extra virgin olive oil exerts its valuable protective and therapeutic effects against neurodegeneration and other peripheral inflammatory and NDs including AD. Moreover, the noteworthy protective role of OLE reflected in significant amelioration of pathological "hallmarks" which originated from stress situations like oxidative stress, an immoderate inflammatory response, and the existence of amassed fibrillary matter of Aβ and hyper-phosphorylated tau triggering neuro-cytotoxicity [670].

The effects produced by nutritional administration of two OLE doses, (12.5 or 0.5 mg/kg of diet) in TgCRND8 (Tg) mice models, were investigated. In parallel, to exploit the abundant content of olive mill wastewater in the mix of polyphenols, a dose as high as 50 mg/kg of diet has administered. The findings showed a significant amelioration of cognitive operation of Tg mice after OLE supplementation at 12.5 mg/kg of diet and the mix of polyphenols. It is notable that OLE affects importantly the Aß42, the pE-3Aß plaque area and number, which have been diminished in the cortex by OLE and in both the cortex and hippocampus by the mixture of polyphenols, exerting a neuroprotective role. However, conclusively, despite that the consequences of OLE were recorded on behavioral efforts, and on neuropathological situation are dose-dependent, however, they are not closely related to OLE by itself [669].

A number of both *in vivo* and *in vitro* studies carried out in the meantime, and data have been emerged concerning the important potentiality of the phenolic ingredients of EVOO (mostly OLE and oleocanthal) in confronting amyloid deposition and neurotoxicity, emphasizing especially on the pathways implicated in the emergence and advancement of AD: βAPP processing, Aβ and tau assemblage, autophagy dysfunction and neuro-inflammation [671].

In the sequence of events for occurrence of the cell death in brain of AD patients that initiates with Aβ accumulation, the enzyme poly(ADP-ribose) polymerase-1 (PARP1) activation was critically correlated as contributor. Recent data highlight the beneficial effect of OLE, which when administered to 6-month-old TgCRND8 mice at dose of 50 mg/kg of diet for duration of 2 months, restored the levels of PARP1 activation and the levels of its product PAR, to these of control values [672].

Moreover, in *in vitro* and *in vivo* studies, the OLE-promoted decrease of PARP1 activation was co-occurred by the over expression of metabolic sensor Sirtuin1 (Sirt1), and, *in vivo*, by a diminution of NF-κB and the pro-apoptotic marker p53. Conclusively, OLE therapy contravenes neuronal injury by modulating the interaction between PARP1 and SIRT1. It should be noted that Sirtuin1 (Sirt1), a NAD^+-dependent deacetylase is influenced by dietary factors, environmental stress, and also plays crucial roles in metabolic health by de-acetylating proteins in many tissues, as well as in the complexity of the hypothalamus. Owing its dependency on NAD+, Sirt1 also operates as a nutrient/redox sensor, which participates in the maturation process of hypothalamic peptide hormones by regulation of specific nuclear transcription factors [673].

(-)- Epigallocatechin-3-gallate
Green Tea

The principal constituent of green tea, with clinical importance, is epigallocatechin gallate (EGCG) known for its therapeutic action in health and disease. Other foods rich EGCG is carob flour, nuts, peaches, avocados, blackberries, strawberries, raspberries, plums, and onions. The relation that link oxidative stress and inflammation is well-established. A number of properties were ascribed to EGCG, that are associated with anti-AD, anti-aging or anti-tumor activities, and amelioration of the oxido-reduction situation of tissues by impeding structural destruction exerted by its powerful antioxidant potential [674].

Collectively, the chemical structure of compound found as constituents in natural foods exhibiting beneficial effects in AD as well as their biological activities are summarized in (Table **3**).

Table 3. Natural food-constituents with beneficial effects in AD.

Name	Chemical Structure	Foods Found in	Biological Activities	Refs.
Crocin	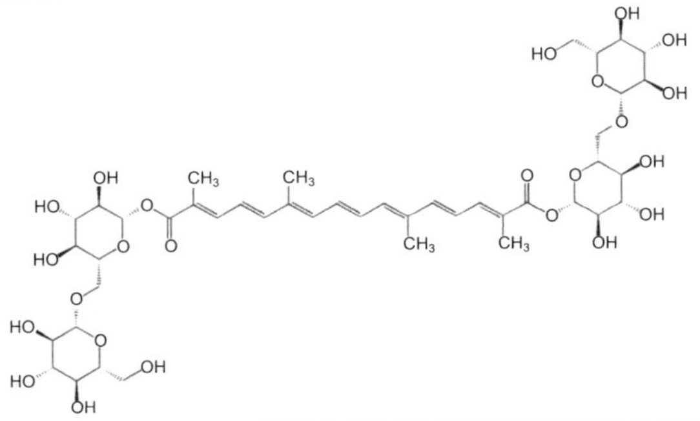	Plant *Croccus sativus*	Anti-amyloidogenic, anti-oxidative, anti-inflammatory neuroprotective anti-proliferative activities	[535 - 546]
Crocetin	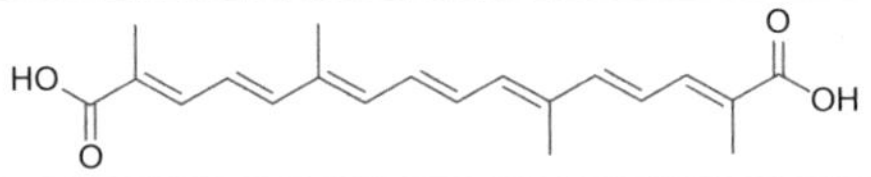	Plant *Croccus sativus*	Similar activities	
Picrocrocin	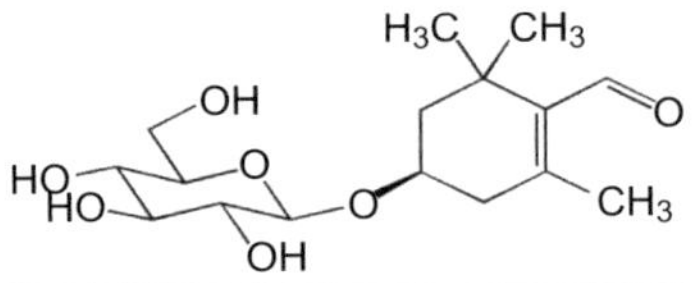	Plant *Croccus sativus*	Similar activities	
Safranal	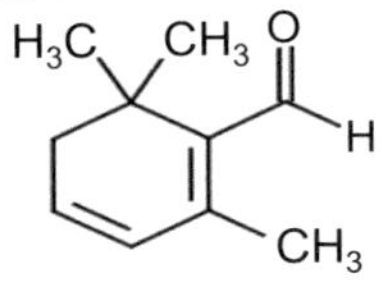	Plant *Croccus sativus*	Anti-inflammatory Anti-AD	[535 - 546]
Rosmarinic acid	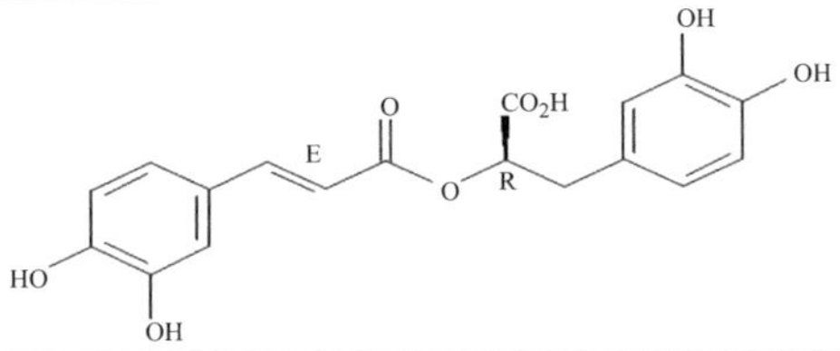	Rosemary, basil, holy basil, lemon balm, marjoram, sage, thyme and peppermint	anti-oxidative	[549, 550, 562, 565, 568]

(Table 3) contd.....

Name	Chemical Structure	Foods Found in	Biological Activities	Refs.
Quercetin	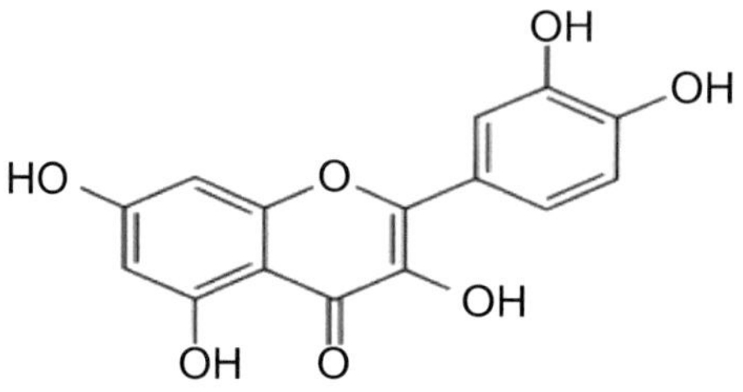	Red or white wines, raw spinach, sweet peppers, beans and broccoli, green chile peppers, lettuce, kale, asparagus, chicory greens capers, onions, cranberries, black plums, blueberries, chokeberries, black currants, apples and cherries	Anti-amyloidogenic, anti-oxidant, anti-inflammatory, Anti-proliferative, neuroprotective activities	[555, 556, 569]
Isoflavone skeleton Isoflavones (genistein, daidzein, glycitein, biochanin A, formononetin)	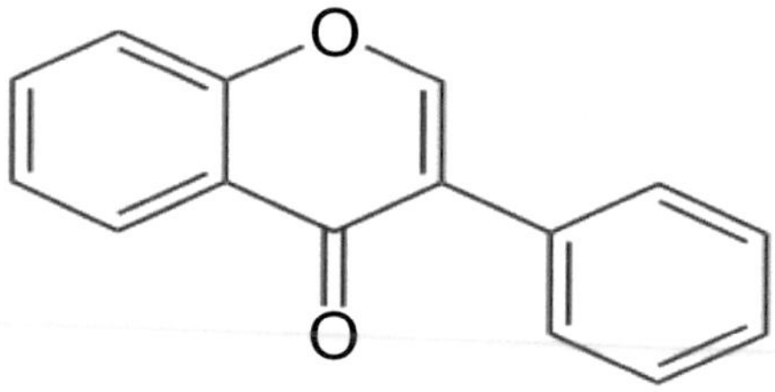	Soy products (soy flour, soybeans, chickpeas, pigeon peas, soya proteins, e.g. tofu, natto), bacon, meatless, nuts, peanuts, green tea	Ameliorative memory and learning ability, NMDA receptor interacting activity Safeguard of synaptic plasticity	[580 - 581]
Resveratrol	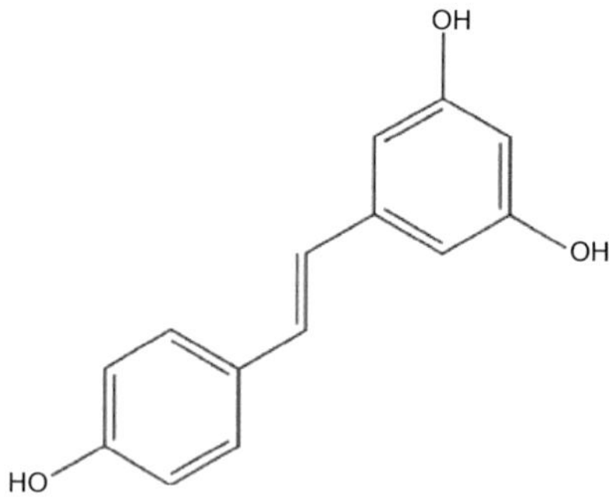	Red wine, red grapes, peanut butter, dark chocolate, blueberries	Anti-amyloidogenic, anti-oxidant, neuroprotective activities	[582, 584, 588, 592, 597 - 599, 605, 606, 609]
Curcumin	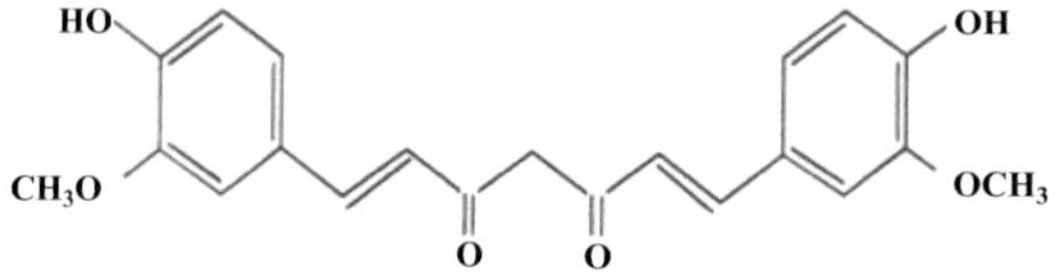	Turmeric, curry powders, mango ginger	Anti-amyloidogenic, anti-oxidant, anti-inflammatory	[661 - 622, 624, 628, 633, 634]

(Table 3) contd.....

Name	Chemical Structure	Foods Found in	Biological Activities	Refs.
Caffeic acid	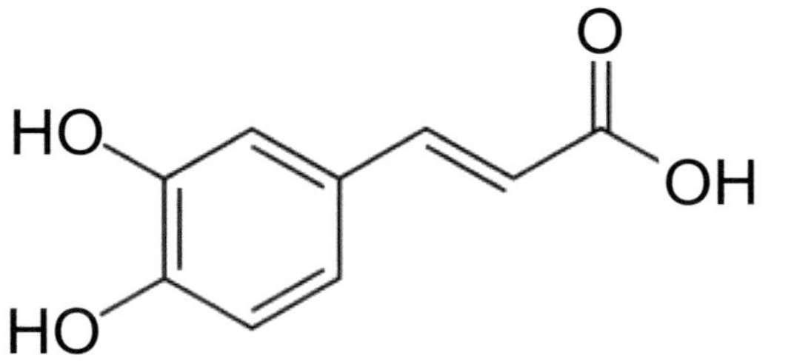	Coffee, green and black tea, ginger, olive oil and olive leaf extract, cucumbers, artichoke, potatoes, radishes, bell peppers, cabbage, apples, grapefruit, pear, basil, thyme, celery, oregano, tarragon, cayenne, curcumin	anti-oxidant, anti-inflammatory and anti-bacterial activities	[638, 639]
Cinnamic acid	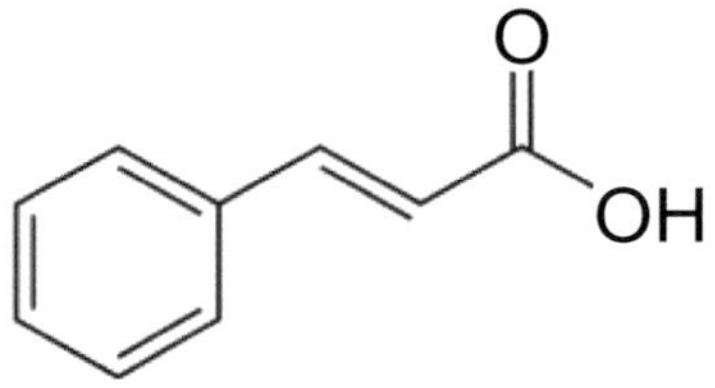	Olives green and black, extra virgin olive oil, cinnamon, orange (blood), berries (raw lingonberries, strawberries)	Anti-oxidative activity Anti-apoptotic activity, anti-inflammatory, diminution of Aβ, safeguard of memory and learning	[640 - 642]
Hydrolyzable tannins (Ellagitannins) Carbohydrate with Gallic acid and/or Ellagic acid	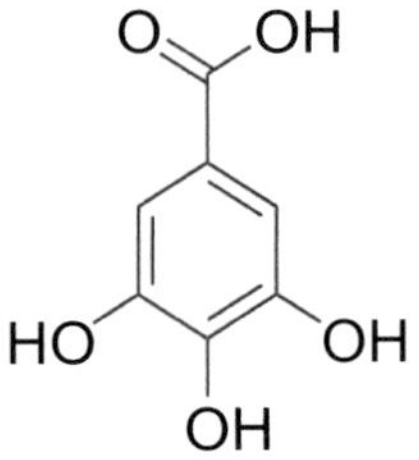 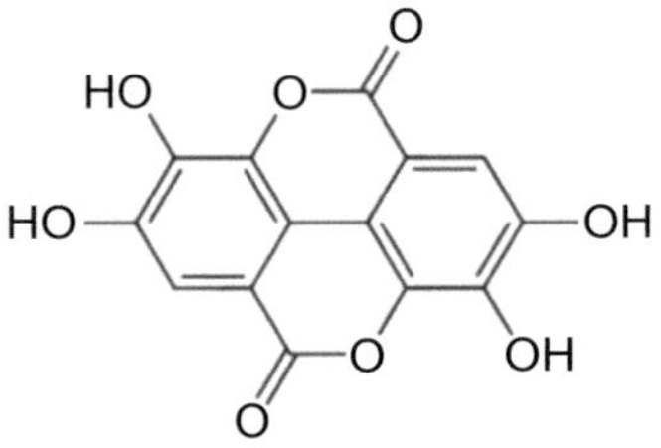	Pomegranate, raspberry, cloudberry, rose hip, strawberry, sea buckthorn, nuts species, oak-aged wines, walnuts, pecans, meaty mushroom, exotic fruits	Anti-inflammatory, anti-AD	[643 - 645]
Anthocyanins	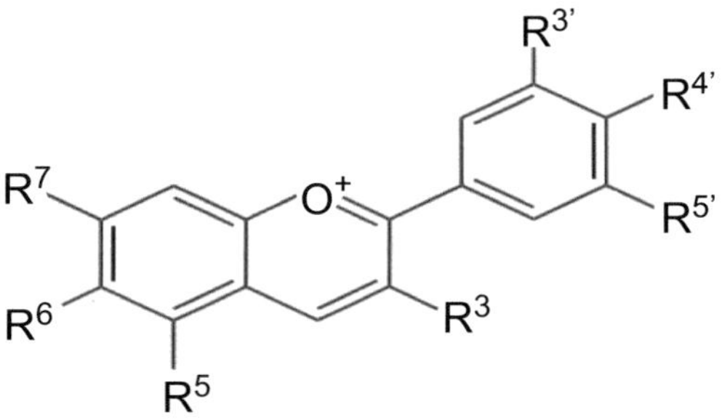	Blackberry, red and black raspberries, blueberries, bilberries, cherries, currants, blood orange, elderberries, grapes, and vegetables such as: red onion, radish, red cabbage, red lettuce, egg-plant, red-skinned potato and purple sweet potatoes.	Anti-inflammatory, anti-AD	[646]

(Table 3) contd.....

Name	Chemical Structure	Foods Found in	Biological Activities	Refs.
Hydroxy-tyrosol	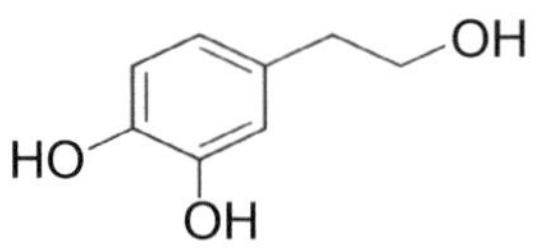	Virgin olive oil, olives black and green	anti-AD	[647]
Oleocanthal	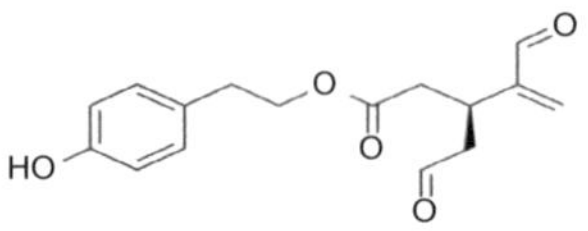	Extra virgin olive oil, olives black and green	anti-oxidant, anti-inflammatory, anti-AD	[647, 650, 651, 653]
Oleoporein	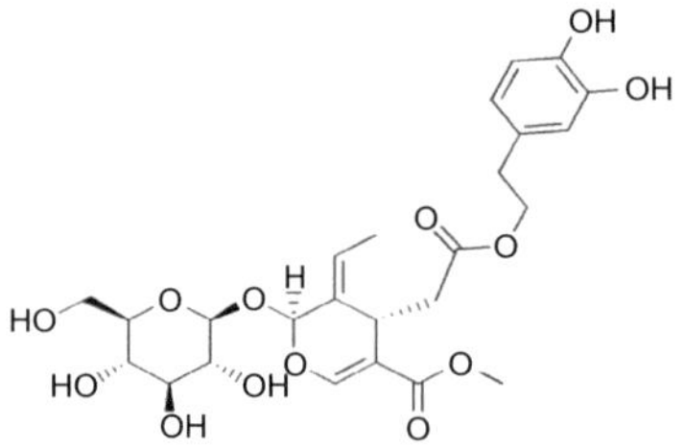	Virgin olive oil, olives black and green, olive leaves	anti-AD	[654 - 658]
(-)-Epigallo catechin-3-gallate	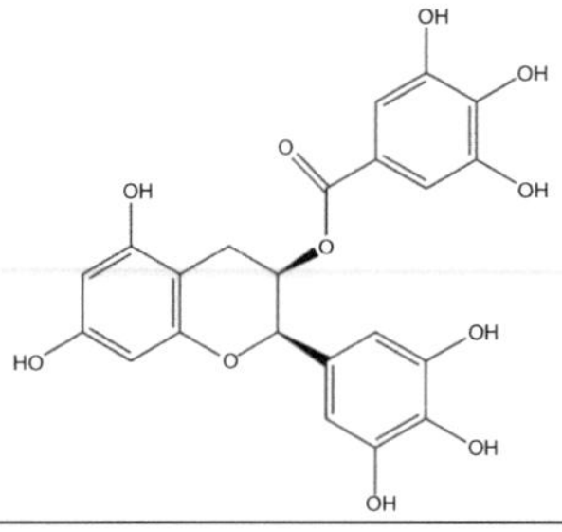	Green tea, carob flour, nuts, peaches, avocados, blackberries, strawberries, raspberries, plums, onions	Anti-oxidative activity	[659]

6.3. Mediterranean Diet (MeDi) and Asian Diet (AsDi)

MeDi and AsDi are nowadays regarded as the healthiest traditionary nutritional practices, efficacious against the hazard of senescence-related diseases, especially cardiovascular and neurodegenerative. The MeDi is an exhortation of contemporary alimentary habits, originally inspired by the traditional dietary footprints of Greece, Southern Italy, and Spain and other Mediterranean countries in the 1940s and 1950s [675, 676].

The principal features of these two regimens, MeDi and AsDi, include predominantly high consumption of food abundant in legumes, unrefined cereals, fruits, and vegetables, moderate to high consumption of fish, moderate consumption of dairy products (mostly as cheese and yogurt), moderate red wine consumption, and low consumption of non-fish meat products [677 - 679], and beverages of plant origin (green tea, extra virgin olive oil, red wine, condiments or seasoning, various berries, and fragrant herbs) that are considered responsible for the observed beneficial effects of aromatic herbs, thereby providing high quantities of plant bioactive constituents including polyphenols, glucosinolates, and antioxidant vitamins.

Furthermore, the oily fish, which is abundant in omega-3 fatty acids, is an important and common feature of the MeDi and of the AsDi (*e.g.*, Japanese). Both diets are enriched in particular plant bioactives, which occur in preponderance in the MeDi (*e.g.*, resveratrol from red wine, hydroxyl-tyrosol, and oleuropein from olive oil) and in the AsDi (*e.g.*, isoflavones from soybean and epigallocatechin gallate from green tea), shown in Fig. (**2**) [678]. It was suggested the recently so-called "MediterrAsian" diet that combines the sirtuin-activating foods (=sirtfoods) of the MeDi and AsDi, which may be a promising dietary tactic in prolepsis of chronic diseases, thereby ensuring health and healthy ageing. It is also notable that, when compared to calorie restriction which has been repeatedly shown to expand health span, these polyphenols activate similar molecular targets such as Sirt1 [678].

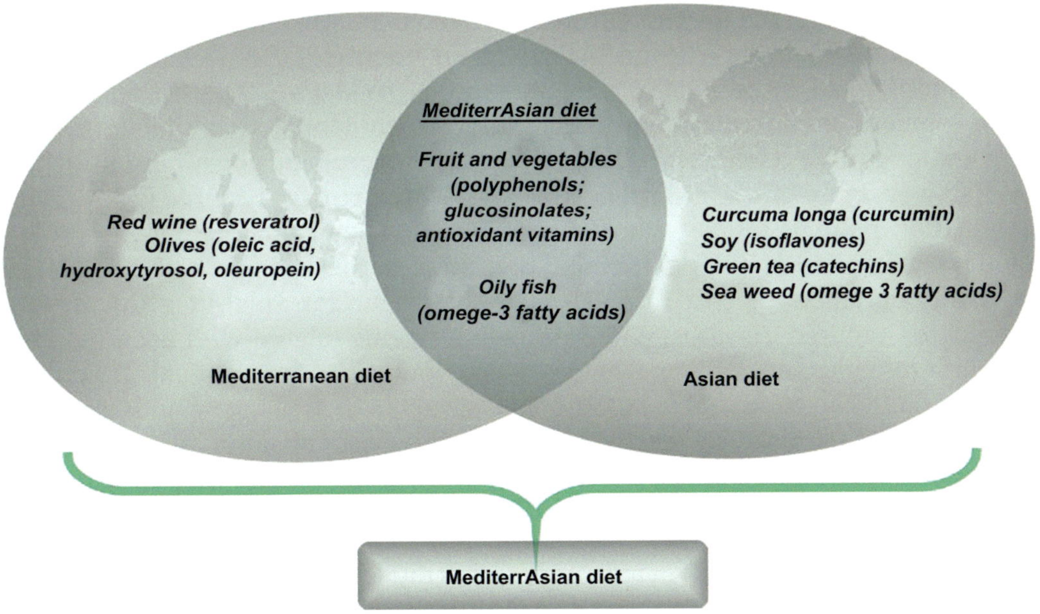

Fig. (2). Important food items and their corresponding constituents in the Mediterranean, Asian, and socalled MediterrAsian diet. Scheme kindly granted from [678]; Pallauf *et al.*, 2013, PMID: 24069505, http://dx.doi.org/10.1155/2013/707421.

The various kinds of NDs constitute a principal worldwide provocation and their social encumbrance increase with senescence of population. Taken into account the absence of efficient pharmaceutical therapies for habitual kinds of dementia comprising AD and vascular dementia, a growing research interest turns in different lifestyle changes, that will be able to impedes, slow down the clinical syndrome or retard the evolution of dementia. Higher adherence to a MeDi is linked with a considerable amelioration in health state, as observed by a notable decrease in the total death rate (9%), from various diseases including AD that reached (13%) [680]. It was suggested that these findings appeared to be clinically significant for public health, especially to embolden a MeDi-like alimentary model for the fundamental prolepsis of serious chronic diseases [680].

Recent predictable studies provided evidence that higher dedication (loyalty) to a MeDi-type could be correlated with delay of cognitive decline, decreased hazard of evolution from MCI to AD, diminished danger of AD, and generally decrease in all reasons of mortality in AD patients. The greater adaptation to a MeDi-type was connected with decreased cognitive decline only recently albeit the MeDi incorporates several foods, micro- and macronutrients although already separately each of them has proposed as potential protective agents against dementia and pre-dementia syndromes [681, 682]. Despite the fact that vascular parameters are probably to be involved in the causative route that joins MeDi and dementia syndromes and should be assumed as powerful intermediaries, some other non-vascular biological mechanisms (*i.e.*, metabolic, oxidative, and inflammatory) may be recruited in order to interpret the multiplex epidemiological liaison linking MeDi and cognitive decline [681]. However, high levels of consumption of fats from fish, vegetable oils, non-farinaceous vegetables, small glycemic index fruits, and nutrition poor in foods with added sugars and with moderate wine intake, should be emboldened. Epidemiological data suggest that the phenolic component remarkably-enriched in these foods play an important role in reducing the incidence of amyloid diseases, pathological situations related with accumulation of toxic proteinaceous aggregates in tissue, culpable for gradual functional deterioration [679]. In fact, this nutritional counsel is in symphony with guidance for reducing the risk of cardiovascular diseases, obesity, diabetes, and hypertension and might open new avenues for the prolepsis and administration of cognitive enfeeblement and dementia [682].

According to a systematic review, strict nutritional adherence to a MeDi is connected with a reduced danger of AD and slower cognitive decline [683]. Whereas another one conducted out by screening 664 studies to estimate the eventual association between the MeDi and cognitive impairment, has reached in similar conclusions, and found a negative relationship between high adherences to a MeDi with the risk of advancing from MCI to AD [684].

Much ink has been spent in the literature in recent years, galloping on the effects of polyphenols, from experiments in animal models and clinical trials to patients. The emerging attractiveness of these compounds for AD prevention and cure is localized in their broad spectrum of beneficial properties that ascribed them, including its anti-amyloidogenic capacity that is executed by inhibition of βAPP hydrolysis, antioxidant ability, and inflammation decrease and autophagy activation. A new notion was noted, which it should not consider natural polyphenols only as antioxidants or anti-amyloidogenic ingredients but as multi-potential targeting drugs. However, the principal pre-occupation focused on amelioration of their bioavailability, which seems to be low, using various strategies like encapsulation techniques *etc.* [684].

Several epidemiological studies demonstrated the correlation between MeDi and the diminished danger for AD. Furthermore, another study investigated the effect of the great dedication to MeDi and the structural alterations of brain atrophy observed in crucial areas for AD, in cognitively normal subjects, with and sans danger factors for AD, by comparing the total intracranial volume, as deduced by MRI [10]. Individuals who followed the MeDi possessed thicker cortex than those who did not follow, and the differences were significant, especially in the sensitive for AD areas of left hemisphere, as entorhinal cortex (EC), inferior parietal lobe, middle temporal gyrus, orbitofrontal cortex (OFC) and posterior cingulate cortex (PCC) Conclusively, MeDi exerts a protective role against the brain tissue loss [685].

A recent review centered on epidemiological evidence on the effects of MeDi on the prolepsis of dementia, that originated from cross-sectional and long-term studies with successive cognitive estimations, performed in Me and non-Me countries. Various dietary models were assayed for their influence on cognitive function ending up that the MeDi exhibited encouraging outcomes. It is notable that these findings have been also repeated in the frame of one recent randomized-controlled clinical trial, and the apparent mechanisms of action that may be responsible for the eventual protective role of MeDi on cognitive decline, were developed. Although the liaison among MeDi and cognitive decline has been only investigated last decade, evidence concerning the effectiveness is quickly galloping, and justifies the optimism for MeDi establishment, as an alternative prophylactic therapy for dementia [686]. A review also evaluates proofs on the comportment linked to the Me manner of life that have been proved to be correlated with cognition, namely the social interplay, the contribution in entertainment and somatic activities, as well as the sleep quality [687].

Several investigations have considered various dietary exemplars, notably the MeDi and the called DASH (Dietary Approaches to Stop Hypertension); however, they were not adapted to include nutrients and foods assigned as neuroprotective. A novel diet named MIND (Mediterranean-DASH Intervention for Neurodegenerative Delay) combines numerous constituents of the Me nutrition and DASH, but includes modifications that mirror present indications for their involvement in brain neuroprotection. However, the data supporting the correlation of diverse nutrients and the MeDi to dementia has been inconsequent, due to the trial design or to the inattention of the nutrients/food intake levels [688].

6.3.1. Diet Composition

6.3.1.1. Polyunsaturated Fatty Acids (PUFAs)

PUFAs constitute a significant member of membrane components, which affect membrane function *via* competition with n-6 PUFAs, the precursors molecules mediated in inflammatory process, and they exert improvement of brain disorders, by modulating neuro-immune and apoptotic mechanisms [689]. The consumption of fishes is considered a significant source of their PUFAs. Plethora of epidemiological studies evidenced the negative effects caused by the increased saturated fatty acids on age-related cognitive decline (ARCD) and MCI, whereas in contrast the augmented fish consumption providing high intake in mono-unsaturated fatty acids (MUFAs) and PUFAs respectively, particularly n-3 PUFAs, which influences in the reduction of risk for cognitive decline [690].

Epidemiological results showed that high PUFAs intake seems to have borderline non-considerable tendency for a protective upshot against the development of MCI. A number of assumptions, could be explicate the relationship between dietary UFAs and cognitive functioning, comprising the mechanisms through the concomitant existence of anti-oxidant constituents in food clusters abundant in fatty acids, *via* atherosclerosis, thrombosis, inflammation, or deposition of Aβ or also *via* an influence in structural integrity maintenance of neuronal membranes, specifying the fluidness of synaptosomal membranes that thereby arrange neuronal transmission [691].

In addition, recent data from clinical studies with n-3 PUFAs supplementation showed effectiveness on depressive symptoms only in non-apolipoprotein E (APOE) epsilon4 carriers, and on cognitive symptoms only in very mild AD subgroups, MCI patients, and cognitively unimpaired subjects non-APOE epsilon4 carriers. Collectively, these data support a probable role of fatty acid intake in preserving sufficient cognitive operation, and presumably in the prolepsis and administration of cognitive decline and dementia, but it seems to be not valid in case that the AD evolution process has already undertaken over [690].

Diet with abundant saturated fatty acids could negatively influences on both cognitive decline and MCI, whereas several epidemiological studies supported the correlation between the MUFAs and PUFAs (particularly, n-3 PUFAs) from fish intake, and the diminished danger of cognitive decline and dementia. Slight to modest alcohol consumption may be reflected to a decreased hazard of dementia occurrence and AD, while only a protective action is currently evidenced for vascular dementia, cognitive decline, and pre-dementia syndromes. Similarly, a protective effect against cognitive decline, dementia, and AD was associated with fruit and vegetable consumption. These findings suggested that adherence to the MeDi may affect not only the risk for AD, but also for pre-dementia syndromes and their progression to apparent dementia. Nonetheless, at present, no definitive dietary recommendations are possible [682].

Generally, it is commonly accepted that diets based in high content in fat affect body weight as well increase the danger of AD development. A comparative study was carried out for diets with different composition concerning a high content in fat against a high protein, or against high carbohydrates, with the same colorimetric value, in respect of their effect in development of cognitive impairment and brain pathology, in wild-type and Tg AD models mice. It was demonstrated that prolonged period of nutritional administration with equilibrated diets containing analogue calorimetric value but with essential variations in the source of calories, exerts negative influence on cognition when compared to the control diet, and that this result is more emphasized in Tg animals with AD pathology [692].

Various studies were carried out that exhort different diets in order to prevent or to better administrate AD, by adopting certain dietary habits or practices, strongly emphasizing the MeDi and the Japanese-style diet, both of which are abundant in fish and vegetables that are rich in vitamin E, carotenes, antioxidant flavonoids, vitamin B12, folate, and n-3PUFAs. It is proposed the administration of supplements of folate (to reach in serum <12 nmol/L) and of vitamin E daily to be <6.1 mg that may act protectively against cognitive decline of old people's. Conclusively, the nutritional recommendations in order to prevent and manage AD include a high intake of fish, vegetables, and low glycemic index fruits; a moderate quantity of meat and milk products; and a lower amount of carbohydrates and refined sugar [693].

An important nutritional issue concerning the relationship between diet and dementia is the link of type-2 diabetes and hyper-insulinemia with AD. The malfunction of insulin signaling pathway could directly reflect to disturbed utilization of glucose in the AD brain as supported from expression array data obtained in the Hisayama study. In this case the medium-chain length triglyceride ketone bodies might be used in place of improper utilization of glucose, constituting an alternative resource of energy for the AD brain [694].

A recent article reviews the association between AD and type 2-diabetes, strongly supported by epidemiologic evidence and common molecular mechanisms. It claims that in both diseases, common features occur, like local inflammation and amyloidosis that are associated with periodontitis and the presence of various infectious agents, providing also evidence for the presence of bacteria in diabetes type 2 and discussing the interactions host-pathogen during chronic inflammatory disorders. It also records some bacteria, like *Chlamydophyla pneumoniae, Helicobacter pylori* and spirochetes that are demonstrated to be associated with dementia and brain lesions in AD, and with islet lesions in diabetes type 2. The presence of various pathogens in host stimulates immune responses through TLRs signaling pathways, described previously in this review. Evasion of pathogens from complement-mediated attack ends in tenacious infection, inflammation and amyloidosis. Aβ and the pancreatic amyloid, named amylin, are connected to lipid bilayers and cause Ca ($^{2+}$) inflow and bacteriolysis. In a similar way with AD, cumulation of amylin deposits in diabetes type 2 may originate from an inherent immune response to protracted bacterial infections, which are linked with amyloidosis [693].

Recent studies have promoted the consumption of seafood, thanks to their high content in α-linolenic acid (18:3 n-3), and because it is associated with the appearance of lesser features of AD neuropathology such as the lower compactness of neuritic plaques, less intense and widely-extended neurofibrillary tangles. Nevertheless, high levels of the neurotoxic mercury implicated in the brain, and they are not associated with elevated levels of brain neuropathology. This effect is not due to fish oil supplementation, since it was not correlated positively with any markers of neuropathology. Moreover, it is notable the report that higher intake of α-linolenic acid (18:3 n-3) levels were associated with lower odds of cerebral macro-infarctions [688].

For many years, taken into account experimental and clinical studies for n--PUFAs, (mainly eicosapentaenoic acid (EPA) and docosahexaenoic acid (DHA; 22:6 n-3), were considered as significant dietary constituents involved in prevention or amelioration of NDs [689]. However, the manner of action in order to exert their beneficial role is not yet elucidated. DHA (its trivial name is cervonic acid) is an omega-3 long-chain polyunsaturated fatty acid (LCPUFA), which is a fundamental structural component of the human brain and cerebral cortex, and constitutes an undivided piece of structural phospholipids of neurons membrane that affects brain operation, whereas the potential roles of DHA in the mechanisms of AD are under active research [695].

The DHA daily intake (a 0.1-g/day) was suggested as a significant n-3 PUFAs of marine provenance due to its association with lower risk for MCI, dementia or

AD. Significant curvilinear relations between fish consumption and risk of AD and between total PUFAs and risk of MCI (both P-nonlinearity < 0.001), were observed. Marine-derived DHA was associated with lower risk of dementia and AD but without a linear dose-response relation [696].

Recent evidence concerning the ameliorative effects of n-3-PUFAs, of EPA and DHA-on the treatment of major depression and AD, as well as an approach to the cellular and molecular mechanisms, by which these fatty acids alone or in combination, exert these beneficial effects on these diseases, were discussed. It is also emphasized their synergistic capacity on contributing on anti-inflammatory, anti-oxidant and neurotrophic pathways in the brain [689].

The dietary supplementation with the n-3 PUFAs, DHA and EPA; 20:5 n-3, affects positively cognitive operation, by means of an eventual mechanism of modulating the cerebral hemodynamics, as demonstrated recently by numerous trials performed in normal both young and old individuals. It is noteworthy that a recent investigation, that has performed tests either DHA alone or in combination as constituent of multi-nutrient supplement including Gingko biloba, phosphatidylserine and vitamins B_9 and B_{12}) showed that it does not modulate cerebral hemodynamics or cognitive operation in healthy elderly adults [697].

In the diet, it is also important to having an optimal DHA/EPA ratio. The effects of n-3 PUFAs on cardiovascular disease are controversial, while recent results suggest that achieving an n6/n3 ratio of 4:1 is beneficial. Experiments were performed in model apolipoprotein E knockout (apoE−/−) mice, by variation of high-fat diets (HFD) that were partially replaced with fish and algal oils reflecting in the DHA/EPA ratio (DHA/EPA 2:1, 1:1 and 1:2), and/or plant oils enriched in linoleic and alpha-linolenic acids with an n6/n3 ratio of 4:1. Results showed that n3PUFAs from animals had more potent athero-protective effects than that from plants. Supplementation involving higher DHA/EPA ratios and an n6/n3 ratio of 4:1 was beneficial for reducing serum "bad cholesterol" and a 1:1 DHA/EPA ratio with an n6/n3 ratio of 4:1 was beneficial for improving serum "good cholesterol" [698].

The benefits of EPA and DHA supplementations on cognition in dementia and/or AD elderly were explored. Administration of EPA and/or DHA ameliorated oral fluency and attention in patients who had only very mild dementia or AD or displayed APOEε4 negative genotype. However, supplementation of EPA and/or DHA did not restrict the rates of cognitive decline in cases of elderly patients with advanced AD, neither affect scores obtained on the cognitive tests [699]. Observation-based studies support an advantageous correlation between intake/blood levels of DHA/EPA and memory function in elderly adults.

Supplementation of the DHA/EPA combination at dose higher than 1 g/day ameliorated remarkably episodic cognitive issues of elderly individuals expressing mild subjective memory grievances [700].

7. THERAPEUTIC/PREVENTIVE INTERVENTIONS

AD is a debilitating condition, and the search for an effective treatment is ongoing. Currently, no effective treatment exists that can slow, reverse or prevent sporadic AD. Yet, this disease is presently incurable and treatable only in terms of modest delay of symptomatic progression. The need for more effective pharmacological intervention is becoming more pronounced as the patient population increases.

Reviews focusing on the possibility of finding a cure for AD indicate that it is highly unlikely that a cure will ever be available for this dementia [11]. The main reason for this conclusion is that dead or mortally damaged neurons which govern mental activities such as memory, language and intellect, cannot be brought back to health or replaced with transplanted healthy neurons (even if that were possible) because it would entail forming a new individual, that is, a new mind. The alternative option is to search for ways to prevent or delay the appearance of severe cognitive decline before AD conversion to occurs.

7.1. Future Medications

7.1.1. Anti-Inflammatory Drugs

During the past few years, there has been an increase in the use of targeted therapies for different kinds of inflammatory disorders. Most of these drugs, including etanercept – a TNFα inhibitor, have a high molecular weight, which prohibits them from passing the BBB. This is not a problem when treating diseases such as rheumatoid arthritis, but it becomes an obstacle when the brain is the primary focus of inflammation. The latter is presumed to be the case in brain injury in AD. It is suspected that inflammation, as a consequence of amyloid deposition, plays an important role in the cognitive decline in AD and that the intensity of this inflammatory reaction influences the speed of cognitive decline in individual patients [12]. There is lack of proof that perispinal injection of drugs like etanercept would lead to effective concentrations in the brain. Before this technique can be recommended for treatment in patients with AD and other neurologic diseases, proof of concept is needed. However, the vertebral venous system being an anatomical route to bypass the BBB can deliver high molecular drugs to the CNS. Based on the literature, and the now available new data, it is suggested that there is even insufficient basis to propose a randomized controlled trial at this point [13].

7.1.2. Anti-Amyloid Treatment

In this chapter, we hypothesize that bacterial products can possibly increase the probability for an individual to develop sporadic AD. Therefore, what follows are some experimental suggestions regarding treatments against bacterial and other amyloids. Investigating the full, complicated spectrum of amyloids production and metabolism in human cells, is beyond the scope of this project and thus no reference for interventions to the eukaryotic amyloids biosynthesis will be made.

7.1.2.1. Disrupting Bacterial Amyloid Biogenesis

Bacterial functional amyloids, (*e.g.* chaplin, curli and tafin), are, as previously stated, essential for the establishment of their biofilm and therefore for the microbial installment and viability at the host tissue and abiotic structures [701]. Although, amyloids can prove toxic if the production is not under strict control from the cell, bacteria are capable of controlling their biogenesis by employing several control-points. For instance, curli production is the result of the orchestrated expression of seven different genes (curli specific genes A-G – csgA-G), which are incorporated into two different operons (csgDEFG and csgBAC). The expression of curli is csgD-dependent, as the CsgD protein is the regulator of csgBAC operon. CsgG, after transported to the outer membrane, acts as an anchor for the polymerization of the main component of curli – CsgA and the secondary CsgB. CsgC, CsgE and CsgF are also utilized during this process as main effectors for the secretion and localization of curli. Especially CsgE can act as a CsgA-chaperone, inhibiting the polymerization *in vitro* [187].

Curlicides are a class of organic compounds, described in 2009 by Cegelski *et al.*, inspired by pilicides (*i.e.* compounds targeting bacterial pili). They are ring-fused 2-pyridones that differ in their phenyl ring modifications or in the position of naphthyl substitution. Researchers found that the employment of two of these peptidomimetics, namely FN075 and BibC6, at concentrations of 1.0 and 2.5 mM respectively, was enough to block curli biosynthesis *in vivo* from two different E. coli strains (avirulent MC4100 and uropathogenic UTI89). 2.5 mM of another member of these derivatives, VA028, also decreased the production. These results were attributed to a dose-dependent, selective inhibition of CsgA polymerization *in vitro*, while a concomitant CsgB reduction has also been noticed when dosing with FN075 and BibC6 at 2.5 mM. Finally, pretreatment of UTI89 strain with FN075 disabled the virulence ability of the bacteria to colonize mice bladder and prevented the development of intracellular bacterial communities. FN075 compound has been proven both a pilicide and curlicide, thus proving the importance of pili and curli at the virulence of bacteria [702]. The same research group also presented a vast array of additional compounds to be tested as curlicides and pilicides in the future [703].

Recently, Arita-Morioka *et al.* presented a different approach for impeding curli formation. They tested several compounds, namely myricetin, pancuronium bromide, telmisartan and zafirlukast [704], which have been reported to disturb DnaK – a HSP70-bacterial analogue – functions *in vitro* [705]. DnaK has been proven to be crucial for the formation of curli, although the molecular mechanism could not be elucidated. However, researchers speculated that DnaK may control quality and/or quantity of the curli main regulator - CsgD and the sigma factor RpoS, both of which are essential for curli-dependent biofilm formation. In addition, they proved that myricetin, a polyphenolic compound found in vegetables, fruits, nuts, berries, tea and red wine, can disrupt DnaK cellular functions *in vivo*, leading to defective curli biosynthesis and biofilm formation [704].

7.1.2.2. B-sheet Breakers and Other Inhibitors of Amyloid Fibrilization

It is now well-known that the self-assembly of amyloidogenic proteins generally occurs through the following steps: (i) formation of misfolded intermediates, (ii) self-assembly of misfolded intermediates into oligomers and (iii) fibrillization of oligomers into mature fibrils with oligomers functioning as seeds [706]. Mature fibrils are characterized by rich β-sheet structures, recognized with electron microscopy, NMR and X-ray fiber diffraction [707], and dyed by substances like Thioflavin T [708] and Congo Red [709]. Two predominant models have been proposed for the protein self-assembly process. One involves π–π interaction, in which the aromatic residues of amyloidogenic proteins interact *via* π-stacking, resulting in amyloid formation. Amyloid monomers are rich in aromatic residues (especially phenylalanine and tryptophan), thus proving this model plausible [710]. A second model involves fibrilization by hydrophobic interactions [711].

B-sheet breakers are substances designed to inhibit the fibrillogenesis of amyloidogenic proteins. They are usually short peptides, peptide-mimetics or other organic compounds that possess the ability to interfere to the fibrilization procedure. Some of these compounds are resembling amyloids and can interact with them, but are not able to promote further polymerization, thus preventing the amyloidogenic aggregation [712]. Soto *et al.* were the first to describe this class of molecules in 1996, hypothesizing that the Aβ analogues could impede fibrilization of AD amyloid. Indeed, focusing on a highly hydrophobic region (LVFFA), scientists synthesized an 11-amino acid peptide (termed iAβ1). iAβ1 was unable of self-aggregation and could inhibit concentration-dependently the *in vitro* amyloidation of Aβ40 and Aβ42. The inhibitor was also able to induce the disintegration of amyloid fibers after 2 days. Furthermore, shorter derivatives of iAβ1 and D-amino-acids-alternatives, are reported as similar or better inhibitors than iAβ1 and more stable against proteolysis [713]. In 1998, researchers used iAβ5 peptide (LPFFD), employing rat models and neuroblastoma cells. The compound was able to reverse the neurotoxic effects of administrated Aβ42 at the cell lines, and impede the formation of dense plaques in rats dosed with Aβ42 directly into the amygdala [712]. Also, researchers reported *in vivo* reduction of amyloid deposition and of cerebral damage in a double transgenic animal model of AD, treated with an iAβ5 derivative. The product was resistant against proteolytic degradation and able to be taken up by the brain [714]. Similar peptides have also been reported and studied for various other proteins [707].

Β-sheet conformation is based on hydrogen bonds. Consequently, interfering specifically with these bonds should be enough for disturbing amyloid formation. Indeed, Rijkers *et al.* demonstrated that the employment of oligopeptides based on $amylin_{20\text{-}29}$ structure, with L-Ser28 substituted with D-Ser28, could delay the amylin gelation for two hours, as proved by EM and FTIR studies. Further modification on the amide bond near that Ser delayed the gelation more than 24 hours. Replacing Ser with other amino acids, like proline, inhibited the gelation almost completely, proving that the hydrogen donor at the amide bond is essential for β-sheet interactions and fibrillization [715].

N-methylation is a modification that disrupts hydrogen bonding due to steric effects. Therefore, N-methylated peptides (known as "memtides") have been examined as inhibitors of amyloidogenesis. The process involves the methylation of the short region amides that are crucial for the hydrogen bonding and the amyloid aggregation. This modification induces a Janus-like behavior to the monomer – one side is able for interactions, while the other is not, disrupting fibrillization process [716]. Hughes *et al.* first described this approach in 2000, designing six N-methylated derivatives of $A\beta_{25\text{–}35}$. NMeGly33 has been proven the most effective, disrupting aggregated *Aβ* fibrils, inhibiting polymerization of monomers and ameliorating *Aβ* toxicity at rat pheochromocytoma (PC12) cells. Authors also speculated that the detoxifying ability of NMeGly33 is probably attributed to the inhibition of neurotoxic proto-filaments and that N-methylated peptides are exerting their inhibitory effects *via* these elements rather than fully formed fibrils [717].

Several other teams had successfully synthesized and used oligopeptides that could inhibit the aggregation of amyloidogenic proteins. El-Agnaf *et al.* produced a peptide that could interact with full-length α-synuclein (PD-associated amyloid) and block its assembly into both early oligomers and mature amyloid-like fibrils. Also, this peptide could pass through membranes and abolish DNA damage from Fe(II) in neuronal cells transfected with α-syn(A53T) - a familial PD-associated mutation [718].

Hughes' team efforts were pioneering and more followed. Gordon *et al.* experimented with Aβ40, synthesizing nemtides based on $A\beta_{17\text{-}22}$ region. N-Methyl amino acids were utilized in the design of these peptides and two of them, namely Aβ16-22m and Aβ16-22mR, inhibit *in vitro* fibrillogenesis of full-length Aβ40 in a dose-dependent manner. They are also able to cause disassembly of preformed Aβ40 fibrils. These peptides are soluble and resistant to proteolysis – important properties for medicinal applications [719]. The same research team, one year later, produced a truncated analogue (named Aβ16–20m) to their previous nemtides, in order to introduce a positive charge to the peptide and render it membrane-permeable. In addition to its fibrinolytic activity, the nemtides were indeed able to cross through artificial and wild lipid bilayers and also proved resistant to various denaturing agents [720]. Kokkoni *et al.* have synthesized and studied a great variety of N-methylated peptides in order to optimize the structure. They found that that nemtides should contain only D-amino acids, have a free N-terminus but an amidated C-terminus and have large, branched hydrophobic side chains [721].

A double N-methylated peptidomimetic (termed IAPP-IG) has been utilized by Yan *et al.* against the fibrillization of islet amyloid polypeptide (IAPP) – a protein that acts as a neuroendocrine regulator of glucose homeostasis and is found to promote β-cells' death through aggregation, in diabetes mellitus. IAPP-GI is a highly soluble, non-amyloidogenic, and non-cytotoxic. IAPP-GI binds IAPP with high affinity and effectively blocks IAPP cytotoxic self-assembly and fibrillogenesis in low nanomolar concentrations. Furthermore, IAPP-GI dissociates cytotoxic IAPP oligomers and fibrils and is able to reverse their cytotoxicity [722].

Several natural products (extensively reviewed previously in this chapter), are recognized as possible inhibitors of amyloid fibrillization. Natural polyphenols (*e.g.* β-carotene, curcumin, resveratrol, myricetin, caffeic acid), as well as non-phenolic aromatic compounds, are rich in aromatic rings, which can interfere in the specific π-stacking between amyloid monomers and therefore block the self-assembly process. It should be of notice that certain polyphenols mostly inhibit the elongation phase of fibril assembly or the assembly of large oligomers. Indeed, reports argue that polyphenols do not interact with the amyloidogenic monomers but preferably with the amyloidogenic structures, in a conformation-dependent manner. In addition, the aromatic hydroxide groups of polyphenols may inhibit polymerization by interacting with hydrophobic residues [707, 723]. Table **4** summarizes some of the most effective β-sheet harnessers mentioned above.

Table 4. Major amyloid-disruptors studied.

Compound	Molecular Structure	Reference
FN075	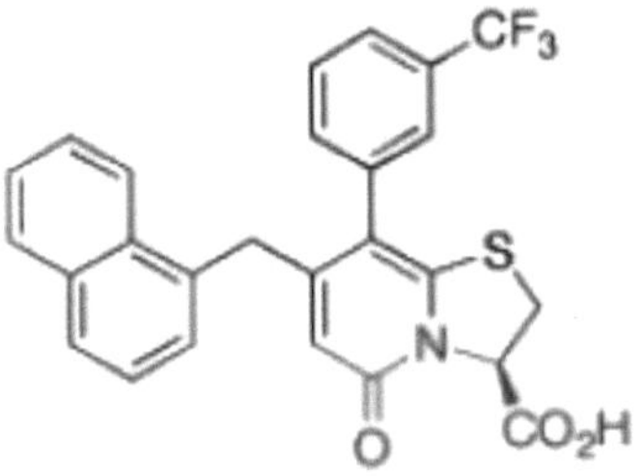	[687]
BibC6	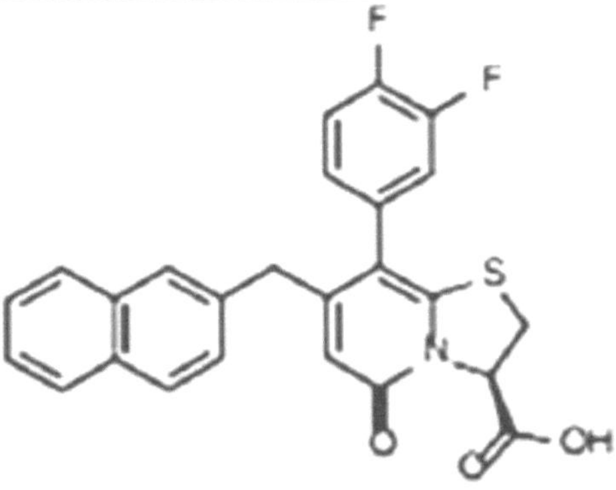	[687]
Myricetin	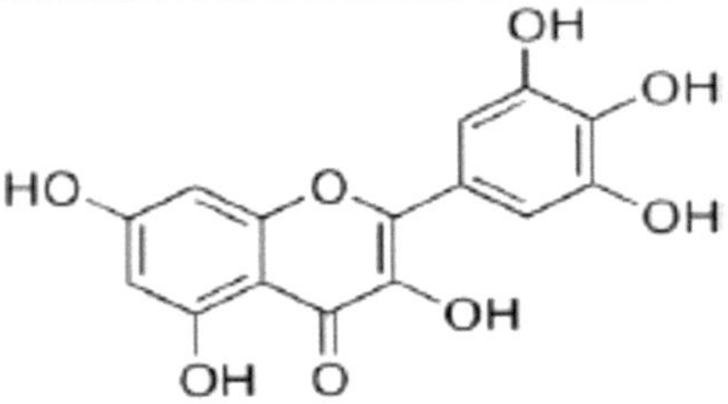	[689]
iAβ5 (LPFFD)	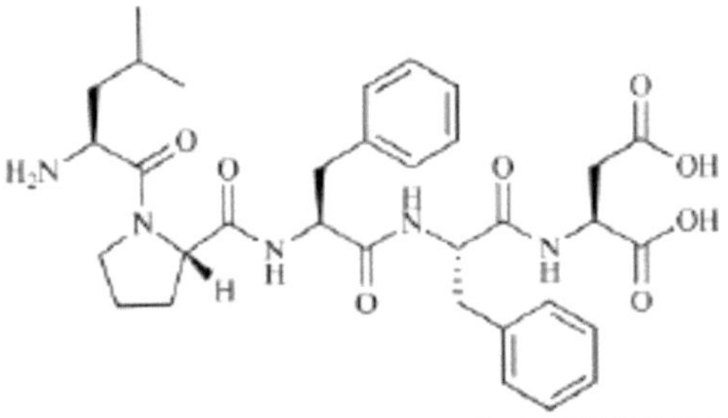	[697]

Though no strategy has been described to this moment targeting curli and other amyloidogenic bacterial products, it is proposed here that it is of great value to proceed in such an effort. It is believed that i) designing special β-sheet interfering agents against bacterial and other microbial amyloids and ii) exploiting crucial dietary agents, could be a way to confront both infectious agents and possibly lessen the risk for developing sporadic, amyloid-relevant pathology (*e.g.* AD, PD and other NDs). To our knowledge, there are but a little clinical researches aiming at the aforementioned options and we urge scientific community for it.

7.1.2.3. Monoclonal Antibodies (mAbs) in the Treatment of AD

Several companies have developed drugs that act against Aβ plaques, only to see them falter in late-stage clinical trials. In fact, some have questioned whether Aβ plaque is the right target for treatment drugs [724]. Current available drugs against AD, target towards cholinergic and glutamatergic neurotransmissions without affecting the underlying disease process. So, current therapies to treat AD are focused on ameliorating symptoms instead of treating the underlying causes of AD [725]. Vaccination has been proposed as a therapeutic approach for NDs, and clinical evaluations of some candidates for AD and multiple sclerosis are ongoing.-Moreover, mAbs for passive immunotherapy are under evaluation for AD [726], synucleinopathies [727], and multiple sclerosis [728]. Experiments, in which AD model mice were immunized actively and passively with Aβ, demonstrated clearance of the Aβ aggregation and amelioration of memory and learning. Despite that the initial human trials were paused due to autoimmune encephalitis, however, it was demonstrated that the immunization with Aβ also has removed the amyloid deposition [729] with human's clinical profit. Putative disease-modifying medicaments are in evolution that target towards Aβ peptide and tau protein, the essential neuro-pathological hallmarks of the disease. Areas covered: Phase III clinical studies of emerging anti-Aβ drugs for the therapy of AD were demanded in clinical trial databases of US and EU as well as in the medical literature until May 2016.

Drugs, in Phase III clinical development for AD, include one inhibitor of the BACE (verubecestat) [730], three anti-Aβ mAbs (solanezumab [34], gantenerumab [731], and aducanumab [732]), an inhibitor of receptor for advanced glycation end products (RAGE) (azeliragon) and the therapeutic scheme of cromolyn sodium and ibuprofen (ALZT-OP1) [733]. These medications mostly must be administrated in AD patients either in the premature stages or at preclinical stages of AD or yet in asymptomatic patients with high hazard of progressing AD. The expectation is to interpose in the pathological process of disease before its further progression. Precedent clinical studies, however, were ended with failures with anti-Aβ medicaments and due to the absence of complete comprehension of the patho-physiological involvement of Aβ in the AD progression, set the novel drugs at essential possibility of failure [35].

They have been developed in this chapter the outcomes of mAbs only in clinical or pre-clinical trials, and it was concluded by supplying a synopsis of other modern and auspicious immunotherapeutic approaches based on antibodies, that they merit further interest for the efficacious AD therapy in the future.

7.1.2.3.1. mAbs that Target Aβ for Treatment of AD

There are different polymorphisms of Aβ species, including three different groups, comprising monomers, soluble oligomers, and insoluble fibrils, with every group enclosing several constructions of Aβ aggregates. Their toxicities are different in relation to the characterized epitopes of anti-Aβ mAb candidates under development. Oligomerization of Aβ42 is an early event in AD. The accumulation of Aβ oligomers, whether by an augmentation in generation or by a reduction in clearance, has been depicted as the seed that initiates the pathological cascade in AD [35].

In the past decades, extensive research focusing on the development of immunotherapy using mAbs as potential "disease-modifying drugs", has shown promise in inhibiting or clearing the formation of toxic Aβ species, the suspected causative agents of AD. As a result, these potential life-saving drugs could interrupt the cataract of toxic amyloid signaling, cease neurodegeneration, and impede more the cognitive decline and somatic function. Passive anti-Aß immunotherapy has been shown to clear brain Aß deposits. Two humanized mAbs, bapineuzumab and solanezumab, directed one against the N-terminal end and the other against the intermediate (middle) domain of Aβ, respectively, were recently tried in large, long-term Phase III trials in patients with mild-to-moderate AD. Results from phase III clinical trials in mild-to-moderate AD patients with these two mAbs and intravenous immunoglobulin have been disappointing [34, 734].

Developing therapies to target these species is a vital step in improving AD treatment. Several mAbs for the treatment of AD have been in development over the last decade. Immunotherapy with mAbs that directed towards Aβ has been examined as a therapy for AD patients. Aβ-immunotherapy, especially passive immunotherapy, is a promising approach to reduce the Aβ encumbrance.- Heretofore, a number of mAbs have been put to the clinical trials on humans, but none of them have advanced to Phase III. Perhaps these tests are not crowned with success because patients were recruited with mild-to-moderate AD, and thus treatment may have been too late to be effective. Therefore, many ongoing clinical trials are being conducted in patients at the prodromal stage. New constructions based on antibody fragments have been designed and engineered targeting to ameliorate safety and efficacy. Antibody-based immunotherapy against Aβ to trigger its clearance or mitigate its neurotoxicity has so far been unsuccessful [26].

Bapinauzumab

The long-term safety and tolerability of intravenous-administered bapineuzumab in patients with AD, was evaluated in apolipoprotein E ε4 allele non-carriers (Study 3002, extension of Study 3000) and apolipoprotein E ε4 allele carriers (Study 3003, extension of Study 3001). Patients treated with bapineuzumab in the initial study continued at the same dose; if receiving placebo, patients began bapineuzumab. Bapineuzumab doses were 0.5 mg/kg in both studies and also 1.0 mg/kg in the non-carrier study. Clinical effectiveness of bapineuzumab was also evaluated in various exploratory analyses. The (11)C-PiB-PET imaging results displayed decrease of fibrillary Aβ accumulation in AD patients subjected in bapineuzumab treatment; however, since no clinical benefit was observed, the results are in accordance with the hypotheses that bapineuzumab may not have been administrated fairly untimely in the disease course: either because the doses were inadequate, or the crucial Aβ species were unsuccessfully treated [735].

Due to the absence of effectiveness in two other phase 3 trials, the initial protocols were paused soon. A number of 694 (492 and 202) patients in total were registered in studies 3003 and 3002, respectively and as a result, the aforementioned studies 3002 and 3003 were also ended. In apolipoprotein E ε4 carriers (Study 3003), treatment-emergent unfavorable consequences occurred in 70.7% of the patients, who originally received placebo and 66.9% of those, who originally received bapineuzumab.

AAB-003

In the First-In-Human (FIH), 39-week, randomized, adaptive design study, safety, tolerability, pharmacokinetics and biomarkers were measured in patients with mild-to-moderate AD after infusion of a humanized mAb to Aβ, AAB-003 (NCT01193608; registered 19 August 2010). AAB-003 was developed by modifying bapineuzumab to reduce Fc-receptor-mediated effector function, as a strategy to reduce the removal of amyloid from vessel walls associated with amyloid-related imaging abnormalities with edema/effusions (ARIA-E), without diminishing overall amyloid clearance. The results from the FIH and extension study showed AAB-003 was safe and well tolerated up to 8 mg/kg for up to 91 weeks (First-In-Human study and its open label extension) in patients with mild to moderate AD. Asymptomatic and resolvable ARIA-E was observed after the first or second infusion of AAB-003, which is similar to bapineuzumab. In contrast, the AAB-003 dose, at which ARIA-E was observed, was considerably higher compared to bapineuzumab, a finding that supports the hypothesis that reducing

Fc-receptor effector function may reduce the risk of ARIA, associated with monoclonal antibodies targeting cerebral amyloid [736].

Solanezumab

EXPEDITION and EXPEDITION2 were identically designed placebo-controlled phase 3 studies assessing effects of solanezumab, an anti-Aβ mAb binding soluble Aβ peptide, on cognitive and functional decline over 80 weeks in patients with mild-to-moderate AD. Primary findings for both studies have been published. Secondary analyses of efficacy, biomarker, and safety endpoints in the pooled (EXPEDTION and EXPEDITION2) mild AD population were performed. In the mild AD population, less cognitive and functional decline was observed with solanezumab (n = 659) *versus* placebo (n = 663), measured by AD Assessment Scale Cognitive subscale (ADAS-cog), Mini-Mental State Examination, and AD Cooperative Study-Activities of Daily Living functional scale Instrumental ADLs. Baseline-to-endpoint changes did not differ between treatment groups for AD Cooperative Study-Activities of Daily Living functional scale, basic items of the ADCS-ADL, and Clinical Dementia Rating Sum of Boxes. Plasma/cerebrospinal fluid biomarker findings indicated target engagement by solanezumab. Solanezumab demonstrated acceptable safety. Efficacy findings for the moderate AD population are also provided. These findings describe solanezumab effects on efficacy/safety measures in a mild AD population. Another phase 3 study, EXPEDITION3, will investigate solanezumab's effects in a mild AD population [734].

Subsequent analysis of pooled data from both phase III trials with solanezumab showed a reduction in cognitive decline, in patients with mild AD. Solanezumab and new mAbs are being tested in patients with prodromal and preclinical AD in search for a disease-modifying treatment. Although solanezumab which recognizes Aβ monomer turned out ineffective in the primary endpoint, it showed significant beneficial effect in mild AD cases in the secondary outcome. Solanezumab showed some beneficial cognitive effects in mildly affected AD patients. This subgroup of AD patients is currently being tested in another Phase III trial to confirm previous encouraging observations. If it turns out that it is effective, it will be the first disease-modifying drug for AD in a few years. Solanezumab is also being tested in a prevention study in asymptomatic older subjects, who have positive positron emission tomography scans for brain amyloid deposits [734].

Aducanumab

Aducanumab is a human mAb that selectively targets aggregated Aβ. In a transgenic mouse model of AD, aducanumab is shown to enter the brain, bind parenchymal Aβ, and to reduce soluble and insoluble Aβ in a dose-dependent manner. The multicenter, randomized, double-blind, placebo-controlled study involved people with prodromal or mild AD who were, on average, between 70 and 74 years of age and were confirmed to have Aβ plaques using a florbetapir positron emission tomography (PET) scan. A number of 146 subjects were randomized into 1 of 5 treatment groups (placebo, 1 mg/kg, 3 mg/kg, 6 mg/kg, and 10 mg/kg of aducanumab) for 52 weeks. Reduction in amyloid plaque, as measured by the Standard Uptake Value Ratio (SUVR) of florbetapir, was seen at 26 weeks with further reductions at 54 weeks. With the mean baseline SUVR value between 1.4 and 1.5 among all the study arms, the mean composite SUVR in the highest dose arm was about 1.175 by Week 54 (in healthy people, SUVR is <1.13). Importantly, in addition to the significant reduction in amyloid plaque measurements, aducanumab was also associated with a slower rate of cognitive decline, as measured by the Mini-Mental State Examination (MMSE) and Clinical Dementia Rating Scale-sum of boxes (CDR-sb) scores [732]. So, in patients with prodromal or mild AD, one year of monthly intravenous infusions of aducanumab reduces brain Aβ in a dose- and time-dependent manner. The main safety and tolerability findings are amyloid-related imaging abnormalities. These results justify further development of aducanumab for the treatment of AD. Should the slowing of clinical decline be confirmed in ongoing phase 3 clinical trials, it would provide compelling support for the amyloid hypothesis. The phase 3 trial has been designed to include more than 1,000 patients. The failures of other Aβ drugs are recent enough to guard against unbridled optimism. But if aducanumab were to make it to market, it would be a major advance to have a disease-modifying drug for AD.

BAN2401 (mAb that Selectively Binds Soluble Aβ Protofibrils)

Safety and tolerability were investigated in mild to moderate AD in the first clinical study with BAN2401, a mAb that selectively binds soluble Aβ protofibrils. A study design was used with staggered parallel single and multiple ascending doses, from 0.1 mg/kg as a single dose to 10 mg/kg biweekly for four months. The presence of amyloid related imaging abnormalities (ARIA) was assessed with magnetic resonance imaging (MRI). CSF and plasma samples were analyzed to investigate pharmacokinetics (PK) and effects on biomarkers.

The incidence of ARIA-E/H (E for edema, H for hemorrhage) on MRI was comparable to that of placebo. BAN2401 exposure was approximately dose proportional, with a serum terminal elimination half-life of ~7 days. Only a slight increase of plasma Aβ1-40 was observed but there were no measurable effects of BAN2401 on CSF biomarkers. On the basis of these findings Phase 2b efficacy study has been initiated in early AD. BAN2401 was well-tolerated across all doses. The PK profile has guided us for selecting dose and dose regimens in the ongoing phase 2b study. There was no clear guidance for an effective dose based on biomarkers [737].

mAbs for Human APP in Transgenic Mice

As rodents do not normally develop Aβ pathology, as a consequence, various transgenic animal models of AD were designed to over-express human APP with mutations favoring its amyloidogenic processing. However, these mouse models display tremendous differences in the spatial and temporal appearance of Aβ deposits, synaptic dysfunction, neurodegeneration and the manifestation of learning deficits, which may be caused by age-related and brain region-specific differences in APP transgenic levels. Consequentially, a comparative temporal and regional analysis of the pathological effects of Aβ in mouse brains is difficult, complicating the validation of therapeutic AD treatment strategies in different mouse models.

To date, no antibodies are available that properly discriminate endogenous rodent and transgenic human APP in brains of APP-transgenic animals. Höfling's team has developed and characterized rat mAbs by immuno-histochemistry and Western blot analysis able to detect human but not murine APP in brains of three APP-transgenic mouse and one APP-transgenic rat models. Using this antibody, they observed significant differences in expression levels and brain region-specific expression of human APP, among the investigated transgenic mouse lines. This may explain the differences between APP-transgenic models mentioned above. These new antibodies specifically detect endogenous human APP in immuno-histochemistry, FACS and immuno-precipitation, and may serve as an important tool for monitoring expression of endogenous or transfected APP in human cells and APP expression in transgenic animals [738].

Gantenerumab and Crenezumab

Gantenerumab and crenezumab are fully human anti-Aβ mAbs with a high capacity to bind and remove Aβ plaques in the brain. Gantenerumab (currently undergoing Phase III clinical trial), represents a promising agent with a disease-modifying potential in AD. Gantenerumab is the first fully human anti-Aβ mAb, which preferentially binds to fibrillary Aβ, directed to both N-terminal and central regions of Aβ, whereas crenezumab preferentially binds to soluble, oligomeric and fibrillary Aβ deposits. A 6-month study with PET in 16 AD patients showed that gantenerumab treatment has reduced dose-dependently Aβ deposition in brain, possibly *via* directing microglia to digest the amyloid plaques. Two ongoing Phase III trials of gantenerumab in patients with prodromal or mild dementia due to AD will determine if any reduction in brain Aβ levels could be accompanied with clinical benefits. Furthermore, there are ongoing secondary prevention trial of gantenerumab and crenezumab in pre-symptomatic subjects with genetic mutations for autosomal-dominant AD, in order to investigate its possible preventive nature that will verify the utility of anti-Aβ mAbs as prevention therapy [731].

7.1.2.3.2. mAbs that Target Tau Pathology in the Treatment of AD

Tauopathies are NDs characterized by accumulation of hyper-phosphorylated tau protein tangles that is a crucial point in AD pathology and certain frontotemporal dementias. Extracellular tau may mediate propagation of amyloid, but no mechanism-of-action has currently be proved [739]. Nevertheless, active and passive vaccination studies against tau, in mouse models, reduce pathology. Intra-cerebro-ventricular administration of three anti-tau mAbs (HJ8.5, HJ9.3, and HJ9.4) reduces pathology in a model over-expressing full-length mutant (P301S) human tau. These effects on tau aggregates have been attributed to its uptake by BV2 microglial-like cells and primary neurons, as heparin blocked antibody-independent tau uptake into BV2 cells, consistent with a previously described role for heparan sulfate proteoglycans. Two alternative therapeutic antibodies (HJ8.5 and HJ9.4) promoted uptake of full-length tau fibrils into microglia *via* Fc receptors. It is surprising that HJ9.3 promoted uptake of fibrils composed of the tau repeat domain or AD-derived tau aggregates, but failed to influence full-length recombinant tau fibrils. Size fractionation of aggregates showed that antibodies preferentially promote uptake of larger oligomers (n ≥ ∼ 20-mer) *versus* smaller oligomers (n ∼ 10-mer) or monomer. It was found that no antibody inhibited uptake of full-length recombinant fibrils into primary neurons, but HJ9.3 blocked neuronal uptake of tau repeat domain fibrils and AD-derived Tau. Collectively, these antibodies may have multiple potential mechanisms, including clearance *via* microglia and blockade of neuronal uptake. However, these effects proved to be epitope- and aggregate size-dependent, and optimization of their effectiveness and elucidation of their mechanism, are peremptory. Demonstrating specific mechanisms of antibody activity *in vitro* may help in designing and optimization of factors that are more effective *in vivo* [740].

Pharmacological manipulation of tau protein in AD included microtubule-stabilizing agents, tau protein kinase inhibitors, tau aggregation inhibitors, active and passive immune-therapies and, more recently, inhibitors of tau acetylation. Animal studies have shown that both, active and passive approaches can remove tau pathology and, in some cases, improve cognitive function. Two active vaccines targeting both non-phosphorylated (AAD-vac1) and phosphorylated tau (ACI-35) have also entered Phase I testing [741]. Not with standing, the recent discontinuation of the mAbs RG7345 for AD, two other anti-tau antibodies,

BMS-986168 and C2N-8E12, are also currently in Phase I testing for progressive supranuclear palsy. After the recent impressive results in animal studies obtained by salsalate, the dimer of salicylic acid, inhibitors of tau acetylation, is being actively pursued.

Conformational changes involving the amino terminus of the tau protein are among the earliest alterations associated with tau pathology in AD and other tauopathies. This region of tau contains a phosphatase-activating domain (PAD) that is aberrantly exposed in pathological forms of the protein, an event that is associated with disruptions in anterograde fast axonal transport. Four antibodies were employed, which recognize the amino terminus of tau, TNT1, TNT2 (a novel antibody), tau12, and tau 13, to further study this significant region. Using scanning alanine mutations in recombinant tau proteins, it has been refined the epitopes of each antibody. To gain insights into some of the mechanistic details of PAD exposure, the antibodies' relative abilities to specifically label pathological tau, were examined in non-denaturing and denaturing assays. Furthermore, to characterize PAD exposure in the context of disease progression, the pattern of tau pathology labeled by each antibody in human hippocampal sections, at various disease stages, was then determined. The features of reactivity for the antibodies are restricted into two groups. TNT1 and TNT2 recognized epitopes within amino acids 7-12 and especially identified recombinant tau aggregates and pathological tau from AD brains in a conformation-dependent way. These antibodies were labeled early in pre-tangle pathology from neurons, in early Braak stages, and co-localized with thiazine red, a marker of fibrillary pathology, in classic neurofibrillary tangles. Whereas, retarded tangles were negative for TNT1 and TNT2 pointing out a loss of the epitope in later stages of tangle evolution. In contrast, tau12 and tau13, both identified discontinuous epitopes in the amino terminus, and were unable to differentiate between normal and pathological tau, in biochemical and tissue immune-histological assays.

Despite the close proximity of these epitopes, the antibodies demonstrated remarkably different abilities to recognize pathological changes in tau pointing out that, detection of conformational alterations involving PAD exposure, is not achieved by all N-terminal tau antibodies, and a relatively discrete region of the N-terminus (*i.e.*, amino acids 7-12, the TNT1 and TNT2 epitope) is central to the differences between normal and pathological tau. The appearance of PAD in early tau pathology and its disappearance in late-stage tangles show toxic forms of tau to be associated with the earliest forms of tau deposits. Collectively, these findings demonstrate that the TNT antibodies are useful markers for early conformational demonstration of PAD, and provide insights concerning conformational changes that have potential involvement in the toxic mechanisms of tau pathology [742].

Traumatic brain injury (TBI), characterized by acute neurological dysfunction, is one of the best known environmental hazard, a well-recognized risk factor for AD chronic traumatic encephalopathy (CTE), and definition of its pathologic features includes tauopathy made of phosphorylated tau (p-tau). However, tauopathy has not been detected in early stages after TBI, and how TBI leads to tauopathy, is unknown. Treating TBI mice with cis-antibody blocks cis-tauosis, prevents tauopathy development, and spreads and restores many TBI-related structural and functional sequelae. Thus, *cis* p-tau is a major early driver after TBI and leads to tauopathy in CTE and AD, and *cis* antibody may be further developed to detect and treat TBI, and prevent progressive neurodegeneration after injury [743].

7.1.2.3.3. mAbs that Target APOE ε4 in the Treatment of AD

Apolipoprotein E ε4 (ApoE ε4) is the most prevalent genetic risk factor for AD and as such is a promising therapeutic target. There is a study, which examined the extent to which the pathological effects of apoE ε4 can be counteracted *in vivo*, utilizing an immunological approach with intraperitoneal-administered antibodies, which are applied peripherally by intraperitoneal injections into apoE ε4-targeted replacement mice. Prerequisites for the successful pursuit of this objective are the availability of antibodies, which that specifically bind brain apoE ε4 and not apoE ε3, and demonstrating that direct application of these antibodies into the brain can counteract the effects of apoE ε4.

Accordingly, it was shown that the anti-apoE ε4 mAb 9D11 binds specifically to brain apoE ε4 and not apoE ε3. Direct intra cerebro ventricular application of mAb 9D11 prevented the apoE ε4-driven accumulation of Aβ in hippocampal neurons, following activation of the amyloid cascade by inhibiting the Aβ-degrading enzyme neprilysin. These findings provide a proof-of-concept that anti-apoE ε4 mAb 9D11, when introduced into the brain, can counteract the apoE ε4 effects *in vivo*. Further experiments, utilizing repeated intraperitoneal injections of mAb 9D11, resulted in the formation of apoE/IgG complexes specifically in apoE ε4 mice. This was associated with reversal of the cognitive impairments of apoE ε4 in the Morris water maze and the novel object recognition test as well as with reversal of key apoE ε4-driven pathologies including the hyper phosphorylated tau and the reduced levels of the apoE ε2 receptor. These results point out that anti-apoE ε4 immunotherapy counteracts the cognitive and brain pathological effects of apoE ε4, and suggest that such an approach could also benefit human apoE ε4 carriers [744].

Recombinant Antibody Fragments

Recombinant antibody fragments are promising alternatives to full-length-immune-globulins (Ig) and offer important advantages compared with conventional mAbs: are characterized by extreme high specificity, higher affinity, superior stability and solubility, reduced immunogenicity in comparison with full-length Ig, as well as easy and inexpensive large-scale production. Different antibody formats, such as single-chain fragment variable (scFv), single-domain antibody fragments (VHHs or sdAbs), bispecific antibodies (bsAbs), intra-bodies and nano-bodies, are currently being studied in pre-clinical models of cancer as well as infectious and autoimmune diseases and many of them are being tested as therapeutics in clinical trials. Immunotherapy approaches, both active immunization and passive, transfer of protective antibodies, have shown therapeutic efficacy in several animal models of AD, PD, dementia with Lewy bodies (DLB), frontotemporal dementia (FTD), HD, transmissible spongiform encephalopathies (TSEs) and multiple sclerosis (MS). Recombinant antibody fragments represent a promising tool for the development of antibody-based immuno-therapeutics for NDs. It has been demonstrated that these fragments may neutralize toxic extra- and intracellular misfolded accumulated proteins involved in the pathogenesis of AD, PD, DLB, FTD, HD or TSEs and may target toxic immune cells participating in the pathogenesis of MS [745].

New Methods for Drugs Administration (Nanoparticles and mAbs) in the Treatment of AD

It is critical to develop technologies for continuous antibody delivery applicable to disease prevention. New drugs, such as peptide iAβ5, capable to inhibit the aggregates associated with AD, are being tested, but the most frequent drawback is to reach the brain in the desired concentrations due to the low BBB permeability-surface area. During the last few decades, several efforts have been reported to design nano-carriers for drug transport through the BBB.

Loureiro' team designed poly-(lactic-co-glycolic acid) (PLGA) nano-particles with surface functionalized with anti-transferrin receptor monoclonal antibody (OX26) and anti-Aβ (DE2B4) to deliver encapsulated iAβ5 into the brain. As a BBB model to evaluate the system efficacy and toxicity porcine brain capillary endothelial cells (PBCECs) were used. As a consequence, they achieved to increase the uptake of immune nano-particles with a controlled delivery of the peptide iAβ5 compared to the nano-particles (NPs) without monoclonal antibody functionalization [746].

Lathuilière's group used a bioactive cellular implant to deliver recombinant anti-Aβ Abs in the subcutaneous tissue. An immune-competent, encapsulating device permeable to macromolecules supports the long-term survival of myogenic Ab-producing cells over more than 10 months in immune-competent allogeneic recipients. The encapsulated cells are genetically engineered to secrete high levels of anti-Aβ Abs. Peripheral implantation leads to continuous antibody delivery to reach plasma levels that exceed the50 μg/ml. When utilized, it was proven that the recombinant Abs produced by this system, penetrate the brain and bind amyloid plaques in two of the AD mouse models pathology. Moreover, when encapsulated cells are implanted before the onset of amyloid plaque deposition in TauPS2APP mice, chronic exposure to anti-Aβ Abs drastically reduced the Aβ40 and Aβ42 levels in the brain, decreased the amyloid plaque encumbrance and prevented phospho-tau pathology in the hippocampus. These findings support the use of encapsulated cell implants for passive immunotherapy against the misfolded proteins, which accumulate in AD and other NDs [747].

Clinical Trials with mAbs in Progress for Prevention

The DIAN observational study compared the pathophysiological markers between mutation carriers and non-carriers for autosomal dominant AD. It has revealed the biomarker changes in the mutation carrier's brain started as early as 20, even 25 years prior to symptoms. The researchers of DIAN started the prevention trial (DIAN-TU) with two monoclonal antibodies. The API study is the clinical trial of the anti-amyloid monoclonal antibody therapy to the kindred of early onset familial AD (EOAD) who carry the PSEN1 E280A mutation. This study has also shown the same biomarker changes that were reported in the DIAN study. Anti-Amyloid Treatment in Asymptomatic AD (A4) is a prevention trial aimed at treating cognitive normal older individuals at risk of developing AD dementia on the basis of having biomarker evidence of amyloid (pre-clinical AD). Solanezumab was selected for the anti-amyloid treatment for A4 [748].

Future Perspectives

Since mAbs antibodies are extremely expensive, less expensive and long acting active immunization will be widely accepted. More effective and sophisticated vaccines such as DNA vaccine [749] and recombinant viral vaccines [750], could be utilized in future as cheaper and possibly more effective alternatives.

8. GENERAL CONCLUSIONS

Arguably, the perception for the influence of nutrition for a single individual to develop the probability of AD has spread, has been accepted and has as arguments many clinical and epidemiological studies. A wide spectrum of dietary ingredients originated from natural products, mainly of MeDi and AsDi were extensively discussed here, for their beneficial neuroprotective activity to fight AD. Conclusively, all these natural bioactive constituents are strongly proposed to disrupt our quotidian habits, and to enrich our diet, as an effective therapeutic alternative to fight AD in the stage of prolepsis than of progression. Pharmaceutical and medical design of novel therapeutic formulations for AD, must be based on the neuro-protective and neuro-therapeutic profit provided by these ingredients.

CONFLICT OF INTEREST

The authors declare no conflict of interest, financial or otherwise.

ACKNOWLEDGEMENTS

Declared none.

REFERENCES

[1] Alzheimers Association. 2015 Alzheimers disease facts and figures. Alzheimers Dement 2015; 11(3): 332-84.
[http://dx.doi.org/10.1016/j.jalz.2015.02.003] [PMID: 25984581]

[2] Baumgart M, Snyder HM, Carrillo MC, Fazio S, Kim H, Johns H. Summary of the evidence on modifiable risk factors for cognitive decline and dementia: A population-based perspective. Alzheimers Dement 2015; 11(6): 718-26.
[http://dx.doi.org/10.1016/j.jalz.2015.05.016] [PMID: 26045020]

[3] Di Fede G, Catania M, Morbin M, *et al.* A recessive mutation in the APP gene with dominant-negative effect on amyloidogenesis. Science 2009; 323(5920): 1473-7.
[http://dx.doi.org/10.1126/science.1168979] [PMID: 19286555]

[4] Prince M, Bryce R, Ferri CP. World Alzheimer Report - The benefits of early diagnosis and intervention World Alzheimer Report Alzeheimer's Dis Int 72. 2011.

[5] Xu W, Tan L, Wang H-F, *et al.* Meta-analysis of modifiable risk factors for Alzheimer's disease. Neurol Neurosurg Psychiatry 2015.
[http://dx.doi.org/jnnp-2015-310548]

[6] Ritchie CW, Molinuevo JL, Truyen L, Satlin A, Van der Geyten S, Lovestone S. European Prevention of Alzheimers Dementia (EPAD) Consortium. Development of interventions for the secondary prevention of Alzheimers dementia: the European Prevention of Alzheimers Dementia (EPAD) project. Lancet Psychiatry 2016; 3(2): 179-86.
[http://dx.doi.org/10.1016/S2215-0366(15)00454-X] [PMID: 26683239]

[7] Norton S, Matthews FE, Barnes DE, Yaffe K, Brayne C. Potential for primary prevention of Alzheimers disease: an analysis of population-based data. Lancet Neurol 2014; 13(8): 788-94.
[http://dx.doi.org/10.1016/S1474-4422(14)70136-X] [PMID: 25030513]

[8] Tayeb HO, Duk H, Price BH, Tarazi FI. Pharmacology & Therapeutics Pharmacotherapies for Alzheimer β€™ s disease : Beyond cholinesterase inhibitors. Pharmacol Ther 2012; 134: 8-25.
[http://dx.doi.org/10.1016/j.pharmthera.2011.12.002] [PMID: 22198801]

[9] Hauss-Wegrzyniak B, Dobrzanski P, Stoehr JD, Wenk GL. Chronic neuroinflammation in rats reproduces components of the neurobiology of Alzheimers disease. Brain Res 1998; 780(2): 294-303.
[http://dx.doi.org/10.1016/S0006-8993(97)01215-8] [PMID: 9507169]

[10] Qiao X, Cummins DJ, Paul SM. Neuroinflammation-induced acceleration of amyloid deposition in the APPV717F transgenic mouse. Eur J Neurosci 2001; 14(3): 474-82.
[http://dx.doi.org/10.1046/j.0953-816x.2001.01666.x] [PMID: 11553297]

[11] Heppner FL, Ransohoff RM, Becher B. Immune attack: the role of inflammation in Alzheimer disease. Nat Rev Neurosci 2015; 16(6): 358-72.
[http://dx.doi.org/10.1038/nrn3880] [PMID: 25991443]

[12] Ruan L, Kang Z, Pei G, Le Y. Amyloid deposition and inflammation in APPswe/PS1dE9 mouse model of Alzheimers disease. Curr Alzheimer Res 2009; 6(6): 531-40. [http://dx.doi.org/10.2174/156720509790147070] [PMID: 19747158]

[13] Lee CY, Landreth GE. The role of microglia in amyloid clearance from the AD brain. J Neural Transm (Vienna) 2010; 117(8): 949-60. [http://dx.doi.org/10.1007/s00702-010-0433-4] [PMID: 20552234]

[14] Malmsten L, Vijayaraghavan S, Hovatta O, Marutle A, Darreh-Shori T. Fibrillar β-amyloid 142 alters cytokine secretion, cholinergic signalling and neuronal differentiation. J Cell Mol Med 2014; 18(9): 1874-88. [http://dx.doi.org/10.1111/jcmm.12343] [PMID: 25109373]

[15] Guerriero F, Sgarlata C, Francis M, *et al.* Neuroinflammation, immune system and Alzheimer disease: searching for the missing link. Aging Clin Exp Res 2016. [http://dx.doi.org/10.1007/s40520-016-0637-z] [PMID: 27718173]

[16] Perlmutter LS, Scott SA, Barrón E, Chui HC. MHC class II-positive microglia in human brain: association with Alzheimer lesions. J Neurosci Res 1992; 33(4): 549-58. [http://dx.doi.org/10.1002/jnr.490330407] [PMID: 1484388]

[17] Dokmeci D. Ibuprofen and Alzheimers disease. Folia Med (Plovdiv) 2004; 46(2): 5-10. [PMID: 15506544]

[18] Rus H, Niculescu F. The complement system in central nervous system diseases. Immunol Res 2001; 24(1): 79-86. [http://dx.doi.org/10.1385/IR:24:1:79] [PMID: 11485211]

[19] McGeer PL, McGeer EG. NSAIDs and Alzheimer disease: epidemiological, animal model and clinical studies. Neurobiol Aging 2007; 28(5): 639-47. [http://dx.doi.org/10.1016/j.neurobiolaging.2006.03.013] [PMID: 16697488]

[20] McGeer PL, Rogers J, McGeer EG. Inflammation, Antiinflammatory Agents, and Alzheimers Disease: The Last 22 Years. J Alzheimers Dis 2016; 54(3): 853-7. [http://dx.doi.org/10.3233/JAD-160488] [PMID: 27716676]

[21] Salloway S, Sperling R, Fox NC, *et al.* Bapineuzumab 301 and 302 Clinical Trial Investigators. Two phase 3 trials of bapineuzumab in mild-to-moderate Alzheimers disease. N Engl J Med 2014; 370(4): 322-33. [http://dx.doi.org/10.1056/NEJMoa1304839] [PMID: 24450891]

[22] Wilcox KC, Lacor PN, Pitt J, Klein WL. Aβ oligomer-induced synapse degeneration in Alzheimers disease. Cell Mol Neurobiol 2011; 31(6): 939-48. [http://dx.doi.org/10.1007/s10571-011-9691-4] [PMID: 21538118]

[23] Benilova I, Karran E, De Strooper B. The toxic Aβ oligomer and Alzheimers disease: an emperor in need of clothes. Nat Neurosci 2012; 15(3): 349-57. [http://dx.doi.org/10.1038/nn.3028] [PMID: 22286176]

[24] Anand K, Sabbagh M. Amyloid Imaging: Poised for Integration into Medical Practice. Neurotherapeutics 2017; 14(1): 54-61. Review [http://dx.doi.org/10.1007/s13311-016-0474-y] [PMID: 27571940]

[25] Murakami K, Tokuda M, Suzuki T, *et al.* Monoclonal antibody with conformational specificity for a toxic conformer of amyloid β42 and its application toward the Alzheimers disease diagnosis. Sci Rep 2016; 6: 29038. [http://dx.doi.org/10.1038/srep29038] [PMID: 27374357]

[26] Montoliu-Gaya L, Villegas S. Aβ-Immunotherapeutic strategies: a wide range of approaches for Alzheimers disease treatment. Expert Rev Mol Med 2016; 18: e13. [http://dx.doi.org/10.1017/erm.2016.11] [PMID: 27357999]

[27] Knopman DS, DeKosky ST, Cummings JL, *et al.* Practice parameter: diagnosis of dementia (an evidence-based review). Report of the Quality Standards Subcommittee of the American Academy of Neurology. Neurology 2001; 56(9): 1143-53.
[http://dx.doi.org/10.1212/WNL.56.9.1143] [PMID: 11342678]

[28] McKhann GM, Knopman DS, Chertkow H, *et al.* The diagnosis of dementia due to Alzheimers disease: recommendations from the National Institute on Aging-Alzheimers Association workgroups on diagnostic guidelines for Alzheimers disease. Alzheimers Dement 2011; 7(3): 263-9.
[http://dx.doi.org/10.1016/j.jalz.2011.03.005] [PMID: 21514250]

[29] Selkoe DJ, Hardy J. The amyloid hypothesis of Alzheimers disease at 25 years. EMBO Mol Med 2016; 8(6): 595-608.
[http://dx.doi.org/10.15252/emmm.201606210] [PMID: 27025652]

[30] Holtzman DM. *In vivo* effects of ApoE and clusterin on amyloid-beta metabolism and neuropathology. J Mol Neurosci 2004; 23(3): 247-54.
[http://dx.doi.org/10.1385/JMN:23:3:247] [PMID: 15181253]

[31] Shankar GM, Li S, Mehta TH, *et al.* Amyloid-beta protein dimers isolated directly from Alzheimers brains impair synaptic plasticity and memory. Nat Med 2008; 14(8): 837-42.
[http://dx.doi.org/10.1038/nm1782] [PMID: 18568035]

[32] Jin M, Shepardson N, Yang T, Chen G, Walsh D, Selkoe DJ. Soluble amyloid beta-protein dimers isolated from Alzheimer cortex directly induce Tau hyperphosphorylation and neuritic degeneration. Proc Natl Acad Sci USA 2011; 108(14): 5819-24.
[http://dx.doi.org/10.1073/pnas.1017033108] [PMID: 21421841]

[33] Hardy J, Selkoe DJ. The amyloid hypothesis of Alzheimers disease: progress and problems on the road to therapeutics. Science 2002; 297(5580): 353-6.
[http://dx.doi.org/10.1126/science.1072994] [PMID: 12130773]

[34] Doody RS, Thomas RG, Farlow M, *et al.* Alzheimers Disease Cooperative Study Steering Committee; Solanezumab Study Group. Phase 3 trials of solanezumab for mild-to-moderate Alzheimers disease. N Engl J Med 2014; 370(4): 311-21.
[http://dx.doi.org/10.1056/NEJMoa1312889] [PMID: 24450890]

[35] Selkoe DJ, Hardy J. The amyloid hypothesis of Alzheimers disease at 25 years. EMBO Mol Med 2016; 8(6): 595-608.
[http://dx.doi.org/10.15252/emmm.201606210] [PMID: 27025652]

[36] Godyń J, Jończyk J, Panek D, Malawska B. Therapeutic strategies for Alzheimers disease in clinical trials. Pharmacol Rep 2016; 68(1): 127-38.
[http://dx.doi.org/10.1016/j.pharep.2015.07.006] [PMID: 26721364]

[37] Microbiology and immunology on line. Edited by Richard Hunt, PhD Available at: http://www.microbiologybook.org/

[38] Yaffe K, Kanaya A, Lindquist K, *et al.* The metabolic syndrome, inflammation, and risk of cognitive decline. JAMA 2004; 292(18): 2237-42.
[http://dx.doi.org/10.1001/jama.292.18.2237] [PMID: 15536110]

[39] Dunn N, Mullee M, Perry VH, Holmes C. Association between dementia and infectious disease: evidence from a case-control study. Alzheimer Dis Assoc Disord 2005; 19(2): 91-4.
[http://dx.doi.org/10.1097/01.wad.0000165511.52746.1f] [PMID: 15942327]

[40] Reitz C, Brayne C, Mayeux R. Epidemiology of Alzheimer disease. Nat Rev Neurol 2011; 7(3): 137-52.
[http://dx.doi.org/10.1038/nrneurol.2011.2] [PMID: 21304480]

[41] Etminan M, Gill S, Samii A. Effect of non-steroidal anti-inflammatory drugs on risk of Alzheimers disease: systematic review and meta-analysis of observational studies. BMJ 2003; 327(7407): 128.
[http://dx.doi.org/10.1136/bmj.327.7407.128] [PMID: 12869452]

[42] Cunningham C, Wilcockson DC, Campion S, Lunnon K, Perry VH. Central and systemic endotoxin challenges exacerbate the local inflammatory response and increase neuronal death during chronic neurodegeneration. J Neurosci 2005; 25(40): 9275-84.
[http://dx.doi.org/10.1523/JNEUROSCI.2614-05.2005] [PMID: 16207887]

[43] Godbout JP, Chen J, Abraham J, *et al.* Exaggerated neuroinflammation and sickness behavior in aged mice following activation of the peripheral innate immune system. FASEB J 2005; 19(10): 1329-31. [PMID: 15919760]

[44] Pott Godoy MC, Tarelli R, Ferrari CC, Sarchi MI, Pitossi FJ. Central and systemic IL-1 exacerbates neurodegeneration and motor symptoms in a model of Parkinsons disease. Brain 2008; 131(Pt 7): 1880-94.
[http://dx.doi.org/10.1093/brain/awn101] [PMID: 18504291]

[45] Relton JK, Rothwell NJ. Interleukin-1 receptor antagonist inhibits ischaemic and excitotoxic neuronal damage in the rat. Brain Res Bull 1992; 29(2): 243-6.
[http://dx.doi.org/10.1016/0361-9230(92)90033-T] [PMID: 1388088]

[46] Balosso S, Maroso M, Sanchez-Alavez M, *et al.* A novel non-transcriptional pathway mediates the proconvulsive effects of interleukin-1beta. Brain 2008; 131(Pt 12): 3256-65.
[http://dx.doi.org/10.1093/brain/awn271] [PMID: 18952671]

[47] Vezzani A, Maroso M, Balosso S, Sanchez M-A, Bartfai T. IL-1 receptor/Toll-like receptor signaling in infection, inflammation, stress and neurodegeneration couples hyperexcitability and seizures. Brain Behav Immun 2011; 25(7): 1281-9.
[http://dx.doi.org/10.1016/j.bbi.2011.03.018] [PMID: 21473909]

[48] Sheng JG, Bora SH, Xu G, Borchelt DR, Price DL, Koliatsos VE. Lipopolysaccharide-induce--neuroinflammation increases intracellular accumulation of amyloid precursor protein and amyloid beta peptide in APPswe transgenic mice. Neurobiol Dis 2003; 14(1): 133-45.
[http://dx.doi.org/10.1016/S0969-9961(03)00069-X] [PMID: 13678674]

[49] Cunningham C, Campion S, Lunnon K, *et al.* Systemic inflammation induces acute behavioral and cognitive changes and accelerates neurodegenerative disease. Biol Psychiatry 2009; 65(4): 304-12.
[http://dx.doi.org/10.1016/j.biopsych.2008.07.024] [PMID: 18801476]

[50] Krstic D, Madhusudan A, Doehner J, *et al.* Systemic immune challenges trigger and drive Alzheimer-like neuropathology in mice. J Neuroinflammation 2012; 9: 151.
[http://dx.doi.org/10.1186/1742-2094-9-151] [PMID: 22747753]

[51] Solana R, Tarazona R, Gayoso I, Lesur O, Dupuis G, Fulop T. Innate immunosenescence: effect of aging on cells and receptors of the innate immune system in humans. Semin Immunol 2012; 24(5): 331-41.
[http://dx.doi.org/10.1016/j.smim.2012.04.008] [PMID: 22560929]

[52] Solana R, Tarazona R, Aiello AE, *et al.* CMV and Immunosenescence: from basics to clinics. Immun Ageing 2012; 9(1): 23.
[http://dx.doi.org/10.1186/1742-4933-9-23] [PMID: 23114110]

[53] Fülöp T, Larbi A, Pawelec G. Human T cell aging and the impact of persistent viral infections. Front Immunol 2013; 4: 271.
[http://dx.doi.org/10.3389/fimmu.2013.00271] [PMID: 24062739]

[54] Stowe RP, Kozlova EV, Yetman DL, Walling DM, Goodwin JS, Glaser R. Chronic herpesvirus reactivation occurs in aging. Exp Gerontol 2007; 42(6): 563-70.
[http://dx.doi.org/10.1016/j.exger.2007.01.005] [PMID: 17337145]

[55] Almanzar G, Schwaiger S, Jenewein B, *et al.* Long-term cytomegalovirus infection leads to significant changes in the composition of the CD8+ T-cell repertoire, which may be the basis for an imbalance in the cytokine production profile in elderly persons. J Virol 2005; 79(6): 3675-83.
[http://dx.doi.org/10.1128/JVI.79.6.3675-3683.2005] [PMID: 15731261]

[56] Westman G, Berglund D, Widén J, *et al.* Increased inflammatory response in cytomegalovirus seropositive patients with Alzheimers disease. PLoS One 2014; 9(5): e96779. [http://dx.doi.org/10.1371/journal.pone.0096779] [PMID: 24804776]

[57] Miklossy J. Emerging roles of pathogens in Alzheimer disease. Expert Rev Mol Med 2011; 13: e30. [http://dx.doi.org/10.1017/S1462399411002006] [PMID: 21933454]

[58] Peila R, Launer LJ. Inflammation and dementia: epidemiologic evidence. Acta Neurol Scand Suppl 2006; 185: 102-6. [http://dx.doi.org/10.1111/j.1600-0404.2006.00693.x] [PMID: 16866918]

[59] Lau FC, Shukitt-Hale B, Joseph JA. Nutritional intervention in brain aging: reducing the effects of inflammation and oxidative stress. Subcell Biochem 2007; 42: 299-318. [http://dx.doi.org/10.1007/1-4020-5688-5_14] [PMID: 17612057]

[60] Schwartz M, Shechter R. Systemic inflammatory cells fight off neurodegenerative disease. Nat Rev Neurol 2010; 6(7): 405-10. [http://dx.doi.org/10.1038/nrneurol.2010.71] [PMID: 20531383]

[61] Schwartz M, Ziv Y. Immunity to self and self-maintenance: a unified theory of brain pathologies. Trends Immunol 2008; 29(5): 211-9. [http://dx.doi.org/10.1016/j.it.2008.01.003] [PMID: 18328784]

[62] Lucin KM, Wyss-Coray T. Immune activation in brain aging and neurodegeneration: too much or too little? Neuron 2009; 64(1): 110-22. [http://dx.doi.org/10.1016/j.neuron.2009.08.039] [PMID: 19840553]

[63] Rubinsztein DC. The roles of intracellular protein-degradation pathways in neurodegeneration. Nature 2006; 443(7113): 780-6. [http://dx.doi.org/10.1038/nature05291] [PMID: 17051204]

[64] Bredesen DE, Rao RV, Mehlen P. Cell death in the nervous system. Nature 2006; 443(7113): 796-802. [http://dx.doi.org/10.1038/nature05293] [PMID: 17051206]

[65] Rivest S. Regulation of innate immune responses in the brain. Nat Rev Immunol 2009; 9(6): 429-39. [http://dx.doi.org/10.1038/nri2565] [PMID: 19461673]

[66] Crutcher KA, Gendelman HE, Kipnis J, *et al.* Debate: is increasing neuroinflammation beneficial for neural repair? J Neuroimmune Pharmacol 2006; 1(3): 195-211. [http://dx.doi.org/10.1007/s11481-006-9021-7] [PMID: 18040798]

[67] Popovich PG, Longbrake EE. Can the immune system be harnessed to repair the CNS? Nat Rev Neurosci 2008; 9(6): 481-93. [http://dx.doi.org/10.1038/nrn2398] [PMID: 18490917]

[68] Tansey MG, McCoy MK, Frank-Cannon TC. Neuroinflammatory mechanisms in Parkinsons disease: potential environmental triggers, pathways, and targets for early therapeutic intervention. Exp Neurol 2007; 208(1): 1-25. [http://dx.doi.org/10.1016/j.expneurol.2007.07.004] [PMID: 17720159]

[69] Block ML, Hong J-S. Microglia and inflammation-mediated neurodegeneration: multiple triggers with a common mechanism. Prog Neurobiol 2005; 76(2): 77-98. [http://dx.doi.org/10.1016/j.pneurobio.2005.06.004] [PMID: 16081203]

[70] McGeer EG, McGeer PL. The role of anti-inflammatory agents in Parkinsons disease. CNS Drugs 2007; 21(10): 789-97. [http://dx.doi.org/10.2165/00023210-200721100-00001] [PMID: 17850169]

[71] Mrak RE, Griffin WS. Glia and their cytokines in progression of neurodegeneration. Neurobiol Aging 2005; 26(3): 349-54. [http://dx.doi.org/10.1016/j.neurobiolaging.2004.05.010] [PMID: 15639313]

[72] Leszek J, Barreto GE, Gąsiorowski K, Koutsouraki E, Ávila-Rodrigues M, Aliev G. Inflammatory

Mechanisms and Oxidative Stress as Key Factors Responsible for Progression of Neurodegeneration: Role of Brain Innate Immune System. CNS Neurol Disord Drug Targets 2016; 15(3): 329-36. [http://dx.doi.org/10.2174/1871527315666160202125914] [PMID: 26831258]

[73] Frank-Cannon TC, Alto LT, McAlpine FE, Tansey MG. Does neuroinflammation fan the flame in neurodegenerative diseases? Mol Neurodegener 2009; 4: 47. [http://dx.doi.org/10.1186/1750-1326-4-47] [PMID: 19917131]

[74] Tansey MG, Wyss-Coray T. Cytokines in CNS inflammation and disease. Central nervous system diseases and inflammation. US: Springer 2008; pp. 59-106. [http://dx.doi.org/10.1007/978-0-387-73894-9_5]

[75] Okamoto T. NF-kappaB and rheumatic diseases. Endocr Metab Immune Disord Drug Targets 2006; 6(4): 359-72. [http://dx.doi.org/10.2174/187153006779025685] [PMID: 17214582]

[76] Walter S, Letiembre M, Liu Y, *et al.* Role of the toll-like receptor 4 in neuroinflammation in Alzheimers disease. Cell Physiol Biochem 2007; 20(6): 947-56. [http://dx.doi.org/10.1159/000110455] [PMID: 17982277]

[77] Goldgaber D, Harris HW, Hla T, *et al.* Interleukin 1 regulates synthesis of amyloid beta-protein precursor mRNA in human endothelial cells. Proc Natl Acad Sci USA 1989; 86(19): 7606-10. [http://dx.doi.org/10.1073/pnas.86.19.7606] [PMID: 2508093]

[78] Del Bo R, Angeretti N, Lucca E, De Simoni MG, Forloni G. Reciprocal control of inflammatory cytokines, IL-1 and IL-6, and beta-amyloid production in cultures. Neurosci Lett 1995; 188(1): 70-4. [http://dx.doi.org/10.1016/0304-3940(95)11384-9] [PMID: 7783982]

[79] Misonou H, Morishima-Kawashima M, Ihara Y. Oxidative stress induces intracellular accumulation of amyloid beta-protein (Abeta) in human neuroblastoma cells. Biochemistry 2000; 39(23): 6951-9. [http://dx.doi.org/10.1021/bi000169p] [PMID: 10841777]

[80] Yan SD, Yan SF, Chen X, *et al.* Non-enzymatically glycated tau in Alzheimers disease induces neuronal oxidant stress resulting in cytokine gene expression and release of amyloid beta-peptide. Nat Med 1995; 1(7): 693-9. [http://dx.doi.org/10.1038/nm0795-693] [PMID: 7585153]

[81] Moreira PI, Smith MA, Zhu X, Nunomura A, Castellani RJ, Perry G. Oxidative stress and neurodegeneration. Ann N Y Acad Sci 2005; 1043: 545-52. [http://dx.doi.org/10.1196/annals.1333.062] [PMID: 16037277]

[82] Nunomura A, Castellani RJ, Zhu X, Moreira PI, Perry G, Smith MA. Involvement of oxidative stress in Alzheimer disease. J Neuropathol Exp Neurol 2006; 65(7): 631-41. [http://dx.doi.org/10.1097/01.jnen.0000228136.58062.bf] [PMID: 16825950]

[83] Okun E, Griffioen KJ, Lathia JD, Tang S-C, Mattson MP, Arumugam TV. Toll-like receptors in neurodegeneration. Brain Res Brain Res Rev 2009; 59(2): 278-92. [http://dx.doi.org/10.1016/j.brainresrev.2008.09.001] [PMID: 18822314]

[84] Lehnardt S. Innate immunity and neuroinflammation in the CNS: the role of microglia in Toll-like receptor-mediated neuronal injury. Glia 2010; 58(3): 253-63. [PMID: 19705460]

[85] Kawai T, Akira S. Toll-like receptor and RIG-I-like receptor signaling. Ann N Y Acad Sci 2008; 1143: 1-20. [http://dx.doi.org/10.1196/annals.1443.020] [PMID: 19076341]

[86] Letiembre M, Hao W, Liu Y, *et al.* Innate immune receptor expression in normal brain aging. Neuroscience 2007; 146(1): 248-54. [http://dx.doi.org/10.1016/j.neuroscience.2007.01.004] [PMID: 17293054]

[87] Arroyo DS, Soria JA, Gaviglio EA, Rodriguez-Galan MC, Iribarren P. Toll-like receptors are key players in neurodegeneration. Int Immunopharmacol 2011; 11(10): 1415-21.

[http://dx.doi.org/10.1016/j.intimp.2011.05.006] [PMID: 21616174]

[88] Bamberger ME, Harris ME, McDonald DR, Husemann J, Landreth GE. A cell surface receptor complex for fibrillar beta-amyloid mediates microglial activation. J Neurosci 2003; 23(7): 2665-74. [PMID: 12684452]

[89] Reed-Geaghan EG, Savage JC, Hise AG, Landreth GE. CD14 and toll-like receptors 2 and 4 are required for fibrillar Abeta-stimulated microglial activation. J Neurosci 2009; 29(38): 11982-92. [http://dx.doi.org/10.1523/JNEUROSCI.3158-09.2009] [PMID: 19776284]

[90] Tang S-C, Lathia JD, Selvaraj PK, *et al.* Toll-like receptor-4 mediates neuronal apoptosis induced by amyloid beta-peptide and the membrane lipid peroxidation product 4-hydroxynonenal. Exp Neurol 2008; 213(1): 114-21. [http://dx.doi.org/10.1016/j.expneurol.2008.05.014] [PMID: 18586243]

[91] Minoretti P, Gazzaruso C, Vito CD, *et al.* Effect of the functional toll-like receptor 4 Asp299Gly polymorphism on susceptibility to late-onset Alzheimers disease. Neurosci Lett 2006; 391(3): 147-9. [http://dx.doi.org/10.1016/j.neulet.2005.08.047] [PMID: 16157451]

[92] Stevens B, Allen NJ, Vazquez LE, *et al.* The classical complement cascade mediates CNS synapse elimination. Cell 2007; 131(6): 1164-78. [http://dx.doi.org/10.1016/j.cell.2007.10.036] [PMID: 18083105]

[93] Boulanger LM. Immune proteins in brain development and synaptic plasticity. Neuron 2009; 64(1): 93-109. [http://dx.doi.org/10.1016/j.neuron.2009.09.001] [PMID: 19840552]

[94] Esquirol E. Mental maladies; a treatise on insanity. Lea and Blanchard 1845.

[95] Hornig M. The role of microbes and autoimmunity in the pathogenesis of neuropsychiatric illness. Curr Opin Rheumatol 2013; 25(4): 488-795. [http://dx.doi.org/10.1097/BOR.0b013e32836208de] [PMID: 23656715]

[96] Kotsopoulos S. Aretaeus the Cappadocian on mental illness. Compr Psychiatry 1986; 27(2): 171-9. [http://dx.doi.org/10.1016/0010-440X(86)90026-X] [PMID: 3514115]

[97] Miller AH, Haroon E, Raison CL, Felger JC. Cytokine targets in the brain: impact on neurotransmitters and neurocircuits. Depress Anxiety 2013; 30(4): 297-306. [http://dx.doi.org/10.1002/da.22084] [PMID: 23468190]

[98] McCusker RH, Kelley KW. Immune-neural connections: how the immune systems response to infectious agents influences behavior. J Exp Biol 2013; 216(Pt 1): 84-98. [http://dx.doi.org/10.1242/jeb.073411] [PMID: 23225871]

[99] Nicholson JK, Holmes E, Kinross J, *et al.* Host-Gut Microbiota Metabolic Interactions. Science (80-) 2012; 336: 1262-7.

[100] Turnbaugh PJ, Ley RE, Hamady M, Fraser-Liggett CM, Knight R, Gordon JI. The human microbiome project. Nature 2007; 449(7164): 804-10. [http://dx.doi.org/10.1038/nature06244] [PMID: 17943116]

[101] Round JL, Mazmanian SK. The gut microbiota shapes intestinal immune responses during health and disease. Nat Rev Immunol 2009; 9(5): 313-23. [http://dx.doi.org/10.1038/nri2515] [PMID: 19343057]

[102] Sampson TR, Mazmanian SK. Control of brain development, function, and behavior by the microbiome. Cell Host Microbe 2015; 17(5): 565-76. [http://dx.doi.org/10.1016/j.chom.2015.04.011] [PMID: 25974299]

[103] O'Mahony SM, Clarke G, Borre YE, Dinan TG, Cryan JF. Serotonin, tryptophan metabolism and the brain-gut-microbiome axis. Behav Brain Res 2015; 277: 32-48. [http://dx.doi.org/10.1016/j.bbr.2014.07.027] [PMID: 25078296]

[104] Cryan JF, Dinan TG. Mind-altering microorganisms: the impact of the gut microbiota on brain and

behaviour. Nat Rev Neurosci 2012; 13(10): 701-12.
[http://dx.doi.org/10.1038/nrn3346] [PMID: 22968153]

[105] Koren O, Spor A, Felin J, *et al.* Human oral, gut, and plaque microbiota in patients with atherosclerosis. Proc Natl Acad Sci USA 2011; 108 (Suppl. 1): 4592-8.
[http://dx.doi.org/10.1073/pnas.1011383107] [PMID: 20937873]

[106] Howitt MR, Garrett WS. A complex microworld in the gut: gut microbiota and cardiovascular disease connectivity. Nat Med 2012; 18(8): 1188-9.
[http://dx.doi.org/10.1038/nm.2895] [PMID: 22869188]

[107] Karlsson FH, Fåk F, Nookaew I, *et al.* Symptomatic atherosclerosis is associated with an altered gut metagenome. Nat Commun 2012; 3: 1245.
[http://dx.doi.org/10.1038/ncomms2266] [PMID: 23212374]

[108] Hansen TH, Gøbel RJ, Hansen T, Pedersen O. The gut microbiome in cardio-metabolic health. Genome Med 2015; 7(1): 33.
[http://dx.doi.org/10.1186/s13073-015-0157-z] [PMID: 25825594]

[109] Collins SM, Bercik P. The relationship between intestinal microbiota and the central nervous system in normal gastrointestinal function and disease. Gastroenterology 2009; 136(6): 2003-14.
[http://dx.doi.org/10.1053/j.gastro.2009.01.075] [PMID: 19457424]

[110] Drennan M. What is "Sterile Blood"? Br Med J 1942; 2(4269): 526.

[111] Proal AD, Albert PJ, Marshall TG. Inflammatory disease and the human microbiome. Discov Med 2014; 17(95): 257-65.
[PMID: 24882717]

[112] Wilson ML, Weinstein MP. General principles in the laboratory detection of bacteremia and fungemia. Clin Lab Med 1994; 14(1): 69-82.
[PMID: 8181235]

[113] Weinstein MP. Current blood culture methods and systems: clinical concepts, technology, and interpretation of results. Clin Infect Dis 1996; 23(1): 40-6.
[http://dx.doi.org/10.1093/clinids/23.1.40] [PMID: 8816127]

[114] Schroeter J, Wilkemeyer I, Schiller RA, Pruss A. Validation of the Microbiological Testing of Tissue Preparations Using the BACTEC™ Blood Culture System. Transfus Med Hemother 2012; 39(6): 387-90.
[http://dx.doi.org/10.1159/000345812] [PMID: 23801426]

[115] Valencia-Shelton F, Loeffelholz M. Nonculture techniques for the detection of bacteremia and fungemia. Future Microbiol 2014; 9(4): 543-59.
[http://dx.doi.org/10.2217/fmb.14.8] [PMID: 24810352]

[116] Gill VJ, Fedorko FD, Witebsky FG. The clinicians and the microbiology laboratory. In: Mandell G, Bennet J, Dolin R, Eds. Principles and Practice of Infectious Diseases. Philadelphia: Churchill Li vingstone 2000.

[117] Vincent J-L, Rello J, Marshall J, *et al.* EPIC II Group of Investigators. International study of the prevalence and outcomes of infection in intensive care units. JAMA 2009; 302(21): 2323-9.
[http://dx.doi.org/10.1001/jama.2009.1754] [PMID: 19952319]

[118] Eleftheriadis T, Liakopoulos V, Leivaditis K, Antoniadi G, Stefanidis I. Infections in hemodialysis: a concise review - Part 1: bacteremia and respiratory infections. Hippokratia 2011; 15(1): 12-7.
[PMID: 21607029]

[119] Havey TC, Fowler RA, Daneman N. Duration of antibiotic therapy for bacteremia: a systematic review and meta-analysis. Crit Care 2011; 15(6): R267.
[http://dx.doi.org/10.1186/cc10545] [PMID: 22085732]

[120] Montassier E, Batard E, Gastinne T, Potel G, de La Cochetière MF. Recent changes in bacteremia in

patients with cancer: a systematic review of epidemiology and antibiotic resistance. Eur J Clin Microbiol Infect Dis 2013; 32(7): 841-50.
[http://dx.doi.org/10.1007/s10096-013-1819-7] [PMID: 23354675]

[121] Fredricks DN. The human microbiota: How microbial communities affect health and disease. John Wiley & Sons 2013.
[http://dx.doi.org/10.1002/9781118409855]

[122] Robles-Alonso V, Guarner F. From basic to applied research: lessons from the human microbiome projects. J Clin Gastroenterol 2014; 48 (Suppl. 1): S3-4.
[http://dx.doi.org/10.1097/MCG.0000000000000242] [PMID: 25291122]

[123] Morgan XC, Huttenhower C. Metaomic analytic techniques for studying the intestinal microbiome. Gastroenterology 2014; 146(6): 1437-1448.e1.
[http://dx.doi.org/10.1053/j.gastro.2014.01.049] [PMID: 24486053]

[124] ElRakaiby M, Dutilh BE, Rizkallah MR, Boleij A, Cole JN, Aziz RK. Pharmacomicrobiomics: the impact of human microbiome variations on systems pharmacology and personalized therapeutics. OMICS 2014; 18(7): 402-14.
[http://dx.doi.org/10.1089/omi.2014.0018] [PMID: 24785449]

[125] Shoemark DK, Allen SJ. The microbiome and disease: reviewing the links between the oral microbiome, aging, and Alzheimers disease. J Alzheimers Dis 2015; 43(3): 725-38.
[PMID: 25125469]

[126] Nicolson GL. Chronic Bacterial and Viral Infections in Neurodegenerative and Neurobehavioral Diseases. Lab Med 2008; 39: 291-9.
[http://dx.doi.org/10.1309/96M3BWYP42L11BFU]

[127] Roubaud Baudron C, Varon C, Mégraud F, Salles N. [Alzheimers disease: the infectious hypothesis]. Geriatr Psychol Neuropsychiatr Vieil 2015; 13(4): 418-24. [Alzheimer's disease: the infectious hypothesis].
[PMID: 26707559]

[128] Miklossy J. Historic evidence to support a causal relationship between spirochetal infections and Alzheimers disease. Front Aging Neurosci 2015; 7: 46.
[http://dx.doi.org/10.3389/fnagi.2015.00046] [PMID: 25932012]

[129] Singhrao SK, Harding A, Poole S, Kesavalu L, Crean S. Porphyromonas gingivalis Periodontal Infection and Its Putative Links with Alzheimers Disease. Mediators Inflamm 2015; 2015: 137357.
[http://dx.doi.org/10.1155/2015/137357] [PMID: 26063967]

[130] Poole S, Singhrao SK, Kesavalu L, Curtis MA, Crean S. Determining the presence of periodontopathic virulence factors in short-term postmortem Alzheimers disease brain tissue. J Alzheimers Dis 2013; 36(4): 665-77.
[PMID: 23666172]

[131] Miklossy J. Alzheimers disease - a neurospirochetosis. Analysis of the evidence following Kochs and Hills criteria. J Neuroinflammation 2011; 8: 90.
[http://dx.doi.org/10.1186/1742-2094-8-90] [PMID: 21816039]

[132] Brooks GF, Butel JS, Morse SA, Jawetz E. Jawetz, Melnick, & Adelberg's medical microbiology, Lange Medical Books/McGraw-Hill, Medical Pub Division, New York, NY. 2010.

[133] Petra AI, Panagiotidou S, Hatziagelaki E, Stewart JM, Conti P, Theoharides TC. Gut-Microbiota-Brain Axis and Its Effect on Neuropsychiatric Disorders With Suspected Immune Dysregulation. Clin Ther 2015; 37(5): 984-95.
[http://dx.doi.org/10.1016/j.clinthera.2015.04.002] [PMID: 26046241]

[134] Cong X, Henderson WA, Graf J, McGrath JM. Early Life Experience and Gut Microbiome: The Brain-Gut-Microbiota Signaling System. Adv Neonatal Care 2015; 15(5): 314-23.

[135] Dinan TG, Stilling RM, Stanton C, Cryan JF. Collective unconscious: how gut microbes shape human

behavior. J Psychiatr Res 2015; 63: 1-9.
[http://dx.doi.org/10.1016/j.jpsychires.2015.02.021] [PMID: 25772005]

[136] Malaguarnera M, Bella R, Alagona G, Ferri R, Carnemolla A, Pennisi G. Helicobacter pylori and Alzheimers disease: a possible link. Eur J Intern Med 2004; 15(6): 381-6.
[http://dx.doi.org/10.1016/j.ejim.2004.05.008] [PMID: 15522573]

[137] Kountouras J, Zavos C, Boziki M, Gavalas E, Kyriakou P, Deretzi G. Association between Helicobacter pylori infection and Alzheimers disease in Japan. J Neurol 2011; 258(11): 2086.
[http://dx.doi.org/10.1007/s00415-011-6054-5] [PMID: 21516361]

[138] Kountouras J, Gavalas E, Polyzos SA, *et al.* Association between Helicobacter pylori burden and Alzheimers disease. Eur J Neurol 2014; 21(12): e100.
[http://dx.doi.org/10.1111/ene.12563] [PMID: 25393387]

[139] Cong X, Xu W, Romisher R, *et al.* Gut Microbiome and Infant Health: Brain-Gut-Microbiota Axis and Host Genetic Factors. Yale J Biol Med 2016; 89(3): 299-308.
[PMID: 27698614]

[140] Garay PA, Hsiao EY, Patterson PH, McAllister AK. Maternal immune activation causes age- and region-specific changes in brain cytokines in offspring throughout development. Brain Behav Immun 2013; 31: 54-68.
[http://dx.doi.org/10.1016/j.bbi.2012.07.008] [PMID: 22841693]

[141] Meyer U, Feldon J. To poly(I:C) or not to poly(I:C): advancing preclinical schizophrenia research through the use of prenatal immune activation models. Neuropharmacology 2012; 62(3): 1308-21.
[http://dx.doi.org/10.1016/j.neuropharm.2011.01.009] [PMID: 21238465]

[142] Schwarz JM, Bilbo SD. LPS elicits a much larger and broader inflammatory response than Escherichia coli infection within the hippocampus of neonatal rats. Neurosci Lett 2011; 497(2): 110-5.
[http://dx.doi.org/10.1016/j.neulet.2011.04.042] [PMID: 21536105]

[143] Willette AA, Lubach GR, Knickmeyer RC, *et al.* Brain enlargement and increased behavioral and cytokine reactivity in infant monkeys following acute prenatal endotoxemia. Behav Brain Res 2011; 219(1): 108-15.
[http://dx.doi.org/10.1016/j.bbr.2010.12.023] [PMID: 21192986]

[144] Oskvig DB, Elkahloun AG, Johnson KR, Phillips TM, Herkenham M. Maternal immune activation by LPS selectively alters specific gene expression profiles of interneuron migration and oxidative stress in the fetus without triggering a fetal immune response. Brain Behav Immun 2012; 26(4): 623-34.
[http://dx.doi.org/10.1016/j.bbi.2012.01.015] [PMID: 22310921]

[145] Nouel D, Burt M, Zhang Y, Harvey L, Boksa P. Prenatal exposure to bacterial endotoxin reduces the number of GAD67- and reelin-immunoreactive neurons in the hippocampus of rat offspring. Eur Neuropsychopharmacol 2012; 22(4): 300-7.
[http://dx.doi.org/10.1016/j.euroneuro.2011.08.001] [PMID: 21889316]

[146] Baharnoori M, Bhardwaj SK, Srivastava LK. Neonatal behavioral changes in rats with gestational exposure to lipopolysaccharide: a prenatal infection model for developmental neuropsychiatric disorders. Schizophr Bull 2012; 38(3): 444-56.
[http://dx.doi.org/10.1093/schbul/sbq098] [PMID: 20805287]

[147] Malkova NV, Yu CZ, Hsiao EY, Moore MJ, Patterson PH. Maternal immune activation yields offspring displaying mouse versions of the three core symptoms of autism. Brain Behav Immun 2012; 26(4): 607-16.
[http://dx.doi.org/10.1016/j.bbi.2012.01.011] [PMID: 22310922]

[148] Chang EY, Zhang J, Sullivan S, Newman R, Singh I. N-acetylcysteine attenuates the maternal and fetal proinflammatory response to intrauterine LPS injection in an animal model for preterm birth and brain injury. J Matern Fetal Neonatal Med 2011; 24(5): 732-40.
[http://dx.doi.org/10.3109/14767058.2010.528089] [PMID: 21219105]

[149] Dowling O, Chatterjee PK, Gupta M, *et al.* Magnesium sulfate reduces bacterial LPS-induced inflammation at the maternal-fetal interface. Placenta 2012; 33(5): 392-8. [http://dx.doi.org/10.1016/j.placenta.2012.01.013] [PMID: 22341339]

[150] De Miranda J, Yaddanapudi K, Hornig M, Villar G, Serge R, Lipkin WI. Induction of Toll-Like Receptor 3-Mediated Immunity during Gestation Inhibits Cortical Neurogenesis and Causes Behavioral Disturbances. MBio 2010; 1: e00176-10-.

[151] Yaddanapudi K, De Miranda J, Hornig M, Lipkin WI. Toll-like receptor 3 regulates neural stem cell proliferation by modulating the Sonic Hedgehog pathway. PLoS One 2011; 6(10): e26766. [http://dx.doi.org/10.1371/journal.pone.0026766] [PMID: 22046349]

[152] Hsiao EY, McBride SW, Chow J, Mazmanian SK, Patterson PH. Modeling an autism risk factor in mice leads to permanent immune dysregulation. Proc Natl Acad Sci USA 2012; 109(31): 12776-81. [http://dx.doi.org/10.1073/pnas.1202556109] [PMID: 22802640]

[153] Forsythe P, Kunze WA, Bienenstock J. On communication between gut microbes and the brain. Curr Opin Gastroenterol 2012; 28(6): 557-62. [http://dx.doi.org/10.1097/MOG.0b013e3283572ffa] [PMID: 23010679]

[154] Douglas-Escobar M, Elliott E, Neu J. Effect of intestinal microbial ecology on the developing brain. JAMA Pediatr 2013; 167(4): 374-9. [http://dx.doi.org/10.1001/jamapediatrics.2013.497] [PMID: 23400224]

[155] Ait-Belgnaoui A, Durand H, Cartier C, *et al.* Prevention of gut leakiness by a probiotic treatment leads to attenuated HPA response to an acute psychological stress in rats. Psychoneuroendocrinology 2012; 37(11): 1885-95. [http://dx.doi.org/10.1016/j.psyneuen.2012.03.024] [PMID: 22541937]

[156] Singh PK, Chopra K, Kuhad A, Kaur IP. Role of *Lactobacillus*acidophilus loaded floating beads in chronic fatigue syndrome: behavioral and biochemical evidences. Neurogastroenterol Motil 2012; 24(4): 366-e170. [http://dx.doi.org/10.1111/j.1365-2982.2011.01861.x] [PMID: 22296294]

[157] McVey Neufeld KA, Mao YK, Bienenstock J, Foster JA, Kunze WA. The microbiome is essential for normal gut intrinsic primary afferent neuron excitability in the mouse. Neurogastroenterol Motil 2013; 25(2): 183-e88. [http://dx.doi.org/10.1111/nmo.12049] [PMID: 23181420]

[158] Perez-Burgos A, Wang B, Mao Y-K, *et al.* Psychoactive bacteria *Lactobacillus*rhamnosus (JB-1) elicits rapid frequency facilitation in vagal afferents. Am J Physiol Gastrointest Liver Physiol 2013; 304(2): G211-20. [http://dx.doi.org/10.1152/ajpgi.00128.2012] [PMID: 23139216]

[159] Clarke G, Grenham S, Scully P, *et al.* The microbiome-gut-brain axis during early life regulates the hippocampal serotonergic system in a sex-dependent manner. Mol Psychiatry 2013; 18(6): 666-73. [http://dx.doi.org/10.1038/mp.2012.77] [PMID: 22688187]

[160] Persico AM, Napolioni V. Urinary p-cresol in autism spectrum disorder. Neurotoxicol Teratol 2013; 36: 82-90. [http://dx.doi.org/10.1016/j.ntt.2012.09.002] [PMID: 22975621]

[161] Williams BL, Hornig M, Parekh T, Lipkin WI. Application of Novel PCR-Based Methods for Detection, Quantitation, and Phylogenetic Characterization of Sutterella Species in Intestinal Biopsy Samples from Children with Autism and Gastrointestinal Disturbances. MBio 2012; 3: e00261-11.

[162] Williams BL, Hornig M, Buie T, *et al.* Impaired carbohydrate digestion and transport and mucosal dysbiosis in the intestines of children with autism and gastrointestinal disturbances. PLoS One 2011; 6(9): e24585. [http://dx.doi.org/10.1371/journal.pone.0024585] [PMID: 21949732]

[163] Atkinson MA, Chervonsky A. Does the gut microbiota have a role in type 1 diabetes? Early evidence

from humans and animal models of the disease. Diabetologia 2012; 55(11): 2868-77. [http://dx.doi.org/10.1007/s00125-012-2672-4] [PMID: 22875196]

[164] Vaarala O. Is the origin of type 1 diabetes in the gut? Immunol Cell Biol 2012; 90(3): 271-6. [http://dx.doi.org/10.1038/icb.2011.115] [PMID: 22290506]

[165] Yano JM, Yu K, Donaldson GP, *et al.* Indigenous bacteria from the gut microbiota regulate host serotonin biosynthesis. Cell 2015; 161(2): 264-76. [http://dx.doi.org/10.1016/j.cell.2015.02.047] [PMID: 25860609]

[166] Williams BB, Van Benschoten AH, Cimermancic P, *et al.* Discovery and characterization of gut microbiota decarboxylases that can produce the neurotransmitter tryptamine. Cell Host Microbe 2014; 16(4): 495-503. [http://dx.doi.org/10.1016/j.chom.2014.09.001] [PMID: 25263219]

[167] Takaki M, Mawe GM, Barasch JM, Gershon MD, Gershon MD. Physiological responses of guinea-pig myenteric neurons secondary to the release of endogenous serotonin by tryptamine. Neuroscience 1985; 16(1): 223-40. [http://dx.doi.org/10.1016/0306-4522(85)90059-4] [PMID: 2940472]

[168] Julio-Pieper M, OMahony CM, Clarke G, Bravo JA, Dinan TG, Cryan JF. Chronic stress-induced alterations in mouse colonic 5-HT and defecation responses are strain dependent. Stress 2012; 15(2): 218-26. [http://dx.doi.org/10.3109/10253890.2011.607524] [PMID: 21875301]

[169] Aguilera M, Vergara P, Martínez V. Stress and antibiotics alter luminal and wall-adhered microbiota and enhance the local expression of visceral sensory-related systems in mice. Neurogastroenterol Motil 2013; 25(8): e515-29. [http://dx.doi.org/10.1111/nmo.12154] [PMID: 23711047]

[170] Mu C, Yang Y, Zhu W. Gut Microbiota: The Brain Peacekeeper. Front Microbiol 2016; 7: 345. [http://dx.doi.org/10.3389/fmicb.2016.00345] [PMID: 27014255]

[171] Dash SR. The Microbiome and Brain Health: What's the Connection? 2015. http://www.medscape.com/viewarticle/841748

[172] de Theije CG, Wu J, da Silva SL, *et al.* Pathways underlying the gut-to-brain connection in autism spectrum disorders as future targets for disease management. Eur J Pharmacol 2011; 668 (Suppl. 1): S70-80. [http://dx.doi.org/10.1016/j.ejphar.2011.07.013] [PMID: 21810417]

[173] Soto C. Unfolding the role of protein misfolding in neurodegenerative diseases. Nat Rev Neurosci 2003; 4(1): 49-60. [http://dx.doi.org/10.1038/nrn1007] [PMID: 12511861]

[174] Ochoa-Repáraz J, Mielcarz DW, Begum-Haque S, Kasper LH. Gut, bugs, and brain: role of commensal bacteria in the control of central nervous system disease. Ann Neurol 2011; 69(2): 240-7. [http://dx.doi.org/10.1002/ana.22344] [PMID: 21387369]

[175] WHO Library Cataloguing-in-Publication Data. Neurological disorders: public health challenges ISBN 92 4 156336 2 (NLM classifi cation: WL 140) ISBN 978 92 4 1563369 http://www.who.int/mental_health/neurology/neurological_disorders_report_web.pdf

[176] Riccio P. The molecular basis of nutritional intervention in multiple sclerosis: a narrative review. Complement Ther Med 2011; 19(4): 228-37. [http://dx.doi.org/10.1016/j.ctim.2011.06.006] [PMID: 21827937]

[177] Reichelt K-L, Jensen D. IgA antibodies against gliadin and gluten in multiple sclerosis. Acta Neurol Scand 2004; 110(4): 239-41. [http://dx.doi.org/10.1111/j.1600-0404.2004.00303.x] [PMID: 15355487]

[178] Qin L, Wu X, Block ML, *et al.* Systemic LPS causes chronic neuroinflammation and progressive neurodegeneration. Glia 2007; 55(5): 453-62.

[http://dx.doi.org/10.1002/glia.20467] [PMID: 17203472]

[179] Deschamps V, Barberger-Gateau P, Peuchant E, Orgogozo JM. Nutritional factors in cerebral aging and dementia: epidemiological arguments for a role of oxidative stress. Neuroepidemiology 2001; 20(1): 7-15.
[http://dx.doi.org/10.1159/000054752] [PMID: 11174040]

[180] Qiao Y, Sun J, Ding Y, Le G, Shi Y. Alterations of the gut microbiota in high-fat diet mice is strongly linked to oxidative stress. Appl Microbiol Biotechnol 2013; 97(4): 1689-97.
[http://dx.doi.org/10.1007/s00253-012-4323-6] [PMID: 22948953]

[181] Connor B, Young D, Yan Q, Faull RL, Synek B, Dragunow M. Brain-derived neurotrophic factor is reduced in Alzheimers disease. Brain Res Mol Brain Res 1997; 49(1-2): 71-81.
[http://dx.doi.org/10.1016/S0169-328X(97)00125-3] [PMID: 9387865]

[182] Friedland RP. Mechanisms of molecular mimicry involving the microbiota in neurodegeneration. J Alzheimers Dis 2015; 45(2): 349-62.
[PMID: 25589730]

[183] Jacka FN, Cherbuin N, Anstey KJ, Butterworth P. Dietary patterns and depressive symptoms over time: examining the relationships with socioeconomic position, health behaviours and cardiovascular risk. PLoS One 2014; 9(1): e87657.
[http://dx.doi.org/10.1371/journal.pone.0087657] [PMID: 24489946]

[184] Psaltopoulou T, Sergentanis TN, Panagiotakos DB, Sergentanis IN, Kosti R, Scarmeas N. Mediterranean diet, stroke, cognitive impairment, and depression: A meta-analysis. Ann Neurol 2013; 74(4): 580-91.
[http://dx.doi.org/10.1002/ana.23944] [PMID: 23720230]

[185] Steensma DP. Congo red: out of Africa? Arch Pathol Lab Med 2001; 125(2): 250-2.
[PMID: 11175644]

[186] Badtke MP, Hammer ND, Chapman MR. Functional amyloids signal their arrival. Sci Signal 2009; 2(80): pe43-3.
[http://dx.doi.org/10.1126/scisignal.280pe43] [PMID: 19622831]

[187] Blanco LP, Evans ML, Smith DR, Badtke MP, Chapman MR. Diversity, biogenesis and function of microbial amyloids. Trends Microbiol 2012; 20(2): 66-73.
[http://dx.doi.org/10.1016/j.tim.2011.11.005] [PMID: 22197327]

[188] Buxbaum JN, Linke RP. A molecular history of the amyloidoses. J Mol Biol 2012; 421(2-3): 142-59.
[http://dx.doi.org/10.1016/j.jmb.2012.01.024] [PMID: 22321796]

[189] OBrien RJ, Wong PC. Amyloid precursor protein processing and Alzheimers disease. Annu Rev Neurosci 2011; 34: 185-204.
[http://dx.doi.org/10.1146/annurev-neuro-061010-113613] [PMID: 21456963]

[190] Lukiw WJ. Amyloid beta (Aβ) peptide modulators and other current treatment strategies for Alzheimers disease (AD). Expert Opin Emerg Drugs 2012; 17: 43-60.
[http://dx.doi.org/10.1517/14728214.2012.672559] [PMID: 22439907]

[191] Goldschmidt L, Teng PK, Riek R, Eisenberg D. Identifying the amylome, proteins capable of forming amyloid-like fibrils. Proc Natl Acad Sci USA 2010; 107(8): 3487-92.
[http://dx.doi.org/10.1073/pnas.0915166107] [PMID: 20133726]

[192] Zhao Y, Bhattacharjee S, Jones BM, *et al.* Regulation of TREM2 expression by an NF-κB-sensitive miRNA-34a. Neuroreport 2013; 24(6): 318-23.
[http://dx.doi.org/10.1097/WNR.0b013e32835fb6b0] [PMID: 23462268]

[193] Ferrera D, Mazzaro N, Canale C, Gasparini L. Resting microglia react to Aβ42 fibrils but do not detect oligomers or oligomer-induced neuronal damage. Neurobiol Aging 2014; 35(11): 2444-57.
[http://dx.doi.org/10.1016/j.neurobiolaging.2014.05.023] [PMID: 24973120]

[194] Jones BM, Bhattacharjee S, Dua P, Hill JM, Zhao Y, Lukiw WJ. Regulating amyloidogenesis through the natural triggering receptor expressed in myeloid/microglial cells 2 (TREM2). Front Cell Neurosci 2014; 8: 94.
[http://dx.doi.org/10.3389/fncel.2014.00094] [PMID: 24744699]

[195] Bhattacharjee S, Lukiw WJ. Alzheimers disease and the microbiome. Front Cell Neurosci 2013; 7: 153.
[http://dx.doi.org/10.3389/fncel.2013.00153] [PMID: 24062644]

[196] Hill JM, Clement C, Pogue AI, Bhattacharjee S, Zhao Y, Lukiw WJ. Pathogenic microbes, the microbiome, and Alzheimers disease (AD). Front Aging Neurosci 2014; 6: 127.
[PMID: 24982633]

[197] Lin CS, Chang CJ, Lu CC, *et al.* Impact of the gut microbiota, prebiotics, and probiotics on human health and disease. Biomed J 2014; 37(5): 259-68.
[http://dx.doi.org/10.4103/2319-4170.138314] [PMID: 25179725]

[198] Hattori M, Taylor TD. The human intestinal microbiome: a new frontier of human biology. DNA Res 2009; 16(1): 1-12.
[http://dx.doi.org/10.1093/dnares/dsn033] [PMID: 19147530]

[199] Schwartz K, Boles BR. Microbial amyloidsfunctions and interactions within the host. Curr Opin Microbiol 2013; 16(1): 93-9.
[http://dx.doi.org/10.1016/j.mib.2012.12.001] [PMID: 23313395]

[200] Syed AK, Boles BR. Fold modulating function: bacterial toxins to functional amyloids. Front Microbiol 2014; 5: 401.
[http://dx.doi.org/10.3389/fmicb.2014.00401] [PMID: 25136340]

[201] Asti A, Gioglio L. Can a bacterial endotoxin be a key factor in the kinetics of amyloid fibril formation? J Alzheimers Dis 2014; 39(1): 169-79.
[PMID: 24150108]

[202] Zhou ZD, Chan CH, Ma QH, Xu XH, Xiao ZC, Tan E-K. The roles of amyloid precursor protein (APP) in neurogenesis: Implications to pathogenesis and therapy of Alzheimer disease. Cell Adhes Migr 2011; 5(4): 280-92.
[http://dx.doi.org/10.4161/cam.5.4.16986] [PMID: 21785276]

[203] Marques F, Sousa JC, Sousa N, Palha JA. Blood-brain-barriers in aging and in Alzheimers disease. Mol Neurodegener 2013; 8: 38.
[http://dx.doi.org/10.1186/1750-1326-8-38] [PMID: 24148264]

[204] Oakley R, Tharakan B. Vascular hyperpermeability and aging. Aging Dis 2014; 5(2): 114-25.
[PMID: 24729937]

[205] Van Broeck B, Van Broeckhoven C, Kumar-Singh S. Current insights into molecular mechanisms of Alzheimer disease and their implications for therapeutic approaches. Neurodegener Dis 2007; 4(5): 349-65.
[http://dx.doi.org/10.1159/000105156] [PMID: 17622778]

[206] Zhang H, Ma Q, Zhang YW, Xu H. Proteolytic processing of Alzheimers β-amyloid precursor protein. J Neurochem 2012; 120 (Suppl. 1): 9-21.
[http://dx.doi.org/10.1111/j.1471-4159.2011.07519.x] [PMID: 22122372]

[207] Alexandrov PN, Pogue A, Bhattacharjee S, Lukiw WJ. Retinal amyloid peptides and complement factor H in transgenic models of Alzheimers disease. Neuroreport 2011; 22(12): 623-7.
[http://dx.doi.org/10.1097/WNR.0b013e3283497334] [PMID: 21734608]

[208] Teng PK, Anderson NJ, Goldschmidt L, Sawaya MR, Sambashivan S, Eisenberg D. Ribonuclease A suggests how proteins self-chaperone against amyloid fiber formation. Protein Sci 2012; 21(1): 26-37.
[http://dx.doi.org/10.1002/pro.754] [PMID: 22095666]

[209] Armstrong RA. Plaques and tangles and the pathogenesis of Alzheimers disease. Folia Neuropathol 2006; 44(1): 1-11.
[PMID: 16565925]

[210] Cui J-G, Hill JM, Zhao Y, Lukiw WJ. Expression of inflammatory genes in the primary visual cortex of late-stage Alzheimers disease. Neuroreport 2007; 18(2): 115-9.
[http://dx.doi.org/10.1097/WNR.0b013e32801198bc] [PMID: 17301674]

[211] Boutajangout A, Wisniewski T. The innate immune system in Alzheimers disease. Int J Cell Biol 2013; 2013: 576383.
[http://dx.doi.org/10.1155/2013/576383] [PMID: 24223593]

[212] Furukawa Y, Nukina N. Functional diversity of protein fibrillar aggregates from physiology to RNA granules to neurodegenerative diseases. *Biochim. Biophys. Acta - Mol.* Basis Dis 2013; 1832: 1271-8.
[http://dx.doi.org/10.1016/j.bbadis.2013.04.011]

[213] Serpente M, Bonsi R, Scarpini E, Galimberti D. Innate immune system and inflammation in Alzheimers disease: from pathogenesis to treatment. Neuroimmunomodulation 2014; 21(2-3): 79-87.
[http://dx.doi.org/10.1159/000356529] [PMID: 24557039]

[214] Takeda S, Sato N, Morishita R. Systemic inflammation, blood-brain barrier vulnerability and cognitive/non-cognitive symptoms in Alzheimer disease: relevance to pathogenesis and therapy. Front Aging Neurosci 2014; 6: 171.
[http://dx.doi.org/10.3389/fnagi.2014.00171] [PMID: 25120476]

[215] Colangelo V, Schurr J, Ball MJ, Pelaez RP, Bazan NG, Lukiw WJ. Gene expression profiling of 12633 genes in Alzheimer hippocampal CA1: transcription and neurotrophic factor down-regulation and up-regulation of apoptotic and pro-inflammatory signaling. J Neurosci Res 2002; 70(3): 462-73.
[http://dx.doi.org/10.1002/jnr.10351] [PMID: 12391607]

[216] Hammer ND, Wang X, McGuffie BA, Chapman MR. Amyloids: friend or foe? J Alzheimers Dis 2008; 13(4): 407-19.
[PMID: 18487849]

[217] Dasari M, Espargaro A, Sabate R, *et al.* Bacterial inclusion bodies of Alzheimers disease β-amyloid peptides can be employed to study native-like aggregation intermediate states. ChemBioChem 2011; 12(3): 407-23.
[http://dx.doi.org/10.1002/cbic.201000602] [PMID: 21290543]

[218] Zhou Y, Blanco LP, Smith DR, Chapman MR. Bacterial amyloids. Methods Mol Biol 2012; 849: 303-20.
[http://dx.doi.org/10.1007/978-1-61779-551-0_21] [PMID: 22528099]

[219] Zhao Y, Dua P, Lukiw WJ. Microbial Sources of Amyloid and Relevance to Amyloidogenesis and Alzheimers Disease (AD). J Alzheimers Dis Parkinsonism 2015; 5(1): 177.
[PMID: 25977840]

[220] Hill JM, Bhattacharjee S, Pogue AI, Lukiw WJ. The gastrointestinal tract microbiome and potential link to Alzheimers disease. Front Neurol 2014; 5: 43.
[http://dx.doi.org/10.3389/fneur.2014.00043] [PMID: 24772103]

[221] Via A, Uyar B, Brun C, Zanzoni A. How pathogens use linear motifs to perturb host cell networks. Trends Biochem Sci 2015; 40(1): 36-48.
[http://dx.doi.org/10.1016/j.tibs.2014.11.001] [PMID: 25475989]

[222] Hayashi M. Anti-basal ganglia antibody. Brain Nerve 2013; 65(4): 377-84.
[PMID: 23568985]

[223] Roubaud Baudron C, Franceschi F, Salles N, Gasbarrini A. Extragastric diseases and Helicobacter pylori. Helicobacter 2013; 18 (Suppl. 1): 44-51.
[http://dx.doi.org/10.1111/hel.12077] [PMID: 24011245]

[224] Bu X-L, Yao X-Q, Jiao S-S, *et al.* A study on the association between infectious burden and Alzheimers disease. Eur J Neurol 2015; 22(12): 1519-25.
[http://dx.doi.org/10.1111/ene.12477] [PMID: 24910016]

[225] Lavelle EC, Murphy C, O'Neill LA, Creagh EM. The role of TLRs, NLRs, and RLRs in mucosal innate immunity and homeostasis. Mucosal Immunol 2010; 3(1): 17-28.
[http://dx.doi.org/10.1038/mi.2009.124] [PMID: 19890268]

[226] Atarashi K, Tanoue T, Oshima K, *et al.* Treg induction by a rationally selected mixture of Clostridia strains from the human microbiota. Nature 2013; 500(7461): 232-6.
[http://dx.doi.org/10.1038/nature12331] [PMID: 23842501]

[227] Lathrop SK, Bloom SM, Rao SM, *et al.* Peripheral education of the immune system by colonic commensal microbiota. Nature 2011; 478(7368): 250-4.
[http://dx.doi.org/10.1038/nature10434] [PMID: 21937990]

[228] Li J, Lee DS, Madrenas J. Evolving Bacterial Envelopes and Plasticity of TLR2-Dependent Responses: Basic Research and Translational Opportunities. Front Immunol 2013; 4: 347.
[http://dx.doi.org/10.3389/fimmu.2013.00347] [PMID: 24191155]

[229] Nishimori JH, Newman TN, Oppong GO, *et al.* Microbial amyloids induce interleukin 17A (IL-17A) and IL-22 responses *via* Toll-like receptor 2 activation in the intestinal mucosa. Infect Immun 2012; 80(12): 4398-408.
[http://dx.doi.org/10.1128/IAI.00911-12] [PMID: 23027540]

[230] Tükel C, Nishimori JH, Wilson RP, *et al.* Toll-like receptors 1 and 2 cooperatively mediate immune responses to curli, a common amyloid from enterobacterial biofilms. Cell Microbiol 2010; 12(10): 1495-505.
[http://dx.doi.org/10.1111/j.1462-5822.2010.01485.x] [PMID: 20497180]

[231] Czirr E, Wyss-Coray T. The immunology of neurodegeneration. J Clin Invest 2012; 122(4): 1156-63.
[http://dx.doi.org/10.1172/JCI58656] [PMID: 22466657]

[232] Bechmann I, Priller J, Kovac A, *et al.* Immune surveillance of mouse brain perivascular spaces by blood-borne macrophages. Eur J Neurosci 2001; 14(10): 1651-8.
[http://dx.doi.org/10.1046/j.0953-816x.2001.01793.x] [PMID: 11860459]

[233] Saresella M, Marventano I, Calabrese E, *et al.* A complex proinflammatory role for peripheral monocytes in Alzheimers disease. J Alzheimers Dis 2014; 38(2): 403-13.
[PMID: 23979026]

[234] Trudler D, Farfara D, Frenkel D. Toll-like receptors expression and signaling in glia cells in neuro-amyloidogenic diseases: towards future therapeutic application. Mediators Inflamm 2010; 2010: 1-12.
[http://dx.doi.org/10.1155/2010/497987] [PMID: 20706642]

[235] Palaga T, Buranaruk C, Rengpipat S, *et al.* Notch signaling is activated by TLR stimulation and regulates macrophage functions. Eur J Immunol 2008; 38(1): 174-83.
[http://dx.doi.org/10.1002/eji.200636999] [PMID: 18085664]

[236] McGeer PL, McGeer EG. Local neuroinflammation and the progression of Alzheimers disease. J Neurovirol 2002; 8(6): 529-38.
[http://dx.doi.org/10.1080/13550280290100969] [PMID: 12476347]

[237] Akiyama H, Barger S, Barnum S, *et al.* Inflammation and Alzheimers disease. Neurobiol Aging 2000; 21(3): 383-421.
[http://dx.doi.org/10.1016/S0197-4580(00)00124-X] [PMID: 10858586]

[238] Béraud D, Maguire-Zeiss KA. Misfolded α-synuclein and Toll-like receptors: therapeutic targets for Parkinsons disease. Parkinsonism Relat Disord 2012; 18 (Suppl. 1): S17-20.
[http://dx.doi.org/10.1016/S1353-8020(11)70008-6] [PMID: 22166424]

[239] Richard KL, Filali M, Préfontaine P, Rivest S. Toll-like receptor 2 acts as a natural innate immune

receptor to clear amyloid beta 142 and delay the cognitive decline in a mouse model of Alzheimers disease. J Neurosci 2008; 28(22): 5784-93.
[http://dx.doi.org/10.1523/JNEUROSCI.1146-08.2008] [PMID: 18509040]

[240] Wlodarska M, Thaiss CA, Nowarski R, *et al.* NLRP6 inflammasome orchestrates the colonic host-microbial interface by regulating goblet cell mucus secretion. Cell 2014; 156(5): 1045-59.
[http://dx.doi.org/10.1016/j.cell.2014.01.026] [PMID: 24581500]

[241] Raby A-C, Le Bouder E, Colmont C, *et al.* Soluble TLR2 reduces inflammation without compromising bacterial clearance by disrupting TLR2 triggering. J Immunol 2009; 183(1): 506-17.
[http://dx.doi.org/10.4049/jimmunol.0802909] [PMID: 19542461]

[242] Rapsinski GJ, Newman TN, Oppong GO, van Putten JP, Tükel Ç. CD14 protein acts as an adaptor molecule for the immune recognition of Salmonella curli fibers. J Biol Chem 2013; 288(20): 14178-88.
[http://dx.doi.org/10.1074/jbc.M112.447060] [PMID: 23548899]

[243] Perry VH, Holmes C. Microglial priming in neurodegenerative disease. Nat Rev Neurol 2014; 10(4): 217-24.
[http://dx.doi.org/10.1038/nrneurol.2014.38] [PMID: 24638131]

[244] Bodea L-G, Wang Y, Linnartz-Gerlach B, *et al.* Neurodegeneration by activation of the microglial complement-phagosome pathway. J Neurosci 2014; 34(25): 8546-56.
[http://dx.doi.org/10.1523/JNEUROSCI.5002-13.2014] [PMID: 24948809]

[245] Smith MA, Perry G, Richey PL, *et al.* Oxidative damage in Alzheimers. Nature 1996; 382(6587): 120-1.
[http://dx.doi.org/10.1038/382120b0] [PMID: 8700201]

[246] Benitez BA, Jin SC, Guerreiro R, *et al.* 3C Study Group; EADI consortium; Alzheimers Disease Genetic Consortium (ADGC); Alzheimers Disease Neuroimaging Initiative (ADNI); GERAD Consortium. Missense variant in TREML2 protects against Alzheimers disease. Neurobiol Aging 2014; 35(6): 1510.e19-.
[http://dx.doi.org/10.1016/j.neurobiolaging.2013.12.010] [PMID: 24439484]

[247] Rayaprolu S, Mullen B, Baker M, *et al.* TREM2 in neurodegeneration: evidence for association of the p.R47H variant with frontotemporal dementia and Parkinsons disease. Mol Neurodegener 2013; 8: 19.
[http://dx.doi.org/10.1186/1750-1326-8-19] [PMID: 23800361]

[248] Verbrugghe P, Kujala P, Waelput W, Peters PJ, Cuvelier CA. Clusterin in human gut-associated lymphoid tissue, tonsils, and adenoids: localization to M cells and follicular dendritic cells. Histochem Cell Biol 2008; 129(3): 311-20.
[http://dx.doi.org/10.1007/s00418-007-0369-4] [PMID: 18097679]

[249] Carare RO, Teeling JL, Hawkes CA, *et al.* Immune complex formation impairs the elimination of solutes from the brain: implications for immunotherapy in Alzheimers disease. Acta Neuropathol Commun 2013; 1: 48.
[http://dx.doi.org/10.1186/2051-5960-1-48] [PMID: 24252464]

[250] Hawkes CA, Carare RO, Weller RO. Amyloid and tau in the brain in sporadic Alzheimers disease: defining the chicken and the egg. Acta Neuropathol 2014; 127(4): 617-8.
[http://dx.doi.org/10.1007/s00401-014-1243-9] [PMID: 24452628]

[251] Savva GM, Wharton SB, Ince PG, Forster G, Matthews FE, Brayne C. Medical Research Council Cognitive Function and Ageing Study. Age, neuropathology, and dementia. N Engl J Med 2009; 360(22): 2302-9.
[http://dx.doi.org/10.1056/NEJMoa0806142] [PMID: 19474427]

[252] Holmes C. Review: systemic inflammation and Alzheimers disease. Neuropathol Appl Neurobiol 2013; 39(1): 51-68.
[http://dx.doi.org/10.1111/j.1365-2990.2012.01307.x] [PMID: 23046210]

[253] McGeer PL, McGeer EG. The amyloid cascade-inflammatory hypothesis of Alzheimer disease: implications for therapy. Acta Neuropathol 2013; 126(4): 479-97. [http://dx.doi.org/10.1007/s00401-013-1177-7] [PMID: 24052108]

[254] Maier M, Peng Y, Jiang L, Seabrook TJ, Carroll MC, Lemere CA. Complement C3 deficiency leads to accelerated amyloid beta plaque deposition and neurodegeneration and modulation of the microglia/macrophage phenotype in amyloid precursor protein transgenic mice. J Neurosci 2008; 28(25): 6333-41. [http://dx.doi.org/10.1523/JNEUROSCI.0829-08.2008] [PMID: 18562603]

[255] Aguzzi A. Neurodegeneration: Alzheimers disease under strain. Nature 2014; 512(7512): 32-4. [http://dx.doi.org/10.1038/512032a] [PMID: 25100477]

[256] Bagriantsev S, Liebman S. Modulation of Abeta42 low-n oligomerization using a novel yeast reporter system. BMC Biol 2006; 4: 32. [http://dx.doi.org/10.1186/1741-7007-4-32] [PMID: 17002801]

[257] Kovacs GG. Can Creutzfeldt-Jakob disease unravel the mysteries of Alzheimer? Prion 2016; 10(5): 369-76. [http://dx.doi.org/10.1080/19336896.2016.1228507] [PMID: 27649940]

[258] Jamieson GA, Maitland NJ, Wilcock GK, Craske J, Itzhaki RF. Latent *herpes simplex virus* type 1 in normal and Alzheimers disease brains. J Med Virol 1991; 33(4): 224-7. [http://dx.doi.org/10.1002/jmv.1890330403] [PMID: 1649907]

[259] Miklossy J. Alzheimers diseasea spirochetosis? Neuroreport 1993; 4(7): 841-8. [http://dx.doi.org/10.1097/00001756-199307000-00002] [PMID: 8369471]

[260] Balin BJ, Gérard HC, Arking EJ, *et al.* Identification and localization of Chlamydia pneumoniae in the Alzheimers brain. Med Microbiol Immunol (Berl) 1998; 187(1): 23-42. [http://dx.doi.org/10.1007/s004300050071] [PMID: 9749980]

[261] Saldanha J, Sutton RN, Gannicliffe A, Farragher B, Itzhaki RF. Detection of HSV1 DNA by *in situ* hybridisation in human brain after immunosuppression. J Neurol Neurosurg Psychiatry 1986; 49(6): 613-9. [http://dx.doi.org/10.1136/jnnp.49.6.613] [PMID: 3016195]

[262] Roos KL. Encephalitis. Neurol Clin 1999; 17(4): 813-33. [http://dx.doi.org/10.1016/S0733-8619(05)70168-7] [PMID: 10517930]

[263] Miklossy J, Khalili K, Gern L, *et al.* Borrelia burgdorferi persists in the brain in chronic lyme neuroborreliosis and may be associated with Alzheimer disease 2004.

[264] Wozniak MA, Mee AP, Itzhaki RF. *Herpes simplex virus* type 1 DNA is located within Alzheimers disease amyloid plaques. J Pathol 2009; 217(1): 131-8. [http://dx.doi.org/10.1002/path.2449] [PMID: 18973185]

[265] Letenneur L, Pérès K, Fleury H, *et al.* Seropositivity to *herpes simplex virus* antibodies and risk of Alzheimers disease: a population-based cohort study. PLoS One 2008; 3(11): e3637. [http://dx.doi.org/10.1371/journal.pone.0003637] [PMID: 18982063]

[266] Mancuso R, Baglio F, Cabinio M, *et al.* Titers of *herpes simplex virus* type 1 antibodies positively correlate with grey matter volumes in Alzheimers disease. J Alzheimers Dis 2014; 38(4): 741-5. [PMID: 24072067]

[267] Lövheim H, Gilthorpe J, Johansson A, Eriksson S, Hallmans G, Elgh F. Herpes simplex infection and the risk of Alzheimers disease: A nested case-control study. Alzheimers Dement 2015; 11(6): 587-92. [http://dx.doi.org/10.1016/j.jalz.2014.07.157] [PMID: 25304990]

[268] Lövheim H, Gilthorpe J, Adolfsson R, Nilsson L-G, Elgh F. Reactivated herpes simplex infection increases the risk of Alzheimers disease. Alzheimers Dement 2015; 11(6): 593-9. [http://dx.doi.org/10.1016/j.jalz.2014.04.522] [PMID: 25043910]

[269] Wyss-Coray T, Rogers J. Inflammation in Alzheimer disease-a brief review of the basic science and clinical literature. Cold Spring Harb Perspect Med 2012; 2(1): a006346-6. [http://dx.doi.org/10.1101/cshperspect.a006346] [PMID: 22315714]

[270] Stefaniak J, O'Brien J. Imaging of neuroinflammation in dementia: a review. J Neurol Neurosurg Psychiatry 2015. [http://dx.doi.org/jnnp-2015-311336]

[271] Mahley RW, Weisgraber KH, Huang Y. Apolipoprotein E: structure determines function, from atherosclerosis to Alzheimers disease to AIDS. J Lipid Res 2009; 50 (Suppl.): S183-8. [http://dx.doi.org/10.1194/jlr.R800069-JLR200] [PMID: 19106071]

[272] Verghese PB, Castellano JM, Holtzman DM. Apolipoprotein E in Alzheimers disease and other neurological disorders. Lancet Neurol 2011; 10(3): 241-52. [http://dx.doi.org/10.1016/S1474-4422(10)70325-2] [PMID: 21349439]

[273] Yu J-T, Tan L, Hardy J. Apolipoprotein E in Alzheimers disease: an update. Annu Rev Neurosci 2014; 37: 79-100. [http://dx.doi.org/10.1146/annurev-neuro-071013-014300] [PMID: 24821312]

[274] Lambert J-C, Heath S, Even G, *et al.* European Alzheimers Disease Initiative Investigators. Genome-wide association study identifies variants at CLU and CR1 associated with Alzheimers disease. Nat Genet 2009; 41(10): 1094-9. [http://dx.doi.org/10.1038/ng.439] [PMID: 19734903]

[275] Porcellini E, Carbone I, Ianni M, Licastro F. Alzheimers disease gene signature says: beware of brain viral infections. Immun Ageing 2010; 7: 16. [http://dx.doi.org/10.1186/1742-4933-7-16] [PMID: 21156047]

[276] Carter CJ. APP, APOE, complement receptor 1, clusterin and PICALM and their involvement in the herpes simplex life cycle. Neurosci Lett 2010; 483(2): 96-100. [http://dx.doi.org/10.1016/j.neulet.2010.07.066] [PMID: 20674675]

[277] Lambert J-C, Zelenika D, Hiltunen M, *et al.* Evidence of the association of BIN1 and PICALM with the AD risk in contrasting European populations. Neurobiol Aging 2011; 32(4): 756.e11-5. [http://dx.doi.org/10.1016/j.neurobiolaging.2010.11.022] [PMID: 21220176]

[278] Licastro F, Carbone I, Ianni M, Porcellini E. Gene signature in Alzheimers disease and environmental factors: the virus chronicle. J Alzheimers Dis 2011; 27(4): 809-17. [PMID: 21891868]

[279] Carter CJ. Susceptibility genes are enriched in those of the *herpes simplex virus* 1/host interactome in psychiatric and neurological disorders. Pathog Dis 2013; 69(3): 240-61. [http://dx.doi.org/10.1111/2049-632X.12077] [PMID: 23913659]

[280] Baker HF, Ridley RM, Duchen LW, Crow TJ, Bruton CJ. Induction of β(A4)-amyloid in primates by injection of Alzheimers disease brain homogenate. Mol Neurobiol 1994; 8: 25-39. [http://dx.doi.org/10.1007/BF02778005] [PMID: 8086126]

[281] Kane MD, Lipinski WJ, Callahan MJ, *et al.* Evidence for seeding of beta -amyloid by intracerebral infusion of Alzheimer brain extracts in beta -amyloid precursor protein-transgenic mice. J Neurosci 2000; 20(10): 3606-11. [PMID: 10804202]

[282] Meyer-Luehmann M. Exogenous Induction of Cerebral -Amyloidogenesis Is Governed by Agent and Host. Science 2006; 313(80): 1781-4.

[283] Stanley LC, Mrak RE, Woody RC, *et al.* Glial cytokines as neuropathogenic factors in HIV infection: pathogenic similarities to Alzheimers disease. J Neuropathol Exp Neurol 1994; 53(3): 231-8. [http://dx.doi.org/10.1097/00005072-199405000-00003] [PMID: 8176406]

[284] Esiri MM, Biddolph SC, Morris CS. Prevalence of Alzheimer plaques in AIDS. J Neurol Neurosurg

Psychiatry 1998; 65(1): 29-33.
[http://dx.doi.org/10.1136/jnnp.65.1.29] [PMID: 9667557]

[285] Green DA, Masliah E, Vinters HV, Beizai P, Moore DJ, Achim CL. Brain deposition of beta-amyloid is a common pathologic feature in HIV positive patients. AIDS 2005; 19(4): 407-11.
[http://dx.doi.org/10.1097/01.aids.0000161770.06158.5c] [PMID: 15750394]

[286] Bearer EL, Woltje R, Donahue JE, Kilpatrick K. Herpes Encephalitis and Abeta Plaques 2013.

[287] Smith DB, Simmonds P, Bell JE. Brain viral burden, neuroinflammation and neurodegeneration in HAART-treated HIV positive injecting drug users. J Neurovirol 2014; 20(1): 28-38.
[http://dx.doi.org/10.1007/s13365-013-0225-3] [PMID: 24420447]

[288] McQuaid S, Allen IV, McMahon J, Kirk J. Association of measles virus with neurofibrillary tangles in subacute sclerosing panencephalitis: a combined *in situ* hybridization and immunocytochemical investigation. Neuropathol Appl Neurobiol 1994; 20(2): 103-10.
[http://dx.doi.org/10.1111/j.1365-2990.1994.tb01168.x] [PMID: 8072641]

[289] Little CS, Hammond CJ, MacIntyre A, Balin BJ, Appelt DM. Chlamydia pneumoniae induces Alzheimer-like amyloid plaques in brains of BALB/c mice. Neurobiol Aging 2004; 25(4): 419-29.
[http://dx.doi.org/10.1016/S0197-4580(03)00127-1] [PMID: 15013562]

[290] Miklossy J, Kis A, Radenovic A, *et al.* Beta-amyloid deposition and Alzheimers type changes induced by Borrelia spirochetes. Neurobiol Aging 2006; 27(2): 228-36.
[http://dx.doi.org/10.1016/j.neurobiolaging.2005.01.018] [PMID: 15894409]

[291] Boelen E, Stassen FR, van der Ven AJ, *et al.* Detection of amyloid beta aggregates in the brain of BALB/c mice after Chlamydia pneumoniae infection. Acta Neuropathol 2007; 114(3): 255-61.
[http://dx.doi.org/10.1007/s00401-007-0252-3] [PMID: 17581756]

[292] Wozniak MA, Frost AL, Itzhaki RF. Alzheimers disease-specific tau phosphorylation is induced by *herpes simplex virus* type 1. J Alzheimers Dis 2009; 16(2): 341-50.
[PMID: 19221424]

[293] Velayudhan L, Gasper A, Pritchard M, Baillon S, Messer C, Proitsi P. Pattern of Smell Identification Impairment in Alzheimers Disease. J Alzheimers Dis 2015; 46(2): 381-7.
[http://dx.doi.org/10.3233/JAD-142838] [PMID: 25757648]

[294] Braak H, Braak E, Bohl J. Staging of Alzheimer-related cortical destruction. Eur Neurol 1993; 33(6): 403-8.
[http://dx.doi.org/10.1159/000116984] [PMID: 8307060]

[295] Ball MJ, Lukiw WJ, Kammerman EM, Hill JM. Intracerebral propagation of Alzheimers disease: strengthening evidence of a *herpes simplex virus* etiology. Alzheimers Dement 2013; 9(2): 169-75.
[http://dx.doi.org/10.1016/j.jalz.2012.07.005] [PMID: 23159044]

[296] Gillet L, Frederico B, Stevenson PG. Host entry by gamma-herpesviruseslessons from animal viruses? Curr Opin Virol 2015; 15: 34-40.
[http://dx.doi.org/10.1016/j.coviro.2015.07.007] [PMID: 26246389]

[297] Mori I, Nishiyama Y, Yokochi T, Kimura Y. Olfactory transmission of neurotropic viruses. J Neurovirol 2005; 11(2): 129-37.
[http://dx.doi.org/10.1080/13550280590922793] [PMID: 16036791]

[298] Little CS, Bowe A, Lin R, *et al.* Age alterations in extent and severity of experimental intranasal infection with *Chlamydophila pneumoniae* in BALB/c mice. Infect Immun 2005; 73(3): 1723-34.
[http://dx.doi.org/10.1128/IAI.73.3.1723-1734.2005] [PMID: 15731073]

[299] Braak H, Del Tredici K. The preclinical phase of the pathological process underlying sporadic Alzheimers disease. Brain 2015; 138(Pt 10): 2814-33.
[http://dx.doi.org/10.1093/brain/awv236] [PMID: 26283673]

[300] Blanc M, Hsieh WY, Robertson KA, *et al.* The transcription factor STAT-1 couples macrophage

synthesis of 25-hydroxycholesterol to the interferon antiviral response. Immunity 2013; 38(1): 106-18. [http://dx.doi.org/10.1016/j.immuni.2012.11.004] [PMID: 23273843]

[301] Liu S-Y, Aliyari R, Chikere K, *et al.* Interferon-inducible cholesterol-25-hydroxylase broadly inhibits viral entry by production of 25-hydroxycholesterol. Immunity 2013; 38(1): 92-105. [http://dx.doi.org/10.1016/j.immuni.2012.11.005] [PMID: 23273844]

[302] Papassotiropoulos A, Lambert J-C, Wavrant-De Vrièze F, *et al.* Cholesterol 25-hydroxylase on chromosome 10q is a susceptibility gene for sporadic Alzheimers disease. Neurodegener Dis 2005; 2(5): 233-41. [http://dx.doi.org/10.1159/000090362] [PMID: 16909003]

[303] Lathe R, Sapronova A, Kotelevtsev Y. Atherosclerosis and Alzheimerdiseases with a common cause? Inflammation, oxysterols, vasculature. BMC Geriatr 2014; 14: 36. [http://dx.doi.org/10.1186/1471-2318-14-36] [PMID: 24656052]

[304] Soscia SJ, Kirby JE, Washicosky KJ, *et al.* The Alzheimers disease-associated amyloid β-protein is an antimicrobial peptide. PLoS One 2010; 5(3): e9505. [http://dx.doi.org/10.1371/journal.pone.0009505] [PMID: 20209079]

[305] White MR, Kandel R, Tripathi S, *et al.* Alzheimers associated β-amyloid protein inhibits influenza A virus and modulates viral interactions with phagocytes. PLoS One 2014; 9(7): e101364. [http://dx.doi.org/10.1371/journal.pone.0101364] [PMID: 24988208]

[306] Bourgade K, Garneau H, Giroux G, *et al.* β-Amyloid peptides display protective activity against the human Alzheimers disease-associated *herpes simplex virus*-1. Biogerontology 2015; 16(1): 85-98. [http://dx.doi.org/10.1007/s10522-014-9538-8] [PMID: 25376108]

[307] Bourgade K, Le Page A, Bocti C, *et al.* Protective Effect of Amyloid-β Peptides Against *herpes simplex virus*-1 Infection in a Neuronal Cell Culture Model. J Alzheimers Dis 2016; 50(4): 1227-41. [http://dx.doi.org/10.3233/JAD-150652] [PMID: 26836158]

[308] Williams WM, Torres S, Siedlak SL, *et al.* Antimicrobial peptide β-defensin-1 expression is upregulated in Alzheimers brain. J Neuroinflammation 2013; 10: 127. [http://dx.doi.org/10.1186/1742-2094-10-127] [PMID: 24139179]

[309] Itzhaki RF, Lin W-R, Shang D, Wilcock GK, Faragher B, Jamieson GA. *herpes simplex virus* type 1 in brain and risk of Alzheimers disease. Lancet 1997; 349(9047): 241-4. [http://dx.doi.org/10.1016/S0140-6736(96)10149-5] [PMID: 9014911]

[310] Itzhaki RF, Wozniak MA. Apolipoprotein E: Microbial Friend or Foe? In: Biomedical N, York N, Eds. Apoprotein research, Penfield LR, Nelson RT. NY 2009; pp. 99-112.

[311] Marques AR, Straus SE, Fahle G, Weir S, Csako G, Fischer SH. Lack of association between HSV-1 DNA in the brain, Alzheimers disease and apolipoprotein E4. J Neurovirol 2001; 7(1): 82-3. [http://dx.doi.org/10.1080/135502801300069773] [PMID: 11519487]

[312] Hemling N, Röyttä M, Rinne J, *et al.* Herpesviruses in brains in Alzheimers and Parkinsons diseases. Ann Neurol 2003; 54(2): 267-71. [http://dx.doi.org/10.1002/ana.10662] [PMID: 12891684]

[313] Beffert U, Bertrand P, Champagne D, Gauthier S, Poirier J. HSV-1 in brain and risk of Alzheimers disease. Lancet 1998; 351(9112): 1330-1. [http://dx.doi.org/10.1016/S0140-6736(05)79057-7] [PMID: 9643802]

[314] Pisa D, Alonso R, Juarranz A, Rábano A, Carrasco L. Direct visualization of fungal infection in brains from patients with Alzheimers disease. J Alzheimers Dis 2015; 43(2): 613-24. [PMID: 25125470]

[315] Alonso R, Pisa D, Rábano A, Carrasco L. Alzheimers disease and disseminated mycoses. Eur J Clin Microbiol Infect Dis 2014; 33(7): 1125-32. [http://dx.doi.org/10.1007/s10096-013-2045-z] [PMID: 24452965]

[316] Alonso R, Pisa D, Marina AI, Morato E, Rábano A, Carrasco L. Fungal infection in patients with Alzheimers disease. J Alzheimers Dis 2014; 41(1): 301-11.
[PMID: 24614898]

[317] Castellani RJ, Siedlak SL, Fortino AE, Perry G, Ghetti B, Smith MA. Chitin-like polysaccharides in Alzheimers disease brains. Curr Alzheimer Res 2005; 2(4): 419-23.
[http://dx.doi.org/10.2174/156720505774330555] [PMID: 16248847]

[318] Sotgiu S, Musumeci S, Marconi S, Gini B, Bonetti B. Different content of chitin-like polysaccharides in multiple sclerosis and Alzheimers disease brains. J Neuroimmunol 2008; 197(1): 70-3.
[http://dx.doi.org/10.1016/j.jneuroim.2008.03.021] [PMID: 18485490]

[319] Castellani RJ, Perry G, Smith MA. The role of novel chitin-like polysaccharides in Alzheimer disease. Neurotox Res 2007; 12(4): 269-74.
[http://dx.doi.org/10.1007/BF03033910] [PMID: 18201954]

[320] Choi J, Lee H-W, Suk K. Plasma level of chitinase 3-like 1 protein increases in patients with early Alzheimers disease. J Neurol 2011; 258(12): 2181-5.
[http://dx.doi.org/10.1007/s00415-011-6087-9] [PMID: 21562723]

[321] Rosén C, Andersson C-H, Andreasson U, *et al.* Increased Levels of Chitotriosidase and YKL-40 in Cerebrospinal Fluid from Patients with Alzheimer's Disease. Dement Geriatr Cogn Dis Extra 2014; 4: 297-304.

[322] Watabe-Rudolph M, Song Z, Lausser L, *et al.* Chitinase enzyme activity in CSF is a powerful biomarker of Alzheimer disease. Neurology 2012; 78(8): 569-77.
[http://dx.doi.org/10.1212/WNL.0b013e318247caa1] [PMID: 22323746]

[323] Wildsmith KR, Schauer SP, Smith AM, *et al.* Identification of longitudinally dynamic biomarkers in Alzheimers disease cerebrospinal fluid by targeted proteomics. Mol Neurodegener 2014; 9: 22.
[http://dx.doi.org/10.1186/1750-1326-9-22] [PMID: 24902845]

[324] Ala TA, Doss RC, Sullivan CJ. Reversible dementia: a case of cryptococcal meningitis masquerading as Alzheimers disease. J Alzheimers Dis 2004; 6(5): 503-8.
[PMID: 15505372]

[325] Hoffmann M, Muniz J, Carroll E, De Villasante J. Cryptococcal meningitis misdiagnosed as Alzheimers disease: complete neurological and cognitive recovery with treatment. J Alzheimers Dis 2009; 16(3): 517-20.
[PMID: 19276545]

[326] Espinosa V, Rivera A. Cytokines and the regulation of fungus-specific CD4 T cell differentiation. Cytokine 2012; 58(1): 100-6.
[http://dx.doi.org/10.1016/j.cyto.2011.11.005] [PMID: 22133343]

[327] Gozalbo D, Maneu V, Gil ML. Role of IFN-gamma in immune responses to Candida albicans infections. *Front. Biosci.* Landmark Ed 2014; 19: 1279-90.
[http://dx.doi.org/10.2741/4281]

[328] Romani L. Immunity to fungal infections. Nat Rev Immunol 2011; 11(4): 275-88.
[http://dx.doi.org/10.1038/nri2939] [PMID: 21394104]

[329] Kim KS. Microbial translocation of the blood-brain barrier. Int J Parasitol 2006; 36(5): 607-14.
[http://dx.doi.org/10.1016/j.ijpara.2006.01.013] [PMID: 16542662]

[330] Somer T, Finegold SM. Vasculitides associated with infections, immunization, and antimicrobial drugs. Clin Infect Dis 1995; 20(4): 1010-36.
[http://dx.doi.org/10.1093/clinids/20.4.1010] [PMID: 7795045]

[331] Younger DS. Vasculitis of the nervous system. Curr Opin Neurol 2004; 17(3): 317-36.
[http://dx.doi.org/10.1097/00019052-200406000-00014] [PMID: 15167068]

[332] Lionakis MS, Netea MG, Holland SM. Mendelian genetics of human susceptibility to fungal infection.

Cold Spring Harb Perspect Med 2014; 4(6): a019638-8.
[http://dx.doi.org/10.1101/cshperspect.a019638] [PMID: 24890837]

[333] Smeekens SP, van de Veerdonk FL, Kullberg BJ, Netea MG. Genetic susceptibility to Candida infections. EMBO Mol Med 2013; 5(6): 805-13.
[http://dx.doi.org/10.1002/emmm.201201678] [PMID: 23629947]

[334] Gronow S, Brade H. Lipopolysaccharide biosynthesis: which steps do bacteria need to survive? J Endotoxin Res 2001; 7(1): 3-23.
[PMID: 11521077]

[335] Kabanov DS, Prokhorenko IR. Structural analysis of lipopolysaccharides from Gram-negative bacteria. Biochemistry (Mosc) 2010; 75(4): 383-404.
[http://dx.doi.org/10.1134/S0006297910040012] [PMID: 20618127]

[336] Bartual SG, Otero JM, Garcia-Doval C, *et al.* Structure of the bacteriophage T4 long tail fiber receptor-binding tip. Proc Natl Acad Sci USA 2010; 107(47): 20287-92.
[http://dx.doi.org/10.1073/pnas.1011218107] [PMID: 21041684]

[337] Miyake K. Innate recognition of lipopolysaccharide by Toll-like receptor 4-MD-2. Trends Microbiol 2004; 12(4): 186-92.
[http://dx.doi.org/10.1016/j.tim.2004.02.009] [PMID: 15051069]

[338] Rietschel ET, Wollenweber HW, Zähringer U, Lüderitz O. Lipid A, the lipid component of bacterial lipopolysaccharides: relation of chemical structure to biological activity. Klin Wochenschr 1982; 60(14): 705-9.
[http://dx.doi.org/10.1007/BF01716559] [PMID: 6750222]

[339] Wiese A, Brandenburg K, Ulmer AJ, Seydel U, Müller-Loennies S. The dual role of lipopolysaccharide as effector and target molecule. Biol Chem 1999; 380(7-8): 767-84.
[http://dx.doi.org/10.1515/BC.1999.097] [PMID: 10494826]

[340] Molinaro A, Holst O, Di Lorenzo F, *et al.* Chemistry of lipid A: at the heart of innate immunity. Chemistry 2015; 21(2): 500-19.
[http://dx.doi.org/10.1002/chem.201403923] [PMID: 25353096]

[341] Alexander C, Rietschel ET. Bacterial lipopolysaccharides and innate immunity. J Endotoxin Res 2001; 7(3): 167-202.
[PMID: 11581570]

[342] Kitchens RL, Wang P, Munford RS. Bacterial lipopolysaccharide can enter monocytes *via* two CD14-dependent pathways. J Immunol 1998; 161(10): 5534-45.
[PMID: 9820530]

[343] Van Amersfoort ES, Van Berkel TJ, Kuiper J. Receptors, mediators, and mechanisms involved in bacterial sepsis and septic shock. Clin Microbiol Rev 2003; 16(3): 379-414.
[http://dx.doi.org/10.1128/CMR.16.3.379-414.2003] [PMID: 12857774]

[344] Crosby HA, Bion JF, Penn CW, Elliott TS. Antibiotic-induced release of endotoxin from bacteria *in vitro*. J Med Microbiol 1994; 40(1): 23-30.
[http://dx.doi.org/10.1099/00222615-40-1-23] [PMID: 8289210]

[345] Bucklin SE, Fujihara Y, Leeson MC, Morrison DC. Differential antibiotic-induced release of endotoxin from gram-negative bacteria. Eur J Clin Microbiol Infect Dis 1994; 13 (Suppl. 1): S43-51.
[http://dx.doi.org/10.1007/BF02390684] [PMID: 7821304]

[346] Holzheimer RG. The significance of endotoxin release in experimental and clinical sepsis in surgical patientsevidence for antibiotic-induced endotoxin release? Infection 1998; 26(2): 77-84.
[http://dx.doi.org/10.1007/BF02767765] [PMID: 9561376]

[347] Lu Y-C, Yeh W-C, Ohashi PS. LPS/TLR4 signal transduction pathway. Cytokine 2008; 42(2): 145-51.
[http://dx.doi.org/10.1016/j.cyto.2008.01.006] [PMID: 18304834]

[348] Zughaier SM, Zimmer SM, Datta A, Carlson RW, Stephens DS. Differential induction of the toll-like receptor 4-MyD88-dependent and -independent signaling pathways by endotoxins. Infect Immun 2005; 73(5): 2940-50.
[http://dx.doi.org/10.1128/IAI.73.5.2940-2950.2005] [PMID: 15845500]

[349] Raetz CR, Whitfield C. Lipopolysaccharide endotoxins. Annu Rev Biochem 2002; 71: 635-700.
[http://dx.doi.org/10.1146/annurev.biochem.71.110601.135414] [PMID: 12045108]

[350] Poltorak A, He X, Smirnova I, *et al.* Defective LPS signaling in C3H/HeJ and C57BL/10ScCr mice: mutations in Tlr4 gene. Science 1998; 282(5396): 2085-8.
[http://dx.doi.org/10.1126/science.282.5396.2085] [PMID: 9851930]

[351] Tobias PS, Soldau K, Gegner JA, Mintz D, Ulevitch RJ. Lipopolysaccharide binding protein-mediated complexation of lipopolysaccharide with soluble CD14. J Biol Chem 1995; 270(18): 10482-8.
[http://dx.doi.org/10.1074/jbc.270.18.10482] [PMID: 7537731]

[352] Kitchens RL, Thompson PA, Viriyakosol S, O'Keefe GE, Munford RS. Plasma CD14 decreases monocyte responses to LPS by transferring cell-bound LPS to plasma lipoproteins. J Clin Invest 2001; 108(3): 485-93.
[http://dx.doi.org/10.1172/JCI200113139] [PMID: 11489942]

[353] Nagai Y, Akashi S, Nagafuku M, *et al.* Essential role of MD-2 in LPS responsiveness and TLR4 distribution. Nat Immunol 2002; 3(7): 667-72.
[PMID: 12055629]

[354] Park BS, Song DH, Kim HM, Choi B-S, Lee H, Lee J-O. The structural basis of lipopolysaccharide recognition by the TLR4-MD-2 complex. Nature 2009; 458(7242): 1191-5.
[http://dx.doi.org/10.1038/nature07830] [PMID: 19252480]

[355] Nijland R, Hofland T, van Strijp JA. Recognition of LPS by TLR4: potential for anti-inflammatory therapies. Mar Drugs 2014; 12(7): 4260-73.
[http://dx.doi.org/10.3390/md12074260] [PMID: 25056632]

[356] Kagan JC, Medzhitov R. Phosphoinositide-mediated adaptor recruitment controls Toll-like receptor signaling. Cell 2006; 125(5): 943-55.
[http://dx.doi.org/10.1016/j.cell.2006.03.047] [PMID: 16751103]

[357] Rowe DC, McGettrick AF, Latz E, *et al.* The myristoylation of TRIF-related adaptor molecule is essential for Toll-like receptor 4 signal transduction. Proc Natl Acad Sci USA 2006; 103(16): 6299-304.
[http://dx.doi.org/10.1073/pnas.0510041103] [PMID: 16603631]

[358] Kawai T, Adachi O, Ogawa T, Takeda K, Akira S. Unresponsiveness of MyD88-deficient mice to endotoxin. Immunity 1999; 11(1): 115-22.
[http://dx.doi.org/10.1016/S1074-7613(00)80086-2] [PMID: 10435584]

[359] Yao X, Li G, Bai Q, Xu H, Lü C. Taraxerol inhibits LPS-induced inflammatory responses through suppression of TAK1 and Akt activation. Int Immunopharmacol 2013; 15(2): 316-24.
[http://dx.doi.org/10.1016/j.intimp.2012.12.032] [PMID: 23333629]

[360] Honda K, Taniguchi T. IRFs: master regulators of signalling by Toll-like receptors and cytosolic pattern-recognition receptors. Nat Rev Immunol 2006; 6(9): 644-58.
[http://dx.doi.org/10.1038/nri1900] [PMID: 16932750]

[361] Banks WA, Gray AM, Erickson MA, *et al.* Lipopolysaccharide-induced blood-brain barrier disruption: roles of cyclooxygenase, oxidative stress, neuroinflammation, and elements of the neurovascular unit. J Neuroinflammation 2015; 12: 223.
[http://dx.doi.org/10.1186/s12974-015-0434-1] [PMID: 26608623]

[362] Streck EL, Comim CM, Barichello T, Quevedo J. The septic brain. Neurochem Res 2008; 33(11): 2171-7.
[http://dx.doi.org/10.1007/s11064-008-9671-3] [PMID: 18461451]

[363] Toborek M, Lee YW, Flora G, *et al.* Mechanisms of the blood-brain barrier disruption in HIV-1 infection. Cell Mol Neurobiol 2005; 25(1): 181-99. [http://dx.doi.org/10.1007/s10571-004-1383-x] [PMID: 15962513]

[364] Kong WX, Chen SW, Li YL, *et al.* Effects of taurine on rat behaviors in three anxiety models. Pharmacol Biochem Behav 2006; 83(2): 271-6. [http://dx.doi.org/10.1016/j.pbb.2006.02.007] [PMID: 16540157]

[365] Kuang Y, Lackay SN, Zhao L, Fu ZF. Role of chemokines in the enhancement of BBB permeability and inflammatory infiltration after rabies virus infection. Virus Res 2009; 144(1-2): 18-26. [http://dx.doi.org/10.1016/j.virusres.2009.03.014] [PMID: 19720239]

[366] Roy A, Phares TW, Koprowski H, Hooper DC. Failure to open the blood-brain barrier and deliver immune effectors to central nervous system tissues leads to the lethal outcome of silver-haired bat rabies virus infection. J Virol 2007; 81(3): 1110-8. [http://dx.doi.org/10.1128/JVI.01964-06] [PMID: 17108029]

[367] Wang T, Town T, Alexopoulou L, Anderson JF, Fikrig E, Flavell RA. Toll-like receptor 3 mediates West Nile virus entry into the brain causing lethal encephalitis. Nat Med 2004; 10(12): 1366-73. [http://dx.doi.org/10.1038/nm1140] [PMID: 15558055]

[368] Xaio H, Banks WA, Niehoff ML, Morley JE. Effect of LPS on the permeability of the blood-brain barrier to insulin. Brain Res 2001; 896(1-2): 36-42. [http://dx.doi.org/10.1016/S0006-8993(00)03247-9] [PMID: 11277970]

[369] Singh AK, Jiang Y, Gupta S. Effects of bacterial toxins on endothelial tight junction *in vitro*: a mechanism-based investigation. Toxicol Mech Methods 2007; 17(6): 331-47. [http://dx.doi.org/10.1080/15376510601077029] [PMID: 20020957]

[370] Mayhan WG, Heistad DD. Permeability of blood-brain barrier to various sized molecules. Am J Physiol 1985; 248(5 Pt 2): H712-8. [PMID: 2581459]

[371] Tsao N, Hsu HP, Wu CM, Liu CC, Lei HY. Tumour necrosis factor-alpha causes an increase in blood-brain barrier permeability during sepsis. J Med Microbiol 2001; 50(9): 812-21. [http://dx.doi.org/10.1099/0022-1317-50-9-812] [PMID: 11549183]

[372] Hartz AM, Bauer B, Fricker G, Miller DS. Rapid modulation of P-glycoprotein-mediated transport at the blood-brain barrier by tumor necrosis factor-alpha and lipopolysaccharide. Mol Pharmacol 2006; 69(2): 462-70. [http://dx.doi.org/10.1124/mol.105.017954] [PMID: 16278373]

[373] Yamauchi A, Dohgu S, Nishioku T, *et al.* An inhibitory role of nitric oxide in the dynamic regulation of the blood-brain barrier function. Cell Mol Neurobiol 2007; 27(3): 263-70. [http://dx.doi.org/10.1007/s10571-007-9139-z] [PMID: 17318383]

[374] Sumi N, Nishioku T, Takata F, *et al.* Lipopolysaccharide-activated microglia induce dysfunction of the blood-brain barrier in rat microvascular endothelial cells co-cultured with microglia. Cell Mol Neurobiol 2010; 30(2): 247-53. [http://dx.doi.org/10.1007/s10571-009-9446-7] [PMID: 19728078]

[375] Matsumoto J, Dohgu S, Takata F, *et al.* Lipopolysaccharide-activated microglia lower P-glycoprotein function in brain microvascular endothelial cells. Neurosci Lett 2012; 524(1): 45-8. [http://dx.doi.org/10.1016/j.neulet.2012.07.004] [PMID: 22801252]

[376] Kacimi R, Giffard RG, Yenari MA. Endotoxin-activated microglia injure brain derived endothelial cells *via* NF-κB, JAK-STAT and JNK stress kinase pathways. J Inflamm (Lond) 2011; 8: 7. [http://dx.doi.org/10.1186/1476-9255-8-7] [PMID: 21385378]

[377] Noh H, Jeon J, Seo H. Systemic injection of LPS induces region-specific neuroinflammation and mitochondrial dysfunction in normal mouse brain. Neurochem Int 2014; 69: 35-40. [http://dx.doi.org/10.1016/j.neuint.2014.02.008] [PMID: 24607701]

[378] Olson JK, Miller SD. Microglia initiate central nervous system innate and adaptive immune responses through multiple TLRs. J Immunol 2004; 173(6): 3916-24. [http://dx.doi.org/10.4049/jimmunol.173.6.3916] [PMID: 15356140]

[379] Tarassishin L, Suh H-S, Lee SC. LPS and IL-1 differentially activate mouse and human astrocytes: role of CD14. Glia 2014; 62(6): 999-1013. [http://dx.doi.org/10.1002/glia.22657] [PMID: 24659539]

[380] Guijarro-Muñoz I, Compte M, Álvarez-Cienfuegos A, Álvarez-Vallina L, Sanz L. Lipopolysaccharide activates Toll-like receptor 4 (TLR4)-mediated NF-κB signaling pathway and proinflammatory response in human pericytes. J Biol Chem 2014; 289(4): 2457-68. [http://dx.doi.org/10.1074/jbc.M113.521161] [PMID: 24307174]

[381] Jansson D, Rustenhoven J, Feng S, *et al.* A role for human brain pericytes in neuroinflammation. J Neuroinflammation 2014; 11: 104. [http://dx.doi.org/10.1186/1742-2094-11-104] [PMID: 24920309]

[382] Singh AK, Jiang Y. How does peripheral lipopolysaccharide induce gene expression in the brain of rats? Toxicology 2004; 201(1-3): 197-207. [http://dx.doi.org/10.1016/j.tox.2004.04.015] [PMID: 15297033]

[383] Skelly DT, Hennessy E, Dansereau M-A, Cunningham C. A systematic analysis of the peripheral and CNS effects of systemic LPS, IL-1β, [corrected] TNF-α and IL-6 challenges in C57BL/6 mice. PLoS One 2013; 8(7): e69123. [http://dx.doi.org/10.1371/journal.pone.0069123] [PMID: 23840908]

[384] Chen G, McCuskey RS, Reichlin S. Blood interleukin-6 and tumor necrosis factor-α elevation after intracerebroventricular injection of Escherichia coli endotoxin in the rat is determined by two opposing factors: peripheral induction by LPS transferred from brain to blood and inhibition of peripheral response by a brain-mediated mechanism. Neuroimmunomodulation 2000; 8(2): 59-69. [http://dx.doi.org/10.1159/000026454] [PMID: 10965230]

[385] Czapski GA, Gajkowska B, Strosznajder JB. Systemic administration of lipopolysaccharide induces molecular and morphological alterations in the hippocampus. Brain Res 2010; 1356: 85-94. [http://dx.doi.org/10.1016/j.brainres.2010.07.096] [PMID: 20696148]

[386] Moss DW, Bates TE. Activation of murine microglial cell lines by lipopolysaccharide and interferon-gamma causes NO-mediated decreases in mitochondrial and cellular function. Eur J Neurosci 2001; 13(3): 529-38. [http://dx.doi.org/10.1046/j.1460-9568.2001.01418.x] [PMID: 11168560]

[387] Xie Z, Smith CJ, Van Eldik LJ. Activated glia induce neuron death *via* MAP kinase signaling pathways involving JNK and p38. Glia 2004; 45(2): 170-9. [http://dx.doi.org/10.1002/glia.10314] [PMID: 14730710]

[388] Xie Z, Wei M, Morgan TE, *et al.* Peroxynitrite mediates neurotoxicity of amyloid beta-peptide142- and lipopolysaccharide-activated microglia. J Neurosci 2002; 22(9): 3484-92. [PMID: 11978825]

[389] Arimoto T, Bing G. Up-regulation of inducible nitric oxide synthase in the substantia nigra by lipopolysaccharide causes microglial activation and neurodegeneration. Neurobiol Dis 2003; 12(1): 35-45. [http://dx.doi.org/10.1016/S0969-9961(02)00017-7] [PMID: 12609487]

[390] Finkel E. The mitochondrion: is it central to apoptosis? Science 2001; 292(5517): 624-6. [http://dx.doi.org/10.1126/science.292.5517.624] [PMID: 11330312]

[391] Su B, Ceponis PJ, Lebel S, Huynh H, Sherman PM. Helicobacter pylori activates Toll-like receptor 4 expression in gastrointestinal epithelial cells. Infect Immun 2003; 71(6): 3496-502. [http://dx.doi.org/10.1128/IAI.71.6.3496-3502.2003] [PMID: 12761134]

[392] Yokota S, Ohnishi T, Muroi M, Tanamoto K, Fujii N, Amano K. Highly-purified Helicobacter pylori

LPS preparations induce weak inflammatory reactions and utilize Toll-like receptor 2 complex but not Toll-like receptor 4 complex. FEMS Immunol Med Microbiol 2007; 51(1): 140-8. [http://dx.doi.org/10.1111/j.1574-695X.2007.00288.x] [PMID: 17645528]

[393] Smith MF Jr, Mitchell A, Li G, *et al.* Toll-like receptor (TLR) 2 and TLR5, but not TLR4, are required for Helicobacter pylori-induced NF-kappa B activation and chemokine expression by epithelial cells. J Biol Chem 2003; 278(35): 32552-60. [http://dx.doi.org/10.1074/jbc.M305536200] [PMID: 12807870]

[394] Jiang Z-L, Cui Y-Q, Gao R, *et al.* Study of TNF-α, IL-1β and LPS levels in the gingival crevicular fluid of a rat model of diabetes mellitus and periodontitis. Dis Markers 2013; 34(5): 295-304. [http://dx.doi.org/10.1155/2013/156798] [PMID: 23478270]

[395] Shaddox LM, Wiedey J, Calderon NL, *et al.* Local inflammatory markers and systemic endotoxin in aggressive periodontitis. J Dent Res 2011; 90(9): 1140-4. [http://dx.doi.org/10.1177/0022034511413928] [PMID: 21730256]

[396] Guo Y, Zhou G, He C, Yang W, He Z, Liu Z. Serum Levels of Lipopolysaccharide and 1,3-β-D-Glucan Refer to the Severity in Patients with Crohns Disease. Mediators Inflamm 2015; 2015: 843089. [http://dx.doi.org/10.1155/2015/843089] [PMID: 26106258]

[397] Kamer AR, Dasanayake AP, Craig RG, Glodzik-Sobanska L, Bry M, de Leon MJ. Alzheimers disease and peripheral infections: the possible contribution from periodontal infections, model and hypothesis. J Alzheimers Dis 2008; 13(4): 437-49. [PMID: 18487851]

[398] Abbayya K, Puthanakar NY, Naduwinmani S, Chidambar YS. Association between Periodontitis and Alzheimers Disease. N Am J Med Sci 2015; 7(6): 241-6. [http://dx.doi.org/10.4103/1947-2714.159325] [PMID: 26199919]

[399] Sparks Stein P, Steffen MJ, Smith C, *et al.* Serum antibodies to periodontal pathogens are a risk factor for Alzheimers disease. Alzheimers Dement 2012; 8(3): 196-203. [http://dx.doi.org/10.1016/j.jalz.2011.04.006] [PMID: 22546352]

[400] Noble JM, Scarmeas N, Celenti RS, *et al.* Serum IgG antibody levels to periodontal microbiota are associated with incident Alzheimer disease. PLoS One 2014; 9(12): e114959. [http://dx.doi.org/10.1371/journal.pone.0114959] [PMID: 25522313]

[401] Roubaud-Baudron C, Krolak-Salmon P, Quadrio I, Mégraud F, Salles N. Impact of chronic Helicobacter pylori infection on Alzheimers disease: preliminary results. Neurobiol Aging 2012; 33(5): 1009.e11-. [http://dx.doi.org/10.1016/j.neurobiolaging.2011.10.021] [PMID: 22133280]

[402] Beydoun MA, Beydoun HA, Shroff MR, Kitner-Triolo MH, Zonderman AB. Helicobacter pylori seropositivity and cognitive performance among US adults: evidence from a large national survey. Psychosom Med 2013; 75(5): 486-96. [http://dx.doi.org/10.1097/PSY.0b013e31829108c3] [PMID: 23697465]

[403] Zhang R, Miller RG, Gascon R, *et al.* Circulating endotoxin and systemic immune activation in sporadic amyotrophic lateral sclerosis (sALS). J Neuroimmunol 2009; 206(1-2): 121-4. [http://dx.doi.org/10.1016/j.jneuroim.2008.09.017] [PMID: 19013651]

[404] Liu Y, Walter S, Stagi M, *et al.* LPS receptor (CD14): a receptor for phagocytosis of Alzheimers amyloid peptide. Brain 2005; 128(Pt 8): 1778-89. [http://dx.doi.org/10.1093/brain/awh531] [PMID: 15857927]

[405] Kitazawa M, Oddo S, Yamasaki TR, Green KN, LaFerla FM. Lipopolysaccharide-induced inflammation exacerbates tau pathology by a cyclin-dependent kinase 5-mediated pathway in a transgenic model of Alzheimers disease. J Neurosci 2005; 25(39): 8843-53. [http://dx.doi.org/10.1523/JNEUROSCI.2868-05.2005] [PMID: 16192374]

[406] DiCarlo G, Wilcock D, Henderson D, Gordon M, Morgan D. Intrahippocampal LPS injections reduce Abeta load in APP+PS1 transgenic mice. Neurobiol Aging 2001; 22(6): 1007-12. [http://dx.doi.org/10.1016/S0197-4580(01)00292-5] [PMID: 11755009]

[407] Erickson MA, Hartvigson PE, Morofuji Y, Owen JB, Butterfield DA, Banks WA. Lipopolysaccharide impairs amyloid β efflux from brain: altered vascular sequestration, cerebrospinal fluid reabsorption, peripheral clearance and transporter function at the blood-brain barrier. J Neuroinflammation 2012; 9: 150. [http://dx.doi.org/10.1186/1742-2094-9-150] [PMID: 22747709]

[408] Jaeger LB, Dohgu S, Sultana R, *et al.* Lipopolysaccharide alters the blood-brain barrier transport of amyloid beta protein: a mechanism for inflammation in the progression of Alzheimers disease. Brain Behav Immun 2009; 23(4): 507-17. [http://dx.doi.org/10.1016/j.bbi.2009.01.017] [PMID: 19486646]

[409] Lee DC, Rizer J, Selenica M-L, *et al.* LPS- induced inflammation exacerbates phospho-tau pathology in rTg4510 mice. J Neuroinflammation 2010; 7: 56. [http://dx.doi.org/10.1186/1742-2094-7-56] [PMID: 20846376]

[410] Gibson GR, Roberfroid MB. Dietary modulation of the human colonic microbiota: introducing the concept of prebiotics. J Nutr 1995; 125(6): 1401-12. [PMID: 7782892]

[411] Reid G, Sanders ME, Gaskins HR, *et al.* New scientific paradigms for probiotics and prebiotics. J Clin Gastroenterol 2003; 37(2): 105-18. [http://dx.doi.org/10.1097/00004836-200308000-00004] [PMID: 12869879]

[412] Gibson GR, Probert HM, Loo JV, Rastall RA, Roberfroid MB. Dietary modulation of the human colonic microbiota: updating the concept of prebiotics. Nutr Res Rev 2004; 17(2): 259-75. [http://dx.doi.org/10.1079/NRR200479] [PMID: 19079930]

[413] Roberfroid M. Prebiotics: the concept revisited. J Nutr 2007; 137(3) (Suppl. 2): 830S-7S. [PMID: 17311983]

[414] Pineiro M, Asp N-G, Reid G, *et al.* FAO Technical meeting on prebiotics. J Clin Gastroenterol 2008; 42 (Suppl. 3 Pt 2): S156-9. [http://dx.doi.org/10.1097/MCG.0b013e31817f184e] [PMID: 18685504]

[415] Gibson GR, Scott KP, Rastall RA, *et al.* Dietary prebiotics: current status and new definition. Food Sci Technol Bull Funct Foods 2010; 7: 1-19. [http://dx.doi.org/10.1616/1476-2137.15880]

[416] Bindels LB, Delzenne NM, Cani PD, Walter J. Towards a more comprehensive concept for prebiotics. Nat Rev Gastroenterol Hepatol 2015; 12(5): 303-10. [http://dx.doi.org/10.1038/nrgastro.2015.47] [PMID: 25824997]

[417] Olle B. Medicines from microbiota. Nat Biotechnol 2013; 31(4): 309-15. [http://dx.doi.org/10.1038/nbt.2548] [PMID: 23563425]

[418] Roberfroid M, Gibson GR, Hoyles L, *et al.* Prebiotic effects: metabolic and health benefits. Br J Nutr 2010; 104 (Suppl. 2): S1-S63. [http://dx.doi.org/10.1017/S0007114510003363] [PMID: 20920376]

[419] Bindels LB, Dewulf EM, Delzenne NM. GPR43/FFA2: physiopathological relevance and therapeutic prospects. Trends Pharmacol Sci 2013; 34(4): 226-32. [http://dx.doi.org/10.1016/j.tips.2013.02.002] [PMID: 23489932]

[420] Fukuda S, Toh H, Hase K, *et al.* *Bifidobacteria* can protect from enteropathogenic infection through production of acetate. Nature 2011; 469(7331): 543-7. [http://dx.doi.org/10.1038/nature09646] [PMID: 21270894]

[421] Seifert S, Watzl B. Inulin and oligofructose: review of experimental data on immune modulation. J

Nutr 2007; 137(11) (Suppl.): 2563S-7S.
[PMID: 17951503]

[422] Blaut M. Relationship of prebiotics and food to intestinal microflora. Eur J Nutr 2002; 41 (Suppl. 1): I11-6.
[http://dx.doi.org/10.1007/s00394-002-1102-7] [PMID: 12420111]

[423] Smith EA, Macfarlane GT. Enumeration of human colonic bacteria producing phenolic and indolic compounds: effects of pH, carbohydrate availability and retention time on dissimilatory aromatic amino acid metabolism. J Appl Bacteriol 1996; 81(3): 288-302.
[http://dx.doi.org/10.1111/j.1365-2672.1996.tb04331.x] [PMID: 8810056]

[424] Mykkänen H, Laiho K, Salminen S. Variations in faecal bacterial enzyme activities and associations with bowel function and diet in elderly subjects. J Appl Microbiol 1998; 85(1): 37-41.
[http://dx.doi.org/10.1046/j.1365-2672.1998.00454.x] [PMID: 9721654]

[425] Nyangale EP, Mottram DS, Gibson GR. Gut microbial activity, implications for health and disease: the potential role of metabolite analysis. J Proteome Res 2012; 11(12): 5573-85.
[http://dx.doi.org/10.1021/pr300637d] [PMID: 23116228]

[426] Macfarlane S, Macfarlane GT, Cummings JH. Review article: prebiotics in the gastrointestinal tract. Aliment Pharmacol Ther 2006; 24(5): 701-14.
[http://dx.doi.org/10.1111/j.1365-2036.2006.03042.x] [PMID: 16918875]

[427] Tuohy KM, Ziemer CJ, Klinder A, Knöbel Y, Pool-Zobel BL, Gibson GR. A Human Volunteer Study to Determine the Prebiotic Effects of Lactulose Powder on Human Colonic Microbiota. Microb Ecol Health Dis 2002; 14: 165-73.
[http://dx.doi.org/10.1080/089106002320644357]

[428] Zentek J, Marquart B, Pietrzak T. Intestinal effects of mannanoligosaccharides, transgalactooligosaccharides, lactose and lactulose in dogs. J Nutr 2002; 132(6) (Suppl. 2): 1682S-4S.
[PMID: 12042492]

[429] Olano-Martin E, Williams MR, Gibson GR, Rastall RA. Pectins and pectic-oligosaccharides inhibit Escherichia coli O157:H7 Shiga toxin as directed towards the human colonic cell line HT29. FEMS Microbiol Lett 2003; 218(1): 101-5.
[http://dx.doi.org/10.1111/j.1574-6968.2003.tb11504.x] [PMID: 12583904]

[430] Saito Y, Takano T, Rowland I. Effects of soybean oligosaccharides on the human gut microflora in *in vitro* culture. Microb Ecol Health Dis 1992; 5: 105-10.
[http://dx.doi.org/10.3109/08910609209141296]

[431] Morgan A, Mul A, Beldman G, Voragen AG. Dietary oligosaccharides - New insights. Agro Food Ind Hi-Tech 1992.

[432] Campbell JM, Fahey GC Jr, Wolf BW. Selected indigestible oligosaccharides affect large bowel mass, cecal and fecal short-chain fatty acids, pH and microflora in rats. J Nutr 1997; 127(1): 130-6.
[PMID: 9040556]

[433] Roberfroid MB. Introducing inulin-type fructans. Br J Nutr 2005; 93 (Suppl. 1): S13-25.
[http://dx.doi.org/10.1079/BJN20041350] [PMID: 15877886]

[434] Gibson GR, Beatty ER, Wang X, Cummings JH. Selective stimulation of *Bifidobacteria* in the human colon by oligofructose and inulin. Gastroenterology 1995; 108(4): 975-82.
[http://dx.doi.org/10.1016/0016-5085(95)90192-2] [PMID: 7698613]

[435] Tako E, Glahn RP, Welch RM, Lei X, Yasuda K, Miller DD. Dietary inulin affects the expression of intestinal enterocyte iron transporters, receptors and storage protein and alters the microbiota in the pig intestine. Br J Nutr 2008; 99(3): 472-80.
[http://dx.doi.org/10.1017/S0007114507825128] [PMID: 17868492]

[436] Lorenzoni AS, Aydos LF, Klein MP, Rodrigues RC, Hertz PF. Fructooligosaccharides synthesis by highly stable immobilized β-fructofuranosidase from Aspergillus aculeatus. Carbohydr Polym 2014;

103: 193-7.
[http://dx.doi.org/10.1016/j.carbpol.2013.12.038] [PMID: 24528719]

[437] Dumitriu S. Polysaccharides: Structural Diversity and Functional Versatility 2004. [http://dx.doi.org/10.1201/9781420030822]

[438] Messaoudi M, Rozan P, Nejdi A, Hidalgo S, Desor D. Behavioural and cognitive effects of oligofructose-enriched inulin in rats. Br J Nutr 2005; 93 (Suppl. 1): S27-30. [http://dx.doi.org/10.1079/BJN20041348] [PMID: 15877891]

[439] Rozan P, Nejdi A, Hidalgo S, *et al.* An oligofructose-enriched inulin diet: cognitive and physical performances in rats. Curr Top Nutraceutical Res 2009; 7: 81-7.

[440] Smith AP. The concept of well-being: relevance to nutrition research. Br J Nutr 2005; 93 (Suppl. 1): S1-5.
[http://dx.doi.org/10.1079/BJN20041351] [PMID: 15877882]

[441] Smith AP, Sutherland D, Hewlett P. An Investigation of the Acute Effects of Oligofructose-Enriched Inulin on Subjective Wellbeing, Mood and Cognitive Performance. Nutrients 2015; 7(11): 8887-96. [http://dx.doi.org/10.3390/nu7115441] [PMID: 26516908]

[442] Hsia C-H, Wang C-H, Kuo Y-W, Ho Y-J, Chen H-L. Fructo-oligosaccharide systemically diminished D-galactose-induced oxidative molecule damages in BALB/cJ mice. Br J Nutr 2012; 107(12): 1787-92.
[http://dx.doi.org/10.1017/S0007114511005150] [PMID: 21929837]

[443] Hsieh H-M, Wu W-M, Hu M-L. Soy isoflavones attenuate oxidative stress and improve parameters related to aging and Alzheimers disease in C57BL/6J mice treated with D-galactose. Food Chem Toxicol 2009; 47(3): 625-32.
[http://dx.doi.org/10.1016/j.fct.2008.12.026] [PMID: 19146912]

[444] Cui X, Zuo P, Zhang Q, *et al.* Chronic systemic D-galactose exposure induces memory loss, neurodegeneration, and oxidative damage in mice: protective effects of R-alpha-lipoic acid. J Neurosci Res 2006; 83(8): 1584-90.
[http://dx.doi.org/10.1002/jnr.20845] [PMID: 16555301]

[445] Zhang Q, Li X, Cui X, Zuo P. D-galactose injured neurogenesis in the hippocampus of adult mice. Neurol Res 2005; 27(5): 552-6.
[http://dx.doi.org/10.1179/016164105X25126] [PMID: 15978184]

[446] Sayre LM, Perry G, Smith MA. Oxidative stress and neurotoxicity. Chem Res Toxicol 2008; 21(1): 172-88.
[http://dx.doi.org/10.1021/tx700210j] [PMID: 18052107]

[447] Hagl S, Berressem D, Grewal R, Sus N, Frank J, Eckert GP. Rice bran extract improves mitochondrial dysfunction in brains of aged NMRI mice. Nutr Neurosci 2016; 19(1): 1-10.
[http://dx.doi.org/10.1179/1476830515Y.0000000040] [PMID: 26241203]

[448] Angus F, Smart C, Shortt S. Prebiotic ingredients with emphasis on galacto-oligosaccharides and fructo-oligosaccharides. In: Tamine A, Ed. Probiotic Dairy Product. Oxford: Blackwell Publishing 2005; pp. 120-37.

[449] Yanahira S, Kobayashi T, Suguri T, *et al.* Formation of oligosaccharides from lactose by Bacillus circulans beta-galactosidase. Biosci Biotechnol Biochem 1995; 59(6): 1021-6.
[http://dx.doi.org/10.1271/bbb.59.1021] [PMID: 7612988]

[450] Yang ST, Silva EM. Novel products and new technologies for use of a familiar carbohydrate, milk lactose. J Dairy Sci 1995; 78(11): 2541-62.
[http://dx.doi.org/10.3168/jds.S0022-0302(95)76884-9] [PMID: 8747342]

[451] Waworuntu R, Hain H, Chang Q, Thiede L, Hanania T, Berg B. Dietary prebiotics improve memory and social interactions while reducing anxiety when provided early in life to normally developing rodents. FASEB J 2014; 28: 637-5.

[452] Waworuntu R, Chichlowski M, Cox S, Berg B. Dietary prebiotics modulate fecal microbiota and impact cognitive functions in developing rodents. FASEB J 2014; 28: LB376.

[453] McEvoy G. AHFS Drug Information. 2003. American Society of Health-System Pharmacists, Bethesda, MD.

[454] Panesar PS, Kumari S. Lactulose: production, purification and potential applications. Biotechnol Adv 2011; 29(6): 940-8.
[http://dx.doi.org/10.1016/j.biotechadv.2011.08.008] [PMID: 21856402]

[455] Lee G-C, Lin C-H, Tao Y-C, *et al.* The potential of lactulose and melibiose, two novel trehalase-indigestible and autophagy-inducing disaccharides, for polyQ-mediated neurodegenerative disease treatment. Neurotoxicology 2015; 48: 120-30.
[http://dx.doi.org/10.1016/j.neuro.2015.03.009] [PMID: 25800379]

[456] Mateos-Aparicio I, Redondo Cuenca A, Villanueva-Suárez MJ, Zapata-Revilla MA. Soybean, a promising health source. Nutr Hosp 2008; 23(4): 305-12.
[PMID: 18604315]

[457] Omoni AO, Aluko RE. Soybean foods and their benefits: potential mechanisms of action. Nutr Rev 2005; 63(8): 272-83.
[http://dx.doi.org/10.1111/j.1753-4887.2005.tb00141.x] [PMID: 16190314]

[458] Oku T. Special physiological functions of newly developed mono- and oligosaccharides. In: Goldberg I, Ed. Functional foods: designer foods, pharma foods, nutraceuticals. London, UK: Chapman and Hall 1994; pp. 202-17.
[http://dx.doi.org/10.1007/978-1-4615-2073-3_10]

[459] Hayakawa K, Mizutani J, Wada K, Masai T, Yoshihara I, Mitsuoka T. Effects of Soybean Oligosaccharides on Human Faecal Flora. Microb Ecol Health Dis 2009; 3(6): 293-303.
[http://dx.doi.org/10.3109/08910609009140252]

[460] Wada K, Watabe J, Mizutani J, Tomoda M, Suzuki H, Saitoh Y. Effects of soybean oligosaccharides in a beverage on human fecal flora and metabolites. Nippon Nogeikagaku Kaishi 1992; 66(6): 127-35.

[461] Ahmad A, Ramasamy K, Jaafar SM, Majeed AB, Mani V. Total isoflavones from soybean and tempeh reversed scopolamine-induced amnesia, improved cholinergic activities and reduced neuroinflammation in brain. Food Chem Toxicol 2014; 65: 120-8.
[http://dx.doi.org/10.1016/j.fct.2013.12.025] [PMID: 24373829]

[462] Feng J-F, He L-L, Li D, *et al.* Antagonizing effects of soybean isoflavones on β-amyloid peptide-induced oxidative damage in neuron mitochondria of rats. Basic Clin Pharmacol Toxicol 2012; 111(4): 248-53.
[PMID: 22551092]

[463] Neese SL, Bandara SB, Doerge DR, Helferich WG, Korol DL, Schantz SL. Effects of multiple daily genistein treatments on delayed alternation and a differential reinforcement of low rates of responding task in middle-aged rats. Neurotoxicol Teratol 2012; 34(1): 187-95.
[http://dx.doi.org/10.1016/j.ntt.2011.09.002] [PMID: 21945133]

[464] Neese SL, Pisani SL, Doerge DR, *et al.* The effects of dietary treatment with S-equol on learning and memory processes in middle-aged ovariectomized rats. Neurotoxicol Teratol 2014; 41: 80-8.
[http://dx.doi.org/10.1016/j.ntt.2013.12.004] [PMID: 24368316]

[465] Qian Y, Guan T, Huang M, *et al.* Neuroprotection by the soy isoflavone, genistein, *via* inhibition of mitochondria-dependent apoptosis pathways and reactive oxygen induced-NF-κB activation in a cerebral ischemia mouse model. Neurochem Int 2012; 60(8): 759-67.
[http://dx.doi.org/10.1016/j.neuint.2012.03.011] [PMID: 22490611]

[466] Rettberg JR, Hamilton RT, Mao Z, *et al.* The effect of dietary soy isoflavones before and after ovariectomy on hippocampal protein markers of mitochondrial bioenergetics and antioxidant activity in female monkeys. Brain Res 2011; 1379: 23-33.

[http://dx.doi.org/10.1016/j.brainres.2011.01.012] [PMID: 21238431]

[467] Bansal N, Parle M. Effect of soybean supplementation on the memory of alprazolam-induced amnesic mice. J Pharm Bioallied Sci 2010; 2(2): 144-7. [http://dx.doi.org/10.4103/0975-7406.67001] [PMID: 21814450]

[468] Bansal N, Parle M. Soybean supplementation helps reverse age- and scopolamine-induced memory deficits in mice. J Med Food 2010; 13(6): 1293-300. [http://dx.doi.org/10.1089/jmf.2010.1132] [PMID: 20954807]

[469] Unno K, Konishi T, Nakagawa A, *et al.* Cognitive dysfunction and amyloid β accumulation are ameliorated by the ingestion of green soybean extract in aged mice. J Funct Foods 2015; 14: 345-53. [http://dx.doi.org/10.1016/j.jff.2015.02.011]

[470] Wang X, Brown IL, Khaled D, Mahoney MC, Evans AJ, Conway PL. Manipulation of colonic bacteria and volatile fatty acid production by dietary high amylose maize (amylomaize) starch granules. J Appl Microbiol 2002; 93(3): 390-7. [http://dx.doi.org/10.1046/j.1365-2672.2002.01704.x] [PMID: 12174036]

[471] Silvi S, Rumney CJ, Cresci A, Rowland IR. Resistant starch modifies gut microflora and microbial metabolism in human flora-associated rats inoculated with faeces from Italian and UK donors. J Appl Microbiol 1999; 86(3): 521-30. [http://dx.doi.org/10.1046/j.1365-2672.1999.00696.x] [PMID: 10196757]

[472] Zhou J, Keenan MJ, Fernandez-Kim SO, *et al.* Dietary resistant starch improves selected brain and behavioral functions in adult and aged rodents. Mol Nutr Food Res 2013; 57(11): 2071-4. [http://dx.doi.org/10.1002/mnfr.201300135] [PMID: 23818307]

[473] Lyte M, Chapel A, Lyte JM, *et al.* Resistant Starch Alters the Microbiota-Gut Brain Axis: Implications for Dietary Modulation of Behavior. PLoS One 2016; 11(1): e0146406. [http://dx.doi.org/10.1371/journal.pone.0146406] [PMID: 26745269]

[474] White LA, Newman MC, Cromwell GL, Lindemann MD. Brewers dried yeast as a source of mannan oligosaccharides for weanling pigs. J Anim Sci 2002; 80(10): 2619-28. [http://dx.doi.org/10.2527/2002.80102619x] [PMID: 12413084]

[475] Jiang RW, Du XG, Zhang X, *et al.* Synthesis and bioassay of β-(1,4)-D-mannans as potential agents against Alzheimers disease. Acta Pharmacol Sin 2013; 34(12): 1585-91. [http://dx.doi.org/10.1038/aps.2013.104] [PMID: 24241344]

[476] Djouzi Z, Andrieux C, Pelenc V, *et al.* Degradation and fermentation of alpha-gluco-oligosaccharides by bacterial strains from human colon: *in vitro* and *in vivo* studies in gnotobiotic rats. J Appl Bacteriol 1995; 79(2): 117-27. [http://dx.doi.org/10.1111/j.1365-2672.1995.tb00924.x] [PMID: 7592106]

[477] Wang P, Liao W, Fang J, *et al.* A glucan isolated from flowers of Lonicera japonica Thunb. inhibits aggregation and neurotoxicity of Aβ42. Carbohydr Polym 2014; 110: 142-7. [http://dx.doi.org/10.1016/j.carbpol.2014.03.060] [PMID: 24906740]

[478] Olano-Martin E, Gibson GR, Rastell RA. Comparison of the *in vitro* bifidogenic properties of pectins and pectic-oligosaccharides. J Appl Microbiol 2002; 93(3): 505-11. [http://dx.doi.org/10.1046/j.1365-2672.2002.01719.x] [PMID: 12174051]

[479] Manderson K, Pinart M, Tuohy KM, *et al.* *In vitro* determination of prebiotic properties of oligosaccharides derived from an orange juice manufacturing by-product stream. Appl Environ Microbiol 2005; 71(12): 8383-9. [http://dx.doi.org/10.1128/AEM.71.12.8383-8389.2005] [PMID: 16332825]

[480] Mandalari G, Nueno Palop C, Tuohy K, *et al.* *In vitro* evaluation of the prebiotic activity of a pectic oligosaccharide-rich extract enzymatically derived from bergamot peel. Appl Microbiol Biotechnol 2007; 73(5): 1173-9. [http://dx.doi.org/10.1007/s00253-006-0561-9] [PMID: 17021882]

[481] Pence BD, Bhattacharya TK, Rytych JL, *et al.* Dietary Fiber and Exercise: Effects on Muscle Function, Cognition, and Short-Chain Fatty Acids in Mice FASEB J 2016; 30: 1287.5.

[482] Marzorati M, Verhelst A, Luta G, *et al. In vitro* modulation of the human gastrointestinal microbial community by plant-derived polysaccharide-rich dietary supplements. Int J Food Microbiol 2010; 139(3): 168-76.
[http://dx.doi.org/10.1016/j.ijfoodmicro.2010.02.030] [PMID: 20362351]

[483] Stancil AN, Hicks LH. Glyconutrients and perception, cognition, and memory. Percept Mot Skills 2009; 108(1): 259-70.
[http://dx.doi.org/10.2466/pms.108.1.259-270] [PMID: 19425467]

[484] Wang C, Szabo JS, Dykman RA. Effects of a carbohydrate supplement upon resting brain activity. Integr Physiol Behav Sci 2004; 39(2): 126-38.
[http://dx.doi.org/10.1007/BF02734278] [PMID: 15759600]

[485] Best T, Kemps E, Bryan J. Saccharide effects on cognition and well-being in middle-aged adults: a randomized controlled trial. Dev Neuropsychol 2010; 35(1): 66-80.
[http://dx.doi.org/10.1080/87565640903325709] [PMID: 20390593]

[486] Best T, Bryan J, Burns N. An investigation of the effects of saccharides on the memory performance of middle-aged adults. J Nutr Health Aging 2008; 12(9): 657-62.
[PMID: 18953465]

[487] Best T, Howe P, Bryan J, Buckley J, Scholey A. Acute effects of a dietary non-starch polysaccharide supplement on cognitive performance in healthy middle-aged adults. Nutr Neurosci 2015; 18(2): 76-86.
[http://dx.doi.org/10.1179/1476830513Y.0000000101] [PMID: 24621069]

[488] Probiotics in food. Health and nutritional properties and guidelines for evaouation (ISSN 0254-4725). . Health and nutritional properties of probiotics in food including powder milk with live lactic acid bacteria Report of a Joint FAO WHO Expert Consultation on Evaluation of Health and Nutritional Properties of Probiotics in Food Including Powder Milk with Live Lactic Acid Bacteria American Córdoba Park Hotel, Córdoba, Argentina, 1 - 4 October 2001.ISBN 92-5-105513-0.
http://www.fao.org/3/a-a0512e.pdf

[489] Hill C, Guarner F, Reid G, *et al.* Expert consensus document. The International Scientific Association for Probiotics and Prebiotics consensus statement on the scope and appropriate use of the term probiotic. Nat Rev Gastroenterol Hepatol 2014; 11(8): 506-14.
[http://dx.doi.org/10.1038/nrgastro.2014.66] [PMID: 24912386]

[490] Metchnikoff II. The prolongation of life: optimistic studies. Springer Publishing Company 2004.

[491] Fuller R. Probiotics in man and animals. J Appl Bacteriol 1989; 66(5): 365-78.
[http://dx.doi.org/10.1111/j.1365-2672.1989.tb05105.x] [PMID: 2666378]

[492] Fuller R. Probiotics in human medicine. Gut 1991; 32(4): 439-42.
[http://dx.doi.org/10.1136/gut.32.4.439] [PMID: 1902810]

[493] Fuller R. Probiotics the scientific thesis. Chapman and Hall, London, UK 1992.

[494] Rijkers GT, de Vos WM, Brummer R-J, Morelli L, Corthier G, Marteau P. Health benefits and health claims of probiotics: bridging science and marketing. Br J Nutr 2011; 106(9): 1291-6.
[http://dx.doi.org/10.1017/S000711451100287X] [PMID: 21861940]

[495] Reid G, Gaudier E, Guarner F, *et al.* International Scientific Association for Probiotics and Prebiotics. Responders and non-responders to probiotic interventions: how can we improve the odds? Gut Microbes 2010; 1(3): 200-4.
[http://dx.doi.org/10.4161/gmic.1.3.12013] [PMID: 21637034]

[496] OHara AM, ORegan P, Fanning A, *et al.* Functional modulation of human intestinal epithelial cell responses by Bifidobacterium infantis and *Lactobacillus* salivarius. Immunology 2006; 118(2): 202-

15.
[http://dx.doi.org/10.1111/j.1365-2567.2006.02358.x] [PMID: 16771855]

[497] Rijkers GT, Bengmark S, Enck P, *et al.* Guidance for substantiating the evidence for beneficial effects of probiotics: current status and recommendations for future research. J Nutr 2010; 140(3): 671S-6S. [http://dx.doi.org/10.3945/jn.109.113779] [PMID: 20130080]

[498] Health Canada, Accepted Claims about the Nature of Probiotic Microorganisms in Food http://www.hc-sc.gc.ca/fn-an/label-etiquet/claims-reclam/probiotics_claims-allegations_probiotiques-eng.php

[499] Hu X, Wang T, Jin F. Alzheimers disease and gut microbiota. Sci China Life Sci 2016; 59(10): 1006-23. [http://dx.doi.org/10.1007/s11427-016-5083-9] [PMID: 27566465]

[500] Gareau MG. Cognitive Function and the Microbiome. Int Rev Neurobiol 2016; 131: 227-46. [http://dx.doi.org/10.1016/bs.irn.2016.08.001] [PMID: 27793221]

[501] Liu X, Cao S, Zhang X. Modulation of Gut Microbiota-Brain Axis by Probiotics, Prebiotics, and Diet. J Agric Food Chem 2015; 63(36): 7885-95. [http://dx.doi.org/10.1021/acs.jafc.5b02404] [PMID: 26306709]

[502] Collins SM, Bercik P. Gut microbiota: Intestinal bacteria influence brain activity in healthy humans. Nat Rev Gastroenterol Hepatol 2013; 10(6): 326-7. [http://dx.doi.org/10.1038/nrgastro.2013.76] [PMID: 23648940]

[503] Schorr GS, Falcone EA, Moretti DJ, Andrews RD. First Long-Term Behavioral Records from Cuvier's Beaked Whales (Ziphius cavirostris) Reveal Record-Breaking Dives. PLoS ONE 2014; 9(3): e92633. [http://dx.doi.org/10.1371/journal.pone.0092633]

[504] Rook GA, Raison CL, Lowry CA. Microbiota, immunoregulatory old friends and psychiatric disorders. Adv Exp Med Biol 2014; 817: 319-56. [http://dx.doi.org/10.1007/978-1-4939-0897-4_15] [PMID: 24997041]

[505] Borre YE, OKeeffe GW, Clarke G, Stanton C, Dinan TG, Cryan JF. Microbiota and neurodevelopmental windows: implications for brain disorders. Trends Mol Med 2014; 20(9): 509-18. [http://dx.doi.org/10.1016/j.molmed.2014.05.002] [PMID: 24956966]

[506] Gareau MG, Wine E, Rodrigues DM, *et al.* Bacterial infection causes stress-induced memory dysfunction in mice. Gut 2011; 60(3): 307-17. [http://dx.doi.org/10.1136/gut.2009.202515] [PMID: 20966022]

[507] Ohland CL, Kish L, Bell H, *et al.* Effects of *Lactobacillus* helveticus on murine behavior are dependent on diet and genotype and correlate with alterations in the gut microbiome. Psychoneuroendocrinology 2013; 38(9): 1738-47. [http://dx.doi.org/10.1016/j.psyneuen.2013.02.008] [PMID: 23566632]

[508] Smith CJ, Emge JR, Berzins K, *et al.* Probiotics normalize the gut-brain-microbiota axis in immunodeficient mice. Am J Physiol Gastrointest Liver Physiol 2014; 307(8): G793-802. [http://dx.doi.org/10.1152/ajpgi.00238.2014] [PMID: 25190473]

[509] Liang S, Wang T, Hu X, *et al.* Administration of *Lactobacillus* helveticus NS8 improves behavioral, cognitive, and biochemical aberrations caused by chronic restraint stress. Neuroscience 2015; 310: 561-77. [http://dx.doi.org/10.1016/j.neuroscience.2015.09.033] [PMID: 26408987]

[510] Ohsawa K, Uchida N, Ohki K, Nakamura Y, Yokogoshi H. *Lactobacillus* helveticus-fermented milk improves learning and memory in mice. Nutr Neurosci 2015; 18(5): 232-40. [http://dx.doi.org/10.1179/1476830514Y.0000000122] [PMID: 24694020]

[511] Emge JR, Huynh K, Miller EN, *et al.* Modulation of the microbiota-gut-brain axis by probiotics in a murine model of inflammatory bowel disease. Am J Physiol Gastrointest Liver Physiol 2016; 310(11):

G989-98.
[http://dx.doi.org/10.1152/ajpgi.00086.2016] [PMID: 27056723]

[512] Yeon S-W, You YS, Kwon H-S, *et al.* Fermented milk of *Lactobacillus* helveticus IDCC3801 reduces beta-amyloid and attenuates memory deficit. J Funct Foods 2010; 2: 143-52.
[http://dx.doi.org/10.1016/j.jff.2010.04.002]

[513] Jung I-H, Jung M-A, Kim E-J, Han MJ, Kim D-H. *Lactobacillus pentosus var. plantarum* C29 protects scopolamine-induced memory deficit in mice. J Appl Microbiol 2012; 113(6): 1498-506.
[http://dx.doi.org/10.1111/j.1365-2672.2012.05437.x] [PMID: 22925033]

[514] Phillips HS, Hains JM, Armanini M, Laramee GR, Johnson SA, Winslow JW. BDNF mRNA is decreased in the hippocampus of individuals with Alzheimers disease. Neuron 1991; 7(5): 695-702.
[http://dx.doi.org/10.1016/0896-6273(91)90273-3] [PMID: 1742020]

[515] Woo J-Y, Gu W, Kim K-A, Jang S-E, Han MJ, Kim D-H. *Lactobacillus pentosus var. plantarum* C29 ameliorates memory impairment and inflammaging in a D-galactose-induced accelerated aging mouse model. Anaerobe 2014; 27: 22-6.
[http://dx.doi.org/10.1016/j.anaerobe.2014.03.003] [PMID: 24657159]

[516] Jeong J-J, Woo J-Y, Kim K-A, Han MJ, Kim D-H. *Lactobacillus pentosus var. plantarum* C29 ameliorates age-dependent memory impairment in Fischer 344 rats. Lett Appl Microbiol 2015; 60(4): 307-14.
[http://dx.doi.org/10.1111/lam.12393] [PMID: 25598393]

[517] Jeong J-J, Kim K-A, Ahn Y-T, *et al.* Probiotic Mixture KF Attenuates Age-Dependent Memory Deficit and Lipidemia in Fischer 344 Rats. J Microbiol Biotechnol 2015; 25(9): 1532-6.
[http://dx.doi.org/10.4014/jmb.1505.05002] [PMID: 25975611]

[518] Liu T-H, Chiou J, Tsai T-Y. Effects of *Lactobacillus plantarum* TWK10-Fermented Soymilk on Deoxycorticosterone Acetate-Salt-Induced Hypertension and Associated Dementia in Rats. Nutrients 2016; 8(5): 8.
[http://dx.doi.org/10.3390/nu8050260] [PMID: 27144579]

[519] Benton D, Williams C, Brown A. Impact of consuming a milk drink containing a probiotic on mood and cognition. Eur J Clin Nutr 2007; 61(3): 355-61.
[http://dx.doi.org/10.1038/sj.ejcn.1602546] [PMID: 17151594]

[520] Phelps EA. Emotion and cognition: insights from studies of the human amygdala. Annu Rev Psychol 2006; 57: 27-53.
[http://dx.doi.org/10.1146/annurev.psych.56.091103.070234] [PMID: 16318588]

[521] Rao AV, Bested AC, Beaulne TM, *et al.* A randomized, double-blind, placebo-controlled pilot study of a probiotic in emotional symptoms of chronic fatigue syndrome. Gut Pathog 2009; 1(1): 6.
[http://dx.doi.org/10.1186/1757-4749-1-6] [PMID: 19338686]

[522] Chung Y-C, Jin H-M, Cui Y, *et al.* Fermented milk of *Lactobacillus helveticus* IDCC3801 improves cognitive functioning during cognitive fatigue tests in healthy older adults. J Funct Foods 2014; 10: 465-74.
[http://dx.doi.org/10.1016/j.jff.2014.07.007]

[523] Wall R, Ross RP, Shanahan F, *et al.* Impact of administered bifidobacterium on murine host fatty acid composition. Lipids 2010; 45(5): 429-36.
[http://dx.doi.org/10.1007/s11745-010-3410-7] [PMID: 20405232]

[524] James MJ, Gibson RA, Cleland LG. Dietary polyunsaturated fatty acids and inflammatory mediator production. Am J Clin Nutr 2000; 71(1) (Suppl.): 343S-8S.
[PMID: 10617994]

[525] Wall R, Marques TM, OSullivan O, *et al.* Contrasting effects of *Bifidobacterium breve* NCIMB 702258 and *Bifidobacterium breve* DPC 6330 on the composition of murine brain fatty acids and gut microbiota. Am J Clin Nutr 2012; 95(5): 1278-87.

[http://dx.doi.org/10.3945/ajcn.111.026435] [PMID: 22492373]

[526] OSullivan E, Barrett E, Grenham S, *et al.* BDNF expression in the hippocampus of maternally separated rats: does *Bifidobacterium breve* 6330 alter BDNF levels? Benef Microbes 2011; 2(3): 199-207.
[http://dx.doi.org/10.3920/BM2011.0015] [PMID: 21986359]

[527] Savignac HM, Tramullas M, Kiely B, Dinan TG, Cryan JF. *Bifidobacteria* modulate cognitive processes in an anxious mouse strain. Behav Brain Res 2015; 287: 59-72.
[http://dx.doi.org/10.1016/j.bbr.2015.02.044] [PMID: 25794930]

[528] Savignac HM, Kiely B, Dinan TG, Cryan JF. *Bifidobacteria* exert strain-specific effects on stress-related behavior and physiology in BALB/c mice. Neurogastroenterol Motil 2014; 26(11): 1615-27.
[http://dx.doi.org/10.1111/nmo.12427] [PMID: 25251188]

[529] Dinan TG, Stanton C, Cryan JF. Psychobiotics: a novel class of psychotropic. Biol Psychiatry 2013; 74(10): 720-6.
[http://dx.doi.org/10.1016/j.biopsych.2013.05.001] [PMID: 23759244]

[530] Leahy SC, Higgins DG, Fitzgerald GF, van Sinderen D. Getting better with *Bifidobacteria.* J Appl Microbiol 2005; 98(6): 1303-15.
[http://dx.doi.org/10.1111/j.1365-2672.2005.02600.x] [PMID: 15916644]

[531] Dinan TG, Cryan JF. Regulation of the stress response by the gut microbiota: implications for psychoneuroendocrinology. Psychoneuroendocrinology 2012; 37(9): 1369-78.
[http://dx.doi.org/10.1016/j.psyneuen.2012.03.007] [PMID: 22483040]

[532] Forsythe P, Kunze WA. Voices from within: gut microbes and the CNS. Cell Mol Life Sci 2013; 70(1): 55-69.
[http://dx.doi.org/10.1007/s00018-012-1028-z] [PMID: 22638926]

[533] Bercik P, Verdu EF, Foster JA, *et al.* Chronic gastrointestinal inflammation induces anxiety-like behavior and alters central nervous system biochemistry in mice. Gastroenterology 2010; 139(6): 2102-2112.e1.
[http://dx.doi.org/10.1053/j.gastro.2010.06.063] [PMID: 20600016]

[534] Bravo JA, Forsythe P, Chew MV, *et al.* Ingestion of *Lactobacillus*strain regulates emotional behavior and central GABA receptor expression in a mouse *via* the vagus nerve. Proc Natl Acad Sci USA 2011; 108(38): 16050-5.
[http://dx.doi.org/10.1073/pnas.1102999108] [PMID: 21876150]

[535] Buwalda B, Kole MH, Veenema AH, *et al.* Long-term effects of social stress on brain and behavior: a focus on hippocampal functioning. Neurosci Biobehav Rev 2005; 29(1): 83-97.
[http://dx.doi.org/10.1016/j.neubiorev.2004.05.005] [PMID: 15652257]

[536] McEwen BS, Sapolsky RM. Stress and cognitive function. Curr Opin Neurobiol 1995; 5(2): 205-16.
[http://dx.doi.org/10.1016/0959-4388(95)80028-X] [PMID: 7620309]

[537] Hyun KJ, Myung CJ, Sanghyun L, Ju CE. Protective effects of purple sweet potato added to *Bacillus subtilis*-fermented soymilk against amyloid beta-induced memory impairment. J Agric Sci 2012; 4: 223-32.

[538] Park S, Kang S, Kim HJ, Kwon DY, Daily J. Standardized chungkookjang, short-term fermented soybeans with Bacillus lichemiformis, improves cognitive function and insulin resistance in β-amyloid-infused diabetic rats. FASEB J 2013; 2: 1079.14.

[539] Davari S, Talaei SA, Alaei H, Salami M. Probiotics treatment improves diabetes-induced impairment of synaptic activity and cognitive function: behavioral and electrophysiological proofs for microbiome-gut-brain axis. Neuroscience 2013; 240: 287-96.
[http://dx.doi.org/10.1016/j.neuroscience.2013.02.055] [PMID: 23500100]

[540] Messaoudi M, Lalonde R, Violle N, *et al.* Assessment of psychotropic-like properties of a probiotic formulation (*Lactobacillus helveticus* R0052 and *Bifidobacterium longum* R0175) in rats and human

subjects. Br J Nutr 2011; 105(5): 755-64.
[http://dx.doi.org/10.1017/S0007114510004319] [PMID: 20974015]

[541] Steenbergen L, Sellaro R, van Hemert S, Bosch JA, Colzato LS. A randomized controlled trial to test the effect of multispecies probiotics on cognitive reactivity to sad mood. Brain Behav Immun 2015; 48: 258-64.
[http://dx.doi.org/10.1016/j.bbi.2015.04.003] [PMID: 25862297]

[542] Beck AT, Alford BA. Depression: Causes and treatment. University of Pennsylvania Press 2009.

[543] Kovacs M, Beck AT. Maladaptive cognitive structures in depression. Am J Psychiatry 1978; 135(5): 525-33.
[http://dx.doi.org/10.1176/ajp.135.5.525] [PMID: 645943]

[544] Abramson LY, Metalsky GI, Alloy LB. Hopelessness depression: A theory-based subtype of depression. Prychological Rev 1989; 36: 129-48.

[545] Haaga DA, Dyck MJ, Ernst D. Empirical status of cognitive theory of depression. Psychol Bull 1991; 110(2): 215-36.
[http://dx.doi.org/10.1037/0033-2909.110.2.215] [PMID: 1946867]

[546] Scher CD, Ingram RE, Segal ZV. Cognitive reactivity and vulnerability: empirical evaluation of construct activation and cognitive diatheses in unipolar depression. Clin Psychol Rev 2005; 25(4): 487-510.
[http://dx.doi.org/10.1016/j.cpr.2005.01.005] [PMID: 15914266]

[547] Ingram RE, Miranda J, Segal ZV. Cognitive vulnerability to depression. Guilford Press 1998.

[548] Tillisch K, Labus J, Kilpatrick L, *et al.* Consumption of fermented milk product with probiotic modulates brain activity 2013.
[http://dx.doi.org/10.1053/j.gastro.2013.02.043]

[549] Wang H, Lee I-S, Braun C, Enck P. Effect of Probiotics on Central Nervous System Functions in Animals and Humans: A Systematic Review. J Neurogastroenterol Motil 2016; 22(4): 589-605.
[http://dx.doi.org/10.5056/jnm16018] [PMID: 27413138]

[550] Hosseinzadeh H, Nassiri-Asl M. Avicennas (Ibn Sina) the Canon of Medicine and saffron (*Crocus sativus*): a review. Phytother Res 2013; 27(4): 475-83.
[http://dx.doi.org/10.1002/ptr.4784] [PMID: 22815242]

[551] Abdullaev FI. Cancer chemopreventive and tumoricidal properties of saffron (*Crocus sativus* L.). Exp Biol Med (Maywood) 2002; 227(1): 20-5.
[PMID: 11788779]

[552] Tarantilis PA, Tsoupras G, Polissiou M. Determination of saffron (*Crocus sativus* L.) components in crude plant extract using high-performance liquid chromatography-UV-visible photodiode-array detection-mass spectrometry. J Chromatogr A 1995; 699(1-2): 107-18.
[http://dx.doi.org/10.1016/0021-9673(95)00044-N] [PMID: 7757208]

[553] Abdullaev Jafarova F, Caballero-Ortega H, Riverón-Negrete L, *et al.* [In vitro evaluation of the chemopreventive potential of saffron]. Rev Invest Clin 2002; 54(5): 430-6. [In vitro evaluation of the chemopreventive potential of saffron].
[PMID: 12587418]

[554] Xiang M, Yang M, Zhou C, Liu J, Li W, Qian Z. Crocetin prevents AGEs-induced vascular endothelial cell apoptosis. Pharmacol Res 2006; 54(4): 268-74.
[http://dx.doi.org/10.1016/j.phrs.2006.06.010] [PMID: 16899372]

[555] Papandreou MA, Kanakis CD, Polissiou MG, *et al.* Inhibitory activity on amyloid-beta aggregation and antioxidant properties of *Crocus sativus* stigmas extract and its crocin constituents. J Agric Food Chem 2006; 54(23): 8762-8.
[http://dx.doi.org/10.1021/jf061932a] [PMID: 17090119]

[556] Stoll G, Jander S. The role of microglia and macrophages in the pathophysiology of the CNS. Prog Neurobiol 1999; 58(3): 233-47.
[http://dx.doi.org/10.1016/S0301-0082(98)00083-5] [PMID: 10341362]

[557] Abe K, Saito H. Effects of saffron extract and its constituent crocin on learning behaviour and long-term potentiation. Phytother Res 2000; 14(3): 149-52.
[http://dx.doi.org/10.1002/(SICI)1099-1573(200005)14:3<149::AID-PTR665>3.0.CO;2-5] [PMID: 10815004]

[558] Hosseinzadeh H, Ziaei T. Effects of *Crocus sativus* stigma extract and its constituents, crocin and safranal, on intact memory and scopolamine-induced learning deficits in rats performing the Morris water maze task. J Med Plants 2006; 5: 40-50.

[559] Zheng Y-Q, Liu J-X, Wang J-N, Xu L. Effects of crocin on reperfusion-induced oxidative/nitrative injury to cerebral microvessels after global cerebral ischemia. Brain Res 2007; 1138: 86-94.
[http://dx.doi.org/10.1016/j.brainres.2006.12.064] [PMID: 17274961]

[560] Hosseinzadeh H, Sadeghnia HR, Ghaeni FA, Motamedshariaty VS, Mohajeri SA. Effects of saffron (*Crocus sativus* L.) and its active constituent, crocin, on recognition and spatial memory after chronic cerebral hypoperfusion in rats. Phytother Res 2012; 26(3): 381-6.
[PMID: 21774008]

[561] Tsolaki M, Karathanasi E, Lazarou I, *et al.* Efficacy and Safety of *Crocus sativus* L. in Patients with Mild Cognitive Impairment: One Year Single-Blind Randomized, with Parallel Groups, Clinical Trial. J Alzheimers Dis 2016; 54(1): 129-33.
[http://dx.doi.org/10.3233/JAD-160304] [PMID: 27472878]

[562] Abe K, Sugiura M, Shoyama Y, Saito H. Crocin antagonizes ethanol inhibition of NMDA receptor-mediated responses in rat hippocampal neurons. Brain Res 1998; 787(1): 132-8.
[http://dx.doi.org/10.1016/S0006-8993(97)01505-9] [PMID: 9518580]

[563] Boskabady MH, Rahbardar MG, Jafari Z, Mohammad HB, Rahbardar MG, Jafari Z. The effect of safranal on histamine (H(1)) receptors of guinea pig tracheal chains. Fitoterapia 2011; 82(2): 162-7.
[http://dx.doi.org/10.1016/j.fitote.2010.08.017] [PMID: 20804826]

[564] Lautenschläger M, Sendker J, Hüwel S, *et al.* Intestinal formation of trans-crocetin from saffron extract (*Crocus sativus* L.) and *in vitro* permeation through intestinal and blood brain barrier. Phytomedicine 2015; 22(1): 36-44.
[http://dx.doi.org/10.1016/j.phymed.2014.10.009] [PMID: 25636868]

[565] Moshiri M, Vahabzadeh M, Hosseinzadeh H. Clinical Applications of Saffron (*Crocus sativus*) and its Constituents: A Review. Drug Res (Stuttg) 2015; 65(6): 287-95.
[PMID: 24848002]

[566] Asai A, Nakano T, Takahashi M, Nagao A. Orally administered crocetin and crocins are absorbed into blood plasma as crocetin and its glucuronide conjugates in mice. J Agric Food Chem 2005; 53(18): 7302-6.
[http://dx.doi.org/10.1021/jf0509355] [PMID: 16131146]

[567] Xi L, Qian Z, Du P, Fu J. Pharmacokinetic properties of crocin (crocetin digentiobiose ester) following oral administration in rats. Phytomedicine 2007; 14(9): 633-6.
[http://dx.doi.org/10.1016/j.phymed.2006.11.028] [PMID: 17215113]

[568] Akhondzadeh S, Shafiee Sabet M, Harirchian MH, *et al.* A 22-week, multicenter, randomized, double-blind controlled trial of *Crocus sativus* in the treatment of mild-to-moderate Alzheimers disease. Psychopharmacology (Berl) 2010; 207(4): 637-43.
[http://dx.doi.org/10.1007/s00213-009-1706-1] [PMID: 19838862]

[569] Pitsikas N. The Effect of *Crocus sativus* L. and Its Constituents on Memory: Basic Studies and Clinical Applications. Evid Based Complement Alternat Med 2015; 2015: 926284.
[http://dx.doi.org/10.1155/2015/926284] [PMID: 25713594]

[570] Geromichalos GD, Lamari FN, Papandreou MA, *et al.* Saffron as a source of novel acetylcholinesterase inhibitors: molecular docking and *in vitro* enzymatic studies. J Agric Food Chem 2012; 60(24): 6131-8.
[http://dx.doi.org/10.1021/jf300589c] [PMID: 22655699]

[571] Ramassamy C, Arseneault M, Nam DT. Free radical–mediated damage to brain in Alzheimer's disease: role of acrolein and preclinical promise of antioxidant polyphenols. In: Bondy S, Maiese K, Eds. Aging and Age-Related Disorders. 2010; pp. 417-37.
[http://dx.doi.org/10.1007/978-1-60761-602-3_21]

[572] Rashedinia M, Lari P, Abnous K, Hosseinzadeh H. Protective effect of crocin on acrolein-induced tau phosphorylation in the rat brain. TL - 75 Acta Neurobiol Exp (Wars) 75 VN-r 2015; 208-19.

[573] Mehri S, Abnous K, Mousavi SH, Shariaty VM, Hosseinzadeh H. Neuroprotective effect of crocin on acrylamide-induced cytotoxicity in PC12 cells. Cell Mol Neurobiol 2012; 32(2): 227-35.
[http://dx.doi.org/10.1007/s10571-011-9752-8] [PMID: 21901509]

[574] Khazdair MR, Boskabady MH, Hosseini M, Rezaee R, M Tsatsakis A. The effects of *Crocus sativus* (saffron) and its constituents on nervous system: A review. Avicenna J Phytomed 2015; 5(5): 376-91.
[PMID: 26468457]

[575] Hosseinzadeh H, Jahanian Z. Effect of *Crocus sativus* L. (saffron) stigma and its constituents, crocin and safranal, on morphine withdrawal syndrome in mice. Phytother Res 2010; 24(5): 726-30.
[PMID: 19827024]

[576] Vahidi H, Kamalinejad M, Sedaghati N. Antimicrobial Properties of *Crocus sativus* s. Iran J Pharm Res 2002; 1: 33-5.

[577] Ansari N, Khodagholi F. Natural products as promising drug candidates for the treatment of Alzheimers disease: molecular mechanism aspect. Curr Neuropharmacol 2013; 11(4): 414-29.
[http://dx.doi.org/10.2174/1570159X11311040005] [PMID: 24381531]

[578] Raskin J, Cummings J, Hardy J, Schuh K, Dean RA. Neurobiology of Alzheimers Disease: Integrated Molecular, Physiological, Anatomical, Biomarker, and Cognitive Dimensions. Curr Alzheimer Res 2015; 12(8): 712-22.
[http://dx.doi.org/10.2174/1567205012666150701103107] [PMID: 26412218]

[579] Cervellati C, Wood PL, Romani A, *et al.* Oxidative challenge in Alzheimers disease: state of knowledge and future needs. J Investig Med 2016; 64(1): 21-32.
[http://dx.doi.org/10.1136/jim-2015-000017] [PMID: 26755810]

[580] Iuvone T, De Filippis D, Esposito G, DAmico A, Izzo AA. The spice sage and its active ingredient rosmarinic acid protect PC12 cells from amyloid-beta peptide-induced neurotoxicity. J Pharmacol Exp Ther 2006; 317(3): 1143-9.
[http://dx.doi.org/10.1124/jpet.105.099317] [PMID: 16495207]

[581] Bulgakov VP, Inyushkina YV, Fedoreyev SA. Rosmarinic acid and its derivatives: biotechnology and applications. Crit Rev Biotechnol 2012; 32(3): 203-17.
[http://dx.doi.org/10.3109/07388551.2011.596804] [PMID: 21838541]

[582] Alkam T, Nitta A, Mizoguchi H, Itoh A, Nabeshima T. A natural scavenger of peroxynitrites, rosmarinic acid, protects against impairment of memory induced by Abeta(2535). Behav Brain Res 2007; 180(2): 139-45.
[http://dx.doi.org/10.1016/j.bbr.2007.03.001] [PMID: 17420060]

[583] Lee AY, Hwang BR, Lee MH, Lee S, Cho EJ. Perilla frutescens var. japonica and rosmarinic acid improve amyloid-β2535 induced impairment of cognition and memory function. Nutr Res Pract 2016; 10(3): 274-81.
[http://dx.doi.org/10.4162/nrp.2016.10.3.274] [PMID: 27247723]

[584] Olthof MR, Hollman PC, Katan MB. Chlorogenic acid and caffeic acid are absorbed in humans. J Nutr 2001; 131(1): 66-71.

[PMID: 11208940]

[585] Kelly GS. Quercetin. Monograph. Altern Med Rev 2011; 16(2): 172-94. [PMID: 21649459]

[586] Ossola B, Kääriäinen TM, Männistö PT. The multiple faces of quercetin in neuroprotection. Expert Opin Drug Saf 2009; 8(4): 397-409. [http://dx.doi.org/10.1517/14740330903026944] [PMID: 19538101]

[587] Russo M, Spagnuolo C, Tedesco I, Bilotto S, Russo GL. The flavonoid quercetin in disease prevention and therapy: facts and fancies. Biochem Pharmacol 2012; 83(1): 6-15. [http://dx.doi.org/10.1016/j.bcp.2011.08.010] [PMID: 21856292]

[588] Bischoff SC. Quercetin: potentials in the prevention and therapy of disease. Curr Opin Clin Nutr Metab Care 2008; 11(6): 733-40. [http://dx.doi.org/10.1097/MCO.0b013e32831394b8] [PMID: 18827577]

[589] Jiménez-Aliaga K, Bermejo-Bescós P, Benedí J, Martín-Aragón S. Quercetin and rutin exhibit antiamyloidogenic and fibril-disaggregating effects *in vitro* and potent antioxidant activity in APPswe cells. Life Sci 2011; 89(25-26): 939-45. [http://dx.doi.org/10.1016/j.lfs.2011.09.023] [PMID: 22008478]

[590] Ansari MA, Abdul HM, Joshi G, Opii WO, Butterfield DA. Protective effect of quercetin in primary neurons against Abeta(142): relevance to Alzheimers disease. J Nutr Biochem 2009; 20(4): 269-75. [http://dx.doi.org/10.1016/j.jnutbio.2008.03.002] [PMID: 18602817]

[591] Tchantchou F, Lacor PN, Cao Z, *et al.* Stimulation of neurogenesis and synaptogenesis by bilobalide and quercetin *via* common final pathway in hippocampal neurons. J Alzheimers Dis 2009; 18(4): 787-98. [PMID: 19661619]

[592] Dhawan S, Kapil R, Singh B. Formulation development and systematic optimization of solid lipid nanoparticles of quercetin for improved brain delivery. J Pharm Pharmacol 2011; 63(3): 342-51. [http://dx.doi.org/10.1111/j.2042-7158.2010.01225.x] [PMID: 21749381]

[593] Wei N, Zhu L-Q, Liu D. ATF4: a Novel Potential Therapeutic Target for Alzheimers Disease. Mol Neurobiol 2015; 52(3): 1765-70. [http://dx.doi.org/10.1007/s12035-014-8970-8] [PMID: 25381575]

[594] Nakagawa T, Itoh M, Ohta K, *et al.* Improvement of memory recall by quercetin in rodent contextual fear conditioning and human early-stage Alzheimers disease patients. Neuroreport 2016; 27(9): 671-6. [http://dx.doi.org/10.1097/WNR.0000000000000594] [PMID: 27145228]

[595] Ding J, Xi Y-D, Zhang D-D, *et al.* Soybean isoflavone ameliorates β-amyloid 142-induced learning and memory deficit in rats by protecting synaptic structure and function. Synapse 2013; 67(12): 856-64. [http://dx.doi.org/10.1002/syn.21692] [PMID: 23766238]

[596] Xi Y-D, Ding J, Han J, *et al.* The effect of soybean isoflavone on the dysregulation of NMDA receptor signaling pathway induced by β-amyloid peptides 142 in rats. Cell Mol Neurobiol 2015; 35(4): 555-62. [http://dx.doi.org/10.1007/s10571-014-0151-9] [PMID: 25563203]

[597] Diaz-Gerevini GT, Repossi G, Dain A, Tarres MC, Das UN, Eynard AR. Beneficial action of resveratrol: How and why? Nutrition 2016; 32(2): 174-8. [http://dx.doi.org/10.1016/j.nut.2015.08.017] [PMID: 26706021]

[598] Mazzanti G, Di Giacomo S. Curcumin and resveratrol in the management of cognitive disorders: what is the clinical evidence? Molecules 2016; 21(9): 21. [http://dx.doi.org/10.3390/molecules21091243] [PMID: 27649135]

[599] Dong W, Wang R. Effects of resveratrol-induced cellular autophagy in control of neurodegenerative diseases. Yao Xue Xue Bao 2016; 51(1): 18-22.

[PMID: 27405156]

[600] Ataie A, Shadifar M, Ataee R. Polyphenolic antioxidants and neuronal regeneration. Basic Clin Neurosci 2016; 7(2): 81-90. [http://dx.doi.org/10.15412/J.BCN.03070201] [PMID: 27303602]

[601] Karthick C, Periyasamy S, Jayachandran KS, Anusuyadevi M. Intrahippocampal administration of ibotenic acid induced cholinergic dysfunction *via* NR2A/NR2B expression: implications of resveratrol against alzheimer disease pathophysiology. Front Mol Neurosci 2016; 9: 28. [http://dx.doi.org/10.3389/fnmol.2016.00028] [PMID: 27199654]

[602] Cheng J, Xia X, Rui Y, *et al.* The combination of 1α,25dihydroxyvitaminD3 with resveratrol improves neuronal degeneration by regulating endoplasmic reticulum stress, insulin signaling and inhibiting tau hyperphosphorylation in SH-SY5Y cells. Food Chem Toxicol 2016; 93: 32-40. [http://dx.doi.org/10.1016/j.fct.2016.04.021] [PMID: 27133915]

[603] Spagnuolo C, Napolitano M, Tedesco I, Moccia S, Milito A, Russo GL. Neuroprotective role of natural polyphenols. Curr Top Med Chem 2016; 16(17): 1943-50. [http://dx.doi.org/10.2174/1568026616666160204122449] [PMID: 26845551]

[604] Chan S, Kantham S, Rao VM, *et al.* Metal chelation, radical scavenging and inhibition of Aβ□□ fibrillation by food constituents in relation to Alzheimers disease. Food Chem 2016; 199: 185-94. [http://dx.doi.org/10.1016/j.foodchem.2015.11.118] [PMID: 26775960]

[605] Ko S-Y, Ko H-A, Chu K-H, *et al.* The possible mechanism of advanced glycation end products (AGEs) for alzheimers disease. PLoS One 2015; 10(11): e0143345. [http://dx.doi.org/10.1371/journal.pone.0143345] [PMID: 26587989]

[606] Venigalla M, Sonego S, Gyengesi E, Sharman MJ, Münch G. Novel promising therapeutics against chronic neuroinflammation and neurodegeneration in Alzheimers disease. Neurochem Int 2016; 95: 63-74. [http://dx.doi.org/10.1016/j.neuint.2015.10.011] [PMID: 26529297]

[607] Cheng X, Wang Q, Li N, Zhao H. Effects of resveratrol on hippocampal astrocytes and expression of TNF-α in Alzheimers disease model rate. Wei Sheng Yan Jiu 2015; 44(4): 610-4. [PMID: 26454959]

[608] Zhao HF, Li N, Wang Q, Cheng XJ, Li XM, Liu TT. Resveratrol decreases the insoluble Aβ142 level in hippocampus and protects the integrity of the blood-brain barrier in AD rats. Neuroscience 2015; 310: 641-9. [http://dx.doi.org/10.1016/j.neuroscience.2015.10.006] [PMID: 26454022]

[609] Tellone E, Galtieri A, Russo A, Giardina B, Ficarra S. Resveratrol: A focus on several neurodegenerative diseases. Oxid Med Cell Longev 2015; 2015: 392169. [http://dx.doi.org/10.1155/2015/392169] [PMID: 26180587]

[610] Turner RS, Thomas RG, Craft S, *et al.* Alzheimers Disease Cooperative Study. A randomized, double-blind, placebo-controlled trial of resveratrol for Alzheimer disease. Neurology 2015; 85(16): 1383-91. [http://dx.doi.org/10.1212/WNL.0000000000002035] [PMID: 26362286]

[611] Koukoulitsa C, Villalonga-Barber C, Csonka R, *et al.* Biological and computational evaluation of resveratrol inhibitors against Alzheimers disease. J Enzyme Inhib Med Chem 2016; 31(1): 67-77. [http://dx.doi.org/10.3109/14756366.2014.1003928] [PMID: 26147348]

[612] Regitz C, Fitzenberger E, Mahn FL, Dußling LM, Wenzel U. Resveratrol reduces amyloid-beta (Aβ1-42)-induced paralysis through targeting proteostasis in an Alzheimer model of Caenorhabditis elegans. Eur J Nutr 2016; 55(2): 741-7. [http://dx.doi.org/10.1007/s00394-015-0894-1] [PMID: 25851110]

[613] Hu J, Lin T, Gao Y, *et al.* The resveratrol trimer miyabenol C inhibits β-secretase activity and β-amyloid generation. PLoS One 2015; 10(1): e0115973. [http://dx.doi.org/10.1371/journal.pone.0115973] [PMID: 25629409]

[614] Ma T, Tan M-S, Yu J-T, Tan L. Resveratrol as a therapeutic agent for Alzheimers disease. BioMed Res Int 2014; 2014: 350516.
[http://dx.doi.org/10.1155/2014/350516] [PMID: 25525597]

[615] El-Sayed NS, Bayan Y. Possible role of resveratrol targeting estradiol and neprilysin pathways in lipopolysaccharide model of Alzheimer disease. Adv Exp Med Biol 2015; 822: 107-18.
[http://dx.doi.org/10.1007/978-3-319-08927-0_12] [PMID: 25416980]

[616] Pasinetti GM, Wang J, Ho L, Zhao W, Dubner L. Roles of resveratrol and other grape-derived polyphenols in Alzheimers disease prevention and treatment. Biochim Biophys Acta 2015; 1852(6): 1202-8.
[http://dx.doi.org/10.1016/j.bbadis.2014.10.006] [PMID: 25315300]

[617] Malar DS, Devi KP. Dietary polyphenols for treatment of Alzheimers disease future research and development. Curr Pharm Biotechnol 2014; 15(4): 330-42.
[http://dx.doi.org/10.2174/1389201015666140813122703] [PMID: 25312617]

[618] Rege SD, Geetha T, Griffin GD, Broderick TL, Babu JR. Neuroprotective effects of resveratrol in Alzheimer disease pathology. Front Aging Neurosci 2014; 6: 218.
[http://dx.doi.org/10.3389/fnagi.2014.00218] [PMID: 25309423]

[619] Sezgin Z, Dincer Y. Alzheimers disease and epigenetic diet. Neurochem Int 2014; 78: 105-16.
[http://dx.doi.org/10.1016/j.neuint.2014.09.012] [PMID: 25290336]

[620] Bastianetto S, Ménard C, Quirion R. Neuroprotective action of resveratrol. Biochim Biophys Acta 2015; 1852(6): 1195-201.
[http://dx.doi.org/10.1016/j.bbadis.2014.09.011] [PMID: 25281824]

[621] Porquet D, Griñán-Ferré C, Ferrer I, *et al.* Neuroprotective role of trans-resveratrol in a murine model of familial Alzheimers disease. J Alzheimers Dis 2014; 42(4): 1209-20.
[PMID: 25024312]

[622] Bigford GE, Del Rossi G. Supplemental substances derived from foods as adjunctive therapeutic agents for treatment of neurodegenerative diseases and disorders. Adv Nutr 2014; 5(4): 394-403.
[http://dx.doi.org/10.3945/an.113.005264] [PMID: 25022989]

[623] Mao F, Yan J, Li J, *et al.* New multi-target-directed small molecules against Alzheimers disease: a combination of resveratrol and clioquinol. Org Biomol Chem 2014; 12(31): 5936-44.
[http://dx.doi.org/10.1039/C4OB00998C] [PMID: 24986600]

[624] Granzotto A, Zatta P. Resveratrol and Alzheimers disease: message in a bottle on red wine and cognition. Front Aging Neurosci 2014; 6: 95.
[http://dx.doi.org/10.3389/fnagi.2014.00095] [PMID: 24860502]

[625] Awasthi M, Singh S, Pandey VP, Dwivedi UN. Alzheimers disease: An overview of amyloid beta dependent pathogenesis and its therapeutic implications along with in silico approaches emphasizing the role of natural products. J Neurol Sci 2016; 361: 256-71.
[http://dx.doi.org/10.1016/j.jns.2016.01.008] [PMID: 26810552]

[626] Chin D, Huebbe P, Pallauf K, Rimbach G. Neuroprotective properties of curcumin in Alzheimers disease merits and limitations. Curr Med Chem 2013; 20(32): 3955-85.
[http://dx.doi.org/10.2174/09298673113209990210] [PMID: 23931272]

[627] Ono K, Hasegawa K, Naiki H, Yamada M. Curcumin has potent anti-amyloidogenic effects for Alzheimers beta-amyloid fibrils *in vitro*. J Neurosci Res 2004; 75(6): 742-50.
[http://dx.doi.org/10.1002/jnr.20025] [PMID: 14994335]

[628] Shytle RD, Bickford PC, Rezai-zadeh K, *et al.* Optimized turmeric extracts have potent anti-amyloidogenic effects. Curr Alzheimer Res 2009; 6(6): 564-71.
[http://dx.doi.org/10.2174/156720509790147115] [PMID: 19715544]

[629] Yang F, Lim GP, Begum AN, *et al.* Curcumin inhibits formation of amyloid beta oligomers and

fibrils, binds plaques, and reduces amyloid *in vivo*. J Biol Chem 2005; 280(7): 5892-901. [http://dx.doi.org/10.1074/jbc.M404751200] [PMID: 15590663]

[630] Garcia-Alloza M, Borrelli LA, Rozkalne A, Hyman BT, Bacskai BJ. Curcumin labels amyloid pathology *in vivo*, disrupts existing plaques, and partially restores distorted neurites in an Alzheimer mouse model. J Neurochem 2007; 102(4): 1095-104. [http://dx.doi.org/10.1111/j.1471-4159.2007.04613.x] [PMID: 17472706]

[631] Lim GP, Chu T, Yang F, Beech W, Frautschy SA, Cole GM. The curry spice curcumin reduces oxidative damage and amyloid pathology in an Alzheimer transgenic mouse. J Neurosci 2001; 21(21): 8370-7. [PMID: 11606625]

[632] Wang YJ, Pan MH, Cheng AL, *et al.* Stability of curcumin in buffer solutions and characterization of its degradation products. J Pharm Biomed Anal 1997; 15(12): 1867-76. [http://dx.doi.org/10.1016/S0731-7085(96)02024-9] [PMID: 9278892]

[633] Dolai S, Shi W, Corbo C, *et al.* Clicked sugar-curcumin conjugate: modulator of amyloid-β and tau peptide aggregation at ultralow concentrations. ACS Chem Neurosci 2011; 2(12): 694-9. [http://dx.doi.org/10.1021/cn200088r] [PMID: 22860163]

[634] Mourtas S, Canovi M, Zona C, *et al.* Curcumin-decorated nanoliposomes with very high affinity for amyloid-β142 peptide. Biomaterials 2011; 32(6): 1635-45. [http://dx.doi.org/10.1016/j.biomaterials.2010.10.027] [PMID: 21131044]

[635] Qin X-Y, Cheng Y, Yu L-C. Potential protection of curcumin against intracellular amyloid beta-induced toxicity in cultured rat prefrontal cortical neurons. Neurosci Lett 2010; 480(1): 21-4. [http://dx.doi.org/10.1016/j.neulet.2010.05.062] [PMID: 20638958]

[636] Ye J, Zhang Y. Curcumin protects against intracellular amyloid toxicity in rat primary neurons. Int J Clin Exp Med 2012; 5(1): 44-9. [PMID: 22328947]

[637] Gouras GK, Tsai J, Naslund J, *et al.* Intraneuronal Abeta42 accumulation in human brain. Am J Pathol 2000; 156(1): 15-20. [http://dx.doi.org/10.1016/S0002-9440(10)64700-1] [PMID: 10623648]

[638] Xiao Z, Lin L, Liu Z, *et al.* Potential therapeutic effects of curcumin: relationship to microtubule-associated proteins 2 in Aβ142 insult. Brain Res 2010; 1361: 115-23. [http://dx.doi.org/10.1016/j.brainres.2010.09.019] [PMID: 20840842]

[639] Srivastava RM, Singh S, Dubey SK, Misra K, Khar A. Immunomodulatory and therapeutic activity of curcumin. Int Immunopharmacol 2011; 11(3): 331-41. [http://dx.doi.org/10.1016/j.intimp.2010.08.014] [PMID: 20828642]

[640] Hsu C-H, Cheng A-L. Clinical studies with curcumin. Adv Exp Med Biol 2007; 595: 471-80. [http://dx.doi.org/10.1007/978-0-387-46401-5_21] [PMID: 17569225]

[641] Marathe SA, Dasgupta I, Gnanadhas DP, Chakravortty D. Multifaceted roles of curcumin: two sides of a coin! Expert Opin Biol Ther 2011; 11(11): 1485-99. [http://dx.doi.org/10.1517/14712598.2011.623124] [PMID: 21942554]

[642] Park S-Y, Kim H-S, Cho E-K, *et al.* Curcumin protected PC12 cells against beta-amyloid-induced toxicity through the inhibition of oxidative damage and tau hyperphosphorylation. Food Chem Toxicol 2008; 46(8): 2881-7. [http://dx.doi.org/10.1016/j.fct.2008.05.030] [PMID: 18573304]

[643] Lin M-S, Hung K-S, Chiu W-T, *et al.* Curcumin enhances neuronal survival in N-methyl-d-aspartic acid toxicity by inducing RANTES expression in astrocytes *via* PI-3K and MAPK signaling pathways. Prog Neuropsychopharmacol Biol Psychiatry 2011; 35(4): 931-8. [http://dx.doi.org/10.1016/j.pnpbp.2010.12.022] [PMID: 21199667]

[644] Mori I. Anti-herpesviral activity of curcumin may attenuate the development of Alzheimers disease.

Med Hypotheses 2015; 84(6): 603.
[http://dx.doi.org/10.1016/j.mehy.2015.03.014] [PMID: 25804240]

[645] McClure R, Yanagisawa D, Stec D, *et al.* Inhalable curcumin: offering the potential for translation to imaging and treatment of Alzheimers disease. J Alzheimers Dis 2015; 44(1): 283-95.
[PMID: 25227316]

[646] Okuda M, Hijikuro I, Fujita Y, *et al.* Design and synthesis of curcumin derivatives as tau and amyloid β dual aggregation inhibitors. Bioorg Med Chem Lett 2016; 26(20): 5024-8.
[http://dx.doi.org/10.1016/j.bmcl.2016.08.092] [PMID: 27624076]

[647] Rubagotti S, Croci S, Ferrari E, *et al.* Affinity of (nat/68)Ga-Labelled Curcumin and Curcuminoid Complexes for β-Amyloid Plaques: Towards the Development of New Metal-Curcumin Based Radiotracers. Int J Mol Sci 2016; 17(9): 17.
[http://dx.doi.org/10.3390/ijms17091480] [PMID: 27608011]

[648] Liu Z-J, Li Z-H, Liu L, *et al.* Curcumin attenuates beta-amyloid-induced neuroinflammation *via* activation of peroxisome proliferator-activated receptor-gamma function in a rat model of alzheimers disease. Front Pharmacol 2016; 7: 261.
[http://dx.doi.org/10.3389/fphar.2016.00261] [PMID: 27594837]

[649] Reddy PH, Manczak M, Yin X, *et al.* Protective effects of a natural product, curcumin, against amyloid β induced mitochondrial and synaptic toxicities in Alzheimers disease. J Investig Med 2016; 64(8): 1220-34.
[http://dx.doi.org/10.1136/jim-2016-000240] [PMID: 27521081]

[650] Rahimi HR, Nedaeinia R, Sepehri Shamloo A, Nikdoust S, Kazemi Oskuee R. Novel delivery system for natural products: Nano-curcumin formulations. Avicenna J Phytomed 2016; 6(4): 383-98.
[PMID: 27516979]

[651] Feng H-L, Dang H-Z, Fan H, *et al.* Curcumin ameliorates insulin signalling pathway in brain of Alzheimers disease transgenic mice. Int J Immunopathol Pharmacol 2016; 29(4): 734-41.
[http://dx.doi.org/10.1177/0394632016659494] [PMID: 27466310]

[652] Ferrari E, Benassi R, Saladini M, Orteca G, Gazova Z, Siposova K. *In vitro* study on potential pharmacological activity of curcumin analogues and their copper complexes. Chem Biol Drug Des 2016.
[http://dx.doi.org/10.1111/cbdd.12847] [PMID: 27569739]

[653] Liu Q-P, Wu Y-F, Cheng H-Y, *et al.* Habitual coffee consumption and risk of cognitive decline/dementia: A systematic review and meta-analysis of prospective cohort studies. Nutrition 2016; 32(6): 628-36.
[http://dx.doi.org/10.1016/j.nut.2015.11.015] [PMID: 26944757]

[654] Kim JH, Wang Q, Choi JM, Lee S, Cho EJ. Protective role of caffeic acid in an Aβ2535-induced Alzheimers disease model. Nutr Res Pract 2015; 9(5): 480-8.
[http://dx.doi.org/10.4162/nrp.2015.9.5.480] [PMID: 26425277]

[655] Modi KK, Roy A, Brahmachari S, Rangasamy SB, Pahan K. Cinnamon and Its Metabolite Sodium Benzoate Attenuate the Activation of p21rac and Protect Memory and Learning in an Animal Model of Alzheimers Disease. PLoS One 2015; 10(6): e0130398.
[http://dx.doi.org/10.1371/journal.pone.0130398] [PMID: 26102198]

[656] Hill JM, Lukiw WJ. Microbial-generated amyloids and Alzheimers disease (AD). Front Aging Neurosci 2015; 7: 9.
[http://dx.doi.org/10.3389/fnagi.2015.00009] [PMID: 25713531]

[657] Modi KK, Jana M, Mondal S, Pahan K. Sodium benzoate, a metabolite of cinnamon and a food additive, upregulates ciliary neurotrophic factor in astrocytes and oligodendrocytes. Neurochem Res 2015; 40(11): 2333-47.
[http://dx.doi.org/10.1007/s11064-015-1723-x] [PMID: 26399250]

[658] Singh RP, Chidambara Murthy KN, Jayaprakasha GK. Studies on the antioxidant activity of pomegranate (Punica granatum) peel and seed extracts using *in vitro* models. J Agric Food Chem 2002; 50(1): 81-6.
[http://dx.doi.org/10.1021/jf010865b] [PMID: 11754547]

[659] Hernández F, Melgarejo P, Tomás-Barberán FA, Artés F. Evolution of juice anthocyanins during ripening of new selected pomegranate (Punica granatum) clones. Eur Food Res Technol 1999; 210: 39-42.
[http://dx.doi.org/10.1007/s002170050529]

[660] Rojanathammanee L, Puig KL, Combs CK. Pomegranate polyphenols and extract inhibit nuclear factor of activated T-cell activity and microglial activation *in vitro* and in a transgenic mouse model of Alzheimer disease. J Nutr 2013; 143(5): 597-605.
[http://dx.doi.org/10.3945/jn.112.169516] [PMID: 23468550]

[661] Burton-Freeman BM, Sandhu AK, Edirisinghe I. Red raspberries and their bioactive polyphenols: cardiometabolic and neuronal health links. Adv Nutr 2016; 7(1): 44-65.
[http://dx.doi.org/10.3945/an.115.009639] [PMID: 26773014]

[662] Cicerale S, Conlan XA, Barnett NW, Sinclair AJ, Keast RS. Influence of heat on biological activity and concentration of oleocanthala natural anti-inflammatory agent in virgin olive oil. J Agric Food Chem 2009; 57(4): 1326-30.
[http://dx.doi.org/10.1021/jf803154w] [PMID: 19166297]

[663] Beauchamp GK, Keast RS, Morel D, *et al.* Phytochemistry: ibuprofen-like activity in extra-virgin olive oil. Nature 2005; 437(7055): 45-6.
[http://dx.doi.org/10.1038/437045a] [PMID: 16136122]

[664] Abuznait AH, Qosa H, Busnena BA, El Sayed KA, Kaddoumi A. Olive-oil-derived oleocanthal enhances β-amyloid clearance as a potential neuroprotective mechanism against Alzheimers disease: *in vitro* and *in vivo* studies. ACS Chem Neurosci 2013; 4(6): 973-82.
[http://dx.doi.org/10.1021/cn400024q] [PMID: 23414128]

[665] Monti MC, Margarucci L, Tosco A, Riccio R, Casapullo A. New insights on the interaction mechanism between tau protein and oleocanthal, an extra-virgin olive-oil bioactive component. Food Funct 2011; 2(7): 423-8.
[http://dx.doi.org/10.1039/c1fo10064e] [PMID: 21894330]

[666] Qosa H, Batarseh YS, Mohyeldin MM, El Sayed KA, Keller JN, Kaddoumi A. Oleocanthal enhances amyloid-β clearance from the brains of TgSwDI mice and *in vitro* across a human blood-brain barrier model. ACS Chem Neurosci 2015; 6(11): 1849-59.
[http://dx.doi.org/10.1021/acschemneuro.5b00190] [PMID: 26348065]

[667] Keiler AM, Djiogue S, Ehrhardt T, *et al.* Oleocanthal modulates estradiol-induced gene expression involving estrogen receptor α. Planta Med 2015; 81(14): 1263-9.
[http://dx.doi.org/10.1055/s-0035-1546194] [PMID: 26166135]

[668] Li R, Cui J, Shen Y. Brain sex matters: estrogen in cognition and Alzheimers disease. Mol Cell Endocrinol 2014; 389(1-2): 13-21.
[http://dx.doi.org/10.1016/j.mce.2013.12.018] [PMID: 24418360]

[669] Pantano D, Luccarini I, Nardiello P, Servili M, Stefani M, Casamenti F. Oleuropein aglycone and polyphenols from olive mill wastewater ameliorate cognitive deficits and neuropathology. Br J Clin Pharmacol 2016.
[PMID: 27131215]

[670] Casamenti F, Grossi C, Rigacci S, Pantano D, Luccarini I, Stefani M. Oleuropein aglycone: A possible drug against degenerative conditions. *in vivo* evidence of its effectiveness against alzheimers disease. J Alzheimers Dis 2015; 45(3): 679-88.
[PMID: 25649656]

[671] Rigacci S. Olive oil phenols as promising multi-targeting agents against alzheimer's disease. Adv Exp Med Biol 2015; 863: 1-20.
[http://dx.doi.org/10.1007/978-3-319-18365-7_1] [PMID: 26092624]

[672] Luccarini I, Pantano D, Nardiello P, *et al.* The polyphenol oleuropein aglycone modulates the PARP1-SIRT1 interplay: an *in vitro* and *in vivo* study. J Alzheimers Dis 2016; 54(2): 737-50.
[http://dx.doi.org/10.3233/JAD-160471] [PMID: 27567859]

[673] Nillni EA. The metabolic sensor Sirt1 and the hypothalamus: Interplay between peptide hormones and pro-hormone convertases. Mol Cell Endocrinol 2016; 438: 77-88.
[http://dx.doi.org/10.1016/j.mce.2016.09.002] [PMID: 27614022]

[674] Afzal M, Safer AM, Menon M. Green tea polyphenols and their potential role in health and disease. Inflammopharmacology 2015; 23(4): 151-61.
[http://dx.doi.org/10.1007/s10787-015-0236-1] [PMID: 26164000]

[675] Swaminathan A, Jicha GA. Nutrition and prevention of Alzheimers dementia. Front Aging Neurosci 2014; 6: 282.
[http://dx.doi.org/10.3389/fnagi.2014.00282] [PMID: 25368575]

[676] Capatti A, Montanari M. Italian cuisine: a cultural history (arts and traditions of the table: perspectives on culinary history. Harvard Medical School, Division of NUTRITION 2003.

[677] Godman H. Adopt a Mediterranean diet now for better health later. Boston: Harvard Health Publications 2016.

[678] Pallauf K, Giller K, Huebbe P, Rimbach G. Nutrition and healthy ageing: calorie restriction or polyphenol-rich MediterrAsian diet? Oxid Med Cell Longev 2013; 2013: 707421.
[http://dx.doi.org/10.1155/2013/707421] [PMID: 24069505]

[679] Stefani M, Rigacci S. Beneficial properties of natural phenols: highlight on protection against pathological conditions associated with amyloid aggregation. Biofactors 2014; 40(5): 482-93.
[http://dx.doi.org/10.1002/biof.1171] [PMID: 24890399]

[680] Sofi F, Cesari F, Abbate R, Gensini GF, Casini A. Adherence to Mediterranean diet and health status: meta-analysis. BMJ 2008; 337: a1344.
[http://dx.doi.org/10.1136/bmj.a1344] [PMID: 18786971]

[681] Frisardi V, Panza F, Seripa D, *et al.* Nutraceutical properties of Mediterranean diet and cognitive decline: possible underlying mechanisms. J Alzheimers Dis 2010; 22(3): 715-40.
[PMID: 20858954]

[682] Solfrizzi V, Frisardi V, Seripa D, *et al.* Mediterranean diet in predementia and dementia syndromes. Curr Alzheimer Res 2011; 8(5): 520-42.
[http://dx.doi.org/10.2174/156720511796391809] [PMID: 21605047]

[683] Lourida I, Soni M, Thompson-Coon J, *et al.* Mediterranean diet, cognitive function, and dementia: a systematic review. Epidemiology 2013; 24(4): 479-89.
[http://dx.doi.org/10.1097/EDE.0b013e3182944410] [PMID: 23680940]

[684] Singh B, Parsaik AK, Mielke MM, *et al.* Association of mediterranean diet with mild cognitive impairment and Alzheimers disease: a systematic review and meta-analysis. J Alzheimers Dis 2014; 39(2): 271-82.
[PMID: 24164735]

[685] Mosconi L, Murray J, Tsui WH, *et al.* Mediterranean diet and magnetic resonance imaging-assessed brain atrophy in cognitively normal individuals at risk for alzheimer's disease. J Prev Alzheimers Dis 2014; 1(1): 23-32.
[PMID: 25237654]

[686] Safouris A, Tsivgoulis G, Sergentanis TN, Psaltopoulou T. Mediterranean diet and risk of dementia. Curr Alzheimer Res 2015; 12(8): 736-44.

[http://dx.doi.org/10.2174/1567205012666150710114430] [PMID: 26159192]

[687] Yannakoulia M, Kontogianni M, Scarmeas N. Cognitive health and Mediterranean diet: just diet or lifestyle pattern? Ageing Res Rev 2015; 20: 74-8. [http://dx.doi.org/10.1016/j.arr.2014.10.003] [PMID: 25461244]

[688] Morris MC. Nutrition and risk of dementia: overview and methodological issues. Ann N Y Acad Sci 2016; 1367(1): 31-7. [http://dx.doi.org/10.1111/nyas.13047] [PMID: 27116239]

[689] Song C, Shieh C-H, Wu Y-S, Kalueff A, Gaikwad S, Su K-P. The role of omega-3 polyunsaturated fatty acids eicosapentaenoic and docosahexaenoic acids in the treatment of major depression and Alzheimers disease: Acting separately or synergistically? Prog Lipid Res 2016; 62: 41-54. [http://dx.doi.org/10.1016/j.plipres.2015.12.003] [PMID: 26763196]

[690] Solfrizzi V, Frisardi V, Capurso C, *et al.* Dietary fatty acids and predementia syndromes. ScientificWorldJournal 2009; 9: 792-810. [http://dx.doi.org/10.1100/tsw.2009.82] [PMID: 19705039]

[691] Solfrizzi V, Frisardi V, Capurso C, *et al.* Dietary fatty acids in dementia and predementia syndromes: epidemiological evidence and possible underlying mechanisms. Ageing Res Rev 2010; 9(2): 184-99. [http://dx.doi.org/10.1016/j.arr.2009.07.005] [PMID: 19643207]

[692] Kadish I, Kumar A, Beitnere U, Jennings E, McGilberry W, van Groen T. Dietary composition affects the development of cognitive deficits in WT and Tg AD model mice. Exp Gerontol 2016; 86: 39-49. [http://dx.doi.org/10.1016/j.exger.2016.05.003] [PMID: 27167583]

[693] Otsuka M. Prevention of Alzheimers Disease and Nutrients. Brain Nerve 2016; 68(7): 809-17. [PMID: 27395465]

[694] Miklossy J, McGeer PL. Common mechanisms involved in Alzheimers disease and type 2 diabetes: a key role of chronic bacterial infection and inflammation. Aging (Albany, NY) 2016; 8(4): 575-88. [http://dx.doi.org/10.18632/aging.100921] [PMID: 26961231]

[695] Cederholm T, Salem N Jr, Palmblad J. ω-3 fatty acids in the prevention of cognitive decline in humans. Adv Nutr 2013; 4(6): 672-6. [http://dx.doi.org/10.3945/an.113.004556] [PMID: 24228198]

[696] Zhang Y, Chen J, Qiu J, Li Y, Wang J, Jiao J. Intakes of fish and polyunsaturated fatty acids and mild-to-severe cognitive impairment risks: a dose-response meta-analysis of 21 cohort studies. Am J Clin Nutr 2016; 103(2): 330-40. [http://dx.doi.org/10.3945/ajcn.115.124081] [PMID: 26718417]

[697] Jackson PA, Forster JS, Bell JG, Dick JR, Younger I, Kennedy DO. DHA Supplementation Alone or in Combination with Other Nutrients Does not Modulate Cerebral Hemodynamics or Cognitive Function in Healthy Older Adults. Nutrients 2016; 8(2): 86. [http://dx.doi.org/10.3390/nu8020086] [PMID: 26867200]

[698] Liu L, Hu Q, Wu H, *et al.* Protective role of n6/n3 PUFA supplementation with varying DHA/EPA ratios against atherosclerosis in mice. J Nutr Biochem 2016; 32: 171-80. [http://dx.doi.org/10.1016/j.jnutbio.2016.02.010] [PMID: 27142749]

[699] de Souza Fernandes DP, Canaan Rezende FA, Pereira Rocha G, De Santis Filgueiras M, Silva Moreira PR, Gonçalves Alfenas RdeC. Effect of eicosapentaenoic acid and docosahexaenoic acid supplementations to control cognitive decline in dementia and Alzheimers disease: a systematic review. Nutr Hosp 2015; 32(2): 528-33. [PMID: 26268080]

[700] Yurko-Mauro K, Alexander DD, Van Elswyk ME. Docosahexaenoic acid and adult memory: a systematic review and meta-analysis. PLoS One 2015; 10(3): e0120391. [http://dx.doi.org/10.1371/journal.pone.0120391] [PMID: 25786262]

[701] Gebbink MF, Claessen D, Bouma B, Dijkhuizen L, Wösten HA. Amyloidsa functional coat for

microorganisms. Nat Rev Microbiol 2005; 3(4): 333-41.
[http://dx.doi.org/10.1038/nrmicro1127] [PMID: 15806095]

[702] Cegelski L, Pinkner JS, Hammer ND, *et al.* Small-molecule inhibitors target Escherichia coli amyloid biogenesis and biofilm formation. Nat Chem Biol 2009; 5(12): 913-9.
[http://dx.doi.org/10.1038/nchembio.242] [PMID: 19915538]

[703] Chorell E, Pinkner JS, Bengtsson C, *et al.* Design and synthesis of fluorescent pilicides and curlicides: bioactive tools to study bacterial virulence mechanisms. Chemistry 2012; 18(15): 4522-32.
[http://dx.doi.org/10.1002/chem.201103936] [PMID: 22431310]

[704] Arita-Morioka K, Yamanaka K, Mizunoe Y, Ogura T, Sugimoto S. Novel strategy for biofilm inhibition by using small molecules targeting molecular chaperone DnaK. Antimicrob Agents Chemother 2015; 59(1): 633-41.
[http://dx.doi.org/10.1128/AAC.04465-14] [PMID: 25403660]

[705] Cesa LC, Patury S, Komiyama T, Ahmad A, Zuiderweg ER, Gestwicki JE. Inhibitors of difficult protein-protein interactions identified by high-throughput screening of multiprotein complexes. ACS Chem Biol 2013; 8(9): 1988-97.
[http://dx.doi.org/10.1021/cb400356m] [PMID: 23819499]

[706] Wisniewski T, Sadowski M. Preventing beta-amyloid fibrillization and deposition: beta-sheet breakers and pathological chaperone inhibitors. BMC Neurosci 2008; 9 (Suppl. 2): S5.
[http://dx.doi.org/10.1186/1471-2202-9-S2-S5] [PMID: 19090993]

[707] Cheng B, Gong H, Xiao H, Petersen RB, Zheng L, Huang K. Inhibiting toxic aggregation of amyloidogenic proteins: a therapeutic strategy for protein misfolding diseases. Biochim Biophys Acta 2013; 1830(10): 4860-71.
[http://dx.doi.org/10.1016/j.bbagen.2013.06.029] [PMID: 23820032]

[708] Krebs MR, Bromley EH, Donald AM. The binding of thioflavin-T to amyloid fibrils: localisation and implications. J Struct Biol 2005; 149(1): 30-7.
[http://dx.doi.org/10.1016/j.jsb.2004.08.002] [PMID: 15629655]

[709] Inouye H, Kirschner DA. Alzheimers beta-amyloid: insights into fibril formation and structure from Congo red binding. Subcell Biochem 2005; 38: 203-24.
[http://dx.doi.org/10.1007/0-387-23226-5_10] [PMID: 15709480]

[710] Gazit E. A possible role for pi-stacking in the self-assembly of amyloid fibrils. FASEB J 2002; 16(1): 77-83.
[http://dx.doi.org/10.1096/fj.01-0442hyp] [PMID: 11772939]

[711] Gazit E. Mechanisms of amyloid fibril self-assembly and inhibition. Model short peptides as a key research tool. FEBS J 2005; 272(23): 5971-8.
[http://dx.doi.org/10.1111/j.1742-4658.2005.05022.x] [PMID: 16302962]

[712] Soto C, Sigurdsson EM, Morelli L, Kumar RA, Castaño EM, Frangione B. Beta-sheet breaker peptides inhibit fibrillogenesis in a rat brain model of amyloidosis: implications for Alzheimers therapy. Nat Med 1998; 4(7): 822-6.
[http://dx.doi.org/10.1038/nm0798-822] [PMID: 9662374]

[713] Soto C, Kindy MS, Baumann M, Frangione B. Inhibition of Alzheimers amyloidosis by peptides that prevent β-sheet conformation. Biochem Biophys Res Commun 1996; 226(3): 672-80.
[http://dx.doi.org/10.1006/bbrc.1996.1413] [PMID: 8831674]

[714] Permanne B, Adessi C, Saborio GP, *et al.* Reduction of amyloid load and cerebral damage in a transgenic mouse model of Alzheimers disease by treatment with a beta-sheet breaker peptide. FASEB J 2002; 16(8): 860-2.
[PMID: 11967228]

[715] Rijkers DT, Höppener JW, Posthuma G, Lips CJ, Liskamp RM. Inhibition of amyloid fibril formation of human amylin by N-alkylated amino acid and α-hydroxy acid residue containing peptides.

Chemistry 2002; 8(18): 4285-91.
[http://dx.doi.org/10.1002/1521-3765(20020916)8:18<4285::AID-CHEM4285>3.0.CO;2-0] [PMID: 12298020]

[716] Amijee H, Madine J, Middleton DA, Doig AJ. Inhibitors of protein aggregation and toxicity. Biochem Soc Trans 2009; 37(Pt 4): 692-6.
[http://dx.doi.org/10.1042/BST0370692] [PMID: 19614577]

[717] Hughes E, Burke RM, Doig AJ. Inhibition of toxicity in the beta-amyloid peptide fragment beta - (2535) using N-methylated derivatives: a general strategy to prevent amyloid formation. J Biol Chem 2000; 275(33): 25109-15.
[http://dx.doi.org/10.1074/jbc.M003554200] [PMID: 10825171]

[718] El-Agnaf OM, Paleologou KE, Greer B, *et al.* A strategy for designing inhibitors of alpha-synuclein aggregation and toxicity as a novel treatment for Parkinsons disease and related disorders. FASEB J 2004; 18(11): 1315-7.
[PMID: 15180968]

[719] Gordon DJ, Sciarretta KL, Meredith SC. Inhibition of beta-amyloid(40) fibrillogenesis and disassembly of beta-amyloid(40) fibrils by short beta-amyloid congeners containing N-methyl amino acids at alternate residues. Biochemistry 2001; 40(28): 8237-45.
[http://dx.doi.org/10.1021/bi002416v] [PMID: 11444969]

[720] Gordon DJ, Tappe R, Meredith SC. Design and characterization of a membrane permeable N-methyl amino acid-containing peptide that inhibits Abeta140 fibrillogenesis. J Pept Res 2002; 60(1): 37-55.
[http://dx.doi.org/10.1034/j.1399-3011.2002.11002.x] [PMID: 12081625]

[721] Kokkoni N, Stott K, Amijee H, Mason JM, Doig AJ. N-Methylated peptide inhibitors of β-amyloid aggregation and toxicity. Optimization of the inhibitor structure. Biochemistry 2006; 45(32): 9906-18.
[http://dx.doi.org/10.1021/bi060837s] [PMID: 16893191]

[722] Yan L-M, Tatarek-Nossol M, Velkova A, Kazantzis A, Kapurniotu A. Design of a mimic of nonamyloidogenic and bioactive human islet amyloid polypeptide (IAPP) as nanomolar affinity inhibitor of IAPP cytotoxic fibrillogenesis. Proc Natl Acad Sci USA 2006; 103(7): 2046-51.
[http://dx.doi.org/10.1073/pnas.0507471103] [PMID: 16467158]

[723] Porat Y, Abramowitz A, Gazit E. Inhibition of amyloid fibril formation by polyphenols: structural similarity and aromatic interactions as a common inhibition mechanism. Chem Biol Drug Des 2006; 67(1): 27-37.
[http://dx.doi.org/10.1111/j.1747-0285.2005.00318.x] [PMID: 16492146]

[724] Herrup K. The case for rejecting the amyloid cascade hypothesis. Nat Neurosci 2015; 18(6): 794-9.
[http://dx.doi.org/10.1038/nn.4017] [PMID: 26007212]

[725] Martorana A, Esposito Z, Koch G. Beyond the Cholinergic Hypothesis : Do Current Drugs Work in Alzheimer' s Disease ? 2010; 16: 235-45.

[726] Wisniewski T, Goñi F. Immunotherapy for Alzheimers disease. Biochem Pharmacol 2014; 88(4): 499-507.
[http://dx.doi.org/10.1016/j.bcp.2013.12.020] [PMID: 24412277]

[727] Bergström A-L, Kallunki P, Fog K. Development of Passive Immunotherapies for Synucleinopathies. Mov Disord 2016; 31(2): 203-13.
[http://dx.doi.org/10.1002/mds.26481] [PMID: 26704735]

[728] Dubey D, Kieseier BC, Hartung HP, Hemmer B, Miller-Little WA, Stuve O. Clinical management of multiple sclerosis and neuromyelitis optica with therapeutic monoclonal antibodies: approved therapies and emerging candidates. Expert Rev Clin Immunol 2015; 11(1): 93-108.
[http://dx.doi.org/10.1586/1744666X.2015.992881] [PMID: 25495182]

[729] Yang C, Xiao S. New developments of clinical trial in immunotherapy for Alzheimers disease. Curr Pharm Biotechnol 2015; 16(6): 484-91.

[http://dx.doi.org/10.2174/1389201016061504071123l9] [PMID: 25860060]

[730] Kennedy ME, Stamford AW, Chen X, *et al.* The BACE1 inhibitor verubecestat (MK-8931) reduces CNS β-amyloid in animal models and in Alzheimers disease patients. Sci Transl Med 2016; 8(363): 363ra150.
[http://dx.doi.org/10.1126/scitranslmed.aad9704] [PMID: 27807285]

[731] Panza F, Solfrizzi V, Imbimbo BP, *et al.* Efficacy and safety studies of gantenerumab in patients with Alzheimers disease. Expert Rev Neurother 2014; 14(9): 973-86.
[http://dx.doi.org/10.1586/14737175.2014.945522] [PMID: 25081412]

[732] Patel KR. Biogens aducanumab raises hope that Alzheimers can be treated at its source. Manag Care 2015; 24(6): 19.
[PMID: 26182718]

[733] Panza F, Seripa D, Solfrizzi V, *et al.* Emerging drugs to reduce abnormal β-amyloid protein in Alzheimers disease patients. Expert Opin Emerg Drugs 2016; 21(4): 377-91.
[http://dx.doi.org/10.1080/14728214.2016.1241232] [PMID: 27678025]

[734] Siemers ER, Sundell KL, Carlson C, *et al.* Phase 3 solanezumab trials: Secondary outcomes in mild Alzheimers disease patients. Alzheimers Dement 2016; 12(2): 110-20.
[http://dx.doi.org/10.1016/j.jalz.2015.06.1893] [PMID: 26238576]

[735] Liu E, Schmidt ME, Margolin R, *et al.* Bapineuzumab 301 and 302 Clinical Trial Investigators. Amyloid-β 11C-PiB-PET imaging results from 2 randomized bapineuzumab phase 3 AD trials. Neurology 2015; 85(8): 692-700.
[http://dx.doi.org/10.1212/WNL.0000000000001877] [PMID: 26208959]

[736] Delnomdedieu M, Duvvuri S, Li DJ, *et al.* First-In-Human safety and long-term exposure data for AAB-003 (PF-05236812) and biomarkers after intravenous infusions of escalating doses in patients with mild to moderate Alzheimers disease. Alzheimers Res Ther 2016; 8(1): 12.
[http://dx.doi.org/10.1186/s13195-016-0177-y] [PMID: 26925577]

[737] Logovinsky V, Satlin A, Lai R, *et al.* Safety and tolerability of BAN2401a clinical study in Alzheimers disease with a protofibril selective Aβ antibody. Alzheimers Res Ther 2016; 8(1): 14.
[http://dx.doi.org/10.1186/s13195-016-0181-2] [PMID: 27048170]

[738] Höfling C, Morawski M, Zeitschel U, *et al.* Differential transgene expression patterns in Alzheimer mouse models revealed by novel human amyloid precursor protein-specific antibodies. Aging Cell 2016; 15(5): 953-63.
[http://dx.doi.org/10.1111/acel.12508] [PMID: 27470171]

[739] Arendt T, Stieler JT, Holzer M. Tau and tauopathies. Brain Res Bull 2016; 126(Pt 3): 238-92.
[http://dx.doi.org/10.1016/j.brainresbull.2016.08.018] [PMID: 27615390]

[740] Funk KE, Mirbaha H, Jiang H, Holtzman DM, Diamond MI. Distinct therapeutic mechanisms of tau antibodies: promoting microglial clearance *versus* blocking neuronal uptake. J Biol Chem 2015; 290(35): 21652-62.
[http://dx.doi.org/10.1074/jbc.M115.657924] [PMID: 26126828]

[741] Panza F, Solfrizzi V, Seripa D, *et al.* Tau-based therapeutics for Alzheimers disease: active and passive immunotherapy. Immunotherapy 2016; 8(9): 1119-34.
[http://dx.doi.org/10.2217/imt-2016-0019] [PMID: 27485083]

[742] Combs B, Hamel C, Kanaan NM. Pathological conformations involving the amino terminus of tau occur early in Alzheimers disease and are differentially detected by monoclonal antibodies. Neurobiol Dis 2016; 94: 18-31.
[http://dx.doi.org/10.1016/j.nbd.2016.05.016] [PMID: 27260838]

[743] Kondo A, Shahpasand K, Mannix R, *et al.* Antibody against early driver of neurodegeneration cis P-tau blocks brain injury and tauopathy. Nature 2015; 523(7561): 431-6.
[http://dx.doi.org/10.1038/nature14658] [PMID: 26176913]

[744] Luz I, Liraz O, Michaelson DM. An anti-apoE4 specific monoclonal antibody counteracts the pathological effects of apoE4 *in vivo.* Curr Alzheimer Res 2016; 13(8): 918-29. [http://dx.doi.org/10.2174/1567205013666160404120817] [PMID: 27040139]

[745] Manoutcharian K, Perez-Garmendia R, Gevorkian G. Recombinant antibody fragments For neurodegenerative diseases. Curr Neuropharmacol 2016. [http://dx.doi.org/10.2174/1570159X01666160930121647] [PMID: 27697033]

[746] Loureiro JA, Gomes B, Fricker G, Coelho MA, Rocha S, Pereira MC. Cellular uptake of PLGA nanoparticles targeted with anti-amyloid and anti-transferrin receptor antibodies for Alzheimers disease treatment. Colloids Surf B Biointerfaces 2016; 145: 8-13. [http://dx.doi.org/10.1016/j.colsurfb.2016.04.041] [PMID: 27131092]

[747] Lathuilière A, Laversenne V, Astolfo A, *et al.* A subcutaneous cellular implant for passive immunization against amyloid-β reduces brain amyloid and tau pathologies. Brain 2016; 139(Pt 5): 1587-604. [http://dx.doi.org/10.1093/brain/aww036] [PMID: 26956423]

[748] Shimada H. Significance and progress of DIAN/A4/API. Nippon Rinsho 2016; 74(3): 417-22. [PMID: 27025079]

[749] Carrera I, Fernandez-Novoa L, Aliev G, Vigo C, Cacabelos R. Validating Immunotherapy in Alzheimers Disease: The EB101 Vaccine. Curr Pharm Des 2016; 22(7): 849-58. [http://dx.doi.org/10.2174/1381612822666151209152204] [PMID: 26648469]

[750] Mouri A, Noda Y, Hara H, Mizoguchi H, Tabira T, Nabeshima T. Oral vaccination with a viral vector containing Abeta cDNA attenuates age-related Abeta accumulation and memory deficits without causing inflammation in a mouse Alzheimer model. FASEB J 2007; 21(9): 2135-48. [http://dx.doi.org/10.1096/fj.06-7685com] [PMID: 17341681]

CHAPTER 2

The Menace of Malaria: An Overview

Satish Agrawal[1,2], **Hafsa Ahmad**[1], **Abhishek Arya**[1,2], **Pankaj Dwivedi**[1] and **Anil Kumar Dwivedi**[1,2,*]

[1] *Division of Pharmaceutics, CSIR-Central Drug Research Institute, Lucknow, (U.P)-226031, India*

[2] *Academy of Scientific and Innovative Research (AcSIR), Chennai-600113, TN, India*

Abstract: Malaria remains one of the most dreadful diseases affecting millions of people across the world. It is an infectious disease spread through the (female anopheles) mosquito caused by the parasitic protozoans belonging to genus Plasmodium. The most lethal species is *Plasmodium falciparum* which if left untreated, may cause organ failures (severe malaria) or may accumulate in brain (cerebral malaria) causing coma and finally leading to the death. The disease is mostly prevalent in Sub-Saharan Africa. Children under the age of 5 years, pregnant women and travellers to the malaria prone area are particularly at higher risk of getting malaria. It is typically diagnosed by microscopic examination of blood using blood film or antigen-based rapid diagnostic tests. The treatment of malaria comprises various synthetic, natural analogues administered orally or parenterally. The choice of therapeutic agents depends on the species of parasite, pattern of resistance and the seriousness of the infection.

Emergence and spread of the multidrug resistant strains of the causative organisms has extremely limited the choice of antimalarial chemotherapeutics. Only limited treatment options are currently available due to the resistant species highlighting the need of efficient research for developing newer broad spectrum antimalarial drugs. The discovery of potent vaccine against malaria still remains a major challenge amongst scientific community, with only limited success achieved till now.

The choice of the delivery system plays a vital role in determining fate of the drug as it's not only important for delivering the right drug at the right site, but also it can minimize the untoward effects of drugs. Nano-carriers or nanosystems are useful tools that are particularly gaining distinctive attention in malaria chemotherapy because of their ability to minimize the side effects, improve bioavailability and the selectivity of the drugs by altering the biopharmaceutics and pharmacokinetic property of the drug molecules.

Discovery of potent drugs like Arteether (ART) and Bulaquin have been some major breakthroughs in antimalarial research. However; the major challenge in management

* **Corresponding author Dr. Anil Kumar Dwivedi:** Division of Pharmaceutics, CSIR-CDRI, Lucknow, (U.P)-226031, India; Tel: +91 522 2772450; Email: anilcdri@gmail.com

Atta-ur-Rahman & M. Iqbal Choudhary (Eds.)

of malaria in the current scenario is to combat drug resistance and to develop new potent drugs in order to completely irradiate this fatal disease. This chapter is intended to highlight on some basic aspects of malaria, challenges in current chemotherapy, current investigations towards malaria chemotherapy and vaccine, and the use of nanotechnology as a promising strategy for malaria treatment.

Keywords: Malaria, *P. falciparum*, *P. vivax*, Artemisinin, Cinchona, Drug-resistance, Malaria vaccine, Nanotechnology, Parasite.

INTRODUCTION

Malaria is one of the most predominant ubiquitous parasitic diseases throughout the globe. The cause of the disease is an apicomplexan protozoan of *Plasmodium (P.)* genus. *P. falciparum* and *P. vivax*, are the major causative organisms. Malarial infection can be found all over the world but it is more common in tropical countries. In 2013, malaria was prevalent in more than 100 countries [1] over hundred million episodes of malaria have been estimated in 2012; in which more than 80% of these cases were reported in Africa, resulting over millions of deaths [2]. This is the statistics, when there was a drop of 50% or more malaria burden in 11 African and 32 of 56 malaria endemic countries outside Africa [3]. In 2015, the number of people infected from malaria have witnessed 21% decline with approximately 212 million malaria cases compared to 2010 because of the increased access to the disease-cutting tools to the needed populations. Approximately 4,29,000 death occurred in 2015 of which 92% deaths occurred in WHO African Region [4]. Among the cases occurring outside Africa, majority of cases were reported in Asian countries including India [1, 4]. The recent figures although show positive trends, there is a lot more to achieve for getting malaria free world.

Among several deaths which occur due to malaria every year, the majority are of children below 5 years of age. The occurrence of malarial infection is so high that most of the children without having acquired adequate immunity went through this infection in the initial years of their lifespan [1, 2, 5, 6]. WHO (World Health Organization) has started several programs to overcome these mortal malarial infections throughout the world, but still there is a lot of need for research and development as the current status of research in not considered being sufficient and there is a need for new therapies and vaccines.

Available malaria chemotherapy has been helpful but not in a significant manner, as these are associated with recurring failures [7]. The unique nature of the disease in relation to its transmission conditions, becomes a significant factor as it is more complex to manage its transmission throughout tropical areas [8]. The complex life cycle of the parasite and development of resistance to the drug are attributed as the principal challenging factors in new drug discovery [9] and causing higher mortality. An alarmingly high incidence of immune-compromised patients suffering from co-infections of malaria and HIV happens to be another crucial factor in new drug discovery [10, 11]. These infections together; account for more than millions of life per year. Moreover, the complex recommended regimen based on combination therapy increases the cost of treatment and brings down patient compliance, due to the associated side effects [7]. Tools and methodologies adopted to detain the prevalent dissemination of malaria include effective disease prevention by abolition of mosquitoes by means of insecticidal spray and providing treatment based on artemisinin combination therapy. The sporadic prophylactic treatment with antimalarial drugs has been used as a last option in case of pregnancy, to lower and reduce the deleterious effects of malaria infection on the fetus. Treatment protocols and regimens for malaria directly correlate to resistance developed by the parasite for the drug, as well as governed by government approach for prevention and control of mortality rate [12]. Taking into consideration the fact that fewer numbers of new antimalarials have been approved since 1990, the search for novel efficient and less toxic antimalarials accomplished with nano-delivery systems assumes significance

The present chapter is aimed to take the brief account of important aspects of malaria including its biology, current malaria chemotherapeutics and the associated problems with them, the current research in the field of antimalarial drug discovery with special focus on nanotechnology. The chapter also covers the role of Central Drug Research Institute (CSIR-CDRI) in the discovery and development of antimalarial drugs.

Methods

The authors made use of search engines and databases such as ScieFinder and Pub-Med and relevant guidelines from World Health Organization, (WHO) for data collection. Data was collected on current global status, statistics, biology and the detailed pathophysiology of malaria. Details about the risk factors, preventive measures, treatment regimens, and the problems associated with the malaria chemotherapy were collected. Detailed information about currents antimalarial leads (from both synthetic and natural sources), research on malaria vaccine, role of CSIR-CDRI in antimalarial research, and the role of nano-formulations in malaria treatment was obtained. The detailed information regarding each topic was collected by narrowing the search by using 2 or more key words. The assimilated data was studied and interpreted, compiled and arranged under different headings covered in this chapter to create a comprehensive insight into the topic and to produce a detailed overview.

MALARIA "A COMPLEX PARASITIC DISEASE"

Life Cycle of the Malaria Parasite

P. falciparum and *P. vivax* are the most widespread *Plasmodium* species causing malaria. *P. falciparum* happens to be the parasite responsible for the severely fatal form of malaria. *P. ovale and P. vivax* are predormant in liver-stage of parasites life cycle *i.e* hypnozoites while *P. malariae* is said to produce long-lasting infections and, when left untreated, it has the ability to persist asymptomatically in the human host for several years, might be a lifetime [8]. When the infected mosquito bites an individual, it marks the start of the life cycle of the malaria parasite in the human host. The inoculated sporozoites move to the liver, thus cause an invasion to the liver cells (hepatocytes) by certain unknown mechanisms (Fig. **1**) [13].

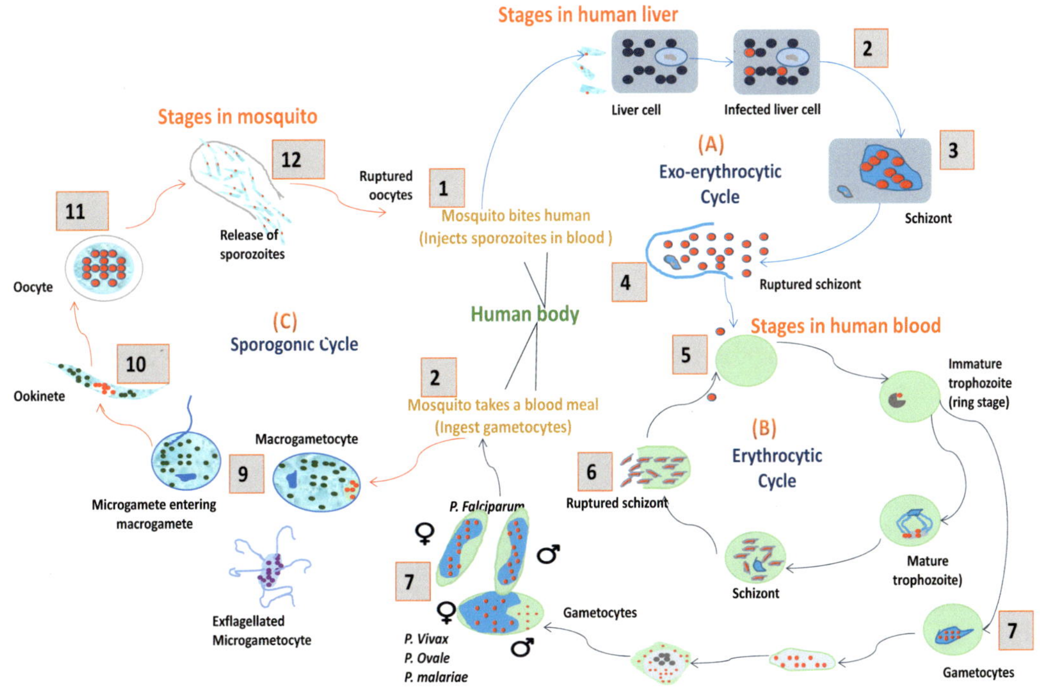

Fig. (1). Life cycle of malaria parasite and its different stages.

One sporozoite is likely to generate approximately thirty thousand new parasites in *P. falciparum* infection and ten thousand new parasites in *P. vivax* infection. *P. vivax* infection induces slow developing sporozoites, called hypnozoites, which might stay in the liver tissues for months. Hypnozoites invariably causes new relapse in malaria for two years after the primary infection. However, the two major asexual blood stages (late trophozoites stage and schizonts stage) are the basic carriers of malaria, resulting in symptoms of infection to appear about fourteen days after the inoculation of mosquito-vectored sporozoite. Thus the asexual intra-erythrocytic stages are probably assumed as the key subject for the development of antimalarials. Invasive forms of the parasite (merozoite) enter the RBCs (red blood cells) and remain there in a metabolically inactive phase for ten to fifteen hours (known as the ring stage). A rapid growth phase is followed for the coming twenty five hours, which constitutes the trophozoite stage; whereby the parasite digests the most of the hemoglobin and grows to increase and occupy more than 50% of the host cell volume. Heme is formed when the hemoglobin is digested in the vacuole. The formed heme now associates with one of the peripheral carboxyl groups *via* the ferric ion of the neighboring heme molecule to result into insoluble hemeozoin. The ending stage of the trophozoite is marked by numerous divisions that parasites undergoes (the schizont stage) prior to lyses of the host cell (48 h after invasion) and after the lyses it releases the new merozoites formed, which further move on with its life cycle. The cell lysis signals the first appearance of the signs and symptoms of classical malaria.

Symptoms

The major symptoms of the malaria are periodic recurrent high fever (every 48–72 h), headache, anemia, myalgia, splenomegaly and hepatitis [9]. In severe case of *P. falciparum* infection the neurological symptoms occur that might lead to death. The cerebral malaria syndrome is the severe form of disease, and affects largely the children inhabiting the tropics causing a neurological handicap [14]. Cerebral malaria pathogenesis is multi-factorial as it is due to parasite sequestration resulting incomplete stoppage of flow of blood to small vessels in the brain, subsequently blockage, sequestration, rosette formation, cerebral edema, cytokines release and high intracranial hypertension [15, 16]. In the absence of promptly instituted treatment, in case of *P. falciparum* induced disease leads to death, especially referring to acute primary infections [17].

Pathophysiology

Malaria is one of the complex diseases. To understand the disease, we need to understand its pathophysiology since it is a vital aspect of any disease as it provides major step to control this disease.

Several studies have suggested that *P. falciparum* is able to adhere with RBCs on the endothelial lining of small blood vessels by modifying its surface so that asexual parasites and gametocytes can adhere there. It causes hurdle in tissue perfusion. This adherence of RBCs on the endothelial lining of small blood vessels provides protection to parasite's from destruction in spleen as well as help to mature parasites which are not adhering on RBCs. Two receptors which are responsible for adherence are CD36 and chondroitin sulphate A. PfEMP1 (*P. falciparum* erythrocytes membrane protein-1) is present in infected RBCs surface which allows parasite binding to various receptors and also helps in recognising the various host. PfEMP1 provides multiple adhesions which are present at extracellular regions [18, 19].

In severe cases of malaria, it leads to higher reduction in deformability of uninfected RBC. It was assumed that it is related with acidosis predominantly lactic acidosis [19]. Malarial patients may also feel dehydrated and hypovolemic. Destruction of RBCs plays an important role in malaria which causes anaemia and causes the reduction in oxygen delivery. Therefore it may lead to hypoxia in some cases [18, 19].

Parasites which are present in the brain area associated with cerebral malaria which involves ICAM-1 (intracellular adhesive molecule 1). In brain endothelium, increased expression of ICAM-1 shows the differences of parasite adhesion in the cerebral malaria. By the support of nonsense mutation in the gene of the adhesion receptors CD36, pathogenic relation was formed between adhesion and host. Binding at multiple receptors by parasite may increase the severity of malaria by showing different properties of adhesion of RBCs such as rosetting and clumping [19 - 21].

Antibodies and cytokines tumour necrosis factor –α and interferon-γ and nitric oxide (NO) may provide defence against an asexual blood stages of malaria. One of the hypothesis also suggested that tumour necrosis factor -α induces brain endothelial cells to express ICAM-1. In cerebral malaria its expression gets increased. It also suggested that in uncomplicated malaria, concentration of NO is higher. Due to increase in concentration of NO in brain, it may result in coma [19]. Infection of *P. falcipuram* causes apoptosis in the mononuclear cells of human body. But still most of hypothesis is unclear [20].

Risk Factors

Risk factors are attributes associated with specific risk. Several risk factors for malaria are:

• Travelling of people from endemic area to malaria free area or from area of low endemicity to hyper-endemicity.

- Interruption in control measures by factors like emergence of resistance or low maintenance of
- Higher population density encouraging mosquito bites.
- Stagnant water
- Inadequate health and services or centres.
- Flooding
- Change in other weather patterns.
- Behavioural factor: Since human behaviour is influenced by socio- economic reasons, it can have greater impact on the risk of malaria, it includes-
  - Poor people in rural areas often cannot afford the housing and bed net that can provide protection from being infected
  - The lack of knowledge to recognize malaria and to treat it in rural areas can also play an important role
  - Increasing domestic animals nearby residential area may play a important role by providing the feast of blood for mosquitoes which will then reduce the human exposure [22, 23].

PREVENTIVE MEASURES

Vector is responsible for transmission of malaria parasite from one host to another. Different vectors may be responsible for transmission of malaria therefore for control over malaria one of the most important target should be control on vectors so as to reduce the transmission [24 - 27]. Various methods for vector control are as per follows-

Insecticide-Treated Mosquito Nets

Insecticide-treated bed nets (ITNs) are one of the ways of personal protection that can reduce malaria sickness, disease severity, and deaths due to malaria. Malaria vectors can be easily controlled by using ITNs. The spread of malaria gets arrested due to avoidance of contact of vectors with the susceptible persons. Most of the malaria endemic countries have adopted policies to promote use of ITNs. However use of ITNs is being increasingly promoted specially in Africa; where the highest population proportion is at risk of malaria. The rise in the percentage of the population sleeping under an ITN has accomplished by increased access to ITNs in the household [28].

The control of mosquito populations with ITNs and indoor residual sprays remains the foundation of malaria reduction and elimination programs [29]. ITNs have been proved to be effective in decreasing malaria morbidity and mortality in many areas. Unfortunately in some regions, malaria has persevered despite the increasing use of ITNs. Recent reports stipulate that human behaviour and mosquito behaviour are potential threats to the efficacy of ITNs [30]. India is the most malaria-endemic country in South-East Asia; therefore malaria has resulted in a high socio-economic burden. As part of an Indian first-aid guideline project, the magnitude of effects of ITNs was investigated in India. It was observed that both treated and untreated nets were able to produce protection from malaria in the Indian context. This effect is more pronounced in India than in other countries [31].

Indoor Residual Spraying

Indoor residual spraying (IRS) is the main vector control programme in malaria elimination. It has potential to reduce malaria transmission from low base line to zero level transmission, in localities where vector population is higher [24, 32]. IRS is the process of spraying of insecticide in the households to kill the malaria vectors. The dilute solution of an insecticide can also be sprayed on the porous walls of house where the parasites dwell. The vectors can be killed or repelled by the IRS thus controlling malaria. It is reported that worldwide about 116 million people were protected by IRS in 2014. This comprised of 50 million people in the WHO Africa region and about 44 million people were in India [28]. For the successful control of malaria vectors, the control of both the larval and adult stages is required. The adult control methods through IRS and utilization of long-lasting insecticidal nets continue to be widely used with some high accounts of success [33].

In the study conducted in Lagos, Nigeria the comparative malariometric indices of children under 5 years of age living in IRS-implementing and non-IRS-implementing communities were determined and it was found that IRS caused reduction in the level of parasitaemia in the study areas [34]. In yet another study conducted in Tororo, Uganda, the impact of IRS on malaria in pregnancy and birth outcomes was determined. In this study, IRS was temporally linked with lower prevalence of malaria parasite during pregnancy and at delivery, and it also improved birth outcomes. Therefore IRS may be a chief tool for defeating malaria in pregnancy and for improving birth outcomes in malaria-endemic regions [33]. The addition of IRS is reported to cause decline in the burden of malaria. However, in highly endemic areas of Africa with widespread pyrethroid resistance, IRS using alternative insecticide formulations may be needed to achieve substantial gains in malaria control [35]. The addition of IRS is reported to cause decline in the burden of malaria. However, in highly endemic areas of Africa with widespread pyrethroid resistance, IRS using alternative insecticide formulations may be needed to achieve substantial gains in malaria control [35].

Larval Control

The larval control of malaria is practiced by at least 48 countries. This type of control involves modification or manipulation of vector habitat, larvicidal and biological control (such as use of larval predator fish) [28]. The interruption of the early and late larval stages can lead to decreased emergence of adult mosquito and low adult mosquito densities. Larviciding may be used to control mosquito vector density by conquering the larval stages thereby reducing adult emergence and malaria risk. In one study, water bodies in the intervention villages were treated using a WHO recommended bio-larvicide, *Bacillus thuringiensis* var. *Israelensis*. It was applied at a rate of 300 g per hectare. There was deduction in the population of the mosquito larvae after using *Bacillus thuringiensis* [36].

TREATMENT OF MALARIA

Chemotherapy strategically reduces the death rate associated with malaria. The choice of most appropriate treatment for a malaria patient should presumably be begin by the identifying the causative *Plasmodium* species, the degree of severity of disease, existence of any pre-infection exposure and determining the patient's clinical condition as well as the response towards the drugs. In current scenario, an effective treatment for malaria by the prevalent species of *Plasmodium i.e. P. vivax* and *P. falciparum* is not possible, because of the differences in the susceptibility of each *Plasmodium* species towards the recommended drugs [37].

The existing antimalarial drugs are broadly categorized into 4 major drug classes a. Quinoline derivatives, b. Antifolates c. Artemisinin derivatives and d. Antimicrobial [38]. The brief account of these classes is discussed in the following sections and Table **1**.

Table 1. Account of some of the major antimalarial drug.

Drug	Class	Uses	Adverse effects	Comments
Mefloquine (MQ)	Quinoline derivatives	long-acting blood schizonticide active against CQ and SP resistant *P. falciparum* cases; highly effective against *P. vivax, P. malariae* [86]	Largely well tolerated [87] but neuropsychiatric adverse reactions [88], dizziness, nausea, vomiting, insomnia and fatigue [86, 87, 89]	It has been used both for prophylaxis and treatment during pregnancy [86]

(Table 1) contd.....

Drug	Class	Uses	Adverse effects	Comments
Amodiaquine	Quinoline derivative	Treatment of infection with some CQ resistant *P. falciparum* strains	Unusual but serious toxic effects like agranulocytosis and hepatoxicity can be observed [90]	Can also used in combination with artesunate [91]
Halofantrine	Quinoline derivative	active against blood stage of all malaria parasites	Rare reports of cardiac toxicity, nausea, vomiting, skin reactions, abdominal pain, diarrhea, convulsions, pruritis, acute intravascular hemolysis [92 - 98]	Reported to be effective against CQ-resistant *P. falciparum* and *P. vivax* [99]
sulfadoxine + pyrimethamine combination	Antifolates	highly effective as blood schizonticides against *P. falciparum* [100]	Generally well tolerated but infrequent and mild adverse effects like abdominal pain, nausea, diarrhoea, headache and itching can occur [101]	Largely ineffective in almost all parts of the Latin America and Southeast Asia [102]
Atovaquone – proguanil combination	Antifolates	Against the blood stage infection of *P. falciparum*, including CQ and MQ resistant strains [103, 104]	Generally well tolerated, though abdominal pain, nausea, vomiting and diarrhea, anaphylaxis are reported [105]	Due to high cost, mainly used for treatment and/or prevention in travellers [86]
Fosmidomycin	Antimicrobials	Fosmidomycin as monotherapy has been shown to be very effective against *P. falciparum*	Generally well tolerated although mild gastrointestinal side effects are reported [106]	Acts through inhibition of 1-deoxy-D-xylulose 5-phosphate reductoisomerase, an enzyme of the nonmevalonate pathway of isoprenoid biosynthesis
Clindamycin	Antimicrobials	Can be used for uncomplicated resistant falciparum malaria in semi-immune patients in the tropics	Generally well tolerated	Fosmidomycin-clindamycin is a promising novel treatment option for malaria [107]

(Table 1) contd.....

Drug	Class	Uses	Adverse effects	Comments
Doxycycline	Antimicrobials	Slow-acting blood schizontocidal agent [108] used in the treatment of CQ-resistant *falciparum* malaria [109, 110]	Fever, headache and dizziness are common [110]	In combination with QN, it can be an excellent candidate for treatment of drug resistant malaria [111]

Breakthrough in Anti-Malarials Agents: History of Cinchona

One of the most captivating epic in the history of medicine and therapeutics is the emergence of the Peruvian bark (Cinchona) and the isolation of pharmacologically active substance, quinine (QN) from it [39]. The revelation of QN's activity to treat malaria in the 17th century brought a revolution to the medical world [40]. QN is a component of the bark of the cinchona (quina-quina) tree which is indigenous to remote mountain areas of Latin America. The tree was referred to as the “Jesuits’ bark,” “sacred bark,” or “cardinal’s bark” in the 17th century [41].

According to a folk tale, an Indian with a high fever was strayed in an Andean forest. Thirsty, he drank water from a pond, but realized that it tasted bitter after perceiving that the water has been contaminated by the surrounding quina-quina tree. He believed that he was poisoned, but to his surprise, his fever was cured. He then shared his experience with the fellow villagers, who thereafter started using the extracts of quina-quina bark for fever treatment [42]. However; there is a different story in Europe regarding finding of antimalarial activity of this plant. It includes the Spanish Countess of Chinchon who, while in Peru, suffered a fever that was cured by the bark of a tree. After coming back to Spain with the bark, she presented QN to Europe in 1638. In 1742, botanist Carl Linnaeus called the tree “Cinchona” in her tribute [41].

Isolation of QN and alkaloids of cinchona was attained in France in the earlier part 19th century and the uncertainties of supply of the bark encouraged efforts to synthesize QN [43]. After this achievement, purified QN replaced the bark for the treatment for malaria [44]. QN and other cinchona alkaloids (quinidine, cinchonine and cinchonidine) are all efficacious against malaria. The antimalarial activity of these four alkaloids was tested in one of the earliest clinical trials, conducted during 1866-1868 in 3600 patients. With the principal outcome measure of “cessation of febrile paroxysms”, all four alkaloids showed comparable cure rates of >98%. QN remained as the main drug of malaria treatment until the 1920s, when more efficacious synthetic anti-malarials became available [41]. Today QN is produced both synthetically and from the tree bark

[40] and it still remains un important antimalarial drug. 2010 WHO guidelines recommend a combination of QN with doxycycline, clindamycin or tetracycline as second-line treatment for uncomplicated malaria (to be used when first-line drug treatment fails or it is not available) and QN plus clindamycin for malaria treatment in the first trimester of pregnancy [45]. Beside malaria, cinchona alkaloids are also having crucial activity against autoimmune disorders such as Lupus and rheumatoid arthritis [40].

Other Antimalarials from Cinchona

Chloroquine

Chloroquine (CQ) is observed to have many pharmacokinetic and pharmacological merits over most other antimalarials, which is evident from its excellent performance for about eight decades in the treatment and management of malaria, in spite of the resistance associated with CQ in various *Plasmodium* strains. The mechanism of action of CQ largely relies on its accumulation in the vacuole of the parasitic agent (lysosomotropic character) which in turn hampers the polymerization of noxious heme monomers [46, 47]. It causes parasite death by heme poisoning. The major beneficial outcome of CQ therapy are its low cost, water solubility, quick action in blood parasitic stages, reduced toxicity, high volume of distribution in the body and good oral bioavailability from various dosage forms.

Primaquine

Primaquine (PQ); a schizontocidal antimalarial is used for the treatment of all forms of malaria; it prevents the basic installation of parasitemia. By large, PQ is available in the present market as the only drug in relapse therapy (terminal prophylaxis). It prevents delayed recurrence due to *P. vivax* and *P. ovale* hypnozoites. PQ provides a radical cure option in patients with *P. vivax* or *P. Ovale* infection [48] and is active against gametocytes in a unit dose (sexual erythrocytic forms) but its high toxicity is a major drawback associated with PQ [11].

Tafenoquine

PQ analogue namely Tafenoquine, is presently under development phase. It was found to be effective in the radical cure of relapse malaria as well as in the prophylaxis of *P. vivax* infections and *P. falciparum* infections. Studies revealed that it showed a protective efficacy of more than ninety percent and has a relatively safe profile for use in malaria patients. Currently it represents a potential alternate to PQ in preventing infection as well as in the treatment and mitigation of malaria [48, 49].

Artemisinin Derivatives

Artemisinin is a sesquiterpene lactone having an endoperoxide bridge which is essential for its antimalarial activity and is a characteristic feature of this class of drugs. Due to solubility issues with the parent drug artemisinin, its carbonyl group was reduced to obtain dihydroartemisinin and its derivatives like the oil soluble artemether and ART and the water-soluble artesunate. These newer derivatives possess greater antimalarial activity. Artemisinins are a potent class of antimalarial agents, and are effective against nearly all asexual and sexual parasite stages [50, 51]. Artemisinins are capable of killing the malaria parasites within minutes (parasite reduction ratio of about 10,000 per RBC cycle) and thus exhibiting rapid clinical responses [52, 53]. Cinchona alkaloids (QN and quinidine) and artemisinins are presently the two classes of compounds being used to manage cases of severe malaria. Several clinical trials have shown that, artemisinins outperform QN on direct comparison basis [54, 55]. When oral therapy of malaria patients is not possible due to impaired consciousness, vomiting, prostration, suppository formulations of artemisinins provide the required additional advantages for easier administration especially in severe malaria [56, 57]. Although artemisinins are the fastest acting drug against all erythrocytic stages of malaria parasites, they have a very short elimination half-life (~1 h), which limits their use. Artemisinin derivatives are promptly bio-transformed into their bioactive metabolite dihydroartemisinin, and subsequently it gets eliminated by glucuronidation [58, 59]. Their metabolism is mediated mainly by the liver cytochrome P450 enzyme CYP2B6. The extent of conversion varies depending on the derivatives: artesunate is transformed to dihydroartemisinin within minutes, however conversion of artemether and ART is relatively slower [60]. Artemisinins auto-induces the CYP450 metabolizing enzymes, which leads to reduced plasma concentrations of the drugs in subsequent administrations [61, 62]. Rapid elimination artemisinins in humans is favoured as it prevents the selection of resistant parasites by remaining concentration of the drugs. The short half-life of artemisinins can be attributed to low cure rates and increased rates of recrudescence (more than 25%) for short courses (3-5 days). Even seven day regimens of artemisinin mono-therapy have been reported to cure only 80–90% of uncomplicated *falciparum* malaria [63, 64]. This is one major reason that combination therapies of artemisinin with a long-lasting drug are recommended for treatment in *falciparum* infections [65].

Mode of Action and Potential Cellular Targets of Artemisinins

Knowledge and understanding of the mode of action is imperative for designing artemisinin derivatives with improved antiparasitic activity and predicting resistance mechanisms. Although tremendous inputs have been put in for research on artemisinin; since its discovery, a debate concerning its mode of action on malaria parasites still remains considerably complex [66, 67]. Studies indicate that artemisinins are prodrugs which get activated to generate carbon-centered free radicals or reactive oxygen species (ROS). Since the O-centered radical produced upon cleavage; is unable to oxidatively cycle, ROS is less significant for artemisinins action [68]. Endoperoxide Bridge in the trioxane pharmacophore of artemisinins, is vital for their anti-malarial activity, as replacing oneperoxidic oxygen with a carbon (1-carba-10-deoxyartemisinin) results in a derivative which shows absence of antimalarial activity. This revelation inspired the design and synthesis of the next generation antimalarial endoperoxides and several trioxanes [69, 70]. Since it's a well known fact that peroxides are sources of ROS, some earlier studies suggest that artemisinins potentially modulated parasite oxidative stress and decreased the antioxidants and glutathione levels in the parasite [71]. In relation to the ring opening of artemisinins during its bio-activation, two models have been postulated that differ in their iron dependency and the role of C-centered radicals. The first theory based on reductive scission model proposes that binding of low-valent transition irons (namely ferrous heme ornonheme, exogenous Fe^{2+}) to artemisinin and the consequent electron transfer induces reductive scission of the peroxide bridge to generate O-centered radical, which then self arranges to produce a C-centered free radical [72]. In comparison, the second theory based on the open peroxide model indicates that the ring opening of artemisinins may be caused by protonation of the peroxide or by complexation with Fe^{2+}. The second model emphasizes upon the intrinsic chemical reactivity of the peroxide group which acts as an oxidant and its ability to form ROS, which is not always dependent on the presence of metal ions. Since the parasite is high on heme iron due to digestion of hemoglobin, it assumes natural obviousness to conjecture involvement of intraparasitic heme in the activation of artemisinins, and this may also explain the reason behind the selective toxicity of artemisinins and the related trioxanes towards malaria parasites [73]. In *in-vitro* conditions, hemin catalyzes the reductive decomposition of artemisinins while *in vivo*, artemisinin binds to intracellular heme, and this binding affinity seems to correlate with their antimalarial activities. Additionally iron chelators are reported to antagonize the activities of artemisinins [74 - 76]. Despite the fact that the heme dependent activation model is well received and follows wide acceptance, it also has been challenged. Haynes *et al.* compared the structure–activity relationships (SAR) of synthetic artemisinin derivatives and were of the opinion that the efficiency of their conversion to C-centered radicals did not logically correlate with their antimalarial activity [77]. Their more recent work suggests that the C-centered radicals are too ephemeral to favorably cause any intermolecular interactions. Moreover, the observable antagonistic effects of iron chelators apply only on some artemisinin derivatives not all, and the *in vitro* observations have yet not been correlated *in vivo* [78]. Secondly, the cidal effects of artemisinins on early ring-stage parasites with little hemozoin content, as well as on parasite species such as Babesia and Toxoplasma which do not form any hemozoin also presents a logical argument against the heme-dependent activation model [79, 80]. Regardless of the debates pertaining, both models may be compatible based on iron-dependent production of ROS species [81], given the probabilities of further reactions of the C- or O-centered radicals with the cellular redox systems or lipids. For instance, reaction with reduced GSH by C-centered primary radicals will lower the GSH levels in the parasite, which may lessen the parasite's capability to deal with oxidative stress. The artemisinin-derived free radicals once produced cause damage to cellular targets in their vicinity *via* alkylation. A combination of both hemin and high concentrations of artemisinin is capable of readily oxidizing the erythrocyte membrane thiols *in vitro*, thus demonstrating the manifested reactivity of artemisinin derived radicals with bio-molecules [82]. The extremely low artemisinin toxicity at therapeutic doses and the tendency of these radicals for intra-molecular reactions strongly indicate that artemisinin-derived radicals, unlike other typical alkyl agents, are selective in action and they selectively damage cellular targets [83].

Besides these drugs, some of the other useful chemotherapeutic agents active against malaria parasites are narrated in Table **1**. These drugs have limited use as they are not effective against MDR malaria, due to the development of *Plasmodium* resistance against these conventional therapies. Although artemisinin derivatives such as ART are more effective against MDR malaria and now are widely used and recommended for the severe condition of malaria and where the entire conventional drug regimen fails, but there are several reports of development of resistance for ART [84, 85] that necessities the development of newer and potent therapeutics against malaria.

PROBLEMS ASSOCIATED WITH MALARIA CHEMOTHERAPY

There has not been a single drug ever discovered or manufactured that is capable of wiping out all strains of the malaria parasites. Therefore the search for the newer drug or drug combinations that can fight malaria effectively still continues [38]. Due to their genetic diversity, the *Plasmodium* strains exhibit a peculiar ability to evade and overcome the unfavorable conditions brought about by drug therapy, and subsequently develop complex mechanisms for drug resistance. Hence, vast numbers of popularly used antimalarial therapies have lost their usefulness in recent times. The most significant challenges in malaria treatment that have surfaced off late remain CQ and MDR. Mutations on the *P. falciparum* multidrug resistance protein-1 gene (pfmdr1) the *P. falciparum* CQ resistance transporter gene, respectively might be the probable reasons for resistance. Two putative protein transporters shown by *P. falciparum*, namely the CQ resistance transporter and the P-glycoprotein homologue 1 are the products of the gene expression, which might be implicated in the CQ-resistance phenomenon. Both these transporters lay on the membrane of the digestive vacuole of *Plasmodium*. *Plasmodium* strains with CQ-resistance accumulate lesser amounts of drug in the digestive vacuole and this protects them against drug damage. On prolonged and continued exposure to drug, the resistant strains turn dominant with time. P-glycoprotein homologue 1 transporter is also implicated *P. falciparum* resistance to MQ, with amplification of the gene encoding this transporter as associated with *in vitro* and *in vivo* resistance to MQ. New strategies and techniques for intracellular delivery of antimalarials assume priority for prevention of drug-resistance. Drugs encapsulated in nano-matrix systems would be successful in bypassing both CQ transporters that are capable to pass through the vacuole membrane through different mechanisms [112]. Reversing CQ-resistance using nano-carriers loaded with CQ and similar approaches could be utilized and exploited.

Another significant aspect in malaria is the route of administration. For clinically uncomplicated malaria the oral route is the preferred choice. But, parenteral therapy is advised in severe cases or in complicated malaria and intravenous administration becomes obligatory in cerebral malaria management. The use of QN or artemisinin, which are effective antimalarials by the parenteral route largely remain the mainstay of cerebral malaria therapy. Certain issues though might crop up with the parenteral route: QN presents increased toxicity and artemisinin derivatives are lipophilic and therefore present short plasma half-lives [113, 114]. Based on these findings, it can be said that developing efficacious intravenous formulations, which present lower side effects of QN with improved solubility and pharmacokinetic profile of artemisinin in the cerebral malaria treatment is the need of the hour. The primary aim of malaria therapy is to provide and promote a high drug concentration in the intracellular parasitophorous vacuole as the *Plasmodium* is hosted there [50].

Malaria Treatment Failure

The treatment against malaria can be failed because of the true antimalarial drug resistance or because of some other reasons. Though drug resistance causes treatment failure, not all treatment failures are because of the drug resistance. There are many factors like incorrect dosing, poor drug quality, non-agreement with the duration of drug regimen. These factors therefore while causing the treatment failure probably may contribute for development of resistance due to increase in the exposure of parasites to suboptimal drug levels.

Antimalarial Drug Resistance

Drug resistance in malaria was initially outlined in 1967 by WHO and they defined it as, "the ability of the parasite strain to survive and/or to multiply despite the administration and absorption of a drug administered in doses equal to or higher than those actually recommended but within the limits of tolerance of the subject [115]. Till now, there are reports of drug resistance in three of the five Plasmodium species that are *P. falciparum, P. vivax* and *P. valariae* [116]. Southeast Asia has witnessed the emergence of resistance in falciparum malaria for chloroquine, sulfadoxine, pyrimethamine, quinine, mefloquine and artemisinins [85].

Drug resistance generally causes delay or failure in clearance of asexual parasites from the blood. It finally enables the production of gametocytes which accounts for the transmission of the resistant genotype [117]. The general mechanism of drug resistance is explained in Fig. (**2**).

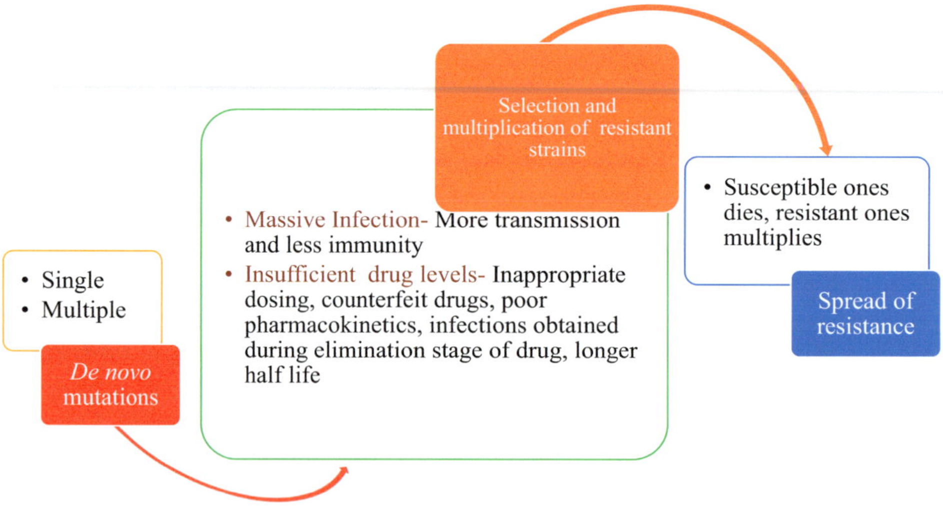

Fig. (2). General mechanisms of antimalarial drug resistance.

Mechanisms of Antimalarial Drug Resistance

CQ, SP and artemisinin class of drugs are widely used as first-line drugs because of their highly effectiveness in eliminating *P. falciparum* infected erythrocytes and their tolerance by human patients [118, 119].

Various factors account for occurrence and massive spread of the resistance. The genetic mutations that lead to emergence of drug resistance are natural and independent of drug effects. The development of resistance to antimalarial drugs due to genetic mutations occurs in two phases. In first phase the initial genetic changes lead to *de novo* mutations (drug resistant mutations) leading to occurrence of drug resistant alleles which gives the parasite survival benefits against the drug. In second phase, the mutated alleles start to multiply, spread to other individuals and finally ends with the parasite population that is no more susceptible to the drug. For few drugs, resistance occurs only after single point mutation while for other drugs multiple point mutations are required to confer the resistance [120]. In such situations, the drug might be able to reduce the parasite population but might not be able to prevent their multiplication or may cause less inhibition of the mutants [121]. The drug will be able to remove the susceptible parasites but the resistant parasites will survive, provided that the mutations are not degenerative for the parasite's survival or reproduction [120]. This heritable drug resistance is further empowered by different mechanisms like reduction in uptake of drug, repudiation of drug activity by change in the form of drug, enhanced expression of drug target, or due to alterations in the protein expressions that cause decrease in the binding capacity of a drug [122]. These heritable phenotypic changes might be the results of the mutations [123]. Following are the some of the typical examples of malaria parasite's resistance against once commonly prescribed antimalarial drugs.

Chloroquine Resistance

Due to digestion of haemoglobin by the malaria parasite, toxic by-products are formed. These are then subsequently polymerized into non-toxic haemazoin (malaria pigment) by the parasite. The resistance in *P. falciparum* for CQ is believed to be because of the increased capacity of the parasite in the efflux of CQ. This leads to decrease in the level of CQ such that it cannot achieve the concentration required for therapeutic activity [124]. The expelling of CQ is about 40-50 times faster in the resistant parasites than the sensitive parasite [125]. This mechanism for CQ resistance is further supported by the fact that CQ resistance can be reverted by the drugs which impedes this efflux system [126]. It is not clear if the parasite resistance to other quinoline antimalarials (MQ, amodiaquine, halofantrine and QN) is because of similar mechanisms [124].

Artemisinin Resistance

Clinical resistance to artemisinin along with its derivatives in malaria parasites collected from patients, is not yet been confirmed but there have been certain sporadic reports claiming clinical failures of artemisinin therapy. In western

Thailand, India and Sierra Leone few cases with reduced response were observed and reported for artemisinins [127 - 129]. Certain clinical parasite isolates from Nigeria-Madagascar exhibit low sensitivity to artemisinins [130]. In the Yunnan province of western China some *in vitro* studies reported detection of decreased susceptibility to artemisinins and drug sensitivity shows geographic variation considerably [131]. Acccording to Jambou *et al.* in French Guiana and Senegal excluding Cambodia, some parasite isolates with IC50 to artemether were observed (30 nM in parasite populations). Reduced efficacy of artesunate-MQ was reported on the Thai-Cambodian border based on three efficacy trials conducted in Cambodia and Thailand having 15-20% recrudescence rates [132, 133]. In a recent study from southern Cambodia, high failure rates of artesunate-MQ therapy were reported indicating that this drug combination is not successful in this area and resistance is not limited to the Thai-Cambodian border [134]. Similar findings were revealed from studies from the Thai-Myanmar border: continuous and regularized deployment of artesunate-MQ therapy (13 years 1995–2007) resulted in significant decrease in 3-day regimen efficacy of this combination therapy [135]. Parasite clearance observed a delayed response, which is associated with high risk of gametocytemia. Although argument is sought that failures in treatment resulted from MQ resistance (increased copy number of pfmdr1) compared to artemisinin resistance, caution should be observed that sensitivities to both drugs are often correlated. Recently a clinical study was undertaken using a 7-day regimen for artesunate therapy (4 mg/kg twice per day) with an aim to explore the potential emergence of artemisinin resistance along the Thai-Cambodian border. Out of 60 *P. falciparum* patients only two were classified as artesunate-resistant and had prolonged parasite clearance time with recrudescence between 21 and 28 days despite of adequate drug plasma concentrations. Parasites from these two patients had a four folds increase in IC50 to dihydroartemisinin when compared to cured patients. It indicate the requirement of four folds higher dose for the achieving the therapeutic action [136]. It was evident from this study that clinical resistance of *P. falciparum* to artemisinin does exist. Although stringent studies on clinical efficacy have not been undertaken in other endemic areas, the data gathered till now marks the intrinsic genetic difference in parasite populations and also provide a scientific rationale for closer and stricter resistance vigil in south-east Asia, where artemisinin resistance is expected to arise.

WHO GUIDELINES FOR THE TREATMENT OF MALARIA

WHO have provided certain guidelines for malaria treatment for reducing the its burden. The guidelines for the treatment of malaria provided in its 3rd edition covers the treatment options for all forms of malaria and these are briefly summarized in following parts [137].

Treatment of Uncomplicated *P. Falciparum* Malaria

A patient showing symptoms of malaria and a positive parasitological test without showing features of severe malaria is defined as having uncomplicated malaria. The important goals of treating uncomplicated malaria are to cleanse the infection as quickly as possible and to stop progression to severe disease. It is recommended that children and adults (except women in their first trimester) should be treated for the 3 days with one of the below mentioned Artemisinin-based combination therapies (*ACTs*).

- Artemether + lumifantrine
- Artesunate + amodiaquine
- Artesunate + MQ
- Dihydroartemesinin + piperaquine
- Artesunate + sulfadoxine-pyrimethamine

ACT is a combination of a rapidly acting artemisinin derivative with a longer-acting *viz.* slowly eliminating partner drug. In 3-days course of the combination therapy, artemisinin component rapidly clears the parasite from blood as it covers 2 asexual cycles; it ensures that only small fraction of the parasites remains for clearance by the partner drug. The shorter courses (less than 3 days) are therefore not preferred, as they are less effective on gametocytes and provide lesser protection to the slowly eliminating partner drug. The partner drug with longer elimination life also provides a period of post-treatment prophylaxis.

Treatment of Recurrent Uncomplicated Falciparum Malaria

Recurrent *falciparum* malaria can result from re-infection or treatment failure. Treatment failure can be due to drug resistance or insufficient exposure of the drug resulting due to sub-optimal dosing, vomiting, unusual pharmacokinetics, poor adherence or substandard medicines. It is important to know this kind of patient's history if he or she has vomited/did not follow the treatment schedule *etc*. Whenever possible, treatment failure must be confirmed parasitologically.

Failure Within 28 Days

The recommended second-line treatment is adherence to alternative ACT treatment regimens (with QN or artesunate, both of which should be co-administered with doxycycline or tetracycline, or clindamycin) for 7 days.

Failure After 28 Days

Recurrence of malaria like symptoms >4 weeks after treatment may be due to either treatment failure or a new infection. Such infections can be treated with first-line ACT. However, the reuse of MQ within 60 days from the first treatment is associated with increased probability of neuropsychiatric reactions, and therefore an alternative ACT should be selected.

Incorrect Approaches of Treatment

- Use of monotherapy
- Incomplete dosing

Treatment of Uncomplicated *P. Falciparum* Malaria in Special Risk Groups

- Females in their first trimester of pregnancy should be treated with 7 days of QN + clindamycin
- Infants less than 5 kg body weight should be treated with ACT at the same mg/kg body weight target dose as for children weighing 5 kg.
- Patients having uncomplicated *P. falciparum* malaria and co-infected with HIV should avoid artesunate + SP if they are receiving co-trimoxazole, and avoid artesunate + amodiaquine if they are also been treated with efavirenz or zidovudine.
- Treat travellers having uncomplicated *P. falciparum* malaria returning to non-endemic regions with ACT.
- The people with *P. falciparum* hyperparasitaemia are at higher risk of therapeutic failure, severe malaria and death therefore they should be monitored closely in addition to ACT administration.

Treatment of Uncomplicated Malaria Caused by *P. Vivax, P. Ovale, P. Malariae* or *P. Knowlesi*

P. ovale, P. malariae or *P. knowlesi* species are all regarded as CQ susceptible, although the CQ resistance was recently reported for *P. malariae*.

Blood Stage Infection

- If malaria species is not known with assurance, then treat as for uncomplicated malaria.
- In CQ-susceptible areas, treat with either an ACT (except women in their first trimester) or CQ.
- In CQ-resistant areas, treat with either ACT (except women in their first trimester).
- Treat pregnant women in their first trimester with QN, who have CQ resistant *P. vivax* malaria.
- For preventing relapse in *P.vivax* or *P.ovale* malaria, PQ may be used. The F6PD (glucose-6-phosphate dehydrogenase) status of the patient should be used as guide for administration of the PQ.

Pregnant and Breast Feeding Women

- In pregnant and breast feeding women, weekly chemoprophylaxis with CQ can be given till delivery and breastfeeding are done, then on the basis of G6PD status, further treatment with PQ may be given to prevent relapse.

Treatment of Severe Malaria

- Severe malaria in adults and children (including infants, pregnant and lactating women) can be treated with intravenous or intramuscular artesunate for at least 24 h administration till they can tolerate oral medication, after which complete treatment with 3 days of an ACT should be given.
- To ensure equivalent exposure to the drug, the children weighing than <20 kg should be treated with a higher dose of artesunate (3 mg/kg bw per dose) compared 2.4 mg/kg bw per dose in larger children and adults.
- In case where parenteral artesunate is not available, artemether can be preferred over QN for treating children and adults with severe malaria [137].

CURRENT LEADS IN MALARIA CHEMOTHERAPY

In 17th century, QN was first used. Over these years, CQ, and 4 -aminoquinoline analogues, semi-synthetic drugs have emerged as antimalarial drugs. Currently, Fixed-dose combinations of artemisinin derivatives is acting as standard for malaria treatment. Synthetic artemisinins like endoperoxides and their derivatives (artesunate, artemether, and dihydroartemisinin) are more effective than CQ. These new antimalarials are having good oral bioavailability, cheaper, and target activity against species of Plasmodium [138]. The emergence of resistance of malaria parasites to currently available drugs makes it crucial for continuous identification of new treatments, including both newer improved analogues of all antimalarial drugs, and the investigation of novel combinations, perfectly with well defined mechanisms of action. Researchers have been working on discovery of new potent antimalarial drugs from plant sources as well as by synthetic chemistry. The following sections summarize the current leads from both synthetic and natural sources.

Leads from Synthetic Chemistry

Currently, new approach of "covalent biotherapy" for antimalarial drug design which involves linking of two active molecules in focus, as it wraps both activities into a single hybrid molecule which will have enhanced efficacy, safety, and/or reduce liability to obtain resistance as compared with the parent drugs [139]. Over the past 20 years, ACT has been used as chemotherapy for malaria, but the poor properties of many artemisinin-derived drugs make them susceptible to quick clearance that reduce their efficacy. In a recent study, for improving physical properties and efficacy, two-carbon-linked, artemisinin derived trioxane dimers were synthesized with known antimalarial drugs. In this system the distinctive conformation places the endoperoxides of each artemisinin unit (required for biological activity) on the outside of a caged structure. This two-carbon-linked dimer system was further functionalized into a sequence of oxime derivatives in an attempt to outdo their *in vivo* behaviour. This new system have demonstrated higher antimalarial activity through single oral dose administration in two 60-day survival studies of *P. berghei* infected mice than artemether [140]. In one other study, semi-synthetic derivatives artemisone and artemiside such as 10- alkylamino-artemisinin and other synthetic peroxides OZ277 and OZ439 displayed potent *ex vivo* activity against the plasmodium species [141].

A new series of pyrazole derivatives were prepared by the hybridization with 5-membered heterocyclic moieties like thiazoles, thiazolidinones, 1,3,4-thiadiazoles and pyrazolines. While *in vitro* and *in vivo* evaluation of these compounds was found to be effective against CQ resistant strain of *P. falciparum* and it exhibited parasitemia suppression by more than 90%. These compounds also had lower IC50 values than CQ [142]. Younis Y *et al.* identified novel series of pyrazine analogues with potent oral antimalarial activity. The replacement of the pyridine core from antimalarial 3,5-Diarylaminopyridines led to synthesis of a novel pyrazine analogues having good *in vitro* antiplasmodial activity, oral *in vivo* efficacy and metabolic stability. The 3,5-diaryl-2 aminopyrazine series showed majestic *in vitro* antiplasmodial activity against the NF54 (sensitive) and K1 (multidrug resistant) strains of *P. falciparum*. However, it was also observed that other changes such as replacement or substitution also lead to loss of activity [143].

Various synthetic quinoline derivatives are still considered to be best candidates for discovery of new drugs. Even after the widespread emergence of resistance to CQ, they act against CQ-resistant strains. The analogues of new 4-aminoquinoline derivatives were prepared and tested for their antimalarial efficacy. These analogues were found to be effective against *P. falciparum*. The synthesis of fluoro amodiaquine, does not form toxic metabolites as in case of amodiaquine due to absence of hydroxyl group although it retains its antimalarial activity against CQ resistant parasites [144].

New antimalarial agents that show multiple activities against drug-resistant strains of malaria parasites denote good beginning points for arising next generation antimalarial therapeutics. To support the progression of such agents into the evolution phase, an image-based parasitological screening technique for defining drug effects on different asexual life cycle stages of *P. falciparum* can be developed. High-throughput screening of a newly collected diversity-oriented synthetic library using this perspective led to the identification of carbohybrid-based 2-aminopyrimidine compounds with fast-acting growth inhibitory activities against three laboratory strains of multi-drug resistant *P. falciparum*. The structure-activity relationship study led to the recognition of two derivatives; 8aA (Fig. **3a**) and 11aA (Fig. **3b**) as the most hopeful antimalarial candidates against all three *P. falciparum* strains, and mouse malaria targeting all major blood stages of multi-drug-resistant *P. falciparum* parasites [145].

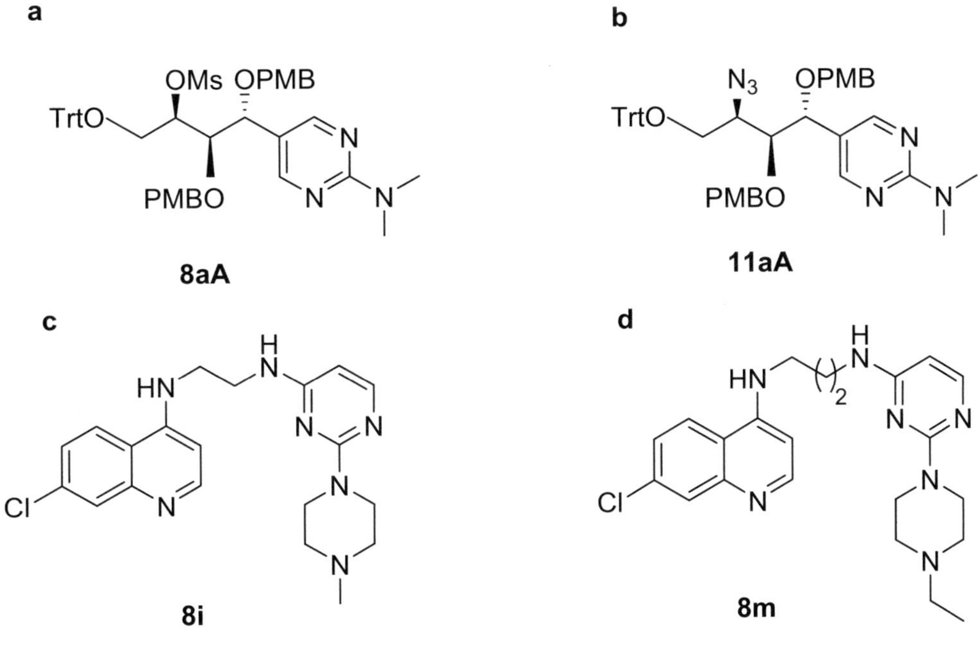

Fig. (3). Chemical structures of some of the antimalarial drug leads.

Manohar *et al.* Synthesized a new class of hybrid molecules that consisted of 4-aminoquinoline and pyrimidine and evaluated these hybrid molecules against both CQ sensitive and CQ resistant strains of *P. falciparum* by *in vitro* assay. Several derivatives of this class exhibited antimalarial activity even more than CQ. Two compounds; 8 i (Fig. **3c**) and 8 m (Fig. **3d**) have shown excellent *in vivo* activity in a mouse model of *P. berghei* without any apparent toxicity [146].

Analogue series of N-alkyl dihydro pyrido quinoxaline were synthesized using Goulde Jacobs reaction, and evaluated their antimalarial activity *in vitro* against CQ sensitive and drug resistant strains of *P. falciparum*. This study revealed that pyrido quinoxalines as a new family of antimalarial agents, and provides a new platform to design novel antimalarial agents other than traditional CQ family [147].

In another study, two biosynthetically engineered fluorinated analogues of pactamycin *viz.* TM-025 and TM-026, were produced by *Streptomyces pactum.* These fluorinated analogues maintained excellent activity and selectivity toward CQ-sensitive and multidrug resistant strains of malarial parasites as the parent compounds [148].

Newer Antimalarials from Natural Sources

The negative conclusions following continual application of synthetic insecticides pointed towards regulation of mosquito populations and have necessitated the effective eco-friendly treatment options. Plant-based compounds have the potential to restrain malaria-transmitting mosquito populations [149]. Plant products have continued to contribute immensely in malaria chemotherapy by either directly providing antimalarial drugs or indirectly by providing important leads for discovery of powerful antimalarial drugs [150]. The vast majority of prescription drugs used today are derived from plants [151] even many of the synthetic antimalarial drugs owe their active chemical moiety to bioactive compounds in plants. The knowledge about native and ethno-pharmacological use of medicines presents a faster perspective to discover new antimalarial drugs. This new approach is now known as reverse pharmacology [152], guarantees to shorten the timing of usual drug discovery process. Hence the plants are under continued research for finding new medicines and beneficial compounds that can be manufactured into new drugs. Presently, many plant remedies are used to treat malaria throughout the malaria prone countries. There are more than 1200 medicinal plants from 160 families reported to be able to treat malaria [153].

It was discovered that ar-curcumene and epi-β-bisabolol from the *Hedychium larsenii* oil (family-Zingiberaceae) exhibited mosquito larvicidal activity [154]. The extract of green tea (*Camellia sinensis* proanthocyanidins) and its active constituents have shown disrupting effects on mosquito larval development [155]. Neem cake can also act as a source of eco-friendly mosquitocides in Anopheline vector control programmes [156]. Black pepper (dried fruit from the vine, *Piper nigrum*), and its principal alkaloid piperine, are reported show the larvicidal properties against insecticide resistant and susceptible strains of Anopheles larvae [157]. The newer and safer natural larvicides from essential oil of Pinaceae plants against malaria mosquito vectors [158]. *Agerantum conyzoides* extracts have demonstrated toxic effects on disease-transmitting mosquitoes and on larvicidal effects on Anopheles gambiae and Anopheles arabiensis larvae [149]. Essential oil of *Zingiber nimmonii* showed the larvicidal and repellent activity against the malaria vector *Anopheles stephensi* [159].

The ethnomedicinal approach in the hunt for new antimalarial drugs from plant sources has demonstrated to be more effective and inexpensive. The leaves of *Aloe pulcherrima* Gilbert and Sebsebe, which is an endemic Ethiopian plant, are used locally for the treatment of malaria and other infectious diseases. In the recent study, two *C*-glycosylated anthrones, nataloin and 7-hydroxyaloin were isolated from the leaf latex of *A. Pulcherrima*. Both these two major constituents and exhibited antimalarial activity in a dose dependant manner [160]. The investigation of the toxicity of *Heracleum sprengelianum* (Apiaceae) leaf essential oil- and its major compounds (lavandulyl acetate & bicyclogermacrene) towards larvae of the malaria vector *Anopheles subpictus* lead to a promising conclusion that it source of eco-friendly larvicides [161].

VACCINES FOR THE PREVENTION OF MALARIA

Malaria vaccine development has been at the major concern [162] and a crucial health priority. Despite enormous research and development efforts since many decades, there is no mercantile malaria vaccine available at the current time [28]. Although many promising experimental vaccines have been developed, the optimistic promise by researchers in the mid-1980s that a successful vaccine against *P. falciparum* would be available has not been yet fulfilled. A malaria vaccine technology roadmap, which is developed by more than 230 experts constituting 100 organizations from 35 countries, has set a strategic aim to develop an effective malaria vaccine by 2025 [163, 164]. A natural malaria infection does not produce much immune protection, and over several years after repetitive and prolonged exposure to the malaria parasites, only partially effective immunity is developed, that too is short-lived and is highly stage- and strain-specific [163]. This immunity is not able to eliminate all parasites and does not provide complete protection against major future challenges [164]. On the basis of their capability to evoke some form of inhibitory immune response against the parasite, some candidates have been chosen and in all these candidates the complete genome sequence of *Plasmodium* has been reported [162]. Backing the sequencing of the entire genome complement of 5300-5500 genes of *P. falciparum,* 579 of annotated *falciparum* genes have been forecasted to encode proteins containing signal peptides but only 197 of these proteins stages are targets of vaccine development: 43 in gametocytes, 57 in sporozoites, and 94 in either the young or late schizonts or merozoites stages. All these proteins are expressed in the life-cycle [165]. In comparison to inactivated or live-attenuated whole sporozoites and whole merozoites, malaria vaccine research strategies using recombinant subunits and/or synthetic peptides have the edges of directing the immune responses toward particular targets [166]. Although, promising protective immunization was observed with some vaccine candidates during initial proof-of-concept studies; they failed in further clinical studies possibly due to their formulation adjuvants [167, 168]. Currently, RTS, S/AS01 (Mosquirix™) is the only vaccine approved against the most fatal form of human malaria, *P. falciparum.* It has got an approval for the active immunization in newborns and children aged 6 weeks to 17 months, with three intramuscular doses administered at 0, 1 and 2 months and a booster dose administered at month 20. The WHO has suggested pilot implementation of RTS,S/AS01 in children ageing 5–17 months prior to its wider scale-up. RTS,S/AS01 has some limitations- it has limited efficacy which wanes over time; and the duration afforded by it remains unclear [169], therefore these drawbacks necessitates the development of more effective malaria vaccine.

More than 20 other vaccine constructs are also being assessed presently in clinical trials or are in advanced preclinical headway [170]. Following are the four important strategies for developing a vaccine against malaria.

Sporozoites and Pre-erythrocytic Vaccines

Vaccines targeting the pre-erythrocytic sporozoite and liver stages have the potential to entirely prevent blood stage infection and disease, as well as onward transmission. Sporozoite surface and secreted proteins are leading candidates for inclusion in a pre-erythrocytic, antibody-based vaccine [171]. The belief that vaccine-induced immune responses against *Plasmodium* sporozoites may provide protective effects by inhibiting the parasite infectivity in the humans [172] and the radiation-attenuated malaria sporozoites may offer immunization, have grabbed the attention of other scientists working in this area. Researchers observed that vaccines aiming at the pre-erythrocytic stages of *P. falciparum* could avert or lessen the counts of parasites reaching the erythrocytic stage that generates the disease [173]. The discovery that immunisation with live radiation attenuated sporozoites generated immune responses provides protection against malaria led to a hunt for subunit vaccines that can reproduce this immunity [174].

This type of vaccines usually target at sporozoites or schizonts which have targeted liver cells and infected them. The goal for preventing infection is achieved by ceasing the step of hepatic stage. These vaccines are intended to produce antibody response in protest of sporozoites and they prevent the entry of sporozoites into hepatocytes. This prevents merozoites release by destroying the infected hepatocytes or by interfering with parasite development. Such vaccine may be highly effective in interrupting the pre-erythrocytic stages if it has to supply sterile immunity in non-immune individuals but the chances of failure are also high. Even a single sporozoite escaping by vaccine-induced immunity may lead to fully pathogenic blood stage infection, as it was found during the clinical trials of the anti-sporozoite RTS, AS vaccine [165]. RTS, S is a pre-erythrocytic vaccine candidate containing *P. falciparum* circumsporozoite surface antigen [175]. This vaccine is formulated with new proprietary Adjuvant Systems - AS01 or AS02 [176]. Promising results with the Phase III trial of RTS,S [175] have demonstrated that a vaccine against malaria can provide partial protection to children in endemic areas [177]. All through its development, increasingly more effectual adjuvants have been a key in enhancing the power of the vaccine. RTS,S-based vaccine formulations proved to be safe, immunogenic, well tolerated, and granted partial efficacy in both malaria-inexperienced and experienced adults as well as children [178]; however its limited efficacy and relatively short window of protection demands more efficacious new generations of vaccines [177].

The Erythrocytic Vaccines

These type of vaccines also referred to as asexual blood-stage vaccines [179], are aimed to target the life-cycle stage that occurs and develops in host erythrocytes, which is linked with disease pathology. Vaccination to block parasite development in host RBCs depends on generation of antibodies to stop erythrocyte capturing by merozoites released from schizonts (of liver or blood origin). Contradictory with pre-erythrocytic vaccine candidates, asexual stage vaccine candidates currently lack a human feigned challenge model and therefore rely on natural challenge in field trials to provide proof-of-concept. Their research is therefore slower and necessitates major commitment, intensive collaborations as well as high-level coordination supported by sufficient funding [180].

Pf66, a synthetic peptide vaccine candidate was the first asexual blood-stage vaccines developed against malaria [173, 181]. It seemed to offer some protection in initial studies but later it failed to produce protection as observed in clinical studies [173, 182 - 184], though it can be a matter of debate that this vaccine could have been done better with potent adjuvants [185]. Later on, many vaccines candidates targeting erythrocytic stage of malaria were attempted. They were designed in such a way to produce antibody responses towards the asexual blood stage of the parasite such as merozoite surface proteins (MSP-1, MSP-2, MSP-3), or at those which contains specialized organelles associated with invasion like the apical membrane antigen (AMA-1) and the glutamate-rich protein (GLURP) [186]. But since this stage, a stage in which merozoites stay outside the red cells is of a very short duration (about 2 minutes); it makes difficult for proposition of such vaccines.

Transmission-Blocking Vaccines

The vaccines are aimed to target sexual stage parasite development [187] and act by interrupting the life-cycle of parasite in the mosquito by producing antibodies which prevent either fertilization of the gametes in the mosquito gut or further growth of the zygote into sporozoites [165]. Pfs25 (*P. falciparum* surface protein) [187], Pfs48/45 and Pfs 230 are leading vaccine candidates for the malaria immunization that have shown transmission blocking immunity [188, 189]. However, none of these have got any marketing approval yet.

Anti-Disease Vaccination

This type of vaccination aims for example to block the sequestration of parasite-affected erythrocytes (that causes much of the dreadful pathology of malaria) by blocking the interaction of the parasite surface protein PfEMP1 with different vascular endothelial cell-surface receptors. A successful vaccine that is not based upon attenuating the complete parasite is likely to have components of the first three categories. Anti-disease vaccination can be of use alone but it would also be a fruitful addition to a polyvalent, multi-component vaccine formulation [165].

CONTRIBUTION OF CDRI IN ANTIMALARIAL RESEARCH

CSIR-CDRI is India's one of the multidisciplinary research laboratories focusing upon biomedical sciences. CDRI is among thirty nine laboratories that are operating under the support of the council of scientific and Industrial Research (CSIR) of India. CDRI has also been one the pioneer institutions in the country which have contributed in developing new treatment regimens against neglected tropical diseases that includes malaria.

Arteether (ART)

ART (Fig. **4a**) α and β enantiomers; 30:70 is an ethyl ether derivative of artemisinin reported to have fast blood schizontocidal action against *P. berghei* [190], *P. knowlesi* [191] and MDR *P. yoelii nigeriensis* [192]. It was reported by Dutta, G. P. *et al* that a MDR *P. Yoelii Nigeriensis* strain having resistance to QN, MQ and CQ is susceptible to ART. The dose found to be curative in Swiss mice by i.m. route was 5 mg/kg × 3 days and artemisinin dosed at 50 mg/kg × seven days exhibited mere suppressive effect against *P. yoelii nigeriensis* [192]. Kar, K. *et al* reported that ART, is useful in cerebral malaria treatment. They have tested ART for pharmacological effects by giving it in a suspension of arachis oil. ART was found to be safe on the central nervous, cardiovascular and urinary systems of the test animals [193]. In yet another study, the comparative activity of intramuscular injectable ART prepared in ground nut oil and artemisinin oil suspension was tested against blood-induced *P. Cynomolgi B* infection in rhesus monkeys. ART showed curative action at comparative lower dose of 5 mg/kg × 3 days verses 10 mg/kg x 7 d or 20 mg/kg x 3 d dose of artemisinin [194]. ART was also evaluated for its gametocytocidal/sporontocidal action against *P. cynomolgi B* infection in the rhesus monkey. It was found to have gametocytocidal action at 2.5-5 mg/kg single intramuscular dose as the complete absence of mosquito infectivity was observed. However, no sporontocial action was observed up to dose 20 mg/kg *i.m* [195].

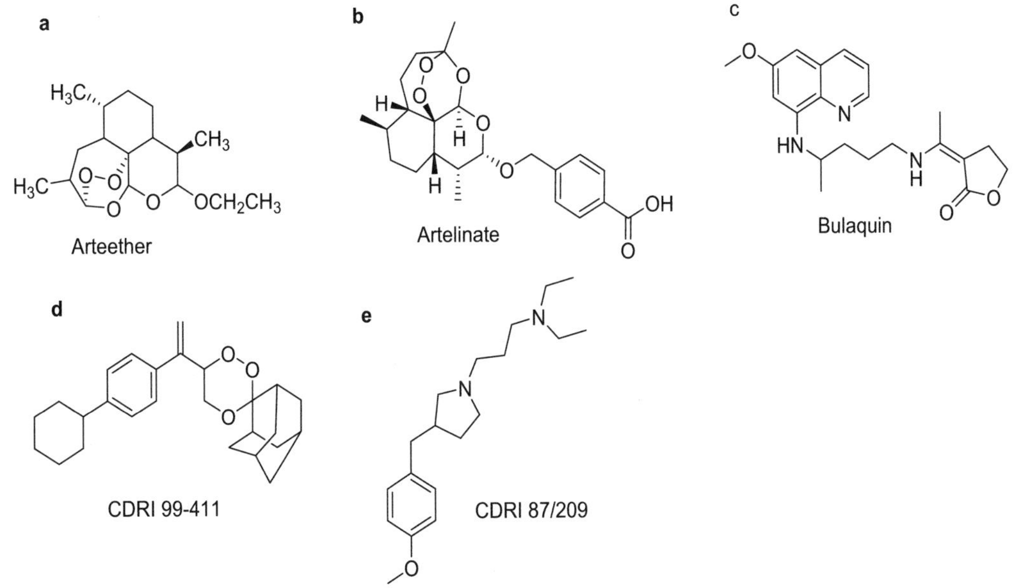

Fig. (4). Chemical structures of CDRI antimalarial drug candidates.

A phase-III clinical trial was conducted on 50 patients (mean age 27.2 years) suffering from acute uncomplicated *falciparum* malaria with mean parasitaemia 0.65% on day 0. The patients were treated with alpha, beta-ART at 150 mg/kg intramuscular dose for 3 consecutive days. The drug was well tolerated and it was able to clear the parasite in 19.94 ±6.87 hours and fever within 37.81 ±21.67 hours. It was concluded that alpha, beta ART is safe, effective and rapidly acting antimalarial drug [196]. In order to combat emerging resistance towards artemisinins, the combination of ART with the fresh root extract of *Vetiver zizanioides* (Linn.) Nash (VET) was studied for their antimalarial potential. There was additive to synergistic antimalarial activity in the combination and the curative dose of ART in the combination was reduced to its one fourth, thereby reducing side effects, if any [197]. The live sporozoites when inoculated with prophylactic antimalarial cover constitute an alternative approach to develop sterile, reproducible and long-term protection against malaria. The immunization activity of ART was evaluated and compared with that of MQ, azithromycin and PQ in the *P. yoelii* sporozoites induced Swiss mice. The results from the study demonstrated that the sporozoite administration under ART, MQ and azithromycin treatment grants powerful protection against subsequent sporozoite infection and the acquired response depends on the presence of liver stage of the parasites [198].

α/β Artelinate

The discovery of new quick-acting water soluble artemisinin derivatives that can be intravenously administered to complex and comatose cerebral malaria cases are still of high priority in global tropical diseases programme [199]. The water-soluble artemisinin analogue [200] α/β artelinate (Fig. **4b**), have been identified as potential fast-acting [199] blood schizontocide [200]. It can be given intravenously so that high blood levels can be quickly achieved. These derivatives have been against *P. Knowlesi (W1)* infection in Rhesus monkey which is considered as one of the experimental models for cerebral malaria. β artelinate showed 100% cure in all the monkeys while α artelinate showed 100% cure in half of the monkeys when tested at 20 mg/kg/day * 3 days. The curative effects of α/β artelinate against MQ resistant *P. Knowlesi (w1)* indicate its potential towards MQ resistant *P. falciparum* infections. Besides fast blood schizontocidal activity, artelinate also exhibits strong gametocytocidal action and could be used to stop malaria transmission [199]. β artelinate was also tested for gametocytocidal action against *P. cynomolgi B* in which a single dose of this compound have been effective gametocytocide by both oral and intravenous routes. It was able to sterilize circulating gametocides in rhesus monkeys thereby resulting in loss of infectivity and oocyte development although no sporontocidal action was observed. The artelinate thus may have dual application in malaria management as fast acting blood schizontocide and as a gametocytocide [200] and it could be a candidate to replace PQ [199].

Bulaquine (CDRI 80/53)

A potential anti-relapse (radical curative) antimalarial compound [201 - 203], an analogue of PQ, CDRI Code 80/53, has shown curative activity against relapsing *P. vivax* malaria [203] and showed causal prophylactic activity against sporozoite induced *P. cynomolgi B* infection in rhesus monkeys [204]. The compound also shows the gametocytocidal action against *P. falciparum* [203]. It is unstable in acidic conditions where it is converted into PQ [205]. Bulaquine (Fig. **4c**) has been cleared as safe drug in regulatory toxicology following administration of the drug for three months [202, 206]. The compound may replace the PQ due to its comparable efficacy [204] but 3.65-fold lower methaemoglobinaemia toxicity and safety in other hematological parameters and liver function tests [202] The code name of Compound 80/53 CDRI has been revised by World Health Organization to bulaquine (=elubaquine) and it has passed through Phase I, II and III clinical trials for anti-relapse efficacy. Aablaquine which is a combination of Bulaquine and CQ is also reported by CDRI for the cure of malaria [203].

CDRI 87/209

The revival of malaria due to resistance against CQ has diminished its value as a potent and safe chemotherapeutic agent in malaria endemic areas [207, 208]. If any agent in combination with CQ can make the resistant parasite susceptible to CQ, then the problem of resistance can be solved [208]. The combination of Ca^{++} channel blockers like verapamil or antidepressants like desipramine with CQ has initiated a strategy to treat CQ resistant malaria [207]. CDRI 87/209, N,N-Diethyl-3-((4-methoxyphenyl)methyl)-1-pyrrolidinepropanamine, (Fig. **4d**) is a class of modulator that reverses CQ resistance in a different manner. CDRI 87/209 (15 mg/kg) when administered in combination with CQ (10 mg/kg) once-a-day for 10 days to chloroquine resistant *P. berghei*/*P. yoelii* (multidrug resistant) infected *Mastomys coucha*/Swiss albino mice respectively, it exhibited potential cure in the test animals. It was also capable of clearing the parasite form the animals [208]. CDRI 87/209 showed contrary mechanism to verapamil and desipramine; it did not restore CQ accumulation in the resistant parasites [207] but it inhibited heme-oxygenase (a heme degrading enzyme) [208]. It thereby indicated that besides proposed blockage of drug efflux there are other mechanisms which are vulnerable targets towards drug resistant malaria treatment [207].

CDRI 99/411

CDRI 99/411 (Fig. **4e**) is a short acting [209] synthetic 1,2,4-trioxane derivative that displayed potent anti-malarial actions against *P. cynomolgi* had and multi drug resistant *P. yoelii nigeriensisin* in preclinical studies [203, 209]. It has been also tested for combination therapy with long-acting prescription antimalarials, lumefantrine and piparaquine. The bioavailability of CDRI 99/411 was increased upon co-administration with lumefantrine and piparaquine. However, the bioavailability of piparaquine was reduced to half while the kinetic profile of lumefantrine remained unchanged upon co-administration. Therefore CDRI 99/411 can be a good alternative for artemisinin derivatives in combination treatment with lumifantrine [209]. The single-pass intestinal perfusion study was performed in rats to predict the human intestinal permeability and the fraction of CDRI 99/411 absorbed after its oral administration. CDRI 99/411 was found to have high permeability and likely complete absorption in human [210]. The metabolic profile of this compound in rat liver microsomes was investigated. The results revealed CYP3A2 mediated metabolism for CDRI 99/411 that was deducted from CYP reaction phenotyping using known powerful inhibitors [211]. The compound has been handed over to IPCA Pharmaceuticals for further Phase I evaluation [203].

ROLE OF NANO-FORMULATIONS IN MALARIA CHEMOTHERAPY

The major disadvantages of traditional malaria chemotherapy are the emergence of multiple drug resistance and the non-specific targeting to intracellular parasites, leading to high dose requirements and the subsequent unbearable toxicity. Moreover, the poor pharmacokinetic profile of drugs due to issues in water solubility and bioavailability limits their use in the malaria chemotherapy. An important factor in the development of drug resistance in *Plasmodium* strains is the use of ineffective and non-rational use of pharmaceutical dosage forms of antimalarials. Nano-carriers or nanosystems are useful tools that are gaining distinctive attention because of their ability to minimize the side effects, improve bioavailability and the selectivity of the drugs by altering the biopharmaceutics and pharmacokinetics property of the drug molecules [212 - 214].

Nano-carriers also provide a better solution and afford an improved therapeutic outcome by drug targeting to specific site of action [215]. Nanotechnology potentially restores the use of old drugs which were relatively toxic by varying and modifying their bio-distribution and thereby minimizing their toxicity. This is particularly advantageous in malaria therapy, since novel dosage forms developed for delivering drugs to specific site *i.e.* parasite infected cells is an urgently need, especially for the antimalarials in clinical use. Nano-carriers not only open an avenue for the use of potentially toxic but effective drugs [216, 217], but they also increase and strengthen the efficacy of the immune responses for vaccine formulations [218]. Several nano-carriers have already tried for malaria diagnosis and treatment [219 - 222], as well as in vaccine formulations [223, 224].

The most promising role of a nanocarrier in the malaria context is its potential to sustain the release of drug in blood stream thereby increasing the interaction of drug with RBCs and parasitic membranes [217]. Other riveting properties of nanocarrier are protection of instable drugs, ability of cell-adhesion, and to be surface modified by conjugation of specific ligands [222, 225]. It is important to note that, for the treatment of cerebral malaria, most of these likely benefits can be attained by colloidal NPs that suit intravenous administration. In case of uncomplicated malaria, non-parenteral routes are favoured due more patient compliance, but they shorten the spectrum of benefits of the use of nanocarriers. Numerous attempts have been tried to implement nanotechnology in the malaria perspective [217, 226 - 229]. The next segments are dedicated to discuss these attempts.

Solid Lipid Nanoparticles (SLN) for Malaria Chemotherapy

The particulate drug carriers worked upon and investigated for several years are liposomes, micro-particles, oil-in-water (O/W) emulsions, and nanoparticles. Somewhere in the fifties, the O/W emulsions successfully reached the clinics from the laboratory bench for parenteral nutrition. This lead to the development and use of drug-containing emulsions like diazepam and etomidate based emulsions [230]. Although these O/W emulsions possess excellent tolerability, the number of products available in the market are still relatively low, which is suggestive of their limited success. An important reason which restricts and prevents the wide-spread use of such emulsions for drug delivery is their physical instability which results from the incorporated drug. Also, the registered oils in use (soybean oil, MCT and LCT and mixtures) demonstrated insufficient solubility for the drugs of choice to be incorporated into emulsion systems.

The scenario for polymeric nanoparticles is even worse, as even more than 30 years of research on this delivery system; it remains practically non-existant. However an exception worth mention is the product Abdoscan produced by Nycomed, although, it is not a formulation for any chronic treatment but a diagnostic agent [231]. The cytotoxicity issues with the use of polymers and the absence of a suitable large scale production method are some of the reasons for such worse scenario. Talking about the nanometer size range with probable a sizes of a few micrometers, the polymer might be internalized by cells like macrophages and their degradation within the cell can often leads to cytotoxicity. According to the results of a study a cent percent mortality was observed in cell cultures when the cells were incubated with 0.5% PLA/GA nanoparticles [232]. Prerequisites for introduction of any product to the pharmaceutical market is the availability of an suitable large scale method of production, method being cost effective and leading to a product of acceptable quality as governed by the regulatory authorities. From the inception of the nineties, various research groups focused on an alternative to polymeric nanoparticles and emulsions; the SLN and thus their emergence as a suitable drug delivery option [233, 234].

SLN are particles composed of solid lipids with an average diameter of about 1 to 1000 nm. SLN have an inner core of lipid that can solubilize lipophilic drug molecules. Surfactants (emulsifiers) are used to stabilize this lipid core. The lipids used for preparation of SLN comprise of triglycerides (*e.g*, trimyristin, tristerin), diglycerides (*e.g.* glycerol bahenate), monoglycerides (*e.g.* glycerol mono-stearate), steroids (*e.g.* cholesterol), fatty acids (*e.g.* stearic acid), and waxes (*e.g.*

cetyl palmitate). Different emulsifiers (with respect to molecular weight and charge) have been used to stabilize the lipid dispersion. It was observed that the combination of emulsifiers can prevent the particle agglomeration more effectively than a single emulsifier [235].

SLN have the advantages of both polymeric NPs and lipid emulsion systems and at the same time they overcome the temporal and *in vivo* stability issues associated with conventional drug delivery systems and polymeric NPs [235]. SLN are reported to have several advantages over types of NPs. They can feasibly incorporate both lipophilic and hydrophilic drugs, avoid use of toxic organic solvents; no biotoxicity; sustain drug release; achieve drug targeting; increase the drug stability and can be produced at large scale without problems [236].

Using solid lipids as a matrix material for nanoparticles as drugs delivery approach can successfully reach the market like the Mucosolvan retard capsules [237]. Mucosolvan retard capsule was the first generation. It was produced by highspeed stirring of a melted lipid phase in a hot surfactant solution obtaining an emulsion. This emulsion was then cooled down to room temperature obtaining the so-called "lipid nanopellets for oral administration" [238, 239]. Those lipids which are well tolerated by the body (*e.g*. glycerides made up of fatty acids as present in emulsions for parenteral nutrition) can be used. SLNs could be produced on a large scale in a cost effective and simple way by using HPH. Additionally SLNs could be produced *via* micro-emulsions [240].

Applications of SLN in Malaria

Aditya P. Nayak *et al.* prepared curcuminoids-loaded lipid nanoparticles with a mean size of 100-250 nm by a nanoemulsion technique employing high-speed homogenizer and ultrasonic probe for parenteral administration. The method had advantages such as easy manufacturing process with mild preparation conditions, use of biocompatible lipids, and production in aqueous media avoiding organic solvents, and high encapsulation parameters. For the production of NPs, tristerin, trimyristin and glyceryl monostearate were selected as solid lipids and medium chain triglyceride as liquid lipid [227, 241]. The *in vivo* pharmacodynamic activity was tested in *P. berghei* induced malaria in Albino mice. Curcuminoids entrapped in lipid nanoparticles showed 2-fold increase in antimalarial activity compared to free curcuminoids at the tested dosage level, thus showing superior activity of SLN [227].

Silver Nanoparticles for Malaria Chemotherapy

Silver nanoparticles (AgNPs) are reported to have anti-fungal [242], anti-bacterial [243], anti-inflammatory [244], and anti-viral activity [245]. Aqueous silver ions can be reduced by aqueous extract of plant parts to produce very stable AgNPs in water [243]. The researchers showed that ionic Ag is very toxic to different freshwater aquatic species with different fatal concentrations depending on the species [246, 247]. Therefore, both ionic Ag and AgNPs are widely investigated for their potential against malaria.

AgNPs Applied in the Control of Malaria

T. Santhoshkumar *et al.* synthesized AgNPs by reduction of the silver ions present in the silver nitrate solution along with the cell free aqueous extract of Nelumbo nucifera leaf. These biologically synthesized nanoparticles and crude methanol and aqueous extracts of N. Nucifera were tested for larvicidal activity. The AgNPs of N. Nucifera were found to have highest activity against Anopheles subpictus Grassi (LC_{90}= 2.15ppm) compared to methanolic exctract (LC_{90}= 28.65 ppm) and aqueous extract (LC_{90}= 36.06 ppm). The LC_{90} values against Culex quinquefasciatus for AgNPs, methanolic extract, and aqueous extract were 28.13, 35.83, and 3.59 ppm respectively. This was the first report on the mosquito larvicidal activity of the plant extracts and synthesized nanoparticles. The results suggested that the green synthesis of AgNPs of N. Nucifera had the highest activity and potential to be used as an ideal eco-friendly approach for the control of the Anopheles subpictus Grassi and Culex quinquefasciatus [248].

Nanoemulsions for Malaria Chemotherapy

Droplet size of ≤300 nm in emulsions are generally termed as nanoemulsions (NEs) [249]. "NE" not only gives an idea of the droplet size being in the nano-scale size range but it is also concise and avoids misinterpretation and confusion with the term micro-emulsion (thermodynamically stable systems) hence it is the preferred term for use in this context. By virtue of their characteristic size, when viewed by the naked eye NEs appear transparent or translucent and they possess stability against sedimentation. These properties make NEs suitable for fundamental studies and practical applications (chemical, pharmaceutical, cosmetic applications).

NEs cannot be formed spontaneously as they are non-equilibrium systems. Thus an energy input generally derived from mechanical devices or through the chemical potential of the components, is a requirement. NEs formation by the dispersion or high-energy emulsification techniques is achieved by the use of high shear stirring, HPH and ultrasound generators. The apparatus which are capable of supplying the available energy in the shortest possible time but providing the most homogeneous flow produces the smallest achievable sizes as reported in literature. Using HPH is one such way which would meet these requirements. This makes them the most widely used emulsifying machines for preparation of NEs [250].

Droplet size could be efficiently reduced by ultrasonic emulsification but it is only suitable for small batches. Recent study [251] demonstrated that the efficiency of the dispersion process depends strongly on the ultra-sonication time at different amplitudes and higher hydrophobicity of the monomer requires a longer the sonication time in terms of preparation of polymerizable NEs.

Stability of NEs

Stability against sedimentation (or creaming) is attributed to the small droplet size of NEs, the reason being the brownian motion and the consequent diffusion rate tends to be higher than the sedimentation rate induced by the gravitational force. Phenomenon of ostwald ripening or molecular diffusion, stems from emulsion poly-dispersity. Solubility differences between small and large size droplets, is the main mechanism for the destabilization of NEs. According to the Lifshitz–Slezov and Wagner (LSW) theory, a linear relationship between the cube of the radius(r^3) and time(t) with the slope being the Ostwald ripening rate is predicted. Postulates of this theory assume that dispersed phasedroplets are spherical, the droplet diameter is smaller than the distance between them and their kinetics is governed by molecular diffusion of the dispersed phase into the continuous phase. The Ostwald ripening rate of O/W emulsions assumes a direct proportionality to the solubility of the oil in the aqueous phase; according to this theory. However the anomalies of this theory are factors such as oil transport due to the presence of micelles and/or micro-emulsion droplets in the aqueous phase, increase in Brownian motion and reduction in the interfacial Gibbs elasticity which have been not taken into account. The Ostwald ripening process could be reduced or controlled by the addition of a small amount of second oil with low solubility in the aqueous phase to the system. According to a recent report, in case of an ethoxylated nonionic surfactant system, the Ostwald ripening rate was decreased by addition of a second surfactant with the same alkyl chain length and higher degree of ethoxylation compared to the primary surfactant.

Advantages of NEs

NE's offer the following advantages in personal care and cosmeceuticals and also in health care [252]:

- No creaming or sedimentation would occur on storage as small droplet size brings about a significant reduction in the gravity force and the Brownian motion which may be sufficient for overcoming gravitational force.
- Flocculation of the droplets is also prevented by small droplet size and this helps the system to remain dispersed without any separation.
- Coalescence is also prevented due to the small droplet size, and these droplets being elastic, surface fluctuations are in turn prevented.

- NEs are suitable for efficient topical delivery of active ingredients. A larger surface area of the emulsion system allows fast and rapid penetration of actives through the skin.
- The transparency of the emulsion system, their fluid character (at reasonable oil concentrations) and absence of any thickeners provides them a pleasant aesthetic character and skin feel.
- Contrary to micro-emulsion systems (requiring a high surfactant concentration, usually 20% and higher), NEs can be produced using reasonable surfactant concentration. A surfactant concentration of 5%-10% may be sufficient to produce a 20% O/W NE. Formulation of NEs utilize surfactants, which are approved for human consumption (GRAS), and can be taken by enteric route.
- Small droplet size enables them to deposit uniformly on substrates. The phenomenon of wetting, spreading and penetration is enhanced due to reduced surface tension of the whole system and the lowered interfacial tension of the O/W droplets.
- NEs find utility in delivery of fragrance, in many personal care products. This is of importance for the formulation of alcohol free perfumes.
- NEs may be substituted for liposomes and vesicular systems (which are much less stable) and in some cases it is possible to build lamellar liquid crystalline phases around the NE droplets.

Disadvantages of NEs

Despite the many advantages there are a number of demerits associated with NEs:

- In many cases preparation of NEs requires special application techniques, like the use of HPHand ultrasonics. These equipments (as the Microfluidiser) became available only recently.
- The requirement of expensive equipment and the use of high emulsifier concentrations increase their cost and make less cost effective from the industry point of view.
- Limited or less understanding into the mechanisms of production of droplets of submicron range and the role played by surfactants and co-surfactants.
- Lack of a rational risk-cost-benefit analysis of NEs over the classical macro-emulsion systems.
- Poor understanding of the interfacial chemistry involved in preparation of NEs.

Applications of NEs in Malaria

O/W NEs have been investigated and known since long; but the water in-oil (W/O) NEs finds the first mention only recently. The NEs based on O/W emulsions having a mean diameter of $\leq$400 nm were also investigated and explored as probable antimalarial carriers. Low cost and availability as oral dosage forms are the two significant advantages that NEs offer over the other colloidal carriers. Based on these merits, a reconstituted artificial chylomicron NEs of PQ were proposed for hepatocyte targeting following *i.v.* injection [253]. In a highly efficient way the PQ was encapsulated into NEs and it remained inside; without any significant release. However on an *i.v.* injection into mice, the PQ-loaded chylomicron NEs exhibited a significantly enhanced accumulation of PQ in the liver, as compared to that following an injection of free PQ. Recently, Miglyol based O/W NEs used to encapsulate PQ for oral administration has been reported [254]. NEs enhanced the antimalarial activity of PQ at a lower dose as compared to the PQ in solution form in miceinfected with *P. berghei.* 25% reduction in the PQ dose level was achieved with NEs dosage form (1.5mg/ Kg/day), which afforded a satisfactory suppression of parasitaemia (about 92.75%) with an average survival time of 34.9 days. Moreover, significantly higher PQ levels were achieved with NEs in the liver following oral administration, corroborating the enhancement in the antimalarial activity of PQ as drug concentration at the site of action was improved.

Our group has also contributed in antimalarial research by preparing ART loaded NE formulation for its improved activity against malaria parasites. ART-NE was formulated by using high pressure homogenization technique with the goal of increasing its solubility and thus its bioavailability. The optimized formulation had 93±7.4% drug loading, 156±10.2nm globule size and -23.3±3.4mV zeta potential. The formulation was able to sustain the release of drug and increased its bioavailability than free ART when administered intramuscularly in young, adult male Sprague-Dawley rats. The formulation was observed to be safe as it caused insignificant cytotoxicity in J774A.1 and caco-2 cells. The antimalarial efficacy and survival studies performed in *P. yoelii nigeriensis* infected mice were treated with ART-NE and free ART at 12.5mg/kg intramuscularly for 5 days. The results demonstrated significantly high antimalarial efficacy and survival rate of mice giving 80% cure rate with ART-NE in comparison to 30% cure rate of free ART. Therefore we concluded that ART-NE can be a promising delivery system for ART, though further much detailed exhaustive research is required to arrive at any final conclusion [226].

Self Micro Emulsifying Drug Delivery Systems (SMEDDS)

SMEDDS are lipid based formulations. An isotropic mixture of drug, oil/lipid, surfactant, and/ or co-surfactant,which on dilution with physiological fluid result in fine emulsion/lipid droplets, in the size ranging from about100 nm- <50 nm is generally termed as SMEDDS. The drug thus remains in solution in the gut, and the dissolution step that limits the rate of absorption of hydrophobic drugs from the crystalline state is bypassed [255].

Excipients Selection

The lipid component might be a fatty acid ester or a medium or long chain saturated, or partially unsaturated hydrocarbon (at room temperature they might be in liquid, semisolid or solid form). Oils like vegetable oil, mineral oil, refined animal oil, silicon oil, lanolin or fatty acids, fatty alcohols, and mono-/di-/t-i-glycerides are the commonly used lipid components. Non-ionic surfactants having a high HLB value are the surfactants most widely recommended. For formation of stable SMEDDS the suitable surfactant concentration lies between 30% and 60% (w/w). SMEDDS which after oral administration rapidly get transformed into micro-emulsions has been recently proposed to be used for treatment of experimental malaria [256]. SMEDDS in hard gelatin capsules may be used as they improve the bioavailability of drugs which are poorly water-soluble. According to recent reports long chain triglycerides have been employed as the oily phase which contained artemeether in a SMEDDS.

The oral bioavailability of a drug may be altered by changing the bio-pharmaceutical properties like increased dissolution rate and solubility in the intestinal fluid, protection against chemical and enzymatic degradation in the oil droplets and lipoproteins formation that promotes lymphatic transport of highly lipophilic drugs; hence it is noteworthy that lipids (triglycerides) affect the oral bio-availability of drugs with respect to these points [257]. For a drug its absorption profile and the blood/lymph distribution depends upon the chain length of the triglyceride, its saturation degree, and total lipid administered (volume). Intestinal lymph process the drugs and they are usually transported to systemic circulation along with the lipid core (lipoproteins). Administration of lipophilic drugs with lipids not only stimulates lymphatic transport but also enhances drug absorption into the portal blood as compared to non-lipid systems [258].

Various factors that affect self-emulsification are the nature of the oil/surfactant pair, oil/surfactant ratio, surfactant concentration and the self emulsification temperature. Few very specific excipients combinations have lead to development of efficient SMEDDS. Drug incorporation efficiency into a SMEDDS depends largely upon the particular physicochemical compatibility of that drug/system. Hence to obtain an optimal formulation design pre-formulation solubility and phase diagram studies are an imperative requirement.

Evaluation of SMEDDS

Self-emulsification is the basic essence of SMEDDS and it can be assessed primarily by visual means. The estimation of self-emulsification efficiency can be made by determination of the emulsification rate and size distribution (of the droplets). The charge possessed by the oil droplets also needs assessment in a

SMEDDS. Polymorphism and melting characteristics of lipid/ drug in these systems may be determined by techniques like X-ray diffraction and differential scanning calorimetry.

Applications of SMEDDS in Malaria

According to recent reports long chain triglycerides have been employed as the oily phase which contained artemeether in a SMEDDS. This artemeether SMEDDS so formed demonstrated a significant improvement in its antimalarial activity against *P. berghei* in mice, (average parasitemia of 35.11 ±4.16 on 20th day of infection in comparison to that of Larither®, a marketed artemeether capsule dosage form, where the average parasitemia of 42.35 ±4.18 ($p<0.05$) was obtained [256].

In another study SMEDDS containing β–Artemether and Lumefantrine was developed by using commercial modified oil and indigenous natural fatty acids. The developed formulations were compared at different doses for *in vivo* anti-malarial activity and efficacy compared with innovator formulation (Coartem®, Novartis pharm., Germany) against *P. berghei* induced male Swiss mice. The percent parasitemia, time-based activity and animal survival probability were examined. On the fourth day of antimalarial studies, both developed SMEDDS and innovator formulation showed zero percent parasitemia even at the half of the normal doses while control showed 33.92 ±6.00% parasitemia. At 1/10th dose both SMEEDS and innovator formulation showed zero percent parasitemia up to 11th day of the studies however the innovator formulation showed recrudescence in 3 mice and 62.5% survival. Conclusively, the SMEDDS formulation exhibited excellent activity with 100% survival probability [259].

CONCLUSIONS

Malaria still remains the significant cause of illness and death in children and adults in areas in which it is endemic. These economies are losing money merely resulting from non-productivity caused by malaria. Majority of the people living in tropical areas are at high risk of getting this disease. The increasing use of preventive measures such as ITS and IRS have provided some protection in prevention but not complete. Numerous chemotherapeutic agents developed for curing malaria initially emerged as highly potent, but later provided lesser relief due to emergence of resistance against them in the malaria vectors. This emergence of resistance to first-line antimalarials including artemisinin has resulted in an increment of malaria cases in many endemic areas, thereby calling urgent need for the development of new therapeutics and technology approaches to battle with the disease and disrupt the drug resistance. Therefore, the biggest challenge across the globe at present is to treat malaria patients with safe and effective medications and to circumvent the decreased sensitivity of antimalarial drugs. In this context, researchers are working upon the following two strategies (1.) to find the exact biology of development of resistance and (2.) search of newer antimalarials based from leads obtained *via* synthetic as well as natural sources. The development of malaria vaccine can also possibly be one of the most sustainable and cost-saving perspective in the malaria prevention and control strategy, although there has been limited success in this field. There are countless challenges lying ahead on the path to accomplish the use of secure, effective, endurable and affordable malaria vaccines. This issue needs to be addressed urgently. Also, the true nature of the protective immune responses *in vivo* in humans remains one of the central unanswered questions in malaria immunology concerns. Therefore, huge progress and better understanding in terms of scientific research and innovation is needed to discover and develop these novel technologies and vaccines to reduce the burden of malaria. Although we are working in the right course steadily and continuing progress, there's still a long way to go to build a malaria-free world.

FUTURE PERSPECTIVES

Experiences in the recent past, post discovery of antimalarial drugs, have given us the lessons and taught that although the conventional interventions of malaria vector control are capable of reducing the disease burden considerably; they however remain unproductive to completely eradicate malaria. If not stopped, a disease like this *i.e* a disease of the underdeveloped tropical nations might become the disease of all nations. Migratory patterns are major stake holders in this regard. As travel patterns expand; the world becomes small and an endemic disease could shape up to be a pandemic one. The only way to stop it is to act now. Positively, at present we have essential knowledge and better comprehension of malaria parasite's biology, disease transmission, and immunology of the host. In addition, the recent advancements in the drug discovery and nanotechnology, modern facilities and straight commitment gives hopes to achieve malaria free world by boosting the development of novel potent antimalarials and prophylactic malaria vaccines.

The WHO: Global Technical Strategy for Malaria 2016-2030 focuses the emergent need to put huge investments across all interventions - including prophylactic measures, diagnostic testing, treatment and disease scrutiny - as well as in harnessing innovation and expanding research. WHO member countries have initiated the courageous vision of a world free of malaria, and set the aspiring new target of reducing the global malaria load by 90% by the year 2030 [260]. To make this dream come true, researches need to discover that magic bullet which can eradicate this fatal curse. The research and development requires the detailed knowledge of the three elements: 1) the physiological, molecular and population biology of the vector; 2) the interaction between vector, parasite and host; and 3) the delivery mechanisms. The synergic combination of these elements may be a crucial factor in eliminating the parasite and eradicsting the disease completely.

CONFLICT OF INTEREST

The author (editor) declares no conflict of interest, financial or otherwise.

ACKNOWLEDGEMENTS

The authors are grateful to the Knowledge Resource Centre, CSIR-CDRI, Lucknow. CDRI Communication No 9488.

REFERENCES

[1] Organization, W.H.O. Malaria control in humanitarian emergencies: an inter-agency field handbook. 2013.

[2] Gardella F, Assi S, Simon F, *et al.* Antimalarial drug use in general populations of tropical Africa. Malar J 2008; 7(124): 124.
[http://dx.doi.org/10.1186/1475-2875-7-124] [PMID: 18611279]

[3] Organization, W.H.O. World malaria report 2010. Geneva: World Health Organization Google Scholar 2014.

[4] Organization, W.H.O. World Malaria Report 2016.

[5] Rathore D, McCutchan TF, Sullivan M, Kumar S. Antimalarial drugs: current status and new developments. Expert Opin Investig Drugs 2005; 14(7): 871-83.
[http://dx.doi.org/10.1517/13543784.14.7.871] [PMID: 16022576]

[6] Smith LA, Jones C, Meek S, Webster J. Review: Provider practice and user behavior interventions to improve prompt and effective treatment of malaria: do we know what works? Am J Trop Med Hyg 2009; 80(3): 326-35.
[PMID: 19270276]

[7] Winstanley P, Ward S. Malaria chemotherapy. Adv Parasitol 2006; 61: 47-76.
[http://dx.doi.org/10.1016/S0065-308X(05)61002-0] [PMID: 16735162]

[8] Krettli AU, Andrade-Neto VF, Brandão MG, Ferrari WM. The search for new antimalarial drugs from plants used to treat fever and malaria or plants randomly selected: a review. Mem Inst Oswaldo Cruz 2001; 96(8): 1033-42.
[http://dx.doi.org/10.1590/S0074-02762001000800002] [PMID: 11784919]

[9] Greenwood BM, Fidock DA, Kyle DE, *et al.* Malaria: progress, perils, and prospects for eradication. J Clin Invest 2008; 118(4): 1266-76.
[http://dx.doi.org/10.1172/JCI33996] [PMID: 18382739]

[10] Skinner-Adams TS, McCarthy JS, Gardiner DL, Andrews KT. HIV and malaria co-infection: interactions and consequences of chemotherapy. Trends Parasitol 2008; 24(6): 264-71.
[http://dx.doi.org/10.1016/j.pt.2008.03.008] [PMID: 18456554]

[11] Krettli AU, Adebayo JO, Krettli LG. Testing of natural products and synthetic molecules aiming at new antimalarials. Curr Drug Targets 2009; 10(3): 261-70.
[http://dx.doi.org/10.2174/138945009787581203] [PMID: 19275562]

[12] Bacon DJ, Jambou R, Fandeur T, *et al.* World Antimalarial Resistance Network (WARN) II: in vitro antimalarial drug susceptibility. Malar J 2007; 6: 120.
[http://dx.doi.org/10.1186/1475-2875-6-120] [PMID: 17822533]

[13] Krettli AU, Miller LH. Malaria: a sporozoite runs through it. Curr Biol 2001; 11(10): R409-12.
[http://dx.doi.org/10.1016/S0960-9822(01)00221-4] [PMID: 11378408]

[14] Mohanty S, Patel DK, Pati SS, Mishra SK. Adjuvant therapy in cerebral malaria. Indian J Med Res 2006; 124(3): 245-60.
[PMID: 17085828]

[15] Coltel N, Combes V, Hunt NH, Grau GE. Cerebral malaria -- a neurovascular pathology with many riddles still to be solved. Curr Neurovasc Res 2004; 1(2): 91-110.
[http://dx.doi.org/10.2174/1567202043480116] [PMID: 16185187]

[16] Pouvelle B, Matarazzo V, Jurzynski C, *et al.* Neural cell adhesion molecule, a new cytoadhesion receptor for Plasmodium falciparum-infected erythrocytes capable of aggregation. Infect Immun 2007; 75(7): 3516-22.
[http://dx.doi.org/10.1128/IAI.01852-06] [PMID: 17485455]

[17] Whitty CJ, Sanderson F. New therapies and changing patterns of treatment for malaria. Curr Opin Infect Dis 1999; 12(6): 579-84.
[http://dx.doi.org/10.1097/00001432-199912000-00008] [PMID: 17035824]

[18] Miller LH, Ackerman HC, Su XZ, Wellems TE. Malaria biology and disease pathogenesis: insights for new treatments. Nat Med 2013; 19(2): 156-67.
[http://dx.doi.org/10.1038/nm.3073] [PMID: 23389616]

[19] Miller LH, Baruch DI, Marsh K, Doumbo OK. The pathogenic basis of malaria. Nature 2002; 415(6872): 673-9.
[http://dx.doi.org/10.1038/415673a] [PMID: 11832955]

[20] Clark IA, Cowden WB. The pathophysiology of falciparum malaria. Pharmacol Ther 2003; 99(2): 221-60.
[http://dx.doi.org/10.1016/S0163-7258(03)00060-3] [PMID: 12888113]

[21] White NJ, Ho M. The pathophysiology of malaria. Adv Parasitol 1992; 31: 83-173.
[http://dx.doi.org/10.1016/S0065-308X(08)60021-4] [PMID: 1496930]

[22] Gallup JL, Sachs JD. The economic burden of malaria. Am J Trop Med Hyg 2001; 64(1-2) (Suppl.): 85-96.
[http://dx.doi.org/10.4269/ajtmh.2001.64.85] [PMID: 11425181]

[23] Ghebreyesus TA, Haile M, Witten KH, *et al.* Household risk factors for malaria among children in the Ethiopian highlands. Trans R Soc Trop Med Hyg 2000; 94(1): 17-21.
[http://dx.doi.org/10.1016/S0035-9203(00)90424-3] [PMID: 10748890]

[24] Okafor(Enugu, N.a.D.I.H.C., Venezuela) H U. Teaching Module for Prevention of Malaria. 1-23.

[25] Welfare N.V.B.D.C.P.D.G.o.H.S.M.o.H.F.. Malaria 2016.

[26] Hall BF, Fauci AS. Malaria control, elimination, and eradication: the role of the evolving biomedical research agenda. J Infect Dis 2009; 200(11): 1639-43.
[http://dx.doi.org/10.1086/646611] [PMID: 19877843]

[27] UNICEF. MALARIA prevention and treatment. UNICEF's Programme Division in cooperation with the World Health Organization United Kingdom 2000.

[28] WHO. World Malaria Report 2015.

[29] Childs LM, Cai FY, Kakani EG, *et al.* Disrupting Mosquito Reproduction and Parasite Development for Malaria Control. PLoS Pathog 2016; 12(12): e1006060.
[http://dx.doi.org/10.1371/journal.ppat.1006060] [PMID: 27977810]

[30] Mangeni JN, Menya D, Obala A, Platt A, O'Meara WP. Development and validation of a rapid assessment tool for malaria prevention. Malar J 2016; 15(1): 544.
[http://dx.doi.org/10.1186/s12936-016-1575-0] [PMID: 27825350]

[31] Van Remoortel H, De Buck E, Singhal M, Vandekerckhove P, Agarwal SP. Effectiveness of insecticide-treated and untreated nets to prevent malaria in India. Trop Med Int Health 2015; 20(8): 972-82.
[http://dx.doi.org/10.1111/tmi.12522] [PMID: 25877758]

[32] Organization, W.H.O. Handbook on vector control in malaria elimination. 2015.

[33] Muhindo MK, Kakuru A, Natureeba P, *et al.* Reductions in malaria in pregnancy and adverse birth outcomes following indoor residual spraying of insecticide in Uganda. Malar J 2016; 15(1): 437.
[http://dx.doi.org/10.1186/s12936-016-1489-x] [PMID: 27566109]

[34] Odugbemi BA, Wright KO, Onajole AT, *et al.* A malariometric survey of under-fives residing in indoor residual spraying-implementing and non-implementing communities of Lagos, Nigeria. Malar J 2016; 15(1): 458.
[http://dx.doi.org/10.1186/s12936-016-1507-z] [PMID: 27604777]

[35] Katureebe A, Zinszer K, Arinaitwe E, *et al.* Measures of Malaria Burden after Long-Lasting Insecticidal Net Distribution and Indoor Residual Spraying at Three Sites in Uganda: A Prospective Observational Study. PLoS Med 2016; 13(11): e1002167.
[http://dx.doi.org/10.1371/journal.pmed.1002167] [PMID: 27824885]

[36] Mpofu M, Becker P, Mudambo K, de Jager C. Field effectiveness of microbial larvicides on mosquito larvae in malaria areas of Botswana and Zimbabwe. Malar J 2016; 15(1): 586.
[http://dx.doi.org/10.1186/s12936-016-1642-6] [PMID: 27923385]

[37] Price RN, Dorsey G, Ashley EA, *et al.* World Antimalarial Resistance Network I: clinical efficacy of antimalarial drugs. Malar J 2007; 6: 119.
[http://dx.doi.org/10.1186/1475-2875-6-119] [PMID: 17822532]

[38] Mishra M, Mishra VK, Kashaw V, *et al.* Comprehensive review on various strategies for antimalarial drug discovery. Eur J Med Chem 2016.
[PMID: 27886547]

[39] Lee MR. Plants against malaria. Part 1: Cinchona or the Peruvian bark. J R Coll Physicians Edinb 2002; 32(3): 189-96.
[PMID: 12434796]

[40] Mates M, Nesher G, Zevin S. Quinines--past and present. Harefuah 2007; 146(7): 560-562, 572.
[PMID: 17803173]

[41] Achan J, Talisuna AO, Erhart A, *et al.* Quinine, an old anti-malarial drug in a modern world: role in the treatment of malaria. Malar J 2011; 10(1): 144.
[http://dx.doi.org/10.1186/1475-2875-10-144] [PMID: 21609473]

[42] Medical Discoveries. Quinine

[43] Greenwood D. The quinine connection. J Antimicrob Chemother 1992; 30(4): 417-27.
[http://dx.doi.org/10.1093/jac/30.4.417] [PMID: 1490916]

[44] Rosenthal PJ. Antimalarial chemotherapy: mechanisms of action, resistance, and new directions in drug discovery. Springer Science & Business Media 2001.
[http://dx.doi.org/10.1385/1592591116]

[45] WHO. Malaria treatment guidelines 2010.

[46] Becker K, Kirk K. Of malaria, metabolism and membrane transport. Trends Parasitol 2004; 20(12): 590-6.
[http://dx.doi.org/10.1016/j.pt.2004.09.004] [PMID: 15522669]

[47] Fidock DA, Eastman RT, Ward SA, Meshnick SR. Recent highlights in antimalarial drug resistance and chemotherapy research. Trends Parasitol 2008; 24(12): 537-44. [http://dx.doi.org/10.1016/j.pt.2008.09.005] [PMID: 18938106]

[48] Vale N, Moreira R, Gomes P. Primaquine revisited six decades after its discovery. Eur J Med Chem 2009; 44(3): 937-53. [http://dx.doi.org/10.1016/j.ejmech.2008.08.011] [PMID: 18930565]

[49] Crockett M, Kain KC. Tafenoquine: a promising new antimalarial agent. Expert Opin Investig Drugs 2007; 16(5): 705-15. [http://dx.doi.org/10.1517/13543784.16.5.705] [PMID: 17461742]

[50] Krishna S, Bustamante L, Haynes RK, Staines HM. Artemisinins: their growing importance in medicine. Trends Pharmacol Sci 2008; 29(10): 520-7. [http://dx.doi.org/10.1016/j.tips.2008.07.004] [PMID: 18752857]

[51] Skinner TS, Manning LS, Johnston WA, Davis TM. In vitro stage-specific sensitivity of Plasmodium falciparum to quinine and artemisinin drugs. Int J Parasitol 1996; 26(5): 519-25. [http://dx.doi.org/10.1016/0020-7519(96)89380-5] [PMID: 8818732]

[52] Woodrow CJ, Haynes RK, Krishna S. Artemisinins. Postgrad Med J 2005; 81(952): 71-8. [http://dx.doi.org/10.1136/pgmj.2004.028399] [PMID: 15701735]

[53] White NJ. Qinghaosu (artemisinin): the price of success. Science 2008; 320(5874): 330-4. [http://dx.doi.org/10.1126/science.1155165] [PMID: 18420924]

[54] Dondorp A, Nosten F, Stepniewska K, Day N, White N. South East Asian Quinine Artesunate Malaria Trial (SEAQUAMAT) group. Artesunate versus quinine for treatment of severe falciparum malaria: a randomised trial. Lancet 2005; 366(9487): 717-25. [http://dx.doi.org/10.1016/S0140-6736(05)67176-0] [PMID: 16125588]

[55] Praygod G, de Frey A, Eisenhut M. Artemisinin derivatives versus quinine in treating severe malaria in children: a systematic review. Malar J 2008; 7(210): 210. [http://dx.doi.org/10.1186/1475-2875-7-210] [PMID: 18928535]

[56] Gomes MF, Faiz MA, Gyapong JO, *et al.* Study 13 Research Group. Pre-referral rectal artesunate to prevent death and disability in severe malaria: a placebo-controlled trial. Lancet 2009; 373(9663): 557-66. [http://dx.doi.org/10.1016/S0140-6736(08)61734-1] [PMID: 19059639]

[57] Gomes M, Ribeiro I, Warsame M, Karunajeewa H, Petzold M. Rectal artemisinins for malaria: a review of efficacy and safety from individual patient data in clinical studies. BMC Infect Dis 2008; 8(39): 39. [http://dx.doi.org/10.1186/1471-2334-8-39] [PMID: 18373841]

[58] Grace JM, Aguilar AJ, Trotman KM, Peggins JO, Brewer TG. Metabolism of beta-arteether to dihydroqinghaosu by human liver microsomes and recombinant cytochrome P450. Drug Metab Dispos 1998; 26(4): 313-7. [PMID: 9531517]

[59] Ilett KF, Ethell BT, Maggs JL, *et al.* Glucuronidation of dihydroartemisinin in vivo and by human liver microsomes and expressed UDP-glucuronosyltransferases. Drug Metab Dispos 2002; 30(9): 1005-12. [http://dx.doi.org/10.1124/dmd.30.9.1005] [PMID: 12167566]

[60] Li QG, Peggins JO, Fleckenstein LL, Masonic K, Heiffer MH, Brewer TG. The pharmacokinetics and bioavailability of dihydroartemisinin, arteether, artemether, artesunic acid and artelinic acid in rats. J Pharm Pharmacol 1998; 50(2): 173-82. [http://dx.doi.org/10.1111/j.2042-7158.1998.tb06173.x] [PMID: 9530985]

[61] Ashton M, Hai TN, Sy ND, *et al.* Artemisinin pharmacokinetics is time-dependent during repeated oral administration in healthy male adults. Drug Metab Dispos 1998; 26(1): 25-7.

[PMID: 9443848]

[62] Simonsson US, Jansson B, Hai TN, Huong DX, Tybring G, Ashton M. Artemisinin autoinduction is caused by involvement of cytochrome P450 2B6 but not 2C9. Clin Pharmacol Ther 2003; 74(1): 32-43.
[http://dx.doi.org/10.1016/S0009-9236(03)00092-4] [PMID: 12844133]

[63] Nosten F, White NJ. Artemisinin-based combination treatment of falciparum malaria. Am J Trop Med Hyg 2007; 77(6) (Suppl.): 181-92.
[PMID: 18165491]

[64] Meshnick SR, Taylor TE, Kamchonwongpaisan S. Artemisinin and the antimalarial endoperoxides: from herbal remedy to targeted chemotherapy. Microbiol Rev 1996; 60(2): 301-15.
[PMID: 8801435]

[65] Mutabingwa TK. Artemisinin-based combination therapies (ACTs): best hope for malaria treatment but inaccessible to the needy! Acta Trop 2005; 95(3): 305-15.
[http://dx.doi.org/10.1016/j.actatropica.2005.06.009] [PMID: 16098946]

[66] Olliaro PL, Haynes RK, Meunier B, Yuthavong Y. Possible modes of action of the artemisinin-type compounds. Trends Parasitol 2001; 17(3): 122-6.
[http://dx.doi.org/10.1016/S1471-4922(00)01838-9] [PMID: 11286794]

[67] Meshnick SR. Artemisinin: mechanisms of action, resistance and toxicity. Int J Parasitol 2002; 32(13): 1655-60.
[http://dx.doi.org/10.1016/S0020-7519(02)00194-7] [PMID: 12435450]

[68] Zhang F, Gosser DK Jr, Meshnick SR. Hemin-catalyzed decomposition of artemisinin (qinghaosu). Biochem Pharmacol 1992; 43(8): 1805-9.
[http://dx.doi.org/10.1016/0006-2952(92)90713-S] [PMID: 1575774]

[69] Meshnick SR, Jefford CW, Posner GH, Avery MA, Peters W. Second-generation antimalarial endoperoxides. Parasitol Today (Regul Ed) 1996; 12(2): 79-82.
[http://dx.doi.org/10.1016/0169-4758(96)80660-0] [PMID: 15275260]

[70] Ploypradith P. Development of artemisinin and its structurally simplified trioxane derivatives as antimalarial drugs. Acta Trop 2004; 89(3): 329-42.
[http://dx.doi.org/10.1016/j.actatropica.2003.10.006] [PMID: 14744559]

[71] Krungkrai SR, Yuthavong Y. The antimalarial action on Plasmodium falciparum of qinghaosu and artesunate in combination with agents which modulate oxidant stress. Trans R Soc Trop Med Hyg 1987; 81(5): 710-4.
[http://dx.doi.org/10.1016/0035-9203(87)90003-4] [PMID: 3329778]

[72] Wu W-M, Wu Y-k, Wu Y-L, *et al.* Unified Mechanistic Framework for the Fe(II)-Induced Cleavage of Qinghaosu and Derivatives/Analogues. The First Spin-Trapping Evidence for the Previously Postulated Secondary C-4 Radical. J Am Chem Soc 1998; 120(14): 3316-25.
[http://dx.doi.org/10.1021/ja973080o]

[73] Stocks PA, Bray PG, Barton VE, *et al.* Evidence for a common non-heme chelatable-iron-dependent activation mechanism for semisynthetic and synthetic endoperoxide antimalarial drugs. Angew Chem Int Ed Engl 2007; 46(33): 6278-83.
[http://dx.doi.org/10.1002/anie.200604697] [PMID: 17640025]

[74] Meshnick SR, Thomas A, Ranz A, Xu CM, Pan HZ. Artemisinin (qinghaosu): the role of intracellular hemin in its mechanism of antimalarial action. Mol Biochem Parasitol 1991; 49(2): 181-9.
[http://dx.doi.org/10.1016/0166-6851(91)90062-B] [PMID: 1775162]

[75] Paitayatat S, Tarnchompoo B, Thebtaranonth Y, Yuthavong Y. Correlation of antimalarial activity of artemisinin derivatives with binding affinity with ferroprotoporphyrin IX. J Med Chem 1997; 40(5): 633-8.
[http://dx.doi.org/10.1021/jm960767v] [PMID: 9057849]

[76] Meshnick SR, Yang YZ, Lima V, Kuypers F, Kamchonwongpaisan S, Yuthavong Y. Iron-dependent free radical generation from the antimalarial agent artemisinin (qinghaosu). Antimicrob Agents Chemother 1993; 37(5): 1108-14.
[http://dx.doi.org/10.1128/AAC.37.5.1108] [PMID: 8517699]

[77] Haynes RK, Ho WY, Chan HW, *et al.* Highly antimalaria-active artemisinin derivatives: biological activity does not correlate with chemical reactivity. Angew Chem Int Ed Engl 2004; 43(11): 1381-5.
[http://dx.doi.org/10.1002/anie.200352343] [PMID: 15368412]

[78] Looareesuwan S, Wilairatana P, Vannaphan S, *et al.* Co-administration of desferrioxamine B with artesunate in malaria: an assessment of safety and tolerance. Ann Trop Med Parasitol 1996; 90(5): 551-4.
[http://dx.doi.org/10.1080/00034983.1996.11813081] [PMID: 8915132]

[79] Jones-Brando L, D'Angelo J, Posner GH, Yolken R. In vitro inhibition of Toxoplasma gondii by four new derivatives of artemisinin. Antimicrob Agents Chemother 2006; 50(12): 4206-8.
[http://dx.doi.org/10.1128/AAC.00793-06] [PMID: 17060514]

[80] Kumar S, Gupta AK, Pal Y, Dwivedi SK. *In-vivo* therapeutic efficacy trial with artemisinin derivative, buparvaquone and imidocarb dipropionate against Babesia equi infection in donkeys. J Vet Med Sci 2003; 65(11): 1171-7.
[http://dx.doi.org/10.1292/jvms.65.1171] [PMID: 14665744]

[81] Mercer AE. The role of bioactivation in the pharmacology and toxicology of the artemisinin-based antimalarials. Curr Opin Drug Discov Devel 2009; 12(1): 125-32.
[PMID: 19152221]

[82] Scott MD, Meshnick SR, Williams RA, *et al.* Qinghaosu-mediated oxidation in normal and abnormal erythrocytes. J Lab Clin Med 1989; 114(4): 401-6.
[PMID: 2794752]

[83] Wu Y, Liu HH. Probing the possible molecular origin of the highly selective toxicity of antimalarial peroxide qinghaosu (artemisinin). Chem Res Toxicol 2003; 16(10): 1202-6.
[http://dx.doi.org/10.1021/tx034133k] [PMID: 14565761]

[84] Imwong M, Suwannasin K, Kunasol C, *et al.* The spread of artemisinin-resistant Plasmodium falciparum in the Greater Mekong subregion: a molecular epidemiology observational study. Lancet Infect Dis 2017; 17(5): 491-7.
[http://dx.doi.org/10.1016/S1473-3099(17)30048-8] [PMID: 28161569]

[85] Fairhurst RM, Dondorp AM. Artemisinin-resistant Plasmodium falciparum malaria. Microbiol Spectr 2016; 4(3)
[PMID: 27337450]

[86] Chattopadhyay R, Mahajan B, Kumar S. Assessment of safety of the major antimalarial drugs. Expert Opin Drug Saf 2007; 6(5): 505-21.
[http://dx.doi.org/10.1517/14740338.6.5.505] [PMID: 17877439]

[87] Nosten F, Price RN. New antimalarials. A risk-benefit analysis. Drug Saf 1995; 12(4): 264-73.
[http://dx.doi.org/10.2165/00002018-199512040-00006] [PMID: 7646825]

[88] Phillips-Howard PA, ter Kuile FO. CNS adverse events associated with antimalarial agents. Fact or fiction? Drug Saf 1995; 12(6): 370-83.
[http://dx.doi.org/10.2165/00002018-199512060-00003] [PMID: 8527012]

[89] Kofi Ekue JM, Ulrich AM, Rwabwogo-Atenyi J, Sheth UK. A double-blind comparative clinical trial of mefloquine and chloroquine in symptomatic falciparum malaria. Bull World Health Organ 1983; 61(4): 713-8.
[PMID: 6354507]

[90] Gil JP. Amodiaquine pharmacogenetics 2008.
[http://dx.doi.org/10.2217/14622416.9.10.1385]

[91] Ouldabdallahi M, Alew I, Salem MS, *et al.* Efficacy of artesunate-amodiaquine for the treatment of acute uncomplicated falciparum malaria in southern Mauritania. Malar J 2014; 13(1): 496. [http://dx.doi.org/10.1186/1475-2875-13-496] [PMID: 25515535]

[92] Karbwang J, Na Bangchang K. Clinical pharmacokinetics of halofantrine. Clin Pharmacokinet 1994; 27(2): 104-19. [http://dx.doi.org/10.2165/00003088-199427020-00003] [PMID: 7955774]

[93] Mojon M, Wallon M, Gravey A, Peaud PY, Sartre J, Peyron F. Intravascular haemolysis following halofantrine intake. Trans R Soc Trop Med Hyg 1994; 88(1): 91. [http://dx.doi.org/10.1016/0035-9203(94)90516-9] [PMID: 8154017]

[94] Gillespie SH, Msaki EP, Ramsay A, Ngowi FI, Fox R. A new micronized formulation of halofantrine hydrochloride in the treatment of acute Plasmodium falciparum malaria. Trans R Soc Trop Med Hyg 1993; 87(4): 467-9. [http://dx.doi.org/10.1016/0035-9203(93)90040-W] [PMID: 8249083]

[95] Vachon F, Fajac I, Gachot B, Coulaud JP, Charmot G. Halofantrine and acute intravascular haemolysis. Lancet 1992; 340(8824): 909-10. [http://dx.doi.org/10.1016/0140-6736(92)93317-G] [PMID: 1357314]

[96] Salako LA, Sowunmi A, Walker O. Evaluation of the clinical efficacy and safety of halofantrine in falciparum malaria in Ibadan, Nigeria. Trans R Soc Trop Med Hyg 1990; 84(5): 644-7. [http://dx.doi.org/10.1016/0035-9203(90)90132-X] [PMID: 2278061]

[97] Coulaud JP, Le Bras J, Matheron S, Moriniere B, Saimot AG, Rossignol JF. Treatment of imported cases of falciparum malaria in France with halofantrine. Trans R Soc Trop Med Hyg 1986; 80(4): 615-7. [http://dx.doi.org/10.1016/0035-9203(86)90158-6] [PMID: 3544361]

[98] Malvy D, Receveur MC, Ozon P, *et al.* Fatal cardiac incident after use of halofantrine. J Travel Med 2000; 7(4): 215-6. [http://dx.doi.org/10.2310/7060.2000.00065] [PMID: 11003738]

[99] Baird JK, Basri H, Subianto B, *et al.* Treatment of chloroquine-resistant Plasmodium vivax with chloroquine and primaquine or halofantrine. J Infect Dis 1995; 171(6): 1678-82. [http://dx.doi.org/10.1093/infdis/171.6.1678] [PMID: 7769318]

[100] Organization, W.H.O. The use of antimalarial drugs Report of a WHO Informal Consultation. Geneva: World Health Organization 2001.

[101] Ekue JM, Phiri DE, Sheth UK, Mukunyandela M. A double-blind trial of a fixed combination of mefloquine plus sulfadoxine-pyrimethamine compared with sulfadoxine-pyrimethamine alone in symptomatic falciparum malaria. Bull World Health Organ 1987; 65(3): 369-73. [PMID: 3311440]

[102] Looareesuwan S, Harinasuta T, Chongsuphajaisiddhi T. Drug resistant malaria, with special reference to Thailand. Southeast Asian J Trop Med Public Health 1992; 23(4): 621-34. [PMID: 1298068]

[103] Looareesuwan S, Wilairatana P, Chalermarut K, Rattanapong Y, Canfield CJ, Hutchinson DB. Efficacy and safety of atovaquone/proguanil compared with mefloquine for treatment of acute *Plasmodium falciparum* malaria in Thailand. Am J Trop Med Hyg 1999; 60(4): 526-32. [http://dx.doi.org/10.4269/ajtmh.1999.60.526] [PMID: 10348224]

[104] Radloff PD, Philipps J, Nkeyi M, Hutchinson D, Kremsner PG. Atovaquone and proguanil for *Plasmodium falciparum* malaria. Lancet 1996; 347(9014): 1511-4. [http://dx.doi.org/10.1016/S0140-6736(96)90671-6] [PMID: 8684102]

[105] Looareesuwan S, Chulay JD, Canfield CJ, Hutchinson DB. Malarone Clinical Trials Study Group. Malarone (atovaquone and proguanil hydrochloride): a review of its clinical development for treatment of malaria. Am J Trop Med Hyg 1999; 60(4): 533-41.

[http://dx.doi.org/10.4269/ajtmh.1999.60.533] [PMID: 10348225]

[106] Lell B, Ruangweerayut R, Wiesner J, *et al.* Fosmidomycin, a novel chemotherapeutic agent for malaria. Antimicrob Agents Chemother 2003; 47(2): 735-8. [http://dx.doi.org/10.1128/AAC.47.2.735-738.2003] [PMID: 12543685]

[107] Borrmann S, Issifou S, Esser G, *et al.* Fosmidomycin-clindamycin for the treatment of Plasmodium falciparum malaria. J Infect Dis 2004; 190(9): 1534-40. [http://dx.doi.org/10.1086/424603] [PMID: 15478056]

[108] Gaillard T, Madamet M, Pradines B. Tetracyclines in malaria. Malar J 2015; 14(1): 445. [http://dx.doi.org/10.1186/s12936-015-0980-0] [PMID: 26555664]

[109] Ponnampalam JT. Doxycycline in the treatment of falciparum malaria among aborigine children in West Malaysia. Trans R Soc Trop Med Hyg 1981; 75(3): 372-7. [http://dx.doi.org/10.1016/0035-9203(81)90095-X] [PMID: 7034311]

[110] Pang L, Limsomwong N, Singharaj P. Prophylactic treatment of vivax and falciparum malaria with low-dose doxycycline. J Infect Dis 1988; 158(5): 1124-7. [http://dx.doi.org/10.1093/infdis/158.5.1124] [PMID: 3053925]

[111] Wilson T. Tetracyclines for malaria. BMJ 1972; 4(5833): 176. [http://dx.doi.org/10.1136/bmj.4.5833.176-b] [PMID: 5078461]

[112] Bareford LM, Swaan PW. Endocytic mechanisms for targeted drug delivery. Adv Drug Deliv Rev 2007; 59(8): 748-58. [http://dx.doi.org/10.1016/j.addr.2007.06.008] [PMID: 17659804]

[113] Newton CR, Krishna S. Severe falciparum malaria in children: current understanding of pathophysiology and supportive treatment. Pharmacol Ther 1998; 79(1): 1-53. [http://dx.doi.org/10.1016/S0163-7258(98)00008-4] [PMID: 9719344]

[114] Mishra SK, Newton CR. Diagnosis and management of the neurological complications of falciparum malaria. Nat Rev Neurol 2009; 5(4): 189-98. [http://dx.doi.org/10.1038/nrneurol.2009.23] [PMID: 19347024]

[115] Organization, W.H.. Chemotherapy of malaria and resistance to antimalarials: report of a WHO scientific group. [meeting held in Geneva from 17 to 24 October 1972]

[116] Organization, W.H.O. Global report on antimalarial drug efficacy and drug resistance: 2000-2010 2010.

[117] Liu DQ, Liu RJ, Ren DX, *et al.* Changes in the resistance of *Plasmodium falciparum* to chloroquine in Hainan, China. Bull World Health Organ 1995; 73(4): 483-6. [PMID: 7554020]

[118] Schlitzer M. Antimalarial drugs - what is in use and what is in the pipeline. Arch Pharm (Weinheim) 2008; 341(3): 149-63. [http://dx.doi.org/10.1002/ardp.200700184] [PMID: 18297679]

[119] Mehlotra RK, Zimmerman PA. Resistance to antimalarial drugs: parasite and host genetic factors Malaria: genetic and evolutionary aspects. Springer 2006; pp. 81-124. [http://dx.doi.org/10.1007/0-387-28295-5_5]

[120] Bloland PB. Drug resistance in malaria. World Health Organization Geneva 2001.

[121] Peters W. The prevention of antimalarial drug resistance. Pharmacol Ther 1990; 47(3): 499-508. [http://dx.doi.org/10.1016/0163-7258(90)90067-C] [PMID: 2290858]

[122] Cowman A. The molecular basis of resistance to the sulfones, sulfonamides, and dihydrofolate reductase inhibitors. Malaria: parasite biology, pathogenesis, and protection 1998; 317-29.

[123] White NJ. Antimalarial drug resistance. J Clin Invest 2004; 113(8): 1084-92. [http://dx.doi.org/10.1172/JCI21682] [PMID: 15085184]

[124] Foley M, Tilley L. Quinoline antimalarials: mechanisms of action and resistance. Int J Parasitol 1997; 27(2): 231-40.
[http://dx.doi.org/10.1016/S0020-7519(96)00152-X] [PMID: 9088993]

[125] Kain KC. Chemotherapy of drug-resistant malaria. Can J Infect Dis 1996; 7(1): 25-33.
[http://dx.doi.org/10.1155/1996/139612] [PMID: 22514413]

[126] Organization WH. World malaria report 2008. World Health Organization 2008.

[127] Luxemburger C, Brockman A, Silamut K, *et al.* Two patients with falciparum malaria and poor in vivo responses to artesunate. Trans R Soc Trop Med Hyg 1998; 92(6): 668-9.
[http://dx.doi.org/10.1016/S0035-9203(98)90807-0] [PMID: 10326118]

[128] Gogtay NJ, Kadam VS, Karnad DR, Kanbur A, Kamtekar KD, Kshirsagar NA. Probable resistance to parenteral artemether in Plasmodium falciparum: case reports from Mumbai (Bombay), India. Ann Trop Med Parasitol 2000; 94(5): 519-20.
[http://dx.doi.org/10.1080/00034983.2000.11813571] [PMID: 10983565]

[129] Sahr F, Willoughby VR, Gbakima AA, Bockarie MJ. Apparent drug failure following artesunate treatment of Plasmodium falciparum malaria in Freetown, Sierra Leone: four case reports. Ann Trop Med Parasitol 2001; 95(5): 445-9.
[http://dx.doi.org/10.1080/00034983.2001.11813658] [PMID: 11487367]

[130] Oduola AM, Sowunmi A, Milhous WK, *et al.* Innate resistance to new antimalarial drugs in Plasmodium falciparum from Nigeria. Trans R Soc Trop Med Hyg 1992; 86(2): 123-6.
[http://dx.doi.org/10.1016/0035-9203(92)90533-I] [PMID: 1440764]

[131] Yang H, Liu D, Yang Y, *et al.* Changes in susceptibility of Plasmodium falciparum to artesunate in vitro in Yunnan Province, China. Trans R Soc Trop Med Hyg 2003; 97(2): 226-8.
[http://dx.doi.org/10.1016/S0035-9203(03)90127-1] [PMID: 14584382]

[132] Denis MB, Tsuyuoka R, Lim P, *et al.* Efficacy of artemether-lumefantrine for the treatment of uncomplicated falciparum malaria in northwest Cambodia. Trop Med Int Health 2006; 11(12): 1800-7.
[http://dx.doi.org/10.1111/j.1365-3156.2006.01739.x] [PMID: 17176344]

[133] Denis MB, Tsuyuoka R, Poravuth Y, *et al.* Surveillance of the efficacy of artesunate and mefloquine combination for the treatment of uncomplicated falciparum malaria in Cambodia. Trop Med Int Health 2006; 11(9): 1360-6.
[http://dx.doi.org/10.1111/j.1365-3156.2006.01690.x] [PMID: 16930257]

[134] Rogers WO, Sem R, Tero T, *et al.* Failure of artesunate-mefloquine combination therapy for uncomplicated Plasmodium falciparum malaria in southern Cambodia. Malar J 2009; 8(10): 10.
[http://dx.doi.org/10.1186/1475-2875-8-10] [PMID: 19138388]

[135] Carrara VI, Zwang J, Ashley EA, *et al.* Changes in the treatment responses to artesunate-mefloquine on the northwestern border of Thailand during 13 years of continuous deployment. PLoS One 2009; 4(2): e4551.
[http://dx.doi.org/10.1371/journal.pone.0004551] [PMID: 19234601]

[136] Noedl H, Se Y, Schaecher K, Smith BL, Socheat D, Fukuda MM. Artemisinin resistance in Cambodia 1 (ARC1) study consortium. Evidence of artemisinin-resistant malaria in western Cambodia. N Engl J Med 2008; 359(24): 2619-20.
[http://dx.doi.org/10.1056/NEJMc0805011] [PMID: 19064625]

[137] Organization WHO. Guidelines for the treatment of malaria. World Health Organization 2006.

[138] Mäser P, Wittlin S, Rottmann M, Wenzler T, Kaiser M, Brun R. Antiparasitic agents: new drugs on the horizon. Curr Opin Pharmacol 2012; 12(5): 562-6.
[http://dx.doi.org/10.1016/j.coph.2012.05.001] [PMID: 22652215]

[139] Pérez BC, Teixeira C, Albuquerque IS, *et al.* N-cinnamoylated chloroquine analogues as dual-stage antimalarial leads. J Med Chem 2013; 56(2): 556-67.

[http://dx.doi.org/10.1021/jm301654b] [PMID: 23273038]

[140] Mott BT, Tripathi A, Siegler MA, Moore CD, Sullivan DJ, Posner GH. Synthesis and antimalarial efficacy of two-carbon-linked, artemisinin-derived trioxane dimers in combination with known antimalarial drugs. J Med Chem 2013; 56(6): 2630-41.
[http://dx.doi.org/10.1021/jm400058j] [PMID: 23425037]

[141] Marfurt J, Chalfein F, Prayoga P, *et al.* Comparative *ex vivo* activity of novel endoperoxides in multidrug-resistant *plasmodium falciparum* and *P. vivax*. Antimicrob Agents Chemother 2012; 56(10): 5258-63.
[http://dx.doi.org/10.1128/AAC.00283-12] [PMID: 22850522]

[142] Bekhit AA, Hassan AM, Abd El Razik HA, El-Miligy MM, El-Agroudy EJ, Bekhit Ael-D. New heterocyclic hybrids of pyrazole and its bioisosteres: design, synthesis and biological evaluation as dual acting antimalarial-antileishmanial agents. Eur J Med Chem 2015; 94: 30-44.
[http://dx.doi.org/10.1016/j.ejmech.2015.02.038] [PMID: 25768697]

[143] Younis Y, Douelle F, González Cabrera D, *et al.* Structure-activity-relationship studies around the 2-amino group and pyridine core of antimalarial 3,5-diarylaminopyridines lead to a novel series of pyrazine analogues with oral in vivo activity. J Med Chem 2013; 56(21): 8860-71.
[http://dx.doi.org/10.1021/jm401278d] [PMID: 24099149]

[144] Singh S, Agarwal D, Sharma K, *et al.* 4-Aminoquinoline derivatives: Synthesis, in vitro and in vivo antiplasmodial activity against chloroquine-resistant parasites. Eur J Med Chem 2016; 122: 394-407.
[http://dx.doi.org/10.1016/j.ejmech.2016.06.033] [PMID: 27394399]

[145] Lee S, Lim D, Lee E, *et al.* Discovery of carbohybrid-based 2-aminopyrimidine analogues as a new class of rapid-acting antimalarial agents using image-based cytological profiling assay. J Med Chem 2014; 57(17): 7425-34.
[http://dx.doi.org/10.1021/jm5009693] [PMID: 25137549]

[146] Manohar S, Rajesh UC, Khan SI, Tekwani BL, Rawat DS. Novel 4-aminoquinoline-pyrimidine based hybrids with improved in vitro and in vivo antimalarial activity. ACS Med Chem Lett 2012; 3(7): 555-9.
[http://dx.doi.org/10.1021/ml3000808] [PMID: 24900509]

[147] Chandra Shekhar A, Shanthan Rao P, Narsaiah B, Allanki AD, Sijwali PS. Emergence of pyrido quinoxalines as new family of antimalarial agents. Eur J Med Chem 2014; 77: 280-7.
[http://dx.doi.org/10.1016/j.ejmech.2014.03.010] [PMID: 24650715]

[148] Almabruk KH, Lu W, Li Y, Abugreen M, Kelly JX, Mahmud T. Mutasynthesis of fluorinated pactamycin analogues and their antimalarial activity. Org Lett 2013; 15(7): 1678-81.
[http://dx.doi.org/10.1021/ol4004614] [PMID: 23521145]

[149] Muema JM, Njeru SN, Colombier C, Marubu RM. Methanolic extract of Agerantum conyzoides exhibited toxicity and growth disruption activities against Anopheles gambiae sensu stricto and Anopheles arabiensis larvae. BMC Complement Altern Med 2016; 16(1): 475.
[http://dx.doi.org/10.1186/s12906-016-1464-7] [PMID: 27876055]

[150] Kumar V, Mahajan A, Chibale K. Synthetic medicinal chemistry of selected antimalarial natural products. Bioorg Med Chem 2009; 17(6): 2236-75.
[http://dx.doi.org/10.1016/j.bmc.2008.10.072] [PMID: 19157883]

[151] Oksman-Caldentey K-M, Inzé D. Plant cell factories in the post-genomic era: new ways to produce designer secondary metabolites. Trends Plant Sci 2004; 9(9): 433-40.
[http://dx.doi.org/10.1016/j.tplants.2004.07.006] [PMID: 15337493]

[152] Chinsembu KC. Model and experiences of initiating collaboration with traditional healers in validation of ethnomedicines for HIV/AIDS in Namibia. J Ethnobiol Ethnomed 2009; 5(1): 30.
[http://dx.doi.org/10.1186/1746-4269-5-30] [PMID: 19852791]

[153] Willcox ML, Bodeker G. Traditional herbal medicines for malaria. BMJ 2004; 329(7475): 1156-9.

[http://dx.doi.org/10.1136/bmj.329.7475.1156] [PMID: 15539672]

[154] AlShebly MM, AlQahtani FS, Govindarajan M, Gopinath K, Vijayan P, Benelli G. Toxicity of ar-curcumene and epi-β-bisabolol from Hedychium larsenii (Zingiberaceae) essential oil on malaria, chikungunya and St. Louis encephalitis mosquito vectors. Ecotoxicol Environ Saf 2017; 137: 149-57. [http://dx.doi.org/10.1016/j.ecoenv.2016.11.028] [PMID: 27918946]

[155] Muema JM, Bargul JL, Nyanjom SG, Mutunga JM, Njeru SN. Potential of Camellia sinensis proanthocyanidins-rich fraction for controlling malaria mosquito populations through disruption of larval development. Parasit Vectors 2016; 9(1): 512. [http://dx.doi.org/10.1186/s13071-016-1789-6] [PMID: 27660043]

[156] Benelli G, *et al.* Neem cake as a promising larvicide and adulticide against the rural malaria vector Anopheles culicifacies (Diptera: Culicidae): a HPTLC fingerprinting approach. Nat Prod Res 2016; 1-6. [PMID: 27552943]

[157] Samuel M, Oliver SV, Coetzee M, Brooke BD. The larvicidal effects of black pepper (Piper nigrum L.) and piperine against insecticide resistant and susceptible strains of Anopheles malaria vector mosquitoes. Parasit Vectors 2016; 9(1): 238. [http://dx.doi.org/10.1186/s13071-016-1521-6] [PMID: 27117913]

[158] Govindarajan M, Rajeswary M, Benelli G. Chemical composition, toxicity and non-target effects of Pinus kesiya essential oil: An eco-friendly and novel larvicide against malaria, dengue and lymphatic filariasis mosquito vectors. Ecotoxicol Environ Saf 2016; 129: 85-90. [http://dx.doi.org/10.1016/j.ecoenv.2016.03.007] [PMID: 26995063]

[159] Govindarajan M, Rajeswary M, Arivoli S, Tennyson S, Benelli G. Larvicidal and repellent potential of Zingiber nimmonii (J. Graham) Dalzell (Zingiberaceae) essential oil: an eco-friendly tool against malaria, dengue, and lymphatic filariasis mosquito vectors? Parasitol Res 2016; 115(5): 1807-16. [http://dx.doi.org/10.1007/s00436-016-4920-x] [PMID: 26792432]

[160] Teka T, Bisrat D, Yeshak MY, Asres K. Antimalarial Activity of the Chemical Constituents of the Leaf Latex of Aloe pulcherrima Gilbert and Sebsebe. Molecules 2016; 21(11): 1415. [http://dx.doi.org/10.3390/molecules21111415] [PMID: 27801850]

[161] Govindarajan M, Benelli G. Eco-friendly larvicides from Indian plants: Effectiveness of lavandulyl acetate and bicyclogermacrene on malaria, dengue and Japanese encephalitis mosquito vectors. Ecotoxicol Environ Saf 2016; 133: 395-402. [http://dx.doi.org/10.1016/j.ecoenv.2016.07.035] [PMID: 27504617]

[162] Alonso PL, Sacarlal J, Aponte JJ, *et al.* Efficacy of the RTS,S/AS02A vaccine against Plasmodium falciparum infection and disease in young African children: randomised controlled trial. Lancet 2004; 364(9443): 1411-20. [http://dx.doi.org/10.1016/S0140-6736(04)17223-1] [PMID: 15488216]

[163] Luke TC, Hoffman SL. Rationale and plans for developing a non-replicating, metabolically active, radiation-attenuated Plasmodium falciparum sporozoite vaccine. J Exp Biol 2003; 206(Pt 21): 3803-8. [http://dx.doi.org/10.1242/jeb.00644] [PMID: 14506215]

[164] Chauhan V. Vaccines for malaria: prospects and promise. Curr Sci 2007; 92: 1525-34.

[165] Waters A. Malaria: new vaccines for old? Cell 2006; 124(4): 689-93. [http://dx.doi.org/10.1016/j.cell.2006.02.011] [PMID: 16497579]

[166] Birkett AJ, Moorthy VS, Loucq C, Chitnis CE, Kaslow DC. Malaria vaccine R&D in the Decade of Vaccines: breakthroughs, challenges and opportunities. Vaccine 2013; 31 (Suppl. 2): B233-43. [http://dx.doi.org/10.1016/j.vaccine.2013.02.040] [PMID: 23598488]

[167] Ellis RD, Sagara I, Doumbo O, Wu Y. Blood stage vaccines for Plasmodium falciparum: current status and the way forward. Hum Vaccin 2010; 6(8): 627-34. [http://dx.doi.org/10.4161/hv.6.8.11446] [PMID: 20519960]

[168] Heppner DG Jr, Kester KE, Ockenhouse CF, *et al.* Towards an RTS, S-based, multi-stage, multi-antigen vaccine against falciparum malaria: progress at the Walter Reed Army Institute of Research. Vaccine 2005; 23(17-18): 2243-50.
[http://dx.doi.org/10.1016/j.vaccine.2005.01.142] [PMID: 15755604]

[169] Keating GM. RTS, S/AS01 malaria vaccine (Mosquirix™): a guide to its use. Drugs Ther Perspect 2016; 32(4): 143-8.
[http://dx.doi.org/10.1007/s40267-016-0290-9]

[170] Organization, W.H.O. World Health Organization Malaria vaccine development 2016.

[171] Steel RW, Sack BK, Tsuji M, *et al.* An opsonic phagocytosis assay for Plasmodium falciparum sporozoites. Clinical and Vaccine Immunology. 2016; pp. CVI. 00445-.

[172] Clyde DF. Immunization of man against falciparum and vivax malaria by use of attenuated sporozoites. Am J Trop Med Hyg 1975; 24(3): 397-401.
[http://dx.doi.org/10.4269/ajtmh.1975.24.397] [PMID: 808142]

[173] Graves P, Gelband H. Vaccines for preventing malaria (SPf66). Cochrane Database Syst Rev 2006; (2): CD005966.
[PMID: 16625647]

[174] Bojang KA, Milligan PJ, Pinder M, *et al.* RTS, S Malaria Vaccine Trial Team. Efficacy of RTS,S/AS02 malaria vaccine against Plasmodium falciparum infection in semi-immune adult men in The Gambia: a randomised trial. Lancet 2001; 358(9297): 1927-34.
[http://dx.doi.org/10.1016/S0140-6736(01)06957-4] [PMID: 11747915]

[175] Agnandji ST, Lell B, Fernandes JF, *et al.* RTS,S Clinical Trials Partnership. A phase 3 trial of RTS,S/AS01 malaria vaccine in African infants. N Engl J Med 2012; 367(24): 2284-95.
[http://dx.doi.org/10.1056/NEJMoa1208394] [PMID: 23136909]

[176] Garcon N. Adjuvant systems and vaccines. Google Patents 2008.

[177] Long CA, Zavala F. Malaria vaccines and human immune responses. Curr Opin Microbiol 2016; 32: 96-102.
[http://dx.doi.org/10.1016/j.mib.2016.04.006] [PMID: 27262417]

[178] Regules JA, Cummings JF, Ockenhouse CF. The RTS,S vaccine candidate for malaria. Expert Rev Vaccines 2011; 10(5): 589-99.
[http://dx.doi.org/10.1586/erv.11.57] [PMID: 21604980]

[179] Girard MP, Reed ZH, Friede M, Kieny MP. A review of human vaccine research and development: malaria. Vaccine 2007; 25(9): 1567-80.
[http://dx.doi.org/10.1016/j.vaccine.2006.09.074] [PMID: 17045367]

[180] Good MF, Kaslow DC, Miller LH. Pathways and strategies for developing a malaria blood-stage vaccine. Annu Rev Immunol 1998; 16(1): 57-87.
[http://dx.doi.org/10.1146/annurev.immunol.16.1.57] [PMID: 9597124]

[181] Patarroyo G, Franco L, Amador R, *et al.* Study of the safety and immunogenicity of the synthetic malaria SPf66 vaccine in children aged 1-14 years. Vaccine 1992; 10(3): 175-8.
[http://dx.doi.org/10.1016/0264-410X(92)90008-8] [PMID: 1557933]

[182] Alonso PL, Smith TA, Armstrong-Schellenberg JR, *et al.* Duration of protection and age-dependence of the effects of the SPf66 malaria vaccine in African children exposed to intense transmission of Plasmodium falciparum. J Infect Dis 1996; 174(2): 367-72.
[http://dx.doi.org/10.1093/infdis/174.2.367] [PMID: 8699068]

[183] Alonso PL, Smith T, Schellenberg JR, *et al.* Randomised trial of efficacy of SPf66 vaccine against Plasmodium falciparum malaria in children in southern Tanzania. Lancet 1994; 344(8931): 1175-81.
[http://dx.doi.org/10.1016/S0140-6736(94)90505-3] [PMID: 7934537]

[184] Beck H-P, Felger I, Huber W, *et al.* Analysis of multiple Plasmodium falciparum infections in

Tanzanian children during the phase III trial of the malaria vaccine SPf66. J Infect Dis 1997; 175(4): 921-6.
[http://dx.doi.org/10.1086/513991] [PMID: 9086150]

[185] Rosas JE, Pedraz JL, Hernández RM, *et al.* Remarkably high antibody levels and protection against P. falciparum malaria in Aotus monkeys after a single immunisation of SPf66 encapsulated in PLGA microspheres. Vaccine 2002; 20(13-14): 1707-10.
[http://dx.doi.org/10.1016/S0264-410X(01)00508-4] [PMID: 11906756]

[186] Woehlbier U, Epp C, Kauth CW, *et al.* Analysis of antibodies directed against merozoite surface protein 1 of the human malaria parasite Plasmodium falciparum. Infect Immun 2006; 74(2): 1313-22.
[http://dx.doi.org/10.1128/IAI.74.2.1313-1322.2006] [PMID: 16428781]

[187] Talaat KR, Ellis RD, Hurd J, *et al.* Safety and Immunogenicity of Pfs25-EPA/Alhydrogel®, a Transmission Blocking Vaccine against Plasmodium falciparum: An Open Label Study in Malaria Naïve Adults. PLoS One 2016; 11(10): e0163144.
[http://dx.doi.org/10.1371/journal.pone.0163144] [PMID: 27749907]

[188] Datta D, *et al.* Immunogenicity and malaria transmission reducing potency of Pfs48/45 and Pfs25 encoded by DNA vaccines administered by intramuscular electroporation. Vaccine 2016.
[PMID: 27912985]

[189] Chaturvedi N, Bharti PK, Tiwari A, Singh N. Strategies & recent development of transmission-blocking vaccines against Plasmodium falciparum. Indian J Med Res 2016; 143(6): 696-711.
[http://dx.doi.org/10.4103/0971-5916.191927] [PMID: 27748294]

[190] Dutta G, Bajpai R, Vishwakarma R. Blood schizontocidal activity of artemisinin (qinghaosu) and a new antimalarial arteether against Plasmodium berghei. Indian J Parasitol 1987; 11: 253-7.

[191] Bajpai R, Dutta GP, Vishwakarma RA. Blood schizontocidal activity of a new antimalarial drug, arteether (α/β), against Plasmodium knowlesi in rhesus monkeys. Trans R Soc Trop Med Hyg 1989; 83(4): 484.
[http://dx.doi.org/10.1016/0035-9203(89)90257-5] [PMID: 2617597]

[192] Dutta GP, Bajpai R, Vishwakarma RA. Antimalarial efficacy of arteether against multiple drug resistant strain of Plasmodium yoelii nigeriensis. Pharmacol Res 1989; 21(4): 415-9.
[http://dx.doi.org/10.1016/1043-6618(89)90159-X] [PMID: 2771860]

[193] Kar K, Nath A, Bajpai R, Dutta GP, Vishwakarma RA. Pharmacology of α/β arteether--a potential antimalarial drug. J Ethnopharmacol 1989; 27(3): 297-305.
[http://dx.doi.org/10.1016/0378-8741(89)90004-4] [PMID: 2615435]

[194] Dutta GP, Bajpai R, Vishwakarma RA. Comparison of antimalarial efficacy of artemisinin (qinghaosu) and arteether against Plasmodium cynomolgi B infection in monkeys. Trans R Soc Trop Med Hyg 1989; 83(1): 56-7.
[http://dx.doi.org/10.1016/0035-9203(89)90704-9] [PMID: 2603208]

[195] Tripathi R, Dutta GP, Vishwakarma RA. Gametocytocidal activity of the antimalarial alpha/beta arteether against Plasmodium cynomolgi B. Am J Trop Med Hyg 1990; 43(6): 571-5.
[http://dx.doi.org/10.4269/ajtmh.1990.43.571] [PMID: 2267960]

[196] Valecha N, Gupta S, Usha D, *et al.* Efficacy of alpha,beta-arteether in acute uncomplicated P. falciparum malaria. Int J Clin Pharmacol Res 1997; 17(1): 11-5.
[PMID: 9403348]

[197] Dhawan S, Gunjan S, Pal A, Tripathi R. Potentiation of antimalarial activity of arteether in combination with Vetiver root extract. Indian J Exp Biol 2016; 54(5): 315-21.
[PMID: 27319050]

[198] Bhardwaj J, Siddiqui AJ, Goyal M, Prakash K, Soni A, Puri SK. Repetitive live sporozoites inoculation under arteether chemoprophylaxis confers protection against subsequent sporozoite challenge in rodent malaria model. Acta Trop 2016; 158: 130-8.

[http://dx.doi.org/10.1016/j.actatropica.2016.02.016] [PMID: 26925772]

[199] Tripathi R, Vishwakarma R, Dutta G. New antimalarial drug development: Pre-clinical status of α and β artelinate as fast acting blood schizontocides. Proc Indian Natn Sci Acad . 2008; 3: pp. 111-7.

[200] Tripathi R, Puri SK, Dutta GP. Sodium β-artelinate--a new potential gametocytocide. Exp Parasitol 1996; 82(3): 251-4.
[http://dx.doi.org/10.1006/expr.1996.0032] [PMID: 8631376]

[201] Pandey VC, Puri SK, Sahni SK, Srivastava P, Dutta GP. Effect of anti-relapse antimalarial compound CDRI 80/53 and primaquine on hepatic mixed function oxidase system of rhesus monkey. Pharmacol Res 1990; 22(6): 701-7.
[http://dx.doi.org/10.1016/S1043-6618(05)80096-9] [PMID: 2075158]

[202] Puri SK, Srivastava R, Pandey VC, Sethi N, Dutta GP. Methemoglobin toxicity and hematological studies on malaria anti-relapse compound CDRI 80/53 in dogs. Am J Trop Med Hyg 1989; 41(6): 638-42.
[http://dx.doi.org/10.4269/ajtmh.1989.41.638] [PMID: 2641641]

[203] Dutta G. New Antimalarial Drug Discovery in India and Future Strategy for Malaria Control. Proceedings of the Indian National Science Academy 2016; 82(1): 31-52.
[http://dx.doi.org/10.16943/ptinsa/2016/v82i1/48391]

[204] Puri SK, Dutta GP. Causal prophylactic activity of a new 8-aminoquinoline derivative against Plasmodium cynomolgi B in rhesus monkeys. Indian J Med Res 1990; 91: 197-9.
[PMID: 2397941]

[205] Paliwal JK, Gupta RC, Grover PK. Simultaneous determination of a new antimalarial agent, CDRI compound 80/53, and its metabolite primaquine in serum by high-performance liquid chromatography. J Chromatogr A 1993; 616(1): 155-60.
[http://dx.doi.org/10.1016/0378-4347(93)80483-K] [PMID: 8376487]

[206] Sethi N, *et al.* Systemic toxicity study of a new schizontocidal antimalarial drug-arteether in rats and monkeys. Indian J Parasitol 1988; 12(2): 223-35.

[207] Walter R, Seth M, Bhaduri A. Reversal of chloroquine resistance in Plasmodium falciparum by CDR 87/209 and analogues. Tropical medicine and parasitology: official organ of Deutsche Tropenmedizinische Gesellschaft and of Deutsche Gesellschaft fur Technische Zusammenarbeit (GTZ) 1993; 44(1): 5-8.

[208] Srivastava R, Pandey V, Bhaduri A. Evaluation of resistant-reversal, CDRI compound 87/209 and its possible mode of action in rodent experimental malaria. Tropical medicine and parasitology: official organ of Deutsche Tropenmedizinische Gesellschaft and of Deutsche Gesellschaft fur Technische Zusammenarbeit (GTZ) 1995; 46(2): 83-7.

[209] Taneja I, Raju KS, Singh SP, Wahajuddin M. Assessment of pharmacokinetic compatibility of short acting CDRI candidate trioxane derivative, 99-411, with long acting prescription antimalarials, lumefantrine and piperaquine. Sci Rep 2015; 5: 17264.
[http://dx.doi.org/10.1038/srep17264] [PMID: 26602250]

[210] Wahajuddin , Singh SP, Patel K, Pradhan T, Siddiqui HH, Singh SK. Prediction of human absorption of a trioxane antimalarial drug (CDRI 99/411) using an in-house validated in situ single-pass intestinal perfusion model. Arzneimittelforschung 2011; 61(9): 532-7.
[http://dx.doi.org/10.1055/s-0031-1296240] [PMID: 22029231]

[211] Mishra S, Manickavasagam L, Jain GK. Determination of metabolic profile of anti-malarial trioxane CDRI 99/411 in rat liver microsomes using HPLC. Biomed Chromatogr 2012; 26(1): 115-22.
[http://dx.doi.org/10.1002/bmc.1635] [PMID: 21503937]

[212] Barratt GM. Therapeutic applications of colloidal drug carriers. Pharm Sci Technol Today 2000; 3(5): 163-71.
[http://dx.doi.org/10.1016/S1461-5347(00)00255-8] [PMID: 10785658]

[213] Vauthier C, Couvreur P. Nanomedicines: A new approach for the treatment of serious diseases. J Biomed Nanotechnol 2007; 3(3): 223-34.
[http://dx.doi.org/10.1166/jbn.2007.038]

[214] Forrest ML, Kwon GS. Clinical developments in drug delivery nanotechnology. Adv Drug Deliv Rev 2008; 60(8): 861-2.
[http://dx.doi.org/10.1016/j.addr.2008.02.013] [PMID: 18358557]

[215] Newton PN, Ward S, Angus BJ, *et al.* Early treatment failure in severe malaria resulting from abnormally low plasma quinine concentrations. Trans R Soc Trop Med Hyg 2006; 100(2): 184-6.
[http://dx.doi.org/10.1016/j.trstmh.2005.01.008] [PMID: 16289166]

[216] Leite EA, Grabe-Guimarães A, Guimarães HN, Machado-Coelho GL, Barratt G, Mosqueira VC. Cardiotoxicity reduction induced by halofantrine entrapped in nanocapsule devices. Life Sci 2007; 80(14): 1327-34.
[http://dx.doi.org/10.1016/j.lfs.2006.12.019] [PMID: 17303179]

[217] Mosqueira VC, Loiseau PM, Bories C, Legrand P, Devissaguet JP, Barratt G. Efficacy and pharmacokinetics of intravenous nanocapsule formulations of halofantrine in Plasmodium berghei-infected mice. Antimicrob Agents Chemother 2004; 48(4): 1222-8.
[http://dx.doi.org/10.1128/AAC.48.4.1222-1228.2004] [PMID: 15047523]

[218] Carcaboso AM, Hernández RM, Igartua M, *et al.* Immune response after oral administration of the encapsulated malaria synthetic peptide SPf66. Int J Pharm 2003; 260(2): 273-82.
[http://dx.doi.org/10.1016/S0378-5173(03)00266-7] [PMID: 12842346]

[219] Sharma MK, Rao VK, Agarwal GS, *et al.* Highly sensitive amperometric immunosensor for detection of Plasmodium falciparum histidine-rich protein 2 in serum of humans with malaria: comparison with a commercial kit. J Clin Microbiol 2008; 46(11): 3759-65.
[http://dx.doi.org/10.1128/JCM.01022-08] [PMID: 18799699]

[220] Wiwanitkit V. Alternative tools for field analysis on malarial infection: a reappraisal. Clin Ter 2009; 160(1): 83-5.
[PMID: 19290416]

[221] Kayser O, Kiderlen AF. Delivery strategies for antiparasitics. Expert Opin Investig Drugs 2003; 12(2): 197-207.
[http://dx.doi.org/10.1517/13543784.12.2.197] [PMID: 12556214]

[222] Date AA, Joshi MD, Patravale VB. Parasitic diseases: Liposomes and polymeric nanoparticles versus lipid nanoparticles. Adv Drug Deliv Rev 2007; 59(6): 505-21.
[http://dx.doi.org/10.1016/j.addr.2007.04.009] [PMID: 17574295]

[223] Alving CR. Design and selection of vaccine adjuvants: animal models and human trials. Vaccine 2002; 20(Suppl 3): S56-64.
[http://dx.doi.org/10.1016/S0264-410X(02)00174-3]

[224] Combadière B, Mahé B. Particle-based vaccines for transcutaneous vaccination. Comp Immunol Microbiol Infect Dis 2008; 31(2-3): 293-315.
[http://dx.doi.org/10.1016/j.cimid.2007.07.015] [PMID: 17915323]

[225] Kayser O, Kiderlen AF. Delivery strategies for antiparasitics. Expert Opin Investig Drugs 2003; 12(2): 197-207.
[http://dx.doi.org/10.1517/13543784.12.2.197] [PMID: 12556214]

[226] Dwivedi P, Khatik R, Chaturvedi P, *et al.* Arteether nanoemulsion for enhanced efficacy against Plasmodium yoelii nigeriensis malaria: an approach by enhanced bioavailability. Colloids Surf B Biointerfaces 2015; 126: 467-75.
[http://dx.doi.org/10.1016/j.colsurfb.2014.12.052] [PMID: 25616971]

[227] Nayak AP, Tiyaboonchai W, Patankar S, Madhusudhan B, Souto EB. Curcuminoids-loaded lipid nanoparticles: novel approach towards malaria treatment. Colloids Surf B Biointerfaces 2010; 81(1):

263-73.
[http://dx.doi.org/10.1016/j.colsurfb.2010.07.020] [PMID: 20688493]

[228] Legrand P, Mosqueira V, Loiseau P, *et al.* Long circulating nanocapsules: interest in the treatment of severe malaria with halofantrine. Annales pharmaceutiques francaises 2003; 61(3): 196-202.

[229] Gupta Y, Jain A, Jain SK. Transferrin-conjugated solid lipid nanoparticles for enhanced delivery of quinine dihydrochloride to the brain. J Pharm Pharmacol 2007; 59(7): 935-40.
[http://dx.doi.org/10.1211/jpp.59.7.0004] [PMID: 17637187]

[230] Müller R, Hildebrand G. Pharmazeutische technologie: moderne Arzneiformen 1998.

[231] MuÈller RH, MaÈder K, Gohla S. Solid lipid nanoparticles (SLN) for controlled drug delivery–a review of the state of the art. Eur J Pharm Biopharm 2000; 50(1): 161-77.
[http://dx.doi.org/10.1016/S0939-6411(00)00087-4] [PMID: 10840199]

[232] Muller RH, Maaben S, Wayhers H, *et al.* Cytotoxicity of magnetite-loaded polylactide, polylactide/glycolide particles and solid lipid nanoparticles. Int J Pharm 1996; 138(1): 85-94.
[http://dx.doi.org/10.1016/0378-5173(96)04539-5]

[233] Muller RH, Mader K, Gohla S. Solid lipid nanoparticles (SLN): an alternative colloidal carrier system for controlled drug delivery. Eur J Pharm Biopharm 1995; 41(1): 62-9.

[234] Müller RH, Mäder K, Gohla S. Solid lipid nanoparticles (SLN) for controlled drug delivery - a review of the state of the art. Eur J Pharm Biopharm 2000; 50(1): 161-77.
[http://dx.doi.org/10.1016/S0939-6411(00)00087-4] [PMID: 10840199]

[235] Mehnert W, Mäder K. Solid lipid nanoparticles: production, characterization and applications. Adv Drug Deliv Rev 2001; 47(2-3): 165-96.
[http://dx.doi.org/10.1016/S0169-409X(01)00105-3] [PMID: 11311991]

[236] Uner M, Yener G. Importance of solid lipid nanoparticles (SLN) in various administration routes and future perspectives. Int J Nanomedicine 2007; 2(3): 289-300.
[PMID: 18019829]

[237] Cegla UH. Long-term therapy over 2 years with ambroxol (Mucosolvan) retard capsules in patients with chronic bronchitis. Results of a double-blind study of 180 patients. Prax Klin Pneumol 1988; 42(9): 715-21.
[PMID: 3141915]

[238] Speiser P. Lipid nano-pellets as excipient system for perorally administered drugs. Google Patents 1989.

[239] Eldem T, Speiser P, Hincal A. Optimization of spray-dried and -congealed lipid micropellets and characterization of their surface morphology by scanning electron microscopy. Pharm Res 1991; 8(1): 47-54.
[http://dx.doi.org/10.1023/A:1015874121860] [PMID: 2014208]

[240] Gasco MR. Method for producing solid lipid microspheres having a narrow size distribution 1991.U.S. Patent, Editor

[241] Oga EF, Singh KK. Exploring nanotechnologies for the effective therapy of malaria using plant-based medicines. Curr Pharm Des 2016; 22(27): 4232-46.
[http://dx.doi.org/10.2174/1381612822666160603014511] [PMID: 27262326]

[242] Kim K-J, Sung WS, Suh BK, *et al.* Antifungal activity and mode of action of silver nano-particles on Candida albicans. Biometals 2009; 22(2): 235-42.
[http://dx.doi.org/10.1007/s10534-008-9159-2] [PMID: 18769871]

[243] Tripathi A, Chandrasekaran N, Raichur AM, Mukherjee A. Antibacterial applications of silver nanoparticles synthesized by aqueous extract of *Azadirachta indica* (Neem) leaves. J Biomed Nanotechnol 2009; 5(1): 93-8.
[http://dx.doi.org/10.1166/jbn.2009.038] [PMID: 20055111]

[244] Nadworny PL, Wang J, Tredget EE, Burrell RE. Anti-inflammatory activity of nanocrystalline silver in a porcine contact dermatitis model. Nanomedicine (Lond) 2008; 4(3): 241-51. [http://dx.doi.org/10.1016/j.nano.2008.04.006] [PMID: 18550449]

[245] Rogers JV, Parkinson CV, Choi YW, *et al.* A preliminary assessment of silver nanoparticle inhibition of monkeypox virus plaque formation. Nanoscale Res Lett 2008; 3(4): 129. [http://dx.doi.org/10.1007/s11671-008-9128-2]

[246] Dethloff GM, Naddy RB, Gorsuch JW. Effects of sodium chloride on chronic silver toxicity to early life stages of rainbow trout (Oncorhynchus mykiss). Environ Toxicol Chem 2007; 26(8): 1717-25. [http://dx.doi.org/10.1897/06-539R.1] [PMID: 17702347]

[247] Naddy RB, Gorsuch JW, Rehner AB, McNerney GR, Bell RA, Kramer JR. Chronic toxicity of silver nitrate to Ceriodaphnia dubia and Daphnia magna, and potential mitigating factors. Aquat Toxicol 2007; 84(1): 1-10. [http://dx.doi.org/10.1016/j.aquatox.2007.03.022] [PMID: 17658626]

[248] Santhoshkumar T, Rahuman AA, Rajakumar G, *et al.* Synthesis of silver nanoparticles using Nelumbo nucifera leaf extract and its larvicidal activity against malaria and filariasis vectors. Parasitol Res 2011; 108(3): 693-702. [http://dx.doi.org/10.1007/s00436-010-2115-4] [PMID: 20978795]

[249] Sonneville-Aubrun O, Simonnet JT, L'Alloret F. Nanoemulsions: a new vehicle for skincare products. Adv Colloid Interface Sci 2004; 108-109: 145-9. [http://dx.doi.org/10.1016/j.cis.2003.10.026] [PMID: 15072937]

[250] Floury J, Desrumaux A, Axelos MAV, *et al.* Effect of high pressure homogenisation on methylcellulose as food emulsifier. J Food Eng 2003; 58(3): 227-38. [http://dx.doi.org/10.1016/S0260-8774(02)00372-2]

[251] Landfester K, Eisenblätter J, Rothe R. Preparation of polymerizable miniemulsions by ultrasonication. JCT Research 2004; 1(1): 65-8.

[252] Tadros T, Izquierdo P, Esquena J, Solans C. Formation and stability of nano-emulsions. Adv Colloid Interface Sci 2004; 108-109(0): 303-18. [http://dx.doi.org/10.1016/j.cis.2003.10.023] [PMID: 15072948]

[253] Dierling AM, Cui Z. Targeting primaquine into liver using chylomicron emulsions for potential vivax malaria therapy. Int J Pharm 2005; 303(1-2): 143-52. [http://dx.doi.org/10.1016/j.ijpharm.2005.07.015] [PMID: 16140485]

[254] Singh KK, Vingkar SK. Formulation, antimalarial activity and biodistribution of oral lipid nanoemulsion of primaquine. Int J Pharm 2008; 347(1-2): 136-43. [http://dx.doi.org/10.1016/j.ijpharm.2007.06.035] [PMID: 17709216]

[255] Hauss DJ. Oral lipid-based formulations. Adv Drug Deliv Rev 2007; 59(7): 667-76. [http://dx.doi.org/10.1016/j.addr.2007.05.006] [PMID: 17618704]

[256] Mandawgade SD, Sharma S, Pathak S, Patravale VB. Development of SMEDDS using natural lipophile: application to β-Artemether delivery. Int J Pharm 2008; 362(1-2): 179-83. [http://dx.doi.org/10.1016/j.ijpharm.2008.06.021] [PMID: 18652886]

[257] Hauss DJ, Fogal SE, Ficorilli JV, *et al.* Lipid-based delivery systems for improving the bioavailability and lymphatic transport of a poorly water-soluble LTB4 inhibitor. J Pharm Sci 1998; 87(2): 164-9. [http://dx.doi.org/10.1021/js970300n] [PMID: 9519148]

[258] Caliph SM, Charman WN, Porter CJ. Effect of short-, medium-, and long-chain fatty acid-based vehicles on the absolute oral bioavailability and intestinal lymphatic transport of halofantrine and assessment of mass balance in lymph-cannulated and non-cannulated rats. J Pharm Sci 2000; 89(8): 1073-84. [http://dx.doi.org/10.1002/1520-6017(200008)89:8<1073::AID-JPS12>3.0.CO;2-V] [PMID: 10906731]

[259] Patil S, Suryavanshi S, Pathak S, Sharma S, Patravale V. Evaluation of novel lipid based formulation of β-Artemether and Lumefantrine in murine malaria model. Int J Pharm 2013; 455(1-2): 229-34. [http://dx.doi.org/10.1016/j.ijpharm.2013.07.033] [PMID: 23886650]

[260] Organization, W.H.O. Global technical strategy for malaria 2016–2030 2016.

CHAPTER 3

Chemical Structures and Classification of Anti-microbial Drugs

F. Zehra Küçükbay[*, 1] and **Hasan Küçükbay**[2]

[1] *Department of Basic Pharmaceutical Sciences, Faculty of Pharmacy, İnönü University, 44280 Malatya, Turkey*

[2] *Department of Chemistry, Faculty of Arts and Science, İnönü University, 44280 Malatya, Turkey*

Abstract: This chapter aims to review the literature on anti-infective (also known as antimicrobial) drugs among the anti-infections drugs, and to highlight recent developments relating to novel antibiotics and their classification. Antibiotic classification is determined according to their structure and mechanism of action; the main groups include β-lactams, macrolides, fluoroquinolones, tetracyclines, and aminoglycosides. Despite significant progress in anti-infective therapies, infectious diseases caused by bacteria and fungi remain a major worldwide health problem due to the rapid development of resistance to existing drugs. This resistance increasingly limits the effectiveness of current anti-infective drugs. To overcome this problem, scientists are searching for novel therapeutic agents that are efficacious against microorganisms and cause limited side-effects. Naturally occuring compounds in plants have previously been used successfully to treat many types of infection and illness. For this reason, it is quite important to understand the chemical composition of natural products and their mechanisms of action, in order to synthesize semi-synthetic or synthetic anti-infective drugs. Indeed, many chemically synthesized drugs originated from natural sources, *e.g.* aspirin (willow plant), opioids such as morphine (opium poppy), atropine (*Atropa belladonna*), and quinine (cinchona). Therefore, nature is a very fruitful source for pharmacy, medicine, biology and chemistry students.

Keywords: Anti-bacterial drugs, Aminoglycosides, Anti-fungal drugs, Anti-infective agents, Antibiotic, Cephalosporins, Chloramphenicol, Classification of antibiotics, Drug research, Drug resistance, Fluoroquinolones, Infectious diseases, Macrolides, Microorganisms, Natural products, Penicillin, Penicillium species, Synthesis, Tetracyclines, β-lactams.

[*] **Corresponding author F. Zehra Küçükbay:** Department of Basic Pharmaceutical Sciences, Faculty of Pharmacy, İnönü University, 44280 Malatya, Turkey; Tel: +90 422 3773881; Fax: +90 422 3410037; E-mail: zkucukbay@inonu.edu.tr

Atta-ur-Rahman & M. Iqbal Choudhary (Eds.)

INTRODUCTION

Infectious diseases are responsible for more deaths worldwide than any other single cause. Their pathology is attributed to microorganisms such as bacteria, viruses, fungi, or parasites that are virulent and can spread between individuals.

Anti-infection Agents

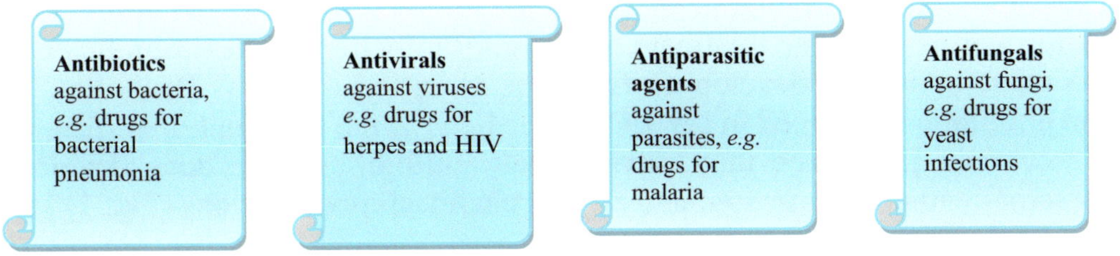

Antibiotics are an important subset of antimicrobial chemotherapeutics. An antibiotic is any therapeutic agent that kills or prevents the reproduction of bacteria in the body. An antimicrobial is a substance composed of natural, semi-synthetic, or synthetic, a broad term for compounds that kill or inhibit the growth of microorganisms but cause little or no damage to the host. Antibiotics are a subset of antimicrobials that specifically treat bacterial infections.

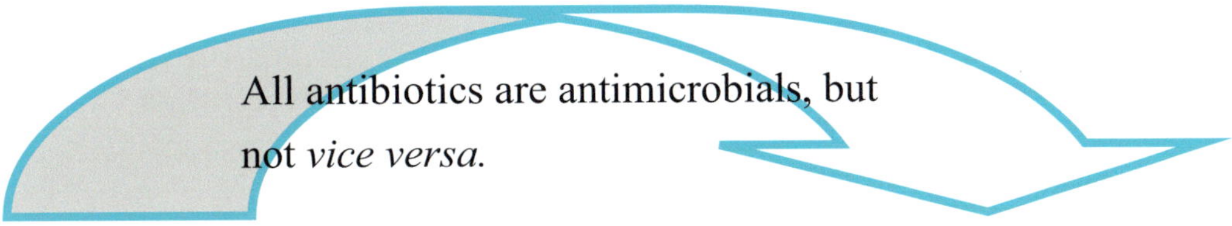

Microorganisms are ubiquitous; they can be found in the air, water, soil, and rocks; many microorganisms also live inside and on the surface of our bodies [1].

Most of the microbes living in our bodies are symbiotic and assist normal bodily function. Many of the drugs available today are derived from compounds first found in microorganisms. However, under certain conditions, some micro-organisms become virulent and cause harmful infections in humans, animals, and plants. Infectious microorganisms can be passed directly between people or indirectly from an infected person to the environment (for example door handles, bedding, toilets, *etc.*) and then to another person who comes in contact with the contaminated source. Some are transmitted by bites from insects or animals, while others are acquired by consuming contaminated food or water. The symptoms and signs of infection vary depending on which part of the body and which type of organism is involved. The first signs of infection are often inflammatory symptoms (fever, pain, swelling, redness, and purulence). Mild infections may respond to rest and home remedies, while life-threatening infections may require hospitalization. The main form of treatment is usually antimicrobial medication. There are several types of anti-infective drugs, depending on the type of organism targeted (such as antibiotics for bacterial infections, antiviral drugs for a limited number of viruses, antifungal medications for fungal infections, and antihelmintic drugs for worms) [2]. The treatment of bacterial infections with antibiotics is one of the most important developments of the twentieth century. Penicillin, a β-lactam antibiotic developed in the 1940s, has been at the forefront of antibacterial drug treatment [3]. Since then, several new antibiotics have been developed, either semi-synthetically or synthetically by chemical modifications (Fig. **1**) [4].

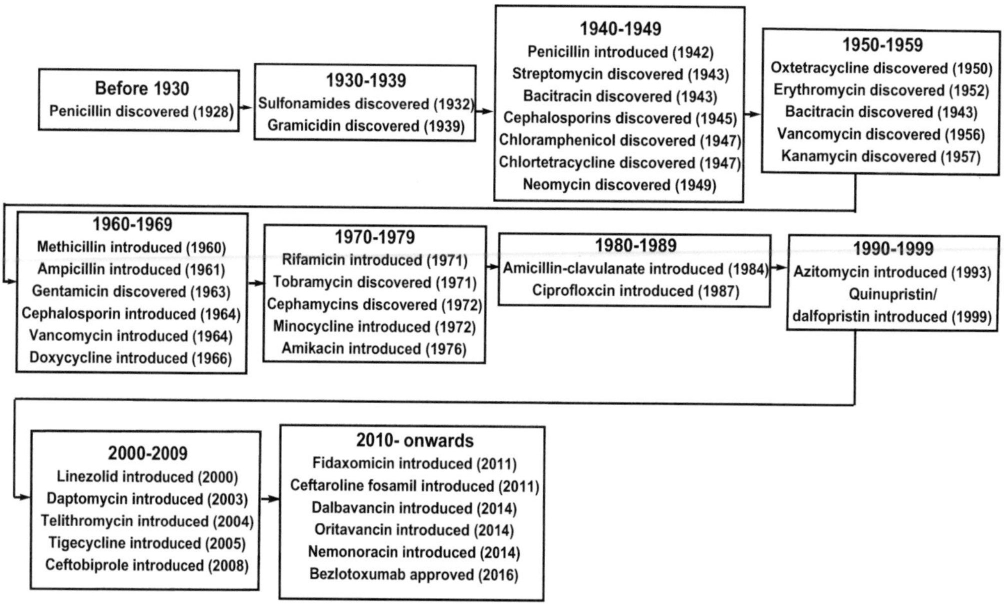

Fig. (1). A timeline of important historical antibiotic discoveries [4].

There was no effective treatment method for infections such as pneumonia, gonorrhea, or rheumatic fever before penicillin. However, the use of antimicrobial agents is known to have been a common practice for at least two millennia. Many ancient Egyptians and Greeks used various molds and plant extracts to fight bacterial infections [5]. Furthermore, ancient Egyptians applied moldy bread to infected wounds for its antibiotic effects. Much later, it was determined that the ssscharacteristic blue-green discoloration seen on moldy bread was the useful antibiotic-producing *Penicillium chrysogenum* mold. In 1928, the active ingredient penicillin was discovered by Alexander Fleming [5, 6]. About a century ago, microbiologists such as Louis Pasteur and Jules Francois Joubert observed an antagonistic effect between different strains of bacteria, and subsequently searched for an application of this knowledge in medicine.

Penicillium notatum and *Penicillium chrysogenum* have been used for the production of penicillin. The *Penicillium* species can grow on different substrates, such as plants, wood, tree bark, cheese, green leather (old boots), cork, animal dung, syrup, seeds, and almost any other organic item. The success of penicillin led scientists to search for other antibiotic-producing microorganisms, particularly those from soil environments. In 1943, streptomycin was discovered from a soil actinomycete, *Streptomyces griseus*. While useful for the treatment of tuberculosis, streptomycin was not as safe as penicillin for general use. Thereafter, chloramphenicol, tetracycline, macrolide, and glycopeptide (*e.g.*, vancomycin) were discovered from soil bacteria and introduced in clinical practice [7]. Although bacteria are being studied extensively for novel metabolites, it is clear that the rate of drug discovery is decreasing, in part due to diminishing returns from traditional resources such as soil bacteria. However, nature continues to be a major source for the discovery of therapeutic compounds. Traditionally, actinomycetes and fungi have provided many important bioactive compounds of high value and they continue to be routinely screened for new bioactive compounds [7]. Every day, new species and taxa of fungi and actinomycetes are being researched. Owing to the fact that drug-resistant strains of pathogens emerge more quickly than the rate of discovery of new drugs and antibiotics, many scientists and pharmaceutical companies are involved in the isolation and screening of actinomycetes from different habitats, in order to identify novel antibiotic substances. Investigation of bacteria from previously unexplored environments have recently yielded many promising new compounds. Marine environments are a potential source of novel drugs; however, the world's oceans, covering more than 70% of the earth's surface, remain relatively unexplored. Environments have recently yielded many promising new compounds. Marine organisms that may produce novel therapeutic compounds include deep-sea sediment actinomycetes, sponges and seaweeds, bacterial symbionts of insects, ascidians, fungi and myxobacteria [8, 9]. Several marine resources have historically been harvested for their useful properties; seaweeds have been used for a long time to fertilize the soil since the ancient ages [10]. However, the first serious investigation of marine organisms started only about fifty years ago [11]. After extensive research, several marine-derived compounds were accepted for clinical trials, particularly as anti-cancer agents, such as mechercharmycins, salinosporamide A, chinikomycins, and lodopyridone [12 - 15]. Marine compounds have also been found to have antibiotic and anti-inflammatory effects, such as glaciapyrroles, frigocyclinone, and pacificanones A and B [16 - 18]. In particular, recent studies have revealed that selected groups of marine actinomycetes are a robust source of new natural products [19].

Antibiotics represent one of the greatest advances in the history of medicine. They enable the treatment of a wide variety of common infections and underlie the delivery of complex care, from cancer treatment to surgery. A wide range of related classes of antibiotics have been identified, including cephalosporins, macrolides, aminoglycosides, and lipopeptides. However, resistance to antibiotics has been rising over time to dangerously high levels in many world regions due to widespread misuse of antibiotics and their increased application in agriculture and livestock. New mechanisms of antibiotic resistance are emerging and spreading globally, and threatening our ability to treat common infectious diseases [20]. Since antibiotic resistance emerges as a part of a natural process in which bacteria evolve, it can only be partially inhibited by scientific and regulatory measures. Resistance to antibiotic is a worldwide health problem and a large financial burden to society. Discussions of antibiotic resistance at the recent G7 summit in Krîn provided a clear reminder of the challenges faced. According to a recent document, "Antibiotic Resistance Threats in the United States" by the U.S. Centers for Disease Control and Prevention (CDC), at least 23,000 people die as a result of antibiotic-resistant bacterial infections each year in the USA alone, and 11,000 of those are caused by methicillin-resistant *Staphylococcus aureus* (MRSA) [21]. Therefore, the need for new antibiotics against resistant bacteria is an ever-pertinent issue. As a result, scientists are attempting to produce and discover new antibiotics to overcome the issue of bacterial resistance to older antibiotics.

In today's modern world, numerous classes of antimicrobial agents are known and classified based on their mechanisms of action [22]. Antimicrobial drugs are compounds that have selective toxicity against microbes; they target microbial cells while leaving the host relatively unharmed. Antibiotics are a subset of antimicrobial drugs, and were originally defined as substances produced by microorganisms that inhibit other microorganisms. Antibiotics (Greek anti, "against" and bios, "life") are chemical compounds produced by living organisms. Dr. Selman A. Waksman, a soil microbiologist, suggested the noun "antibiotic" in 1942 [23]. Dr. Waksman and his colleagues discovered several actinomycetes-derived antibiotics in the following course of time [24].

The nature of antibiotic substances has changed over time, from naturally to synthetically derived. At present, most antibiotics are manufactured synthetically or semi-synthetically, based on the structures originally identified from microorganisms. Semi-synthetic antibiotics are developed by including additional steps that modify naturally produced compounds, while synthetic antibiotics are developed entirely by chemical manufacturing processes [25].

CLASSIFICATION OF ANTIBIOTICS

Antibiotics are classified depending on their origin, chemical structure, bacterial spectrum, or (most commonly) mechanism of action [26]. Some antibiotics inhibit bacterial cell wall biosynthesis (penicillins and cephalosporins); some cause disruption of the cellular membrane (polymyxins); and others inhibit the synthesis of nucleic acids and proteins (rifamycins, lipiarmycins, quinolones, and sulfonamides), disrupting the polymers that constitute bacterial cells (Fig. **2**) [27].

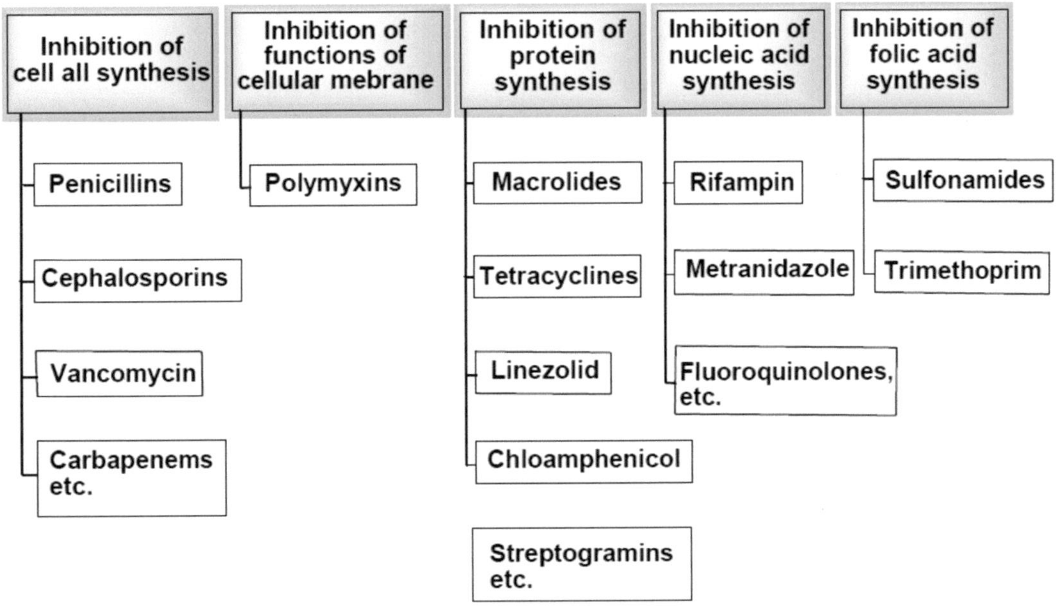

Fig. (2). Mechanism of action of antibiotics agents [28].

Further categorization of antibiotics is based on their target specificity. Some antibiotics act against both Gram-positive and Gram-negative bacteria and are known as "broad-spectrum" antibiotics (tetracyclines, phenicols, and fluoroquinolones, and third-generation and fourth-generation cephalosporins). Others are only effective against particular species of microorganisms and are thus classified as "narrow-spectrum" antibiotics [28, 29]. Aminoglycosides and sulfonamides are only effective against aerobic organisms, while nitroimidazoles are generally only effective against anaerobic microorganisms such as *Trichomonas vaginallis* (Fig. **3**).

Broad Spectrum Antibiotics	Narrow Spectrum Antibiotics
Tetracycline 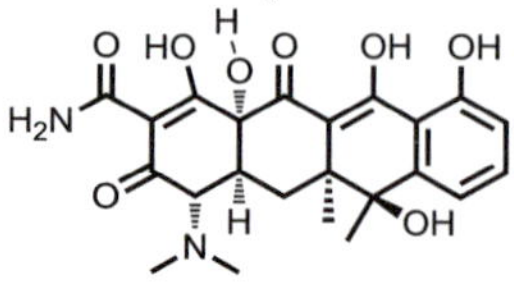	**Penicillin V** 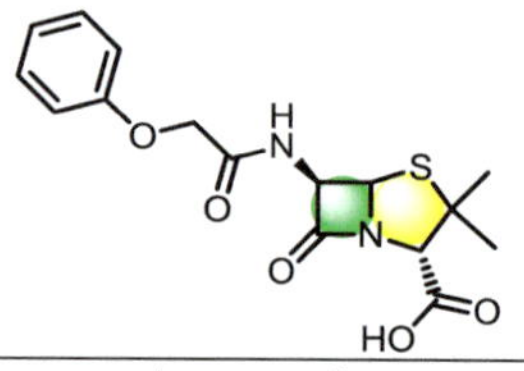
Amoxicillin 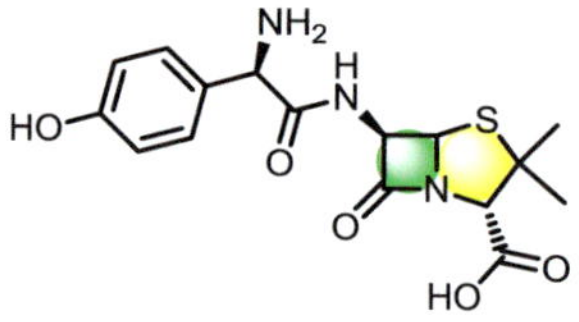	**Aerosporin** 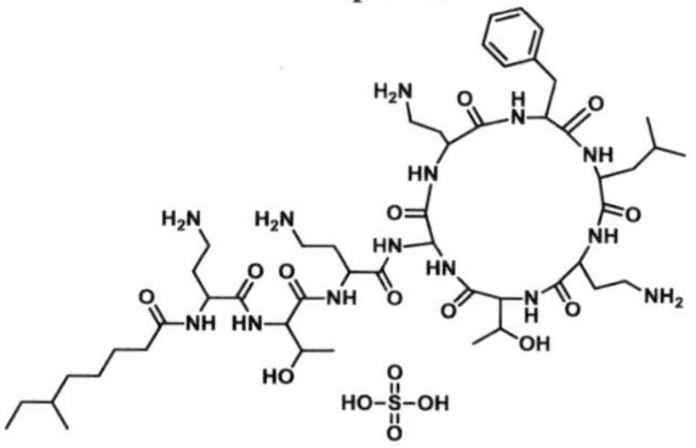
Cefazolin 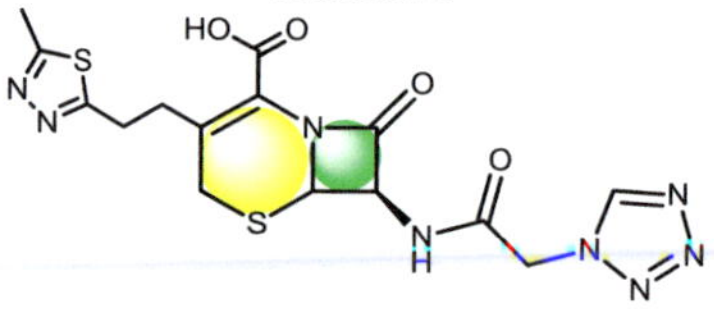	**Clarithromycin** 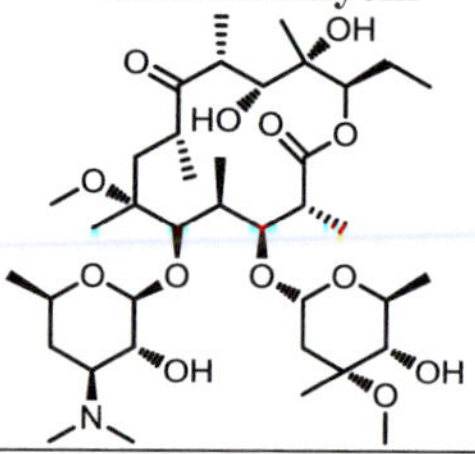
Cefozopran 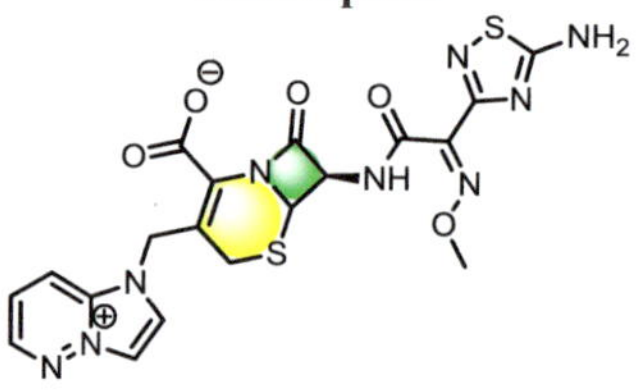	**Tobramycin** 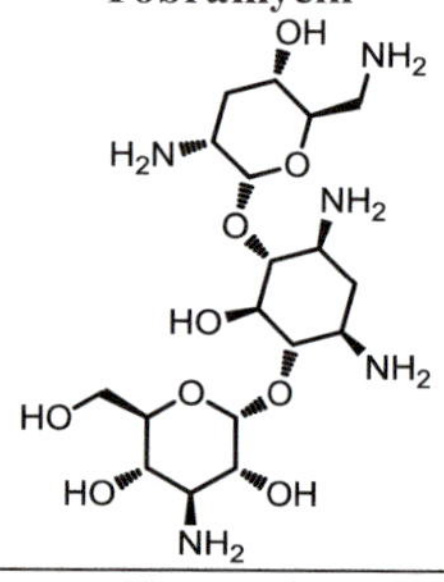
Ciprofloxacin 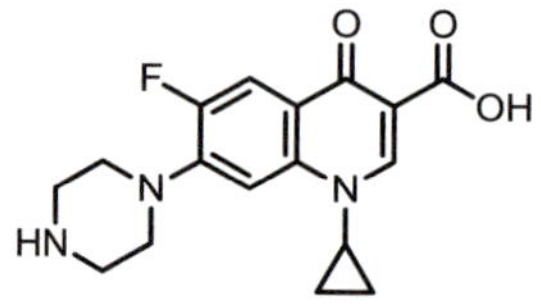	**Neomycin** 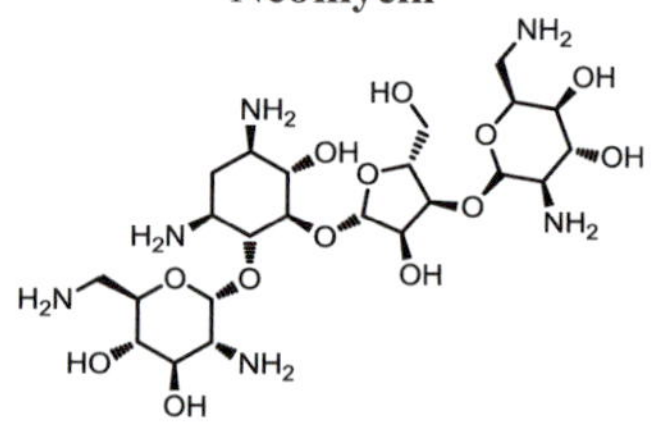

Fig. (3). Therapeutic spectra examples of antibiotics.

In broad terms, antibiotics can be classified as either bactericidal or bacteriostatic. Bactericidal antibiotics kill their target organisms. Aminoglycosides, cephalosporins, penicillins, and quinolones are examples of bactericidal antibiotics. In contrast to bactericidal antibiotics, bacteriostatic antibiotics inhibit or delay bacterial growth and replication. Tetracycline is an example of a bacteriostatic antibiotic. It inhibits the bacterial ribosome, so that no new proteins can be made; however, it does not directly induce cell death. Depending on the dose, duration of exposure, and the state of the invading bacteria, some antibiotics can be both bacteriostatic and bactericidal. For instance, aminoglycosides, fluoroquinolones, and metronidazole exert concentration-dependent characteristics; as the drug concentration increases, their level of cytotoxicity increases. Some common examples of both types of antibiotics are given in Fig. (**4**) [30].

Bactericides antibiotics		**Bacteriostatic antibiotics**	
Daptomycin 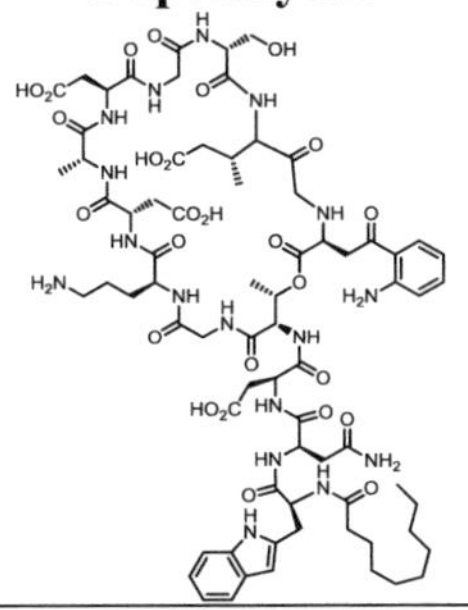	**Fluoroquinolones (Lomefloxacin)** 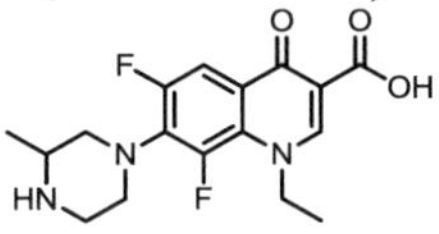	**Tetracyclines (Minocyline)** 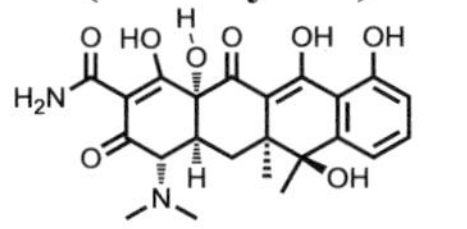	**Sulfonamides (Sulfamethoxazole)** 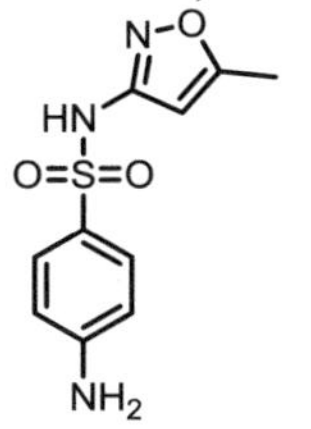
Metronidazole 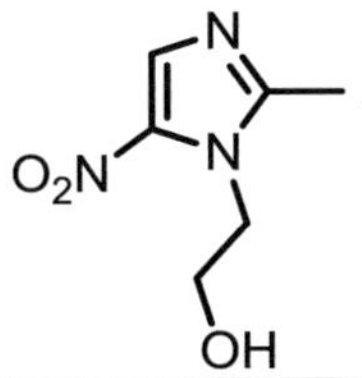	**Nitrofuration** 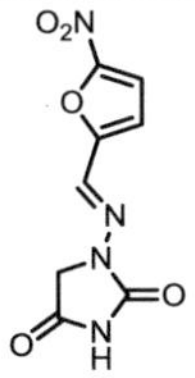	**Spectinomycin** 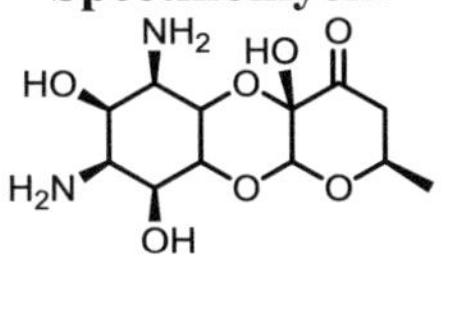	**Trimethoprim** 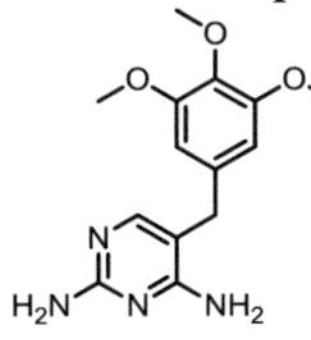
Co-trimoxazole 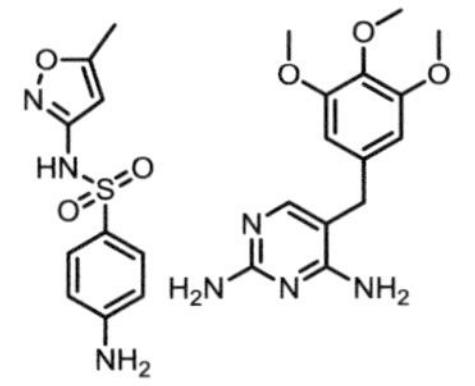	**Telithromycin** 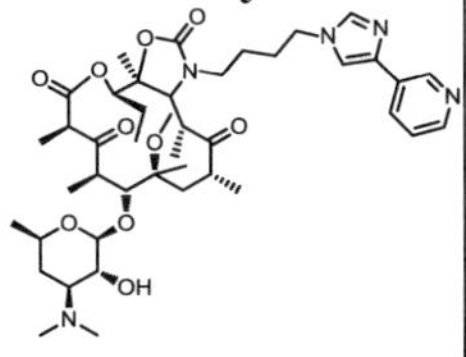	**Chloramphenicol** 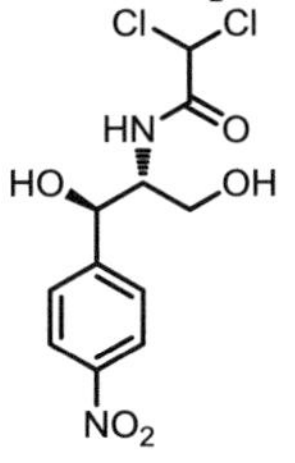	**Macrolides (Erythromycin)** 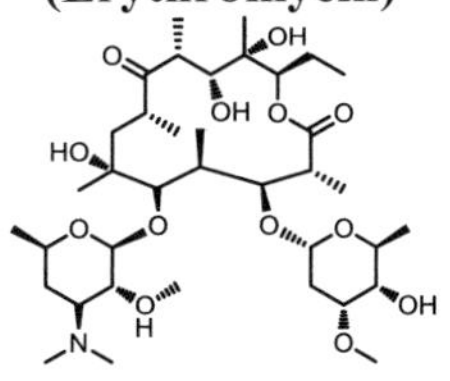

Fig. 4 contd.....

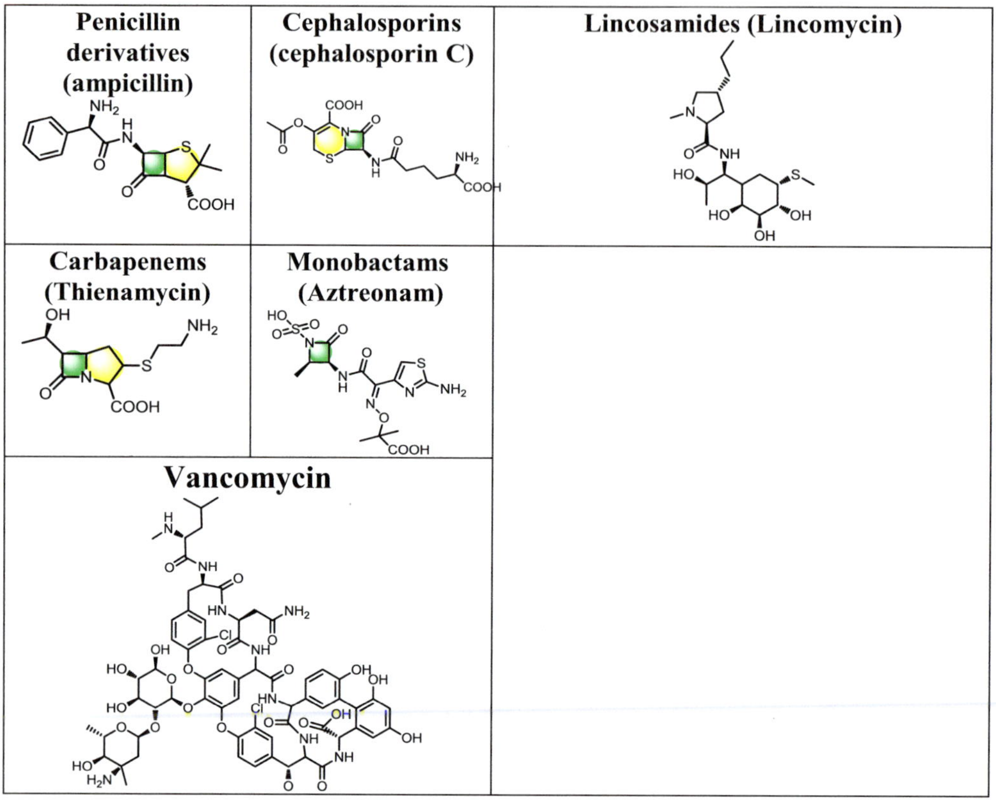

s.

Fig. (4). Some common bactericidal or bacteriostatic antibiotics types.

Based on their origin, antibiotics can also be classified as natural, semi-synthetic, and synthetic (Fig. **5**). A natural antibiotic is a chemical substance produced by a microorganism (bacteria or fungi). Antibiotics from natural sources can be small molecular weight compounds (*e.g.,* penicillins) or large glycopeptides such as teicoplanin; a complex of related natural products isolated from the fermentation broth of a strain of *Actinoplanes teichomyceticus* [31].

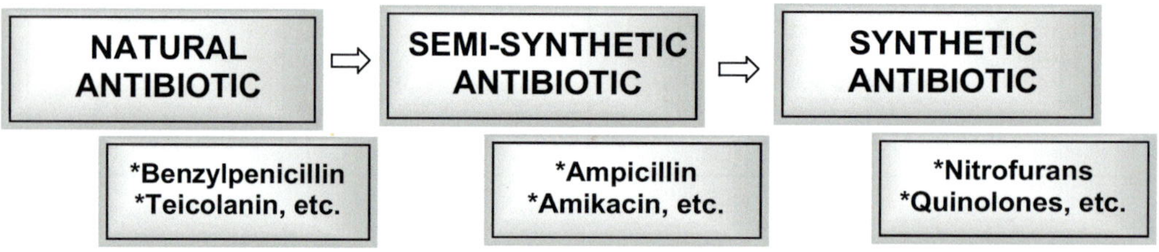

Fig. (5). Antibiotics according to their origin.

Soil microorganisms are a rich source of structurally diverse bioactive substances that interact with various molecular targets [32]. With the improvement of extraction techniques, active components have been isolated from natural materials and structurally characterized. Improvements were later made to naturally occurring antibiotics by synthetic modification, which has subsequently aided clinical outcomes [33]. The preparation of antibacterial drugs using fully synthetic methods has resulted in the discovery and approval of a large number of new antibiotics. Synthetic sulfonamides (also called sulfa or sulpha drugs) were discovered in the 1930s. Sulfonamide drugs were the first antibiotic substances to be used systemically before the discovery of penicillins, and paved the way for revolutionary antibiotic discoveries in medicine [8]. The second class of antibiotics to be fully synthesized were quinolones, discovered in 1962 when Lesher *et al.* made the accidental discovery of nalidixic acid as a by-product of anti-malarial chloroquine synthesis [3]. The third class of synthetic antibiotics to appear was the oxazolidinones, discovered in 1979. However, the first oxazolidinone drug linezolid was not approved for medicinal use until 2000. Currently, the discovery and development of new fully synthetic antibiotics remains an active area of research.

Antibiotics may also be classified on the basis of their chemical structure; as penicillins (penicillin G, penicillin V, ampicillin, amoxicillin, *etc.*), cephalosporins (cefadroxil, cefazolin, cephalexin, *etc.*), aminoglycosides (gentamicin, streptomycin and neomycin), tetracyclines (deoxycycline, minocycline, *etc.*), macrolides (erythromycin, azithromycin, *etc.*), sulfonamides (bactrim, sulfatrim, gantrisin, *etc.*), fluoroquinolones (oflaxacin, levofloxacin, *etc.*), and polypeptides (actinomycin, colistin, polymyxin B, *etc.*) (Fig. **6**) [34].

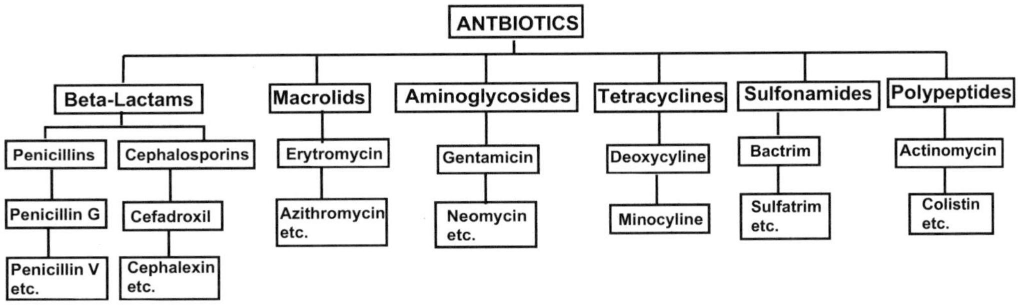

Fig. (6). Classification of antibiotics according to chemical structures.

Although there are several classification schemes for antibiotics, the most useful is based on chemical structure. Antibiotics within a structural class will have, generally display similar patterns of effectiveness, toxicity, and allergic potential.

The main classes of antibiotics can be determined as follows:

- Penicillins
  1. Beta-Lactams
- Cephalosporins
  1. Macrolides
  2. Fluoroquinolones
  3. Tetracyclines
  4. Aminoglycosides

These antibiotics are the most widely used; their various applications are listed in Table **1**.

Table 1. Some common antibiotics with their class and uses.

Class of antibiotic	Antibiotic	Uses
Penicillins	• Amoxicillin • Ampicillin • Bacampicillin • Oxacillin • Penicillin	Used to treat skin infections, dental infections, ear infections, respiratory tract infections, urinary tract infections, gonorrhea.
Cephalosporin	(1) First generation • Cephalothin • Cefazolin • Cephapirin • Cephradine • Cephalexin • Cefadroxil (2) Second generation • Cefaclor • Cefamandole • Cefonicid • Ceforanide • Cefuroxime (3) Third generation • Cefcapene • Cefdaloxime • Cefditoren • Cefetamet • Cefixime • Cefmenoxime • Cefodizime • Cefoperazone • Cefotaxime	Used to treat pneumonia, strep throat, staph infections, tonsillitis, bronchitis, otitis media, various types of skin infections, gonorrhea, urinary tract infections and bone infections.

(Table 1) contd.....

Class of antibiotic	Antibiotic	Uses
Cephalosporin	• Cefpimizole • Cefpodoxime • Ceftibuten • Ceftriaxone (4) Fourth generation • Cefepime • Cefpirome • Cefclidine • Cefluprenam • Cefozopran • Cefquinome	Used to treat pneumonia, strep throat, staph infections, tonsillitis, bronchitis, otitis media, various types of skin infections, gonorrhea, urinary tract infections and bone infections.
Macrolides	• Erythromycin • Clarithromycin • Azithromycin • Dirithromycin • Roxithromycin • Troleandomycin	Used to treat respiratory tract infections (such as pharyngitis, sinusitis, and bronchitis), genital, gastrointestinal tract, and skin infections.
Fluoroquinolones	• Ciprofloxacin • Levofloxacin • Lomefloxacin • Norfloxacin • Sparfloxacin • Clinafloxacin • Gatifloxacin • Ofloxacin • Trovafloxacin	Used to treat urinary tract infections, skin infections, and respiratory infections such as sinusitis, pneumonia, bronchitis.
Tetracyclines	• Tetracycline • Doxycycline • Minocycline • Oxytetracycline	Used in the treatment of infections of the respiratory tract, sinuses, middle ear, urinary tract, skin, intestines, Gonorrhoea, Rocky Mountain spotted fever, lyme disease, typhus.
Aminoglycosides	• Amikacin • Gentamicin • Kanamycin • Neomycin • Streptomycin • Tobramycin	Used to treat infections caused by gram-negative bacteria.

β-Lactam Antibiotics

The β-lactam antibiotics are a large class of diverse compounds applied clinically in both oral and parenteral forms. They are among the most frequently prescribed medications in modern medicine owing to their broad target spectrum and excellent safety [35]. Beta-lactams have a long history in the treatment of infectious, although their use has been confounded by the development of resistance in target organisms. All β-lactam agents share the structural feature of a β-lactam ring. This feature causes the inhibition of bacterial cell wall synthesis [36].

All β-lactam antibiotics are derivatives of a bicyclic ring system. With the exception of 6-aminopenicillanic acid (6-APA) and 7-aminocephalosporanic acid (7-ACA), all β-lactams have an acyl group attached as a side chain to the amino group of a heterocyclic nucleus. The β-lactam antibiotics can be classified as penicillins and cephalosporins, according to their chemical constitution of their ring system. The penicillin ring system contains a four-membered β-lactam ring fused to a five-membered thiazolidine ring. The cephalosporin ring system (Fig. **7**) differs from the penicillins in that it contains an unsaturated six-membered (rather than five-membered) dihydrothiazine ring [37, 38]. Furthermore, penicillins contain a single side-chain at the 6-position, while cephalosporins have two side-chains at the 7- and 3-positions. While all first- and second-generation cephalosporins have similar side-chains to penicillin antibiotics, later generations have structurally different side-chains (Fig. **8**) [37]. β-Lactam antibiotics have been in clinical use for more than half century and are the most frequently used agents in treatment of bacterial infections.

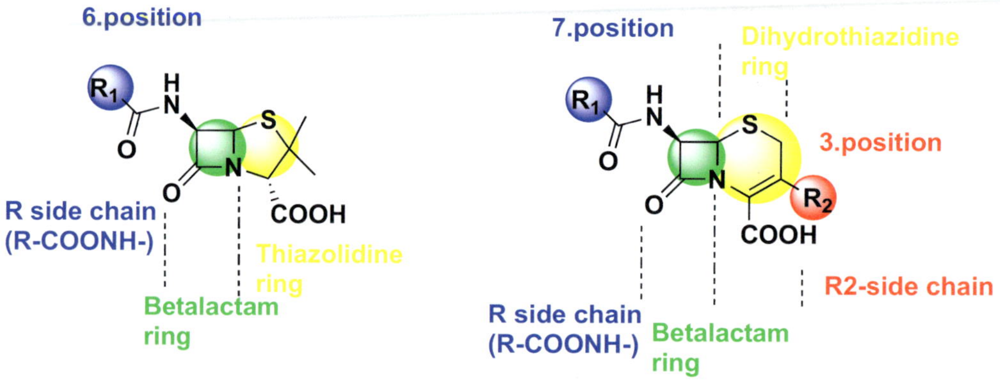

Fig. (7). Penicillins and cephalosporins chemical structures.

The first natural β-lactam antibiotic was penicillin G (benzylpenicillin), discovered unintentionally by Alexander Fleming in 1928 from the fungus *Penicillium chrysogenum* (formerly known as *Penicillium notatum*). The Australian Nobel Laureate Howard Walter Florey later developed penicillin for use as a medicine [39]. Currently, the β-lactam group of compounds is the most successful example of natural product application and chemotherapy.

Amoxicillin	**Cephalexin** **1st generation**	**Cepfrozil** **2nd generation**
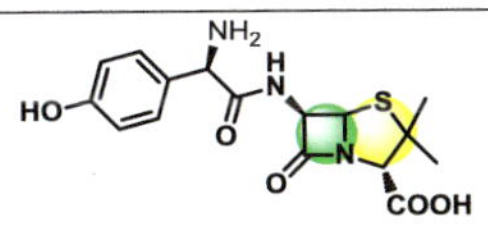 *R₁-side chain*	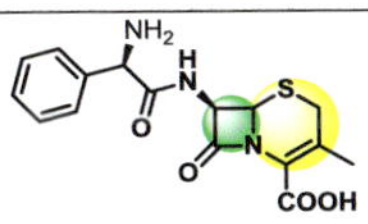 *R₁-side chain*	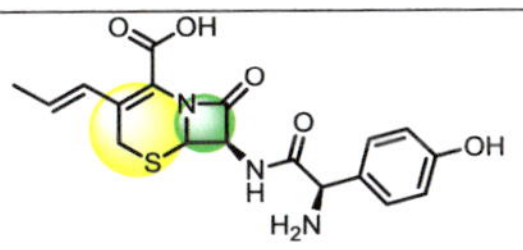 *R₁-side chain*
	Ceftriaxone **3rd generation**	**Cefepime** **4th generation**
	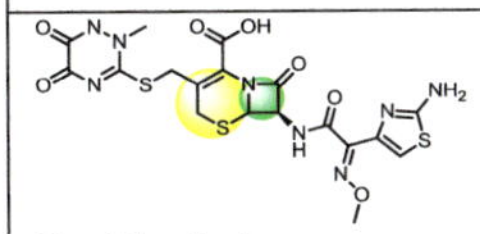 *R₁-side chain*	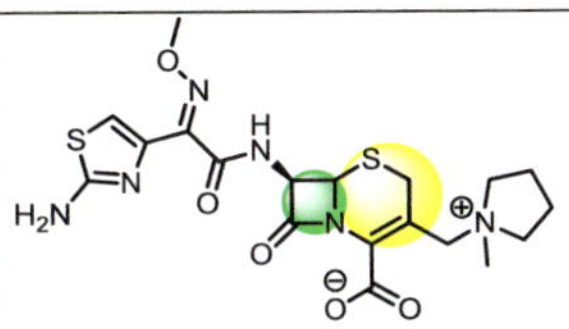 *R₁-side chain*
	Ceftaroline **5th generation**	
	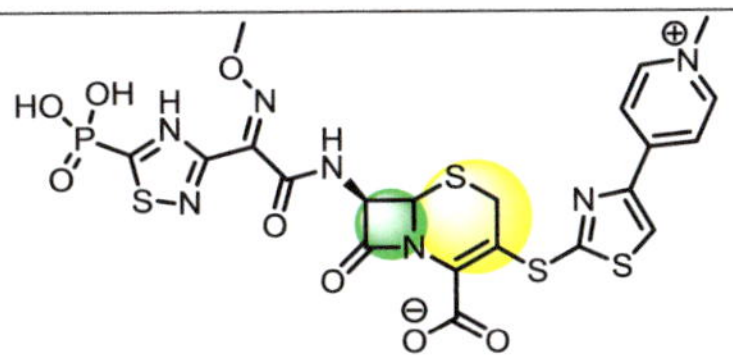 *R₁-side chain*	

Fig. (8). Chemical structures ampicillin and 1st, 2nd, 3rd,4th, 5th generation cephalosporins.

Penicillins, some of the most commonly used β-lactam antibiotics, are composed of three structural features: a fused β-lactam ring, a free carboxylic acid group (also common to penicillin derived antibiotics), and one or more substituted amino acid side chains. Penicillin G, penicillin V, ampicillin, amoxicillin, and methicillin have essentially the same structure and differed only in the R-groups bound to the carbonyl group, shown at the top left of Fig. (**9**) [40].

The penicillin family is composed of both natural and semi-synthetic members. Nevertheless, penicillins are preeminently natural products and their industrial production depends on microbial fermentation. Biosynthetic penicillin is produced directly from the *Penicillium* mold through the process of fermentation. Specific penicillins are synthesized by the addition of different side-chain precursors to the culture medium. The first semi-synthetic penicillins, prepared by chemical substitution of the *p*-hydroxy group of the naturally occurring penicillin X (*p*-hyrdoxybenzylpenicillin). Romansky and Robin [40, 42] found that the two penicillins were equally active. An approach to modify the amino group of *p*-aminobenzylpenicillin was unsuccessful. However, research on this compound led to the critical discovery in 1957 of 6-APA, considered to be the "nucleus" of the penicillin molecule, which has enabled researchers to develop numerous semi-synthetic penicillins. Chemical expansion of 6-APA to 7-ACA generated a number of important orally active cephalosporins such as cephalexin, cephradine, and cefadroxyl [43].

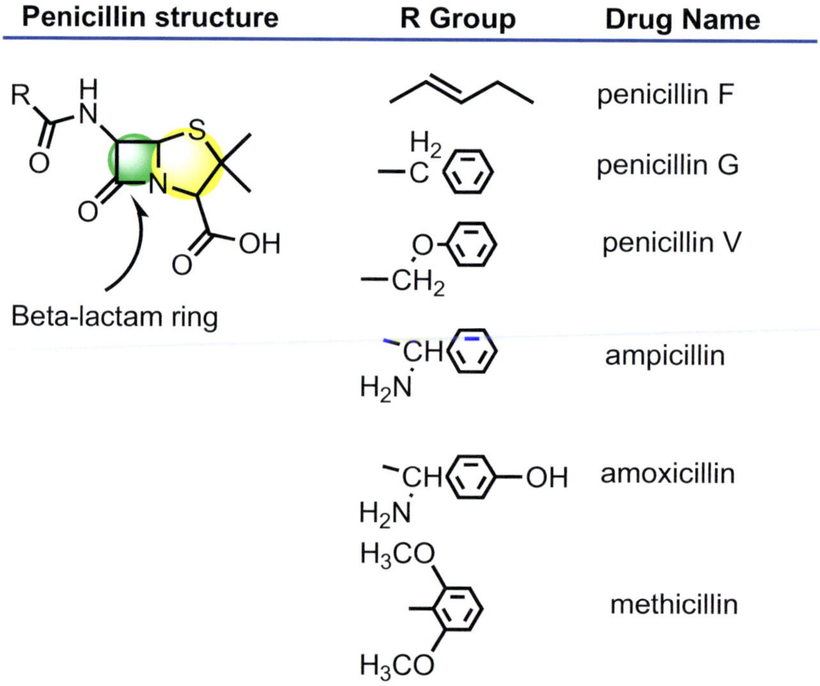

Fig. (9). Penicillin structure and its derivative forms [41].

Most penicillins are semi-synthetic derivatives of 6-APA, prepared by the addition of acyl side-chains at the 6-amino group [44, 45]. The first semi-synthetic penicillin to be introduced into clinical practice was a close analog of penicillin V, namely phenethicillin (or pheneticillin), in 1957 by Sheehan and Henery-Logan [46]. This was followed by methicillin, oxacillin, cloxacillin, dicloxacillin, flucloxacillin, carbenicillin, amoxicillin, and ticarcillin [41]. These β-lactam antibiotics are also known as anti-staphylococcal penicillins, because they target the bacteria *Staphylococcus aureus* [37]. Ampicillin (discovered 1961) and amoxicillin (discovered 1972) were the first antibiotics of the second-generation broad-spectrum penicillins) [47, 48]. Amoxicillin is very closely related to ampicillin, with a similar spectrum of activity and potency. Next generation of penicillins are represented by tircacillin (1971) and piperacillin (1977). These extended-spectrum penicillins (also called antipseudomonals) include both carboxypenicillins (tircacillin) and ureidopenicillins (piperacillin). These antibiotics are active against Gram-positive cocci, anaerobes, and Gram-negative bacteria [37, 40].

Following the extraction of penicillin from *Penicillium chrysogenum,* discoveries by an Italian scientist Giuseppe Brotzu revealed a novel agent cephalosporin from the mold *Cephalosporium acremonium*. Brotzu reportedly isolated this compound from mold identified in a Sardinian sewer in 1948. He noticed these cultures produced substances that were effective against *Salmonella typhi*, responsible for typhoid fever, and that they contained β-lactamase [49]. Scientists Guy Newton and Edward Abraham at the Sir William Dunn School of Pathology at the University of Oxford isolated Cephalosporin C from cultured *Cephalosporium*. By July 1959 Abraham and Newton had synthesized small quantities, containing less than one percent yield of 7-ACA by acid hydrolysis of cephalosporin C, to have any commercial value. However, 7-ACA was soon to become the key semi-synthetic intermediate for production of cephalosporin antibiotics [49].

After a few years, Robert Morin and Bill Jackson (Eli Lily Laboratories) developed a new method to remove the side chain of cephalosporin C, which produced sufficient yields of 7-ACA (40%), substantiating the first semi-synthetic cephalosporins [38]. The 7-ACA nucleus was derived from cephalosporin and is analogous to the 6-ACA penicillin nucleus; however, it was not potent enough for clinical use. Modification of the 7-ACA side chains subsequently produced an efficacious antibiotic compound. Multiple commercial antibiotics used currently were founded on these original semi-synthetic 6-APA and 7-ACA compounds. Approximately 33% of commercial cephalosporins are derivatives of 7-aminodesacetoxycephalosporanic acid (7-ADCA). Due to the lower cost, 7-ADCA is usually produced from penicillin G by ring expansion of a penicillin sulfoxide ester to yield a cephalosporin ester. In this process, the ester group and phenylacetyl side-chain are removed. Overall, 66% of commercial cephalosporins are derived from 7-ACA, which was derived from cephalosporin C by either chemical or enzymatic deacylation [43, 50].

The basic cephalosporin molecule consists of a two-ring system, including a β-lactam ring, which is condensed with a dihydrothiazine ring [51]. Side-chain modification was utilized to create a new class of cephalosporin antibiotics (Fig. **10**), from 1964 to 2000. Cephalosporins are sometimes grouped into "generations" with regard to their spectrum of activity and the order in which they were first identified and isolated [52].

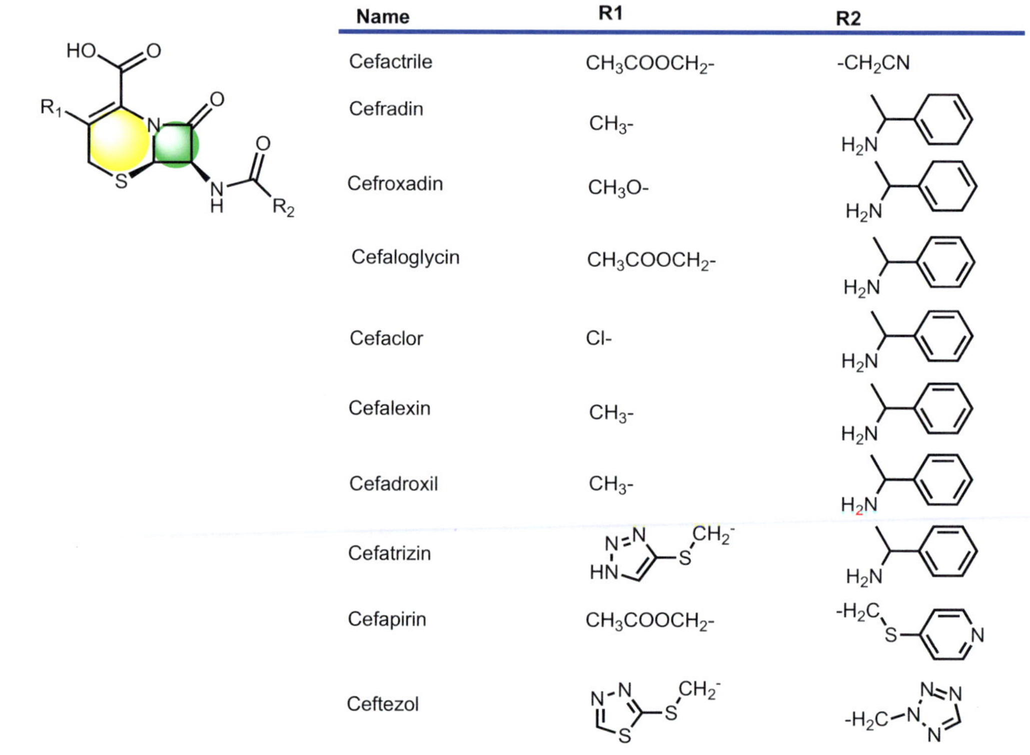

Fig. (10). Structure of the classical cephalosporins.

Extended-spectrum cephalosporins were coined as second-generation antibiotics. Third generation cephalosporins display activity against both Gram-negative and Gram-positive bacteria, although their specificity is more towards the latter. In contrast, fourth-generation cephalosporins have true broad-spectrum activity [52 - 54]. Third- and fourth-generation cephalosporins are currently in use world-wide.

First-generation parenteral cephalosporins cefalotin (cephalothin) and cephalexin, developed by Eli Lilly, and cephaloridine, developed by Glaxo, were approved for medicinal use between 1964 and 1965 [51, 55, 56], and continue to be widely used. Cephalothin exhibits good activity against Gram-positive bacteria, however its activity against Gram-negative bacteria is more moderate. Extended-spectrum antibiotics, namely second-generation cephalosporins such as cefuroxime (Glaxo, approved 1983), display strong action against Gram-negative bacteria but also only moderate activity against Gram-positive bacteria. Third-generation cephalosporins such as ceftazidime were introduced to the field in the early 1980s and approved for medicinal use in 1985 [57]. Until the 1990s, third-generation cephalosporins represented a notable advance in the development of β-lactam antibiotics. As a result of the evolution of bacterial strains that are resistant to third-generation cephalosporins, new β-lactamase-related resistance mechanisms were discovered. Finally, fourth-generation cephalosporins were introduced as therapeutic agents [58]. The third- and fourth-generation cephalosporins are closely related with regard to chemical structure. Their main difference is a positively charged quaternary ammonium group attached to their dihydrothiazone ring; this results in better penetration of the outer membrane of Gram-negative bacteria and a lower affinity for certain chromosomal β-lactamases of Gram-negative bacilli [54]. It has been around more than ten years that cephalosporin antibiotics have been around, and remain a relatively prolific class that continues to be under development. The most recently introduced cephalosporin was ceftaroline (brand name Teflaro), which is a "fifth-generation" agent that is active against methicillin-resistant *Staphylococcus aureus* and *Enterococcus faecalis* [59]. Its activity against other Gram-positive cocci and Gram-negative bacilli is similar to that of third-generation cephalosporins. This novel drug gained FDA approval in September 2010 [59]. Similarly, ceftobiprole is a fifth-generation broad-spectrum cephalosporin that is active against methicillin-resistant *Staphylococcus aureus.* In *in vitro* experiments, ceftobiprole was also active against vancomycin-intermediate *Staphylococcus aureus* (VISA) and vancomycin-resistant *Staphylococcus aureus* (VRSA) [60]. Due to their potential to fight antibiotic-resistant bacterial strains, further development of fifth-generation cephalosporins on-going, as is the search for new classes of antibiotics.

Macrolide Antibiotics

Macrolide antibiotics are a well-established class of antimicrobial agents that have played an important role in the therapy of infectious diseases. The macrolide antibiotics are derived from *Streptomyces bacteria*, and were named according to their characteristic macrocyclic lactone structure [61]. There are three major groups of naturally occurring macrolide antibiotics: the 12-membered, 14-membered and 16-membered, with aglycone components consisting twelve, fourteen and sixteen atom cyclic lactone rings, respectively [3, 62] (Fig. **11**). None of the 12-member macrolides are used clinically. The others are semi-synthetic derivatives that were obtained by chemical or biochemical modifications of macrolides, originally obtained as secondary metabolites from fermentations of certain microorganisms.

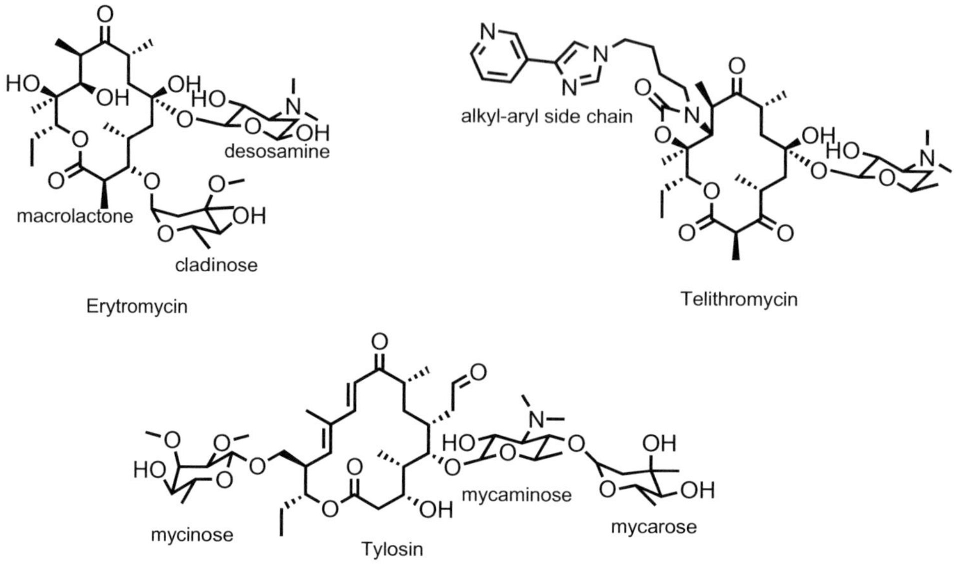

Fig. (11). Chemical structure of representatives of macrolide antibiotics (erythromycin, tylosin) and ketolides (telithromycin).

Macrolides were first discovered in 1950, when scientists isolated erythromycin from the *Streptomyces erythraeus* strain (subsequently renamed "*Saccharo-polyspora erythraea*"), a microorganism first isolated from soil samples from the Philippines [3]. Erythromycin belongs to the 14-membered family and is the most widely used of the macrolide antibiotics. Erythromycin was accepted for use against a variety of Gram-positive bacterial infections but has several drawbacks; for example, it's *in vivo* half-life is short, it has a poor oral bioavailability and acid stability, as well as numerous side effects (gastrointestinal motility, proarrhythmic action, and inhibition of drug metabolism) [26]. In the 1970s and 1980s, the semi-synthetic members of erythromycin, including clarithromycin and azithromycin, were developed as a result of efforts to overcome the acidic stability and oral bioavailability issues of erythromycin [63, 64]. The synthesis of clarithromycin was realized by substituting a methoxy group for the C-6 hydroxyl group of erythromycin. This created a more acid-stable antimicrobial agent, and when compared with erythromycin, this structural change demonstrated better *in vitro* activity against Gram-positive organisms. A new 15-membered macrolide derivative referred to as an "azalide" (azithromycin), with a methylated nitrogen molecule inserted into the lactone ring, displayed inhibitory activity against Gram-negative bacteria [65]. Clarithromycin and azithromycin were approved by the FDA in 1991 and 1992 [66]. Like erythromycin and other macrolides, azithromycin is a bacteriostatic agent. Its major advantages are its absorption rates and prolonged half-life. Because of these reasons, azithromycin is one of the world's best-selling antibiotics. Additionally, other 14-membered macrolides have demonstrated improved chemical, biological, and pharmacokinetic properties. Erythromycin's development and the widespread distribution of its analogs represent the sustained efforts to discover new and potent structural variations of macrolide compounds, and also led to the rediscovery of the 14-membered ring ketolide antibiotics (Fig. **12**).

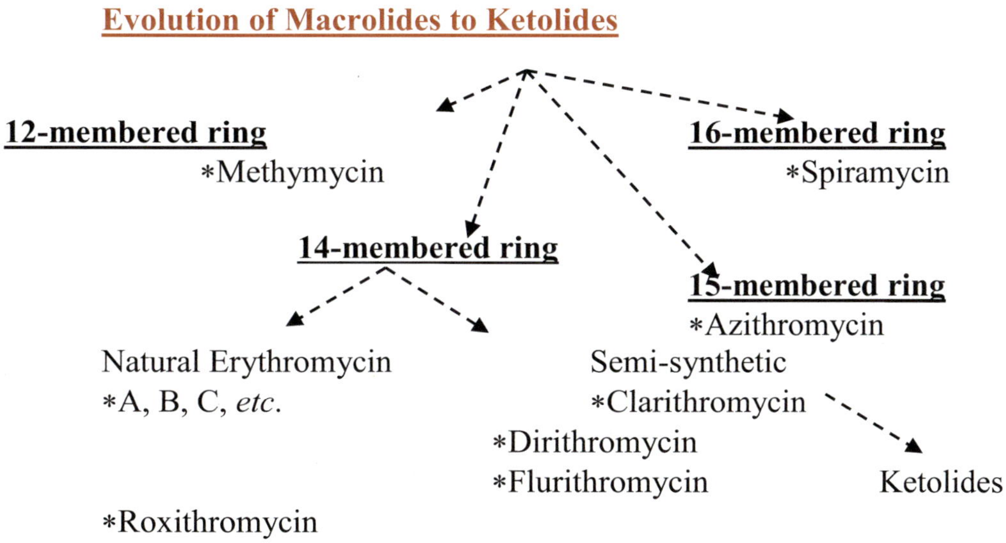

Fig. (12). Evolution of macrolides to ketolides.

Ketolides, like macrolides, are composed of 14-membered rings but are defined by a keto group at C3 of the lactone ring, along with an additional quinolyl ally side chain at C6 of the lactone ring [67]. The ketolides, including telithromycin and cethromycin, which displayed improved activities against macrolide-resistant pathogens (such as *Streptococcus pneumoniae* and *Staphylococcus aureus*), were developed [62]. The FDA approved the first commercial ketolide, namely telithromycin, in 2004 [62]. In order to develop novel, more potent ketolides, several structural modifications of the ketolide core skeleton were performed. The resulting 9-oxime macrolides, 6-O-alkyl ketolides, 13-substituted ketolides, 11,12-cyclic carbamate ketolides, 6,11-bridged ketolides, and desmethyl ketolides displayed excellent inhibitory activities toward numerous macrolide-resistant pathogens [68, 69]. Likewise, leucomycins and their 16-membered derivatives: tylosin, niddamycin, spiramycin I, spiramycin III, and virginiamycin M, constitute another important class of antibiotics of the macrolide family. They were developed in order to overcome a heightening resistance to the 14-membered macrolides. Examples of antimicrobial activity and modification, deriving the 16-membered macrolide antibiotics, such as leucomycin and its analogs, were reported in the literature [70, 71]. Hata *et al.* were the first to isolate leucomycin in 1953 from the fermentation broth of *Streptomyces kitasatoensi* [72]. Their research was later directed towards the creation of numerous analogs and the study of their biological activity [70, 71, 73]. Belonging to the same group, spiramycin was also produced from *Streptomyces ambofaciens* in 1952 and comprises a polyketide lactone, platenolide, to which three deoxyhexose sugars are attached [74]. Chemical modifications of 16-membered macrolides were also explored extensively for their pharmacokinetic and antimicrobial properties. Following these searches, novel macrolide antibiotics (macrolones) were derived, characterized by a macrocycle, linker, and either a free or esterified quinolone moiety [75, 76]. They have since proven to be highly efficacious against erythromycin-resistant pathogens. Synthesis and evaluation of new macrolide antibiotics in ongoing in order to address concerns about microbialresistance.

Quinolones

Quinolones have been of interest to scientists and clinicians alike since their discovery in the early 1960s. An older member of the quinolone class of synthetic antimicrobial agents, nalidixic acid (1-ethyl-1,4-dihydro-7-methyl-4-oxo-1,8-naphthyridine-3-carboxylic acid, Compound **1**), was introduced in 1962 by Lescher and colleagues and approved for clinical use in 1965 [77, 78].

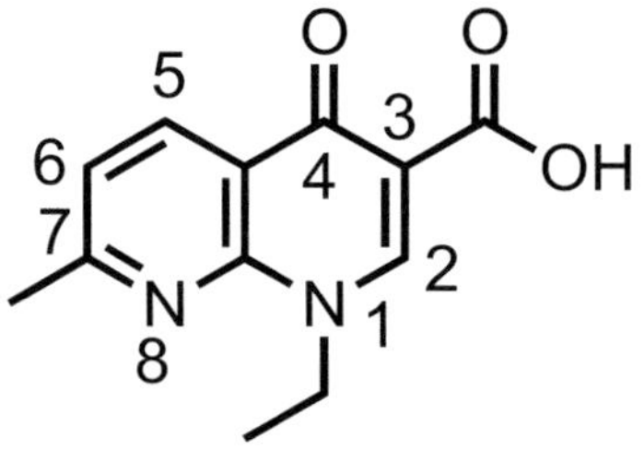

1

Nalidixic acid was widely used in the 1960s and 1970s for the treatment of urinary tract infections caused by Gram-negative pathogens. However, the clinical use of nalidixic acid was limited, due to its narrow spectrum of activity and poor absorption by the gastrointestinal tract [79 - 81]. Several modifications were made to the nucleus in order to improve its pharmacokinetic properties and its antibacterial spectrum. In the 1980s, the novel 4-quinolones (a term referring to the exocyclic oxygen at the fourth position; see Compound **2**), or "fluoro-quinolones," were derived from nalidixic acid by adding a fluorine atom to position 6 of the left-sided ring of the molecule.

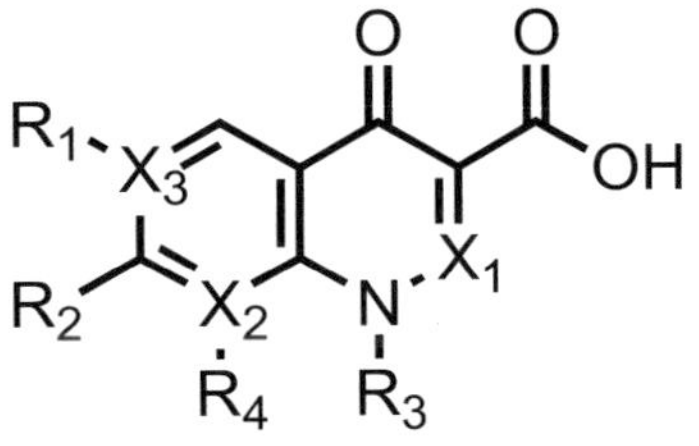

2

The fluoroquinolones contain 6-fluoro substituents, and this greatly broadens their spectrum of activity against both Gram-negative and Gram-positive pathogens; this is attributed to increased tissue penetration and binding to the DNA gyrase enzyme. The presence of fluorine at this position has been shown to induce greater activity than all other halogens or substituents tested [82]. During the 1980s, norfloxacin, ciprofloxacin, and ofloxacin were prepared as novel fluoroquinolone antibiotics. The Kyorin Pharmaceutical Company, Japan, created norfloxacin in 1978, which was characterized by 6-fluoro and 7-piperazinyl chemical moieties [3, 83]. Ofloxacin, a broader-spectrum analog of norfloxacin, is another quinolone developed by scientists at the Daiichi Seiyaku Company in Japan. It was first patented in 1982 (European Patent to Daiichi) and was subsequently approved by the FDA in the 1990s [84]. Later, ciprofloxacin, a fluoroquinolone antibacterial with a chemical structure that differs from norfloxacin by a single carbon atom, was discovered in 1983 by Bayer, Germany [78]. This structural change led to a heightened activity against *Pseudomonas aeruginosa*, a common Gram-negative pathogen, thus making ciprofloxacin one of the most potent drugs against this antibiotic-resistant strain. During the 1990s and 2000s, various fluoroquinolones were introduced, including levofloxacin (1996), grepafloxacin (1996), sparfloxacin (1996), trovafloxacin (1996), moxifloxacin (2000), and gatifloxacin (2000), which displayed an improved activity against several Gram-positive bacterial strains (particularly pneumococci), and also against anaerobes [78, 85, 86]. From the mid-1980s, the major synthetic antibiotics were fluoroquinolones, which were indicated for treatment of Enterobacteriaceae and *Pseudomonas aeruginosa* infections, as well as Gram-positive pathogens including streptococci and staphylococci.

Researchers divide quinolones into several generations based on their antibacterial spectrum. The newer fluoroquinolones have a broad-spectrum of bactericidal activity, high oral bioavailability and cellular absorption, as well as favorable safety and tolerability in patients. The four generations of quinolone antibiotics are described in Table **2** [87, 88].

Table 2. Classification of quinolones.

Generation	Drug Names	Spectrum
First-generation	Nalidixic acid, Cinoxacin, Oxolinic acid	Gram-negative, but not pseudomonas species
Second-generation	Norfloxacin, Ciprofloxacin, Enoxacin, Ofloxacin, Fleroxacin,Lomefloxacin, Rulfloxacin, *etc.*	Gram-negative, (including pseudomonas species) some Gram-positive and atypical.
Third-generation	Levofloxacin, Sparfloxacin, Gatifloxacin, Tosufloxacin, Pazufloxacin, *etc.*	Same as second-generatin with extended Gram-positive and atypical coverage.
Fourth-generation	Trovafloxacin,, Moxifloxacin, Gemifloxacin, Clinafloxacin	Same as third-generatin with broad anaerobic coverage.

Earlier generations of antibiotics, in general, have a narrower spectrum of action. All non-fluorinated quinolone drugs are labeled as first-generation antibiotics (*e.g.*, nalidixic acid). First-generation antibiotics have moderate Gram-negative activity and minimal systemic distribution. Additionally, first generation quinolones are rarely used today due to reported carcinogenic properties, leading to their inclusion on 15 May 1998 to the OEHHA Prop 65 list [89]. Except for alkylation on the distal nitrogen or, less frequently, on ring carbon molecules (second-generation quinolones), the piperazine ring moiety remains relatively undisturbed. Second-generation quinolones (*e.g.*, ciprofloxacin) possess increased systemic and Gram-negative activities [90]. Like sparfloxacin and grepafloxacin, third-generation drugs have expanded activity against Gram-positive bacteria and typical pathogens. Finally, fourth-generation antimicrobial agents (*e.g.*, trovafloxacin and moxifloxacin) have maintained their Gram-negative targeting, improved Gram-positive targeting, and have gained inhibitory activities against anaerobes [91 - 93].

From the time of Lesher's original report, there has been a notable increase in the number of nalidixic acid agents (fluoroquinolones) that have been synthesized, of which a number are currently in development, and to date over 10 000 molecules have been patented [94]. As these novel compounds enter the marketplace, this figure will possibly increase further.

Tetracyclines

Tetracyclines acquired their name because they have four ring moieties (tetra); they occur naturally and are semi-synthetic antimicrobial agents (Compound **3**) [95].

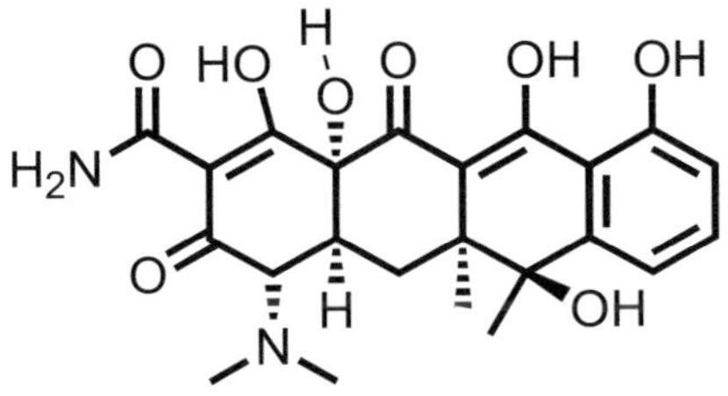

3

Tetracyclines are the third most widely prescribed antibiotic class. Tetracyclines were discovered as natural products from actinomycetes soil bacteria and first reported in scientific literature in 1948. Benjamin Duggar made his discovery of the first tetracycline antibiotic, chlortetracycline (today named aureomycin), from the broth of a novel species of streptomyces, at Lederle Laboratories [96]. Later, more members of this group of antibiotics were isolated by fermentation, thereby establishing tetracyclines as a large family of antimicrobials. In 1955, Conover prepared a deschloro derivative by catalytic hydrogenation of aureomycin, using palladium metal and hydrogen gas. The FDA approved the clinical use of this compound in 1954, as the first novel tetracycline by modification of a natural product, and it came into commercial use in 1978 [96]. A number of semi-synthetic tetracyclines have since entered the market, such as methacycline, doxycycline, and minocycline; currently most antibiotic discoveries are novel derivatives of older compounds [97]. Tetracyclines had marked differences from penicillin and streptomycin, due to their suitability for oral consumption and broad-spectrum efficacy.

Tetracyclines are broad-spectrum antibiotics that prevent bacterial growth by inhibiting protein synthesis, and are widely used in the treatment of bacterial infections occurring in plants, growth factors in veterinary medicine in livestock rearing, in agriculture and in human medicine. Because of their widespread use, resistance to tetracyclines is a frequent occurrence in a variety of bacterial species [98]. New antibiotics are needed to address this challenge. However, new tetracyclines have not been identified within traditional microbial sources. Therefore, structural analogues of known compounds have been derived from the fermentation products, utilizing semi-synthesis to improve pharmacokinetic properties and antimicrobial activity. The second-generation semi-synthetic analogs; which include doxycycline and minocyline, and more recent compounds of the third-generation including semi-synthetic glycylcyclines and methyl-cyclines; indicate the evolution of the tetracycline scaffold to derivatives with increased potency and efficacy against tetracycline-resistant bacteria, along with improved chemical and pharmacokinetic properties [97, 99, 100]. On a chronological basis, tetracyclines are formally divided into three generations (first, second, and third) (Fig. **13**) [101, 102]. The first generation consists of natural and semi-synthetic compounds, including tetracycline, chlortetracycline, oxytetracycline, demeclocycline, and methacycline. The second generation of tetracycline substances consists of semi-synthetic derivatives such as doxycycline and minocyline. The third generation of tetracyclines, namely the glycylcyclines, are currently being developed in order to remedy problems of resistance to earlier tetracyclines [103]. It is likely that future research will focus on the development of new generation tetracycline antibiotics and the investigation of the genetic mechanisms involved in resistance.

1st generation	2nd generation	3rd generation
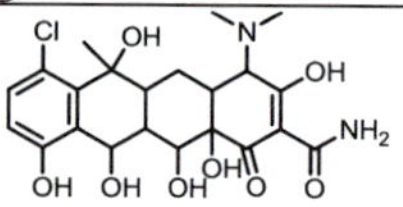 **Chlortetracycline**	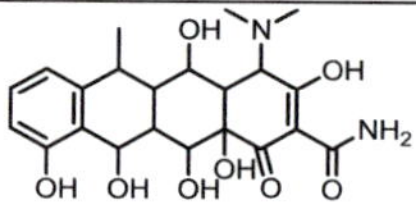 **Doxycycline**	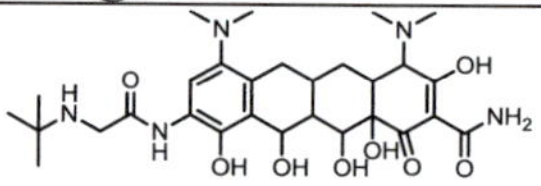 **Tigecycline (Tygacil;Wyeth)**
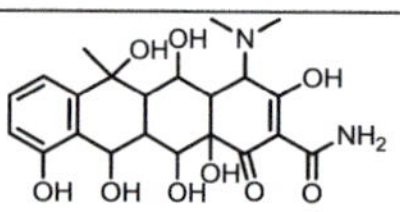 **Oxytetracycline**	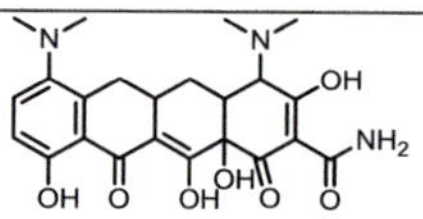 **Minocyline**	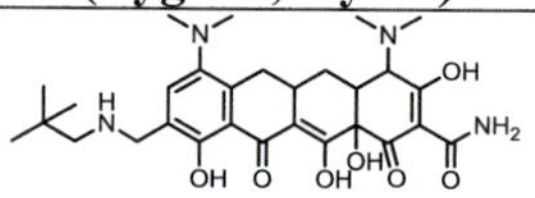 **Omadacycline (formerly known as PTK-0796)**
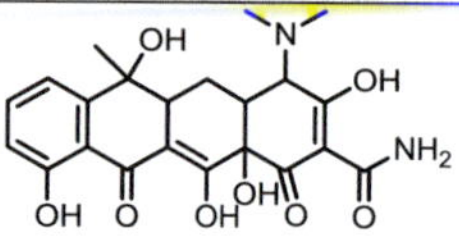 **Tetracycline**	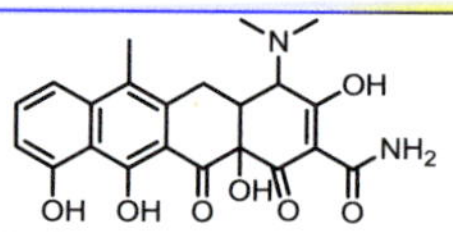 **4-Epianhydrotetracycline**	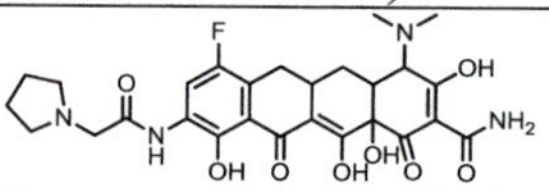 **Eravacycline (TP-434)**
1940s	**1960s** **Time**	**1990s**

Fig. (13). Chemical structures of first, second and third generation tetracyclines and advances in new generation tetracycline development over a period of time.

Tetracyclines may be further divided into so-called typical and atypical groups. Typical tetracyclines compounds, including tetracycline (Pfizer, 1953), chlortetracycline (Lederle, 1948), doxycycline (Pfizer, 1967) and minocyline (Lederle, 1972), act by inhibiting protein synthesis within bacterial cells. Atypical tetracyclines, such as chelocardin, anhydrotetracycline, and 6-thiatetracycline, act by disrupting bacterial membranes [104, 105]. Further classification also applies to tetracyclines according to their method of manufacturing. Those derived as first-generation natural products, which are effective against both Gram-positive and Gram-negative bacterial pathogens, are chlortetracycline, oxytetracycline, and tetracycline. Second- and third-generation semi-synthetic tetracycline derivatives (Fig. **13**) include minocycline, doxycycline, and tigecycline (by Pfizer in 2005), and have been studied and used clinically since the early 1970s. There have since been extensive efforts to investigate tetracyclines and their analogs for the purpose of expanding their application as anti-cancer agents and active tetracycline antibiotics [106, 101].

Aminoglycosides

Antibiotics belonging to the aminoglycoside sub-family are referred to as a "classical," but clinically important class of agents, for example, against *Mycobacterium tuberculosis* [107]. They are natural products and semi-synthetic derivatives obtained from a variety of actinomycetes. Aminoglycoside compounds are a large and diverse class of antibiotics; they characteristically contain two or more amino-sugars linked by glycosidic bonds to an aminocyclitol moiety, hence the name "aminocyclitol" was given. Chemical structures of familiar amino-glycosides are illustrated in Fig. (**14**) [107].

The aminocyclitol antibiotic sub-family members are composed of sugar-derivatives of microbial secondary metabolites that show significant biological activities [108]. Aminoglycoside antibiotics are derived from various species of streptomyces (and given the suffix -mycin, *e.g.* tobramycin) or *Micromonospora* (-micins, *e.g.,* gentamicin).

Amikacin $C_{22}H_{43}N_5O_{13}$	**Spectinomycin** $C_{14}H_{24}N_2O_7$	**Netilmicin** $C_{21}H_{41}N_5O_7$
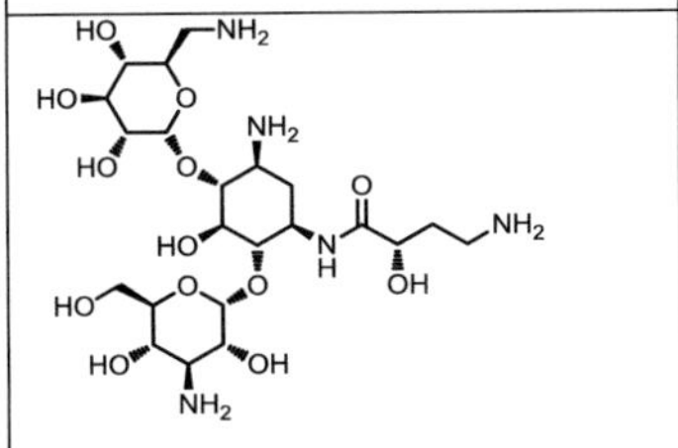	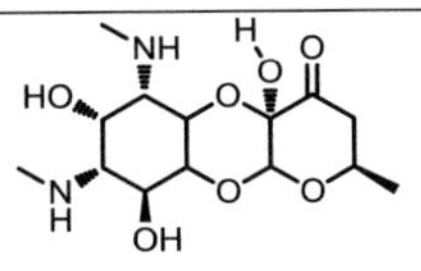	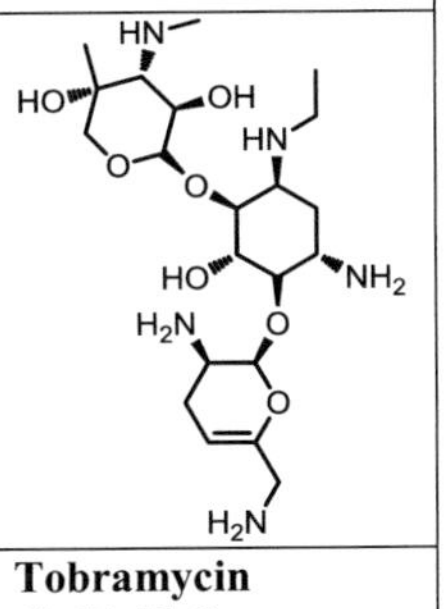
Neomycin $C_{23}H_{46}N_6O_{13}$	**Gentamicin** $C_{21}H_{43}N_5O_7$	**Tobramycin** $C_{18}H_{37}N_5O_9$
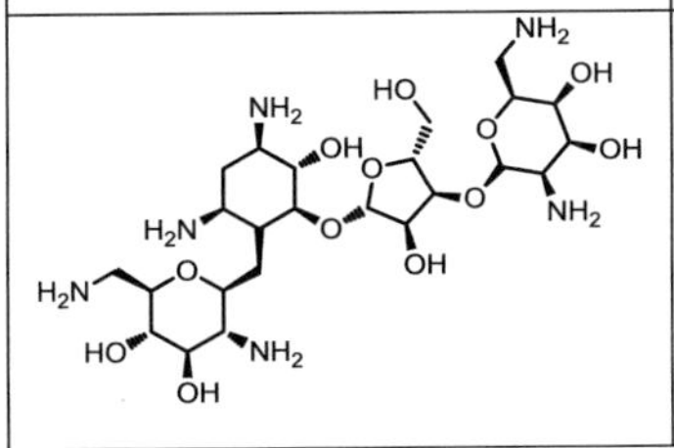	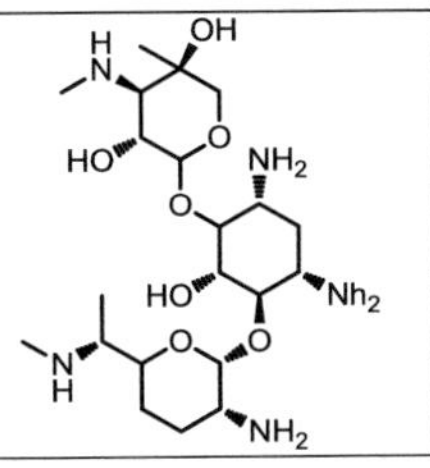	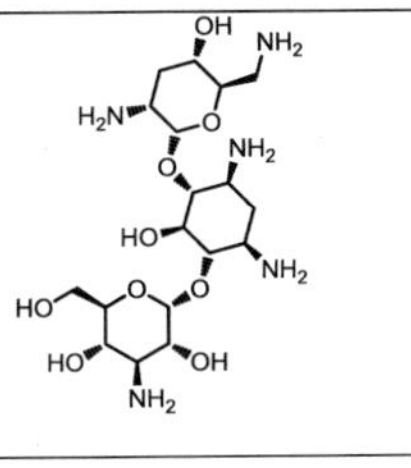

Fig. (14). Chemical structure of aminoglycosides.

In the early 1940s, the research group of Selman Waksman isolated the aminoglycoside antibiotic streptomycin from a fungus named *Streptomyces griseus*, which displayed significant antibacterial activity, particularly against *Mycobacterium tuberculosis* [109]. The discovery of streptomycin contributed significantly to tuberculosis therapy and initiated an era of aminoglycoside antibiotic research. Selman Waksman received the Nobel Prize in Physiology or Medicine in 1952 for his discovery of streptomycin [110]. This was the second antibiotic (after penicillin) to be used clinically. Nowadays, less toxic but equally effective compounds replace the use of streptomycin for bacterial infection; however, it may be applied as a secondary tuberculosis treatment when primary options fail. Additionally, when used in combination with other antimicrobial agents, streptomycin is a first-line antibiotic for the therapy of these life-threatening infective tables [111].

From 1949, additional aminoglycosides were characterized (Fig. **1**). Neomycin, which was isolated from *Streptomyces fradiae* in 1949, had increased activity against aerobic Gram-negative bacilli compared to streptomycin, however, its level of toxicity to humans made it unsafe for use [112, 113]. Kanamycin, isolated in 1957 from *Streptomyces kanamyceticus*, is used primarily against aerobic Gram-negative infections in tissue wounds. In addition to these, paromomycin was first isolated from *Streptomyces krestomuceticus* in the 1950s, and spectinomycin was first isolated from a fermentation broth of *Streptomyces spectabilis* in 1961. Furthermore, gentamicin (also known as garamycin) was isolated from the actinomycete *Micromonospora purpurea* in 1963 at Schering Plough by the research group of Marvin Weinstein, and was successful in the treatment of Gram-negative bacillary infections [114]. Gentamicin is a complex mixture of two compounds, known as gentamicin C1 and gentamicin C2, which differ from each other by a methylation at the 6' position (Fig. **15**). Gentamicin C1 and C2 are closely related in structure and have a similar antibacterial activity. Both substances contain a 2-deoxystreptamine component. The related compound tobramycin was purified in 1967 from products of *Streptomyces tenebrarius* fermentation, and was introduced into clinical use in the 1970s. However, tobramycin can also be obtained through the synthetic modification of kanamycin B [115]. Other aminoglycosides were subsequently developed, including ribostamycin and sisomicin (1970), which have broad-spectrum activity against Gram-positive and –negative bacteria, as well as mycobacteria [116, 117]. Ribostamycin is the precursor of all other family members including neomycin, paromomycin, and lividomycin [118].

The first semi-synthetic aminoglycosides such as dibekacin, amikacin, and netilmicin, created in the 1970s, were developed to overcome an acquired anti-aminoglycoside resistance in bacteria. For example, netilmicin is a synthetic derivative of sisomicin, a naturally occurring aminoglycoside produced by *Micromonospora inyoensis.* Amikacin was derived from kanamycin A by acetylation of an (*S*)-4-amino-2-hydroxybutyryl side chain at the 1-position of its deoxystreptamine moiety, and has a broader antibacterial spectrum than kanamycin [119]. Amikacin is used against numerous nosocomial diseases, and for intestinal and urinary tract diseases [120, 121]. Other than these, butirosin (1971), a water-soluble aminoglycosidic antibiotic complex, was isolated from fermentation filtrates of *Bacillus circulans* by ion exchange [122]. The chemical synthesis of many aminoglycosides has been achieved, however, fermentation remains the most economical means of their production (Table **3**) [120].

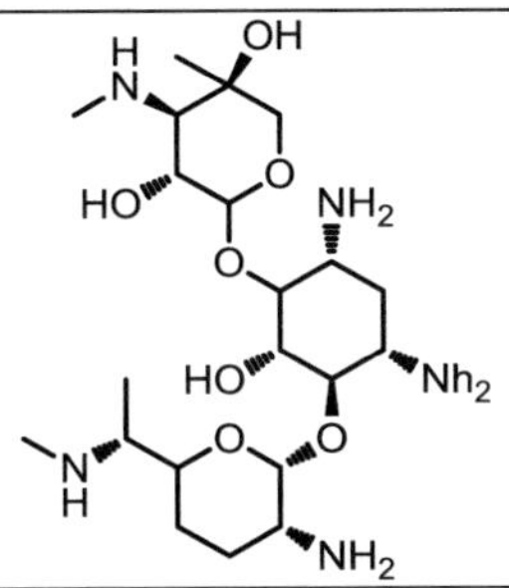	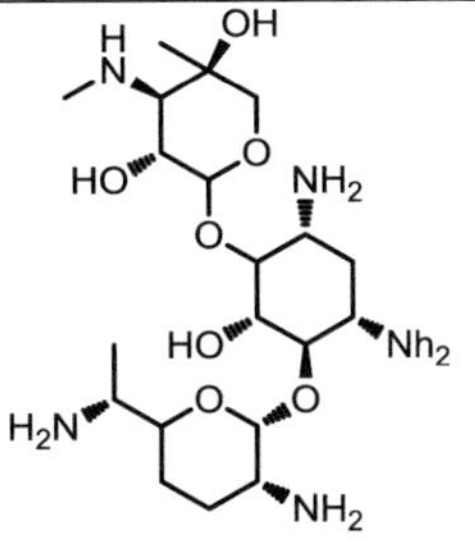
Gentamicin C1 ($C_{21}H_{43}N_5O_7$)	**Gentamicin C2 ($C_{20}H_{41}N_5O_7$)**
Gentamicin C1 is one of the major components of the gentamicin complex. Gentamicin C1 has a methyl group in the 6' position of the 2-amino-hexose ring and is N methylated at the same position.	Gentamicin C2 is one of the major components of the gentamicin complex. Gentamicin C2 has a methyl group at the 6' position of the 2-amino-hexose ring, along with a free amine.

Fig. (15). Chemical structures of gentamicin C1 and gentamicin C2.

Various aminoglycoside antibiotics have been introduced and established as chemotherapeutic agents. However, antibiotic resistance has posed a challenge to their continuing use and development. During the 1970s, efforts to address this problem resulted in the discovery of many novel agents, of which several were successfully developed for therapeutic use. However, because of subsequent introduction of other broad-spectrum antibiotics with fewer side effects, interest in developing new aminoglycosides has slowed [123].

Table 3. Aminoglycoside antibiotic classes and their source organism.

Aminoglycoside	Organism
Streptomycin	*Streptomyces griseus*
Neomycin	Streptomyces fradiae
Kanamycin	Streptomyces kanamyceticus
Paromomycin	*Streptomyces krestomuceticus*
Spectinomycin	*Streptomyces spectabilis*
Gentamicin	*Micromonospora purpurea*
Tobramycin	*Streptomyces tenebrarius*
Sisomicin	*Micromonospora inyoensis*
Ribostamycin	*Streptomyces ribosidificus*
Lividomycins A and B	*Streptomyces lividus*
Fortimicins A and B	*Micromonospora species*
Netilmicin	Semisynthetic derivative of sisomicin
Amikacin	Semisynthetic derivative of kanamycin

Increasing antibiotic resistance has led to a lack of effective antimicrobials for the prevention and treatment of infections. Therefore, clinical interest in aminoglycosides, and in particular their use against serious Gram-negative infections, has been reestablished. The development of novel aminoglycosides depends on an increased understanding of their biosynthetic regulation, and sophisticated metabolic engineering of the producing organisms.

In the following text, recent developments in antibiotics will be discussed according to the following classification scheme.

- Penicillins
  1. Beta-Lactams
- Cephalosporins
  1. Macrolides
  2. Fluoroquinolones
  3. Tetracyclines
  4. Aminoglycosides
  5. Miscellaneous anti-infective drugs

Beta-Lactam Antibiotics and Inhibitors

The β-lactam antibiotics are the most widely used drugs for the treatment of bacterial infections; however, in recent years the emergence of pathogenic bacteria that secrete protective β-lactamases has led to concerns regarding the continuing efficacy of current drugs. The β-lactams can be classified into several groups according to their chemical structures, but their unique structural feature is the presence of the four-membered β-lactam (2-azetidinone) ring. The most popular derivatives of 2-azetidinone are penicillins and cephalosporins; they are the most widely used anti-infectious drugs.

Arjomandi *et al.* first reported the synthesis of *L*-amino acid, and designed several thiol derivatives of this agent, which were investigated for their inhibitory effects against metallo-β-lactamase (MBL). The most potent compound, (*R*)-2--3-mercaptopropanamido)-3-phenylpropanoic acid (compound **4**) derived from *L*-tyrosine, exhibited competitive inhibition, with a K*i* of 86 nM. Additionally, the compound (*S*)-3-(4-(benzyloxy)phenyl)-2-(2-mercaptoacetamido) propanoic acid (compound **5**) found to be same potent inhibitor, with a competitive K*i* of 86 nM. These results may accelerate the further development of potent MBL inhibitors for clinical use [124].

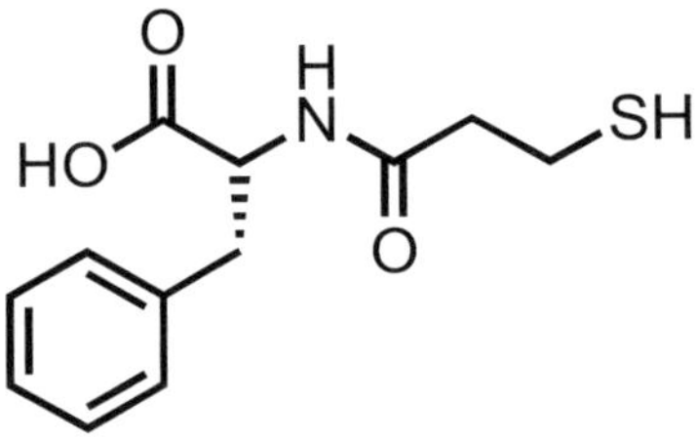

4

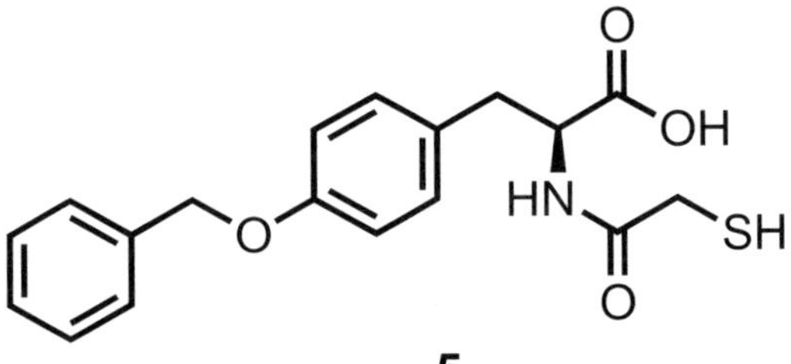

5

Bisht *et al.* reported several methods for the isolation of β-lactam from antibiotic-producing fungi; as well as the processes for the production of penicillin and cephalosporin from *Penicillium chrysogenum* and *Cephalosporium acremonium*, respectively [125].

Deng *et al.* observed synergistic inhibitory effects of AgNPs when combined with β-lactam antibiotics, such as ampicillin and penicillin, or quinolones such as enoxacin or aminoglycosides such as kanamycin A and neomycin or polyketides such as tetracycline, against the multidrug-resistant bacterium *Salmonella typhimurium* DT 104. Their findings are consistent with recent studies that indicate Ag^+ release from AgNPs increases their toxicity [126].

Genç *et al.* synthesized a series of novel β-lactam agents (compounds **6a-k**) from benzylidene-inden derivatives and investigated their inhibitory activities against hCA I and II isoenzymes and AChE. These novel β-lactam derivatives inhibited hCA I and II isoenzymes in the nanomolar range [127].

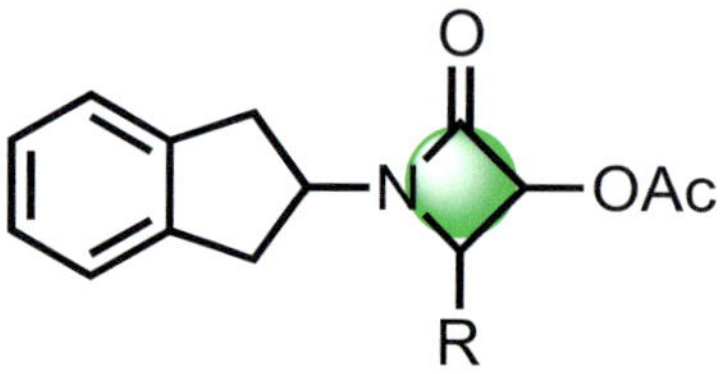

6 (a-k)

	R		R
a	-H	**g**	-*m*Br
b	-*m*OMe	**h**	-*o*Br
c	-*p*Me	**i**	-*p*Br
d	-*m*Me	**j**	-*o*NO_2
e	-*m*Cl	**k**	-*p*F
f	-*m*,*p*-diCl		

Burhanettin *et al.* synthesized five novel N-aryl lactam derivatives (compounds **7a-e**) from the reaction of Schiff base and dichloroketene by using [2+ 2] addition reaction. These compounds showed significant inhibitory activities against AChE enzymes and both hCA isoenzymes, as well as a high affinity for iron(II) metal ions as a chelating ligand [128].

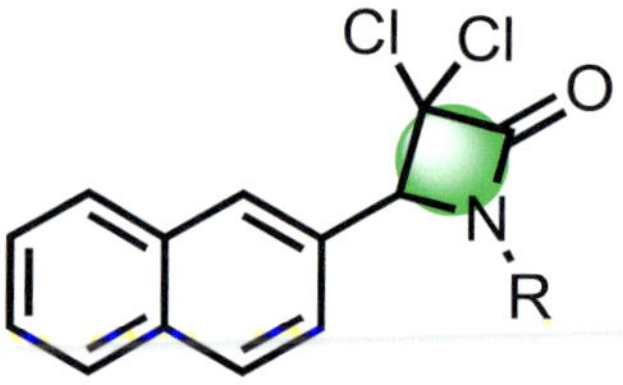

7 (a-e)

	R
a	-Me
b	-Ph
c	-4-MePh
d	-4-EtPh
e	-2,4,6-triMePh

Gonzalez *et al.* synthesized four bisthiazolidine (BTZ) derivatives (compounds **8-11**), of which some resembled the β-lactam scaffold with a metal-binding active site. In *in vitro* experiments, these agents acted as New Delhi metallo-β-lactamase-1 (NDM-1) inhibitors. While all bisthiazolidine derivatives efficiently inhibited NDM-1, one in particular (compound **8**) displayed strong inhibitory activities towards bacterial cells, as well as the ability to restore carbapenem efficacy against NDM-1-producing clinical isolates, at low micromolar concentrations. According to their results, the thiol and carboxylate moieties may play important roles in the inhibitory activities of BTZs [129].

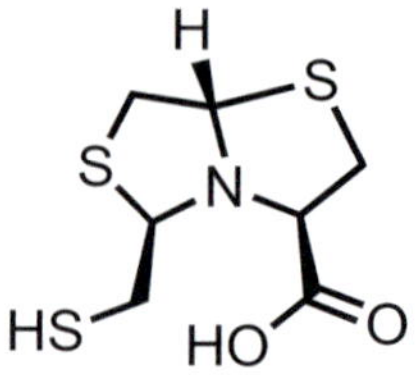

8

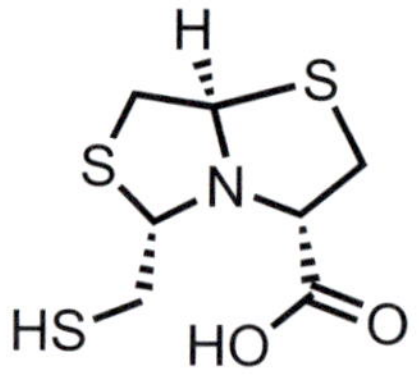

9

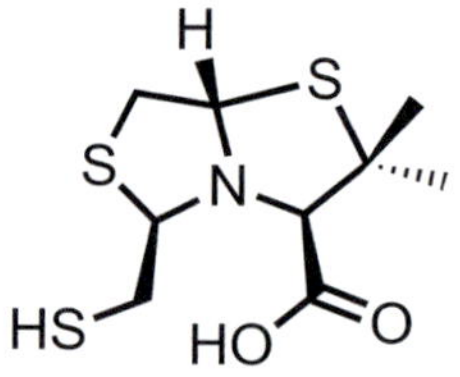

10

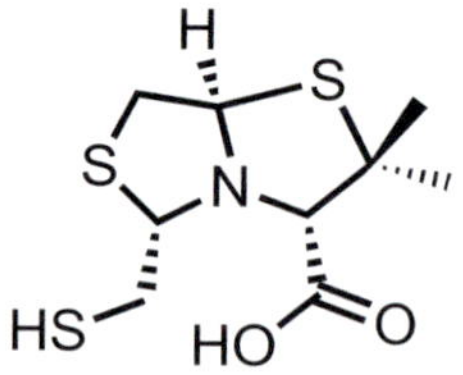

11

Kalita *et al.* first created a preparation of amoxicillin functionalized gold nanoparticles (GNPs), through electrostatic interaction of protonated amino groups and thioether moieties mediated by attractive forces. According to their results, GNP-Amoxicillin hybrid compounds exhibited broad-spectrum bactericidal activity against both Gram-positive and Gram-negative bacteria [130].

Aspergillomarasmine A (AMA) is obtained by a fermentation process utilizing *Aspergillus versicolor*. Koteva *et al.* and Liao *et al.* first synthesized AMA, (compound **12**), and investigated its metallo-β-lacamase inhibitory properties. AMA operates by a zinc-chelation mechanism resulting in an inactive β-lacamase enzyme. New Delhi metallo-β-lactamase (NDM) and Verona integron-encoded metallo-β-lactamase (VIM MBL) are particularly sensitive to the action of AMA. According to their report, AMA in combination with meropenem successfully cured mice infected with a lethal dose of *Klebsiella pneumoniae* harboring the NDM-1 MBL, thus demonstrating the potential of AMA as a candidate MBL inhibitor, complementary to standard β-lactam antibiotics [131, 132]. The activity of compound **12** may result from the *in vivo* formation of β-lactam structures both end of the molecule.

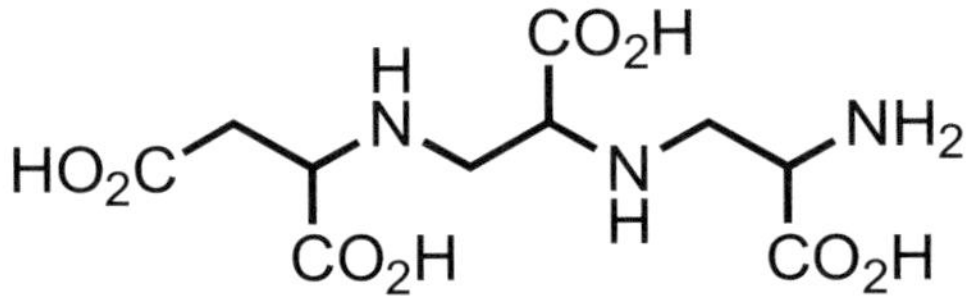

12

Streptomyces clavuligerus simultaneously produces cephamycin C (CephC) and clavulanic acid (CA). Leite *et al.* investigated contributions of both 1,3-diaminopropane and *L*-lysine amino acid to the production of cephamycin and clavulanic acid from *Streptomyces clavuligerus*. According to this study, the low concentrations of 1,3-diaminopropane without *L*-lysine did not promote CephC biosynthesis [133].

Mikolasch *et al.* successfully synthesized a series of cephalosporin (compound **13**) and penicillin (compound **14**) derivatives from the reaction of 1,4-hydroquinone and amino β-lactam. All synthesized cephalosporin and penicillin derivatives have been reported to be stable in aqueous buffers and resistant to β-lactamase. The compounds were found to be effective against various Gram-positive bacterial strains including multidrug-resistant *Staphylococcus aureus* and enterococci, both in agar diffusion and broth micro-dilution assays [134].

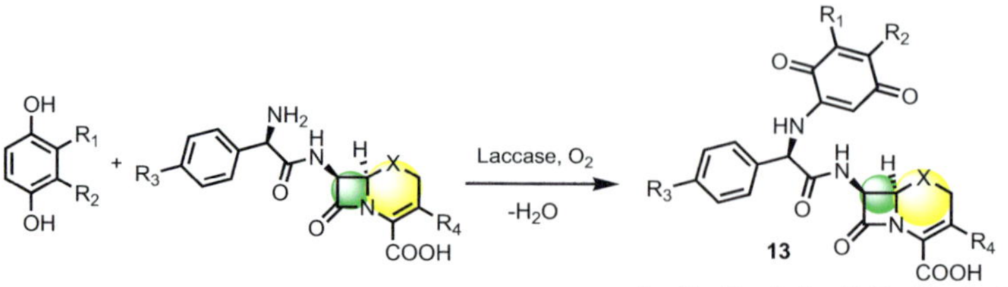

13

a R_1= Me, R_2= H, R_3= H, R_4= Me, X= S
b R_1= H, R_2= Me, R_3= H, R_4= Me, X= S
c R_1= Me, R_2= H, R_3= H*, R_4= Me, X= S
d R_1= H, R_2= CH_3, R_3= H*, R_4= Me, X= S
e R_1= Me, R_2= H, R_3= H, R_4= Cl, X= S
f R_1= H, R_2= CH_3, R_3= H, R_4= Cl, X= S
g R_1= CH_3, R_2= CH_3, R_3= OH, R_4= CH_3, X= S
h R_1= CH_3, R_2= CH_3, R_3= H, R_4= CH_3, X= S
i R_1= CH_3, R_2= CH_3, R_3= H*, R_4= CH_3, X= S
j R_1= CH_3, R_2= CH_3, R_3= H, R_4= Cl, X= S
k R_1= CH_3, R_2= CH_3, R_3= H, R_4= Cl, X= CH_3

* cyclohexa-1,4-dien structure

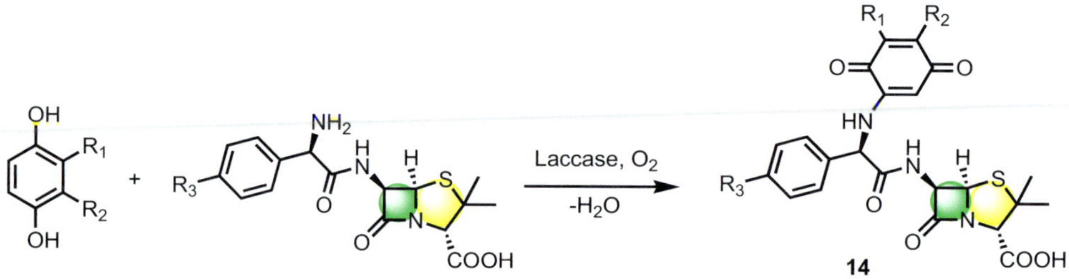

14

a R_1= Me, R_2= H, R_3= OH
b R_1= H, R_2= Me, R_3= OH
c R_1= Me, R_2= H, R_3= H
d R_1= H, R_2= Me, R_3= H
e R_1= Me, R_2= Me, R_3= OH
f R_1= Me, R_2= Me, R_3= OH

Pieczykolan *et al*. reported the synthesis of certain carbapenem derivatives with a high yield (over 90%) by using Tufariello's methodology [135]. According to their report, six-membered ring sugar-derived lactones, and the five-membered nitrone derived from 2-deoxy-ribose were found to be attractive substrates for the synthesis of carbapenems. However, five-membered congeners did not represent attractive substrates for the synthesis of β-lactams using the same methodology, due to possible racemization of the substrate *via* 2-hydroxyfuran stage [136].

Vangala and Pati have described a short and efficient synthesis method for the β-lactam containing α-hydroxy phosphanate esters (compound **15**) under the catalytic effect of cheap tartaric or fumaric acid catalysts [137].

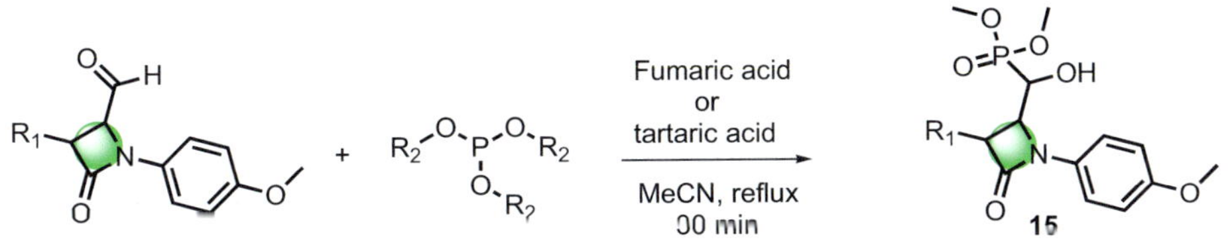

15

a R_1= Me, R_2= Me **e** R_1= Ph, R_2= Me
b R_1= Me, R_2= Et **f** R_1= Ph, R_2= Et
c R_1= *n*-Bu, R_2= Me **g** R_1= PhO, R_2= Me
d R_1= *n*-Bu, R_2= Et **h** R_1= PhO, R_2= Et

Macrolides

Seiple *et al*. recently reported a completely synthetic method to obtain more than 300 macrolide antibiotic candidates by using simple chemical building blocks, enabling the synthesis of diverse structures that could not be produced by traditional semi-synthetic approaches [138].

Domagalska *et al*. reported a number of new C13-triazole-bridged and C13-ether leucomycin analogues with a reduced aldehyde group. Among the newly synthesized compounds, the highest antibacterial [MIC values (*S. epidermidis, S. pneumonia*): ~2-4-mg/mL@1; 2.55-5.09 μm] and cytotoxic [IC50 values (HeLa, KB, MCF-7, A549, HepG2 cells): ~1.35–3.70 mm] potencies were found in those with the best aqueous solubility and that bore a saccharide-triazole arm at the C13 position of the aglycone. According to their findings, increasing the hydrophilic properties at the position of C13 (compounds **16** and **17**) improved the biological activities of the analogues [139].

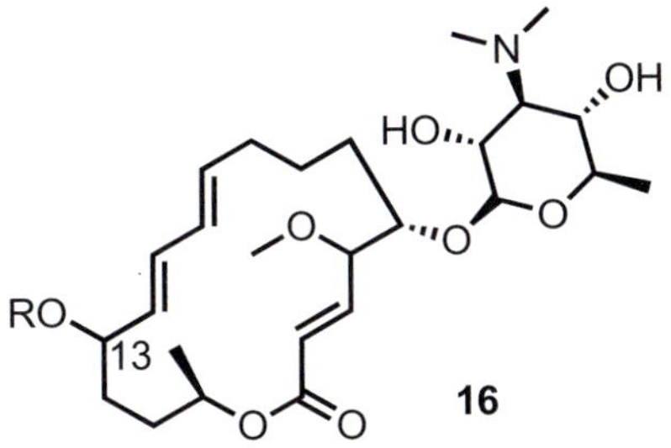

16

R: 2-Fluorabenzyl, 3-fluorabenzyl, 4-trifluoromethyloxybenzyl

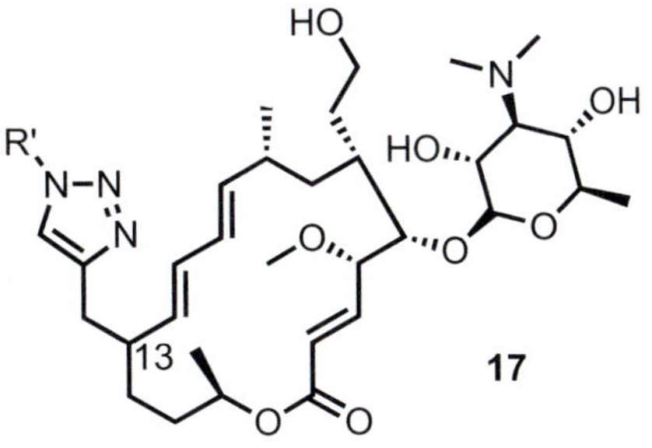

17

R':

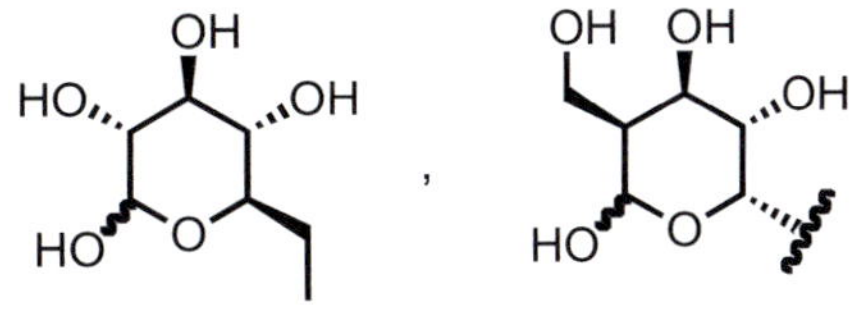

Based on environmental discoveries, Hirama reported the innovative synthesis of structurally complex bioactive natural products, such as avermectin and milbemycin, which are potent anthelmintic macrolides [140].

Klich *et al.* reported the synthesis of novel bicyclic conjugates bearing a reconstructed arm at C(5) of the aglycone, using a combined cascade and click chemistry approach. Antibacterial activity studies subsequently demonstrated that the most active compound of the novel triazole conjugates contained a terminal N-acetylsaccharide moiety (compound **18**). Comparison of the antibacterial activity and physicochemical parameters of this group of macrolides revealed that for antibacterial potency comparable with that of spiramycin (compound **20**), the presence of an aldehyde group was not important. Comparison of cytotoxic data within the group of new triazole conjugates, which contained individually restructured C(5) arms, revealed that the most active (compound **19**) bore hydrophobic and relatively bulky substituents at the end of the arm [141].

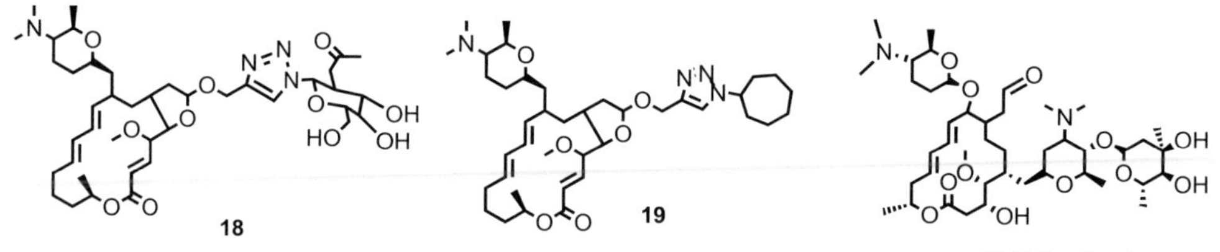

18 **19** **20 (Spiramiycn)**

	18	19	20
S. Pneumoniser:	~1 µM	~93 µM	~0.3 µM
IC_{50}/KBr:	~ 150 µM	~7 µM	~32 µM

Milbemycins, a group of 16-membered macrolides with potent anthelminthic and insecticidal activity and share a common lactone ring moiety with avermectin, are produced by several *streptomyces* bacterium. They have a wide variety of agricultural, medical, and veterinary applications. Milbemycin A3 and A4, the main components produced by *Streptomyces bingchenggensis*, were originally developed as an acaricide to control mites.

Zhang *et al.* was first to report the regulatory mechanism of milbemycin biosynthesis in *S. bingchenggensis* BC04. MilR was subsequently confirmed to be a pathway-specific activator of milbemycin production. Their investigations demonstrated that over-expression of one copy of milR (the gene encoding MilR) is an effective strategy to increase milbemycin production in industrial bacterial strains, and may have practical applications in future bioengineering attempts to improve milbemycin production in *Streptomyces* [142].

Tereshchenkov *et al.* synthesized novel fluorescent derivatives of macrolide antibiotics related to tylosin bearing rhodamine, fluorescein, Alexa Fluor 488, BODIPY FL, and nitrobenzoxadiazole (NBD) residues. They reported that the fluorescent tylosin derivatives containing BODIPY FL and NBD groups could be used to screen the binding of novel antibiotics to bacterial ribosomes in the macrolide-binding site [143].

Walmsley *et al.* synthesized a number of polyene macrolides with potent antifungal agents that have severe side effects. Increased glycosylation of these compounds was shown to improve water solubility and reduce toxicity, and resulted in better antifungal activities of the antibiotics [144].

Fluoroquinolones

Ude *et al.* synthesized 1-cyclopropyl-6-fluoro-4-oxo-7-(piperazin-1-yl)-1,4-dihydroquinoline-3-carboxylic acid (ciprofloxacin) **21**, 1-cyclopropyl-6-fluo-o-4-oxo-7-(4-propionylpiperazin-1-yl)-1,4-dihydroquinoline-3-carboxylic acid **22** and half sandwich rutenium *p*–cymene derivative of compound **23**. The ciprofloxacin ruthenium complex **23** displayed promising cytotoxic activity in the low micromolar range, similar to the clinical drug cisplatin, against the human cancer cell lines A2780, A549, HCT116, and PC3 (of ovarian, lung, colon and prostate origin, respectively). Complex **23** also exhibited moderate and dose-dependent anti-bacterial activity against *E. coli*, one of which was a clinical isolate resistant to first, second and third generation β-lactam antibiotics. These results revealed that the combination of multiple functional moieties into a single drug molecule may improve efficacy and clinical outcomes [145].

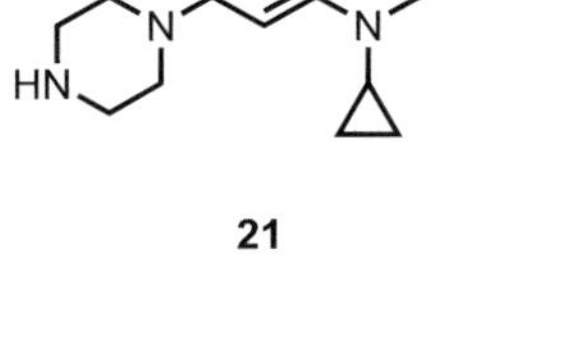

21

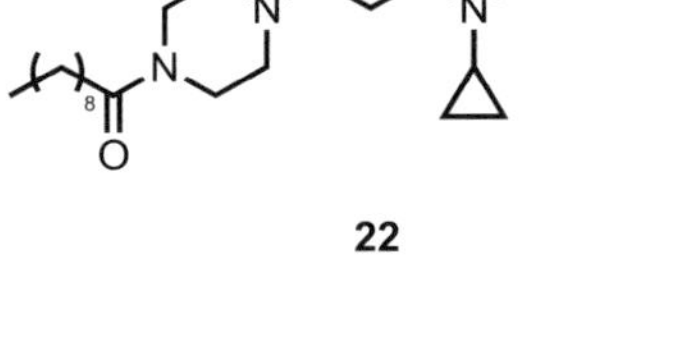

22

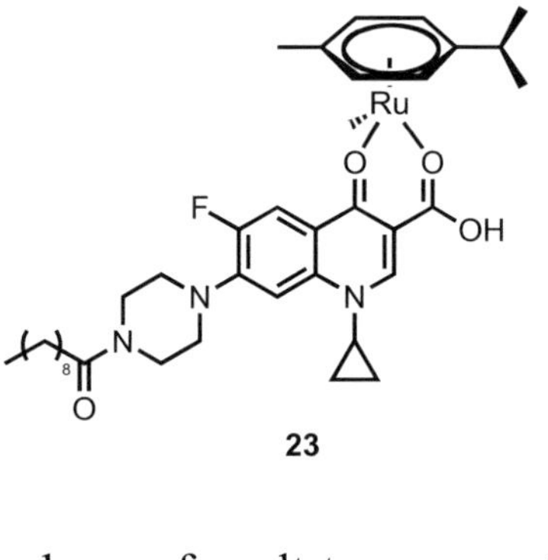

23

Chugunova *et al.* recently synthesized a number of salt-type novel fluoroquinolone derivatives bearing benzofuroxan substituents. The *in vitro* antimicrobial and toxic activities of each compound were also subsequently determined. It was discovered that the fluoroquinolone derivatives had higher antimicrobial activity than parent fluoroquinolones against *Bacillus cereus* 8035. Among the screened compounds, compound **24** exhibited the most pronounced antibacterial activity against *B. cereus* 8035, eight times higher than lomefloxacin (MIC=1.5 mg/mL) [146].

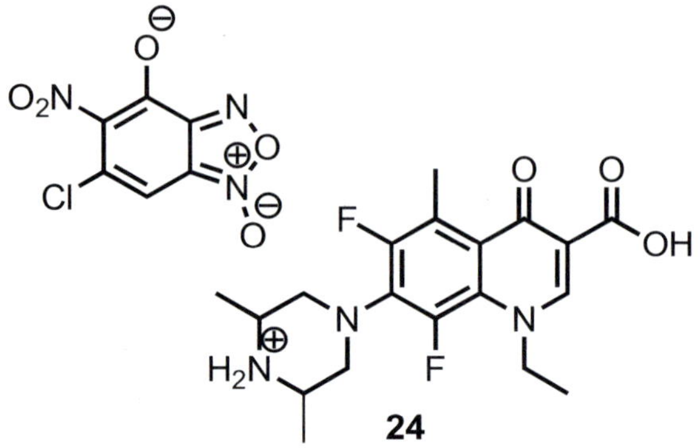

24

Komarnicka *et al*. synthesized four novel copper (I) complexes of fluoroquinolone derivatives (compound **25 a-d**), and investigated their *in vitro* cytotoxic properties against two cancer cell lines (CT26 – mouse colon carcinoma and A549 – human lung adenocarcinoma). The complexes stimulated the generation of reactive oxygen species in the cancer cells, which was examined using two different fluorescent probes. These biological effects contributed to the induction of apoptosis in the cancer cells [147, 148].

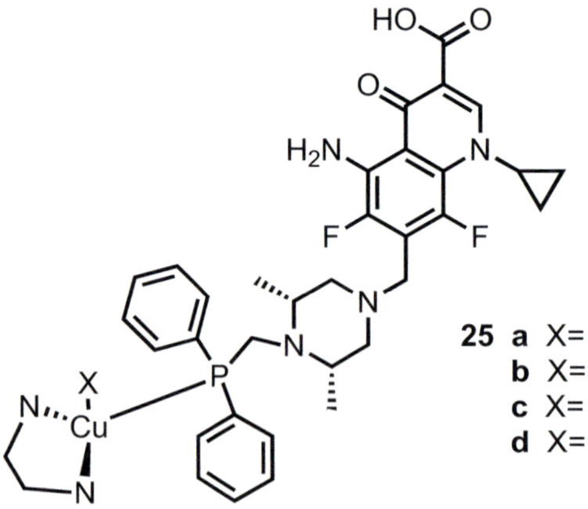

25 **a** X= I, NN= 2,9-Dimethyl-1,10-phenanthroline
b X= NCS, NN= 2,9-Dimethyl-1,10-phenanthroline
c X= I, NN= 2,2'-Biquinoline
d X= NCS, N,N= 2,2'-Biquinoline

Hiltensperger *et al.* have reported the synthesis of novel flouroquinolone derivative bearing morpholine substituted N-benzylamide moiety (compound **26**). These were shown to have high activity against *Trypanosoma brucei*. As the lead compound GHQ168 was unsuccessful in clinical trials due to poor water solubility, the researchers made modifications in order to increase its aqueous solubility while maintaining its *in vitro* anti-trypanosomal activity. The pharmacokinetic parameters of spray-dried GHQ168 and the newly synthesized compounds GHQ242 and GHQ243 were characterized in mice, and had elimination half-lives ranging from 1.5 to 3.5 h after intraperitoneal administration, moderate to strong human serum albumin binding for GHQ168 (80%) and GHQ243 (45%), and very high human serum albumin binding (>99%) for GHQ242 [149].

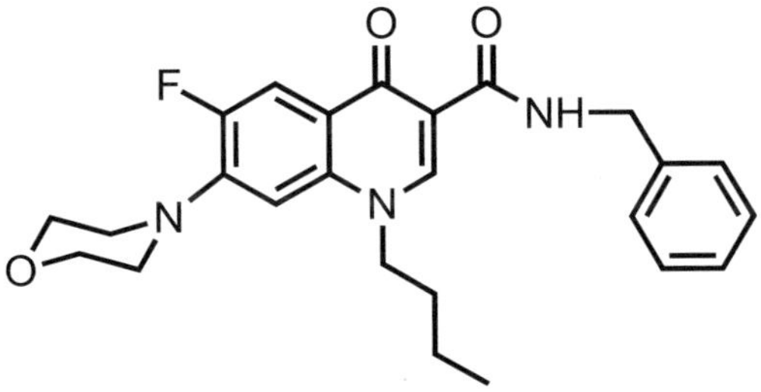

26

Layered nanohybrids represent a new class of materials that have diverse drug release systems. In connection with this concept, Nabipou *et al.* made the intercalation of fluoroquinolone antibiotic gemifloxacin (GEM) anions (compound **27**), into a layered zinc hydroxide (LZH) through an ion-exchange method. They prepared the GEM-LZH/Chitosan nanocomposite coating in alkaline aqueous solution. The thermal stability of the nanohybrid compound was confirmed by thermal analyses [150].

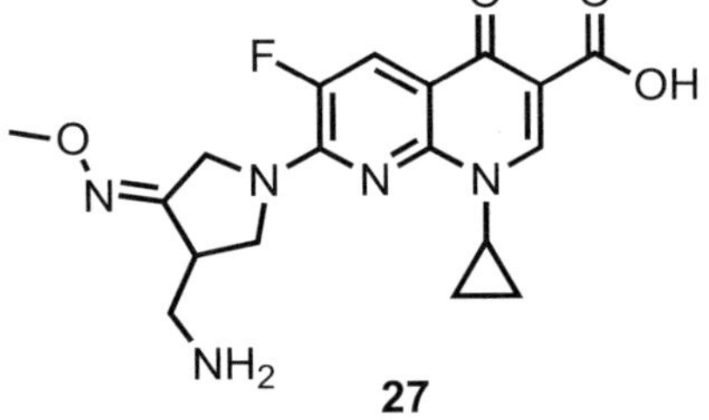

27

Tetracyclines

Tetracyclines are a commonly applied class of broad-spectrum antibiotics. They act to inhibit protein biosynthesis in bacteria by preventing the binding of aminoacyl-tRNAs to the acceptor site of ribosomes [151].

Buszewski *et al.* synthesized silver nanoparticles functionalized with tetracycline *via* synthetic and semi-synthetic methods, and compared their biological activities against a range of Gram-negative bacterial strains such as *Escherichia coli, Pseudomonas aeruginosa* and *Klebsiella pneumoniae*, as well as Gram-positive *Staphylococcus aureus* and *Staphylococcus epidermidis*. Their studies demonstrated that biologically synthesized silver nanoparticles were superior materials for functionalization with tetracycline than chemically obtained nanoparticles stabilized with PVP (poly(N-vinylpyrrolidone), as they absorbed more tetracycline. Further microbiological tests confirmed that functionalized silver nanoparticles exhibited higher antimicrobial activity than unmodified counterparts, thus advancing their use as antibacterial agents [152].

Railean-Plugaru *et al.* reported on the synthesis of bio(AgNPs), and exhibited their significant actions against bacteria in combination with tetracycline, kanamycin, ampicillin, and neomycin, followed by streptomycin and gentamycin against *Escherichia coli*, *Salmonella infantis,* and *Klebsiella pneumoniae* [153].

Devi *et al.* reported a series of novel heterocyclic Schiff base ligands (**28**) 4-hydroxy-3-[1-{(2-hydroxy-aryl)imino}-ethyl]-6-methyl-pyran-2-one; aryl=phenyl, 4-methylphenyl, 4-chlorophenyl or 4-nitrophenyl and their organosilicon (IV) complexes $R_2Si(L)$ (R=Et, Bu, or Ph). They also screened for *in vitro* antimicrobial activity and performed QSAR studies on these compounds. Their studies revealed that the antimicrobial activities of organosilicon (IV) complexes were more potent than their respective ligands [154].

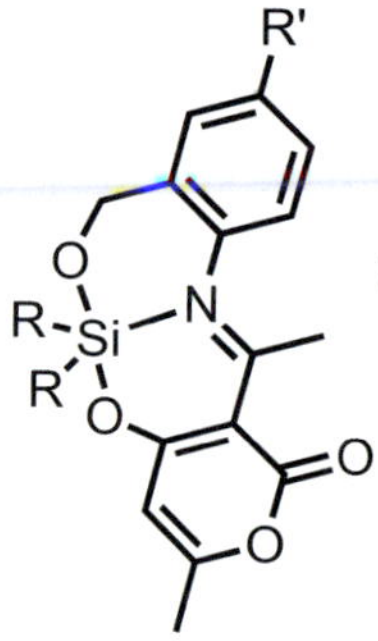

28

Ligand	**R'**
H_2L	H
H_2L_{II}	CH_3
H_2L_{III}	NO_2
H_2L_{IV}	Cl

Mukherjee *et al.* prepared tetracycline-loaded nano-formulations (Tet-CPNPs) using calcium phosphate nanoparticles. After characterization of Tet-CPNPs, they confirmed that the efficiency of tetracycline loading in CPNP was approximately 20%, and the release of antibiotic from Tet-CPNPs was sustainable over a 7-day period. The effectiveness of Tet-CPNPs on multiple-antibiotic-resistant bacteria, such as *Escherichia coli*, *Salmonella kentucky*, and *Shigella flexneri,* was confirmed with an MIC range of 20–40 µg/mL. In comparison, the MIC of free tetracycline was in the range of 150–180 µg/mL. NP-mediated cell filamentation and cell membrane disintegration resulted in bacterial cell death. CPNP alone had no toxic effects on bacteria [155].

Devi *et al.* reported a series of novel heterocyclic Schiff base ligands (compound **28**), 4-hydroxy-3-[1-{(2-hydroxy-aryl)imino}-ethyl]-6-methyl-pyran-2-one; aryl = phenyl, 4-methylphenyl, 4-chlorophenyl or 4-nitrophenyl and their organosilicon(IV) complexes $R_2Si(L)$ (R = Et, Bu or Ph). They also screened for their *in vitro* antimicrobial activities and performed QSAR studies. Their studies revealed that the antimicrobial activities of organosilicon(IV) complexes are more potent than their respective ligands [154].

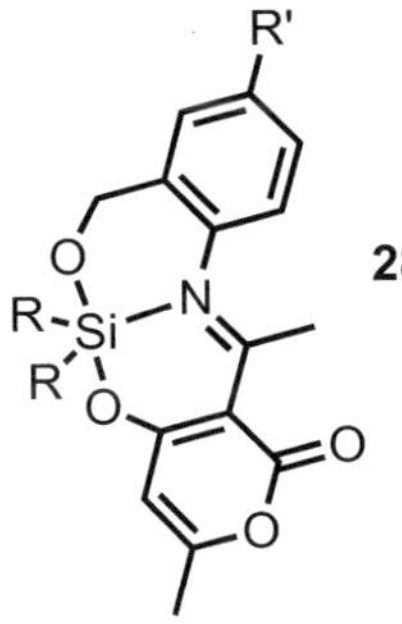

28

Ligand	**R'**
H_2L	H
H_2L_{II}	CH_3
H_2L_{III}	NO_2
H_2L_{IV}	Cl

Mukherjee *et al.* prepared tetracycline-loaded nano-formulations (Tet-CPNPs) using calcium phosphate nanoparticles. After characterization of Tet-CPNPs, they confirmed that efficiency of tetracycline loading in CPNP was about 20% and the release of antibiotic from Tet-CPNPs was sustainable during 7 days. Minimum inhibitory concentration (MIC) of Tet-CPNP on multiple antibiotic (including tetracycline) resistant bacteria like *Escherichia coli*, *Salmonella kentuckey* and *Shigella flexneri* was in the range of 20–40 μg/mL, whereas MIC of free tetracycline was in the range of 150–180 μg/mL. NP-mediated cell filamentation and cell membrane disintegration caused cell killing. CPNP itself had no toxic effect on bacteria as well as on zebrafish [155].

Aminoglycosides

Aminoglycosides (AGs) are a class of broad-spectrum bactericidal antibiotics originally discovered among the arsenal of molecules evolved by soil microbes to wage war on each other. This class of natural and semi-synthetic antibiotics has been highly effective against Gram-positive and Gram-negative pathogens that are difficult to treat and that cause life threatening infections in humans, including the bacterial strains under the "E.S.K.A.P.E." classification (*Escherichia coli*, *Staphylococcus aureus*, *Klebsiella* sp., *Acinetobacter* sp., *Pseudomonas aeruginosa*, and *Enterobacter* sp.) [156]. Maianti and Hanessian, reported the synthesis and systematic evolution of a series of AG hybrid structures (compounds **29-39**) seen in Fig. (**16**). Each of the hybrid analogs in this collection contributes to our understanding of different aspects of the AG structure-antibacterial potency relationships and the requirements for evasion of prevalent AME isoforms.

Chandra *et al.* reported a one-step strategy to synthesize amikacin modified fluorescent carbon dots (CDs@amikacin) for assaying pathogenic bacteria, Escherichia coli. They used amikacin as a binding ligand towards *E. Coli* instead of antibiotic properties. They used it to detect *Escherichia coli* accompanied with a linear range of 3.904 x 10^5 to 7.625 x 10^2 cfu per mL as well as a detection limit of 552 cfu per mL. The prepared amikacin modified fluorescent carbon dots successfully applied to the sensing of *Escherichia coli* in different fruit juice samples like apple, pineapple, and orange [157].

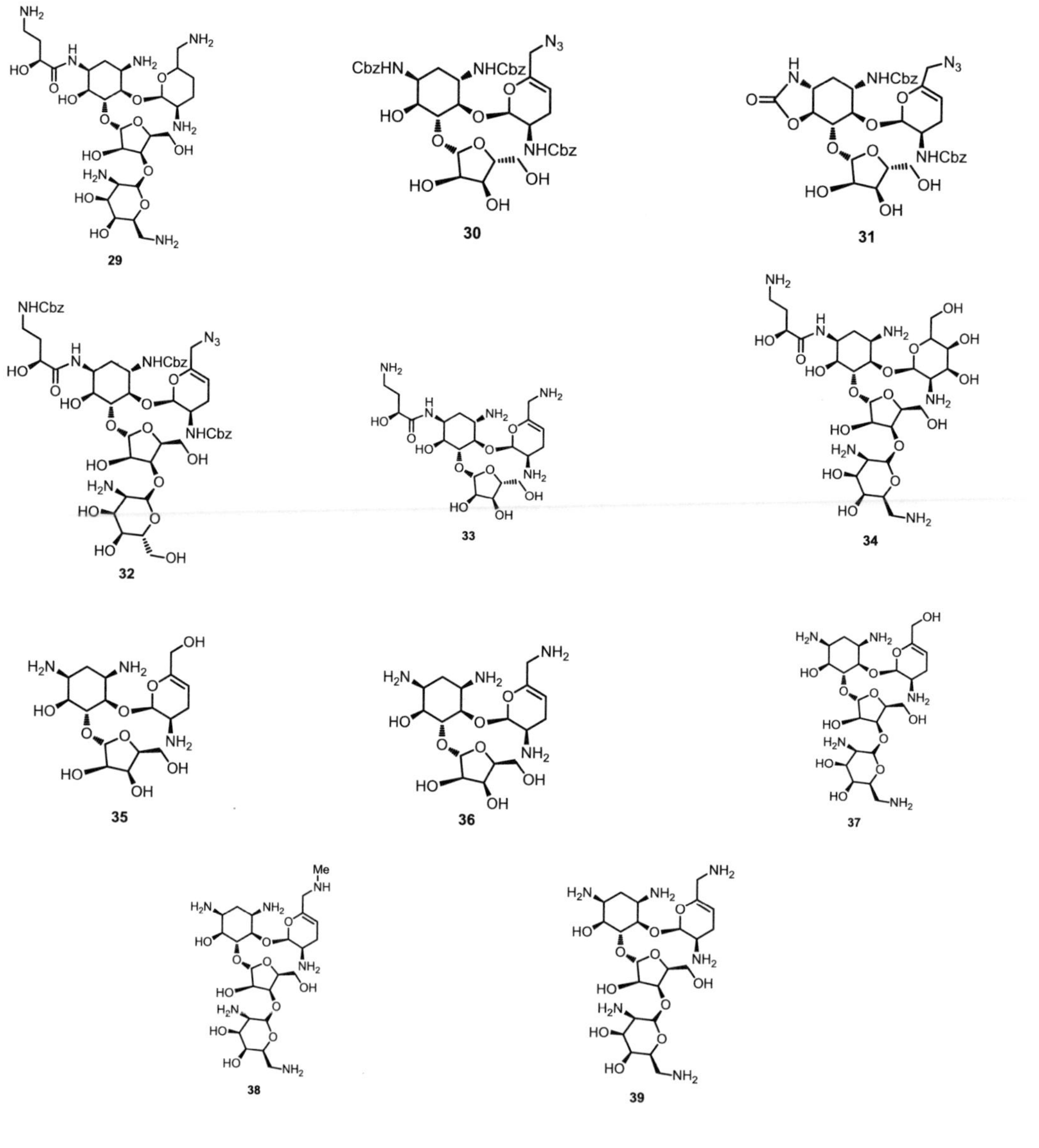

Fig. (16). Structures of hybrid AGs antibiotics.

Junior *et al.* investigated *in vitro* cytoprotective and antagonistic effect of the HEAC (hydroethanol extract of *Annona coriacea* Mart.) in the presence of aminoglycosides. The results obtained in their study show that the *Annona coriacea* Mart. hydroalcoholic extract can be used as a source of natural products derived from this plant, once cytoprotective activity over tested strains is presented *in vitro*, and can also present an antagonistic effect when associated with aminoglycosides, reinforcing the necessity of caution when combining natural products and pharmaceuticals [158].

Kato *et al.* reported efficient chemistry for the modification of the kanamycins (compounds **40-48**) at the 4′- and 4″-positions and investigated their antiribosomal and antimicrobial activities. According to their results, modifications at the 4′-position are fatal to the antiribosomal activity of the already only weakly active kanamycin C and 6′-hydroxylated kanamycin A but lead to only a modest reduction in activity in the kanamycin B series. Modification of kanamycin B at the 4′-position does not afford greater selectivity [159].

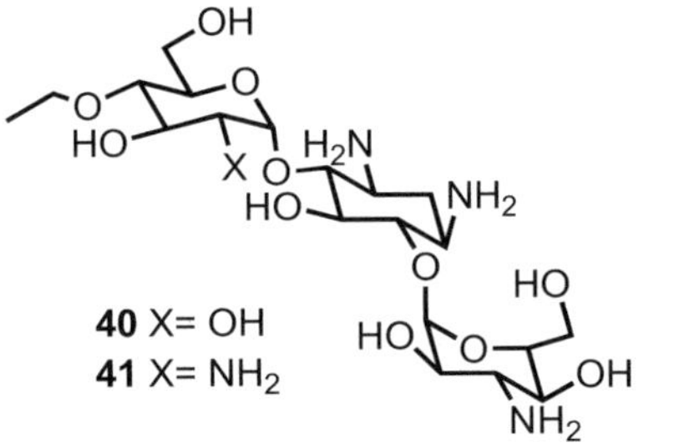

40 X= OH
41 X= NH_2

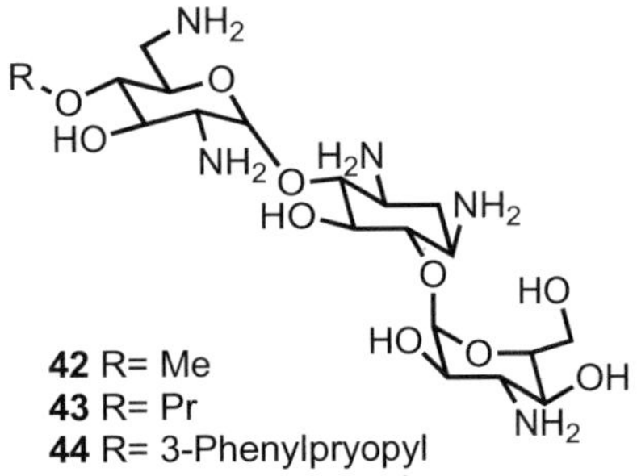

42 R= Me
43 R= Pr
44 R= 3-Phenylpryopyl
45 R= 2-Hydroxyethyl
46 R= 2-(2-Hydroxyethyloxy)ethyl

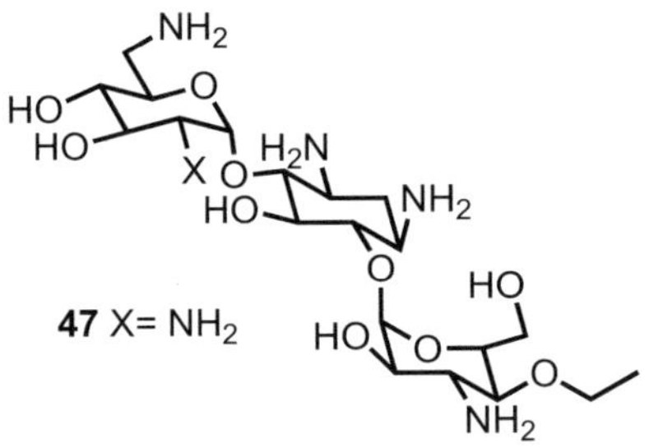

47 X= NH_2

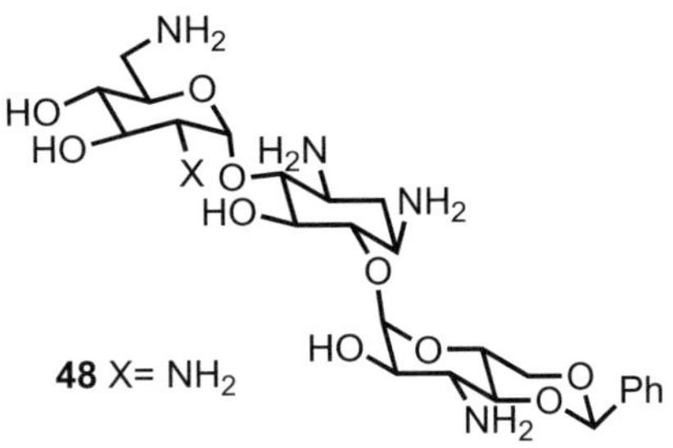

48 X= NH_2

Although fluoroquinolones are first-line agents for the treatment of National Institutes of Health (NIH) category II chronic bacterial prostatitis (CBP), therapy with these agents is not always feasible due to the increasing worldwide resistance of causative uropathogens [160]. In connection with this problem, Magri *et al*, investigated the efficacy aminoglycosides which are the recommended agents for the treatment of category I acute bacterial prostatitis (ABP). According to their results, administration of aminoglycosides eradicated causative pathogens in 79% of patients and significantly decreased the symptoms of the disease, as assessed with the NIH-CPSI (NIH-Chronic Prostatitis Symptom Index) and I-PSS (International Prostate Symptom) questionnaires. Therapy was also effective in significantly decreasing the prostate volume, probably by acting on inflammatory edema. The therapy was in general well tolerated, and genetic testing for mitochondrial mutations predisposing to sensorineural deafness allowed safer administration of the antibiotic in a considerable fraction of patients. But these findings need to be confirmed and further validated in a randomized-controlled setting [160].

Ni *et al.* separated five 3″-N-demethyl-gentamicin C analogues through fermentation broth of *gen*N disruption strains from broth of *Micromonospora echinospora.* Antimicrobial activities of 3″-N-demethyl-gentamicin C components were tested against *Escherichia coli*, *Pseudomonas aeruginosa,* and *Staphylococcus aureus*. The results showed that the 3″-N-demethyl-gentamicin C1a and 3″-N-demethyl-gentamicin C2 have similar activity with C1a. Like gentamicin C1, the 3″-N-demethyl-gentamicin C1 has the most methyl groups, but shows the lowest activity among the 3″-N-demethyl-gentamicin C complex. The antimicrobial activity of the 3″-N-demethyl-gentamicin indicates that 3″-N methylation has negligible impact on the antimicrobial activity, but the 6′-N methylation in gentamicin C1 decreases the antimicrobial activity greatly [161].

Saganappa *et al.* synthesized modified neomycin-sugar conjugates (compound **49**) through an efficient multicomponent domino process. Antimicrobial activities of the synthesized aminoglycoside derivatives were determined against methicillin-resistant *Staphylococcus aureus*, *Klebsiella*, and *Escherichia coli* strains, and their activities were found to be comparable to the parent antibiotics [162].

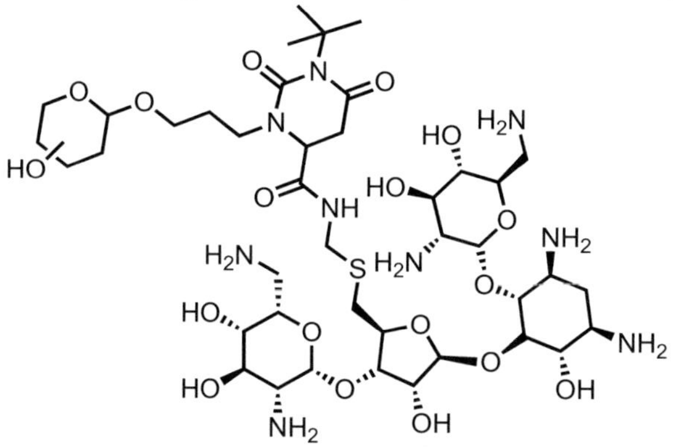

49 (five examples)

Woiwode *et al.* synthesized single labeled gentamicin (GT)-Texas Red (TR) conjugate and purified it using a newly developed semi-preparative MS-compatible HPLC method. Due to the presence of GT components and different primary amino groups for amide coupling with TR-*N*-succinimidyl ester, a number of GTTR-derivatives were detected in the resultant product by UHPLC-ESI-QTOF-MS/MS using information-dependent acquisition scan mode. Aminoglycosides such as GT are efficient antibiotics, but also problematic due to severe side effects such as nephro- and autotoxicity. Fluorescent labeled GT is used to visualize cellular uptake and distribution of the antibiotic to finally understand the mechanisms of serious adverse drug reactions [163].

Zimmermann *et al.* synthesized a series of new amphiphilic 3′,4′-dialkyl neamine derivatives (**50**) and of their smaller analogues in the 6-aminoglucosamine (neosamine) (compounds **51** and **52**) and their antimicrobial activities determined against Gram-negative (*Acinetobacter lwoffi, Escherichia coli,* and *Klebsiella pneumonia*) and/or Gram-positive (*Staphylococcus aureus* and *Pseudomonas aeruginosa)* bacteria with promising results [164].

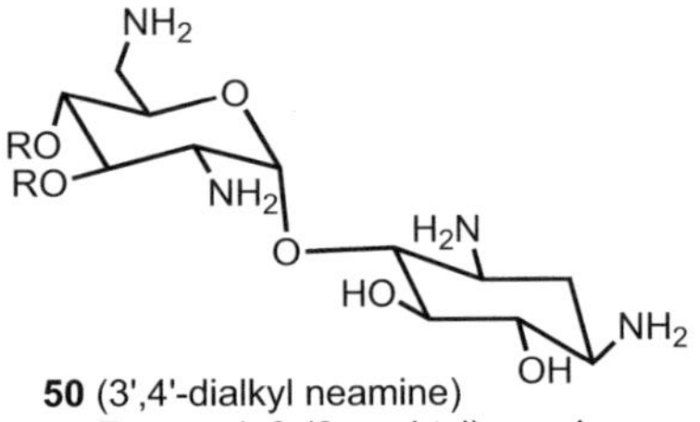

50 (3',4'-dialkyl neamine)
R= nonyl, 3-(2-naphtyl)propyl

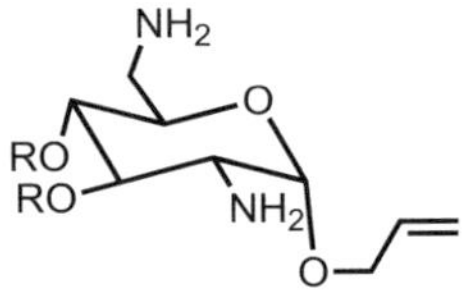

51 (alpha-allyl-3,4,dialkyl neosamine)
R= H, 2-naphtylmethyl

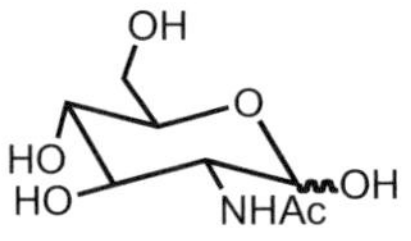

52 (N-acetyl-D-glucosamine)

Miscellaneous Anti-Infective Drugs

Barbaour *et al.* recently reported a series of aza-tricyclic indolines (ATI) synthesis through gold-catalyzed tandem cyclization hope to obtain a novel class of anti-MRSA agents. One of the guanidine-containing aza-tricyclic indoline, (compound **53**) exhibited the improved anti-MRSA activity with lower mammalian toxicity both *in vitro* and *in vivo* studies [21].

Metal-drug complexes have received considerable attention recently because the formation of the complex of biologically-important ligands with metals cause significant changes in their biological properties. Al-Khodira and Refat reported some metal complexes of amoxicylin such as Ca(II), Fe(III), Pd(II), and Au(III) and investigated their antimicrobial activities against *Bacillus subtilis (G+), Escherichia coli (G–), Pseudomonas aeruginosa (G–), and Staphylococcus.* They have obtained promising results particularly from Au(III) and Ca(II) complexes of Amoxicillin (1:1) [165].

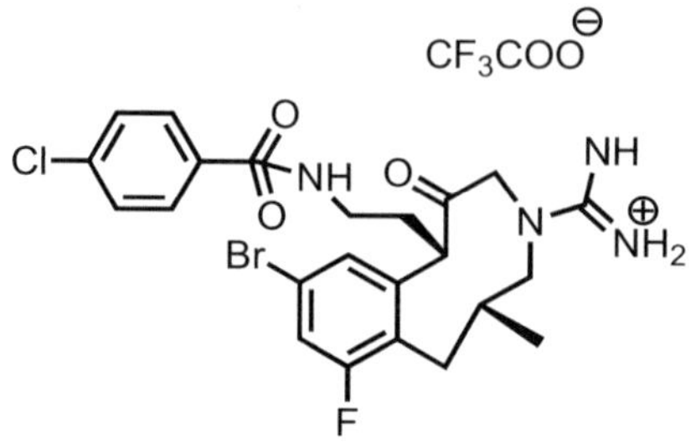

53

Reda *et al.* extracted, purified and identified effective bioactive compound as 2,2-dimethyl-5-((1-(octyloxy)-1-oxodocosan-2-yl)oxy)-5-oxopentanoic acid (compound **54**) produced by *B. amyloliquefaciens* S5I4 strain. They observed that, this compound could be used to reduce the growth of MDR pathogenic bacteria including *S. aureus*, *L. monocytogenes*, *B. cereus*, *E. coli* and *K. pneumonia* [166].

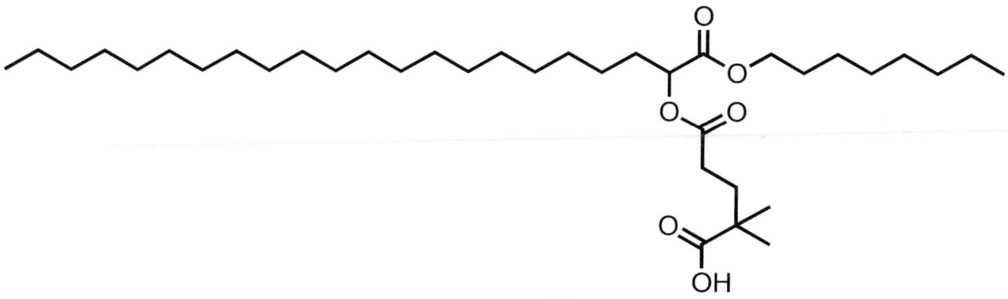

54

Cyclothiazomycin B1 (CTB1) (compound **55**) was isolated from the culture broth of a *Streptomyces* sp. strain as inducing growth inhibition against several filamentous fungi along with morphological changes in hyphae by Mizuhara and his co-workers. They have elucidated the mode of action of an antifungal thiopeptide, cyclothiazomycin B1 (CTB1) and suggested that CTB1 may be a potential candidate antifungal agent with fewer adverse effects [167].

Piper betle L. has traditionally been used in alternative medicine in different countries for several therapeutic purposes, including as an anti-infective agent. Demetrio *et al.* have investigated the antimicrobial activities of its ethanol, methanol, and supercritical CO_2 extracts on clinical isolates of multiple drug resistant bacteria which have been identified by the Infectious Disease Society of America as among the currently more challenging strains in clinical management [168].

Achyrocline bogotensis has been traditionally used to treat skin, respiratory, tract urinary and other infections, but not to treat viral gastrointestinal disease. Téllez *et al.*, have investigated *in vitro* anti-rotavirus and anti-astrovirus properties of *Achyrocline bogotensis* obtained from Colombian-native medicinal plant. Non-toxic concentrations of the fraction obtained exhibited antiviral activity against both viruses characterized by a virucidal effect and by the reduction of the infective particles produced post-infection [169].

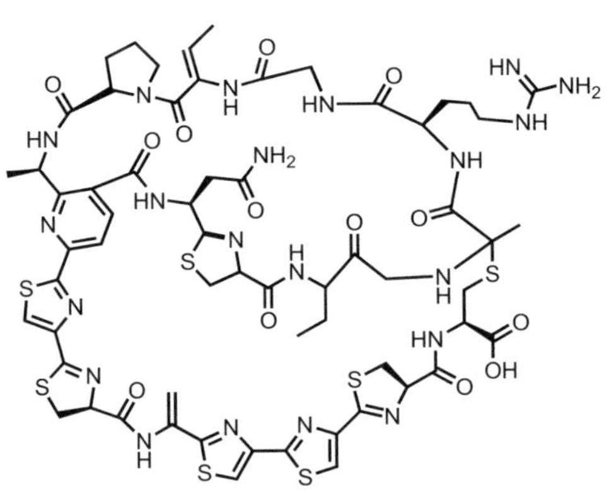

55 Cycothiazomycin B1 (CTB1)

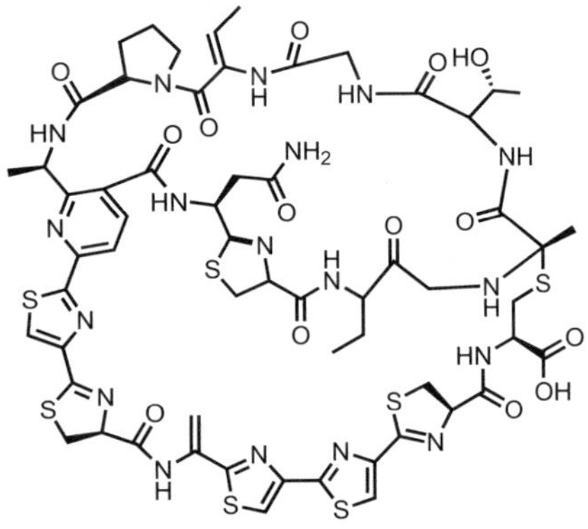

56 Cyclothiazomycin

Zhang *et al.* have reported the synthesis and *in vitro* antibacterial activities against Gram-negative (*E. coli* and *S.aureus*) MRSA and -positive bacteria (*B.subtilis, C.albicans*) of a number of (*S*)-2-(4-tert-butylphenoxy)-3-(benzoxazol-5-yl) propanoic acid derivatives (compound **57**). These compounds were found to exert a broad spectrum of activity against the screened bacteria, but poor MIC values were found for *Candida albicans* fungi. Among the compounds, where R= 4-isopropylphenyl bearing a hydrophobic aromatic tie was the most active derivative against all bacteria studied with MIC values ranging from 0.098 to 0.78 mg/mL. The activity of this compound (R= 4-isopropylphenyl) against *B. subtilis* was 2-fold higher than penicillin, and 8- to 510- fold higher than other control antibiotics such as ceftazidime, cefotaxim, and cefradine antibacterial drugs while antifungal drugs miconazole nitrate and ketoconazole [170].

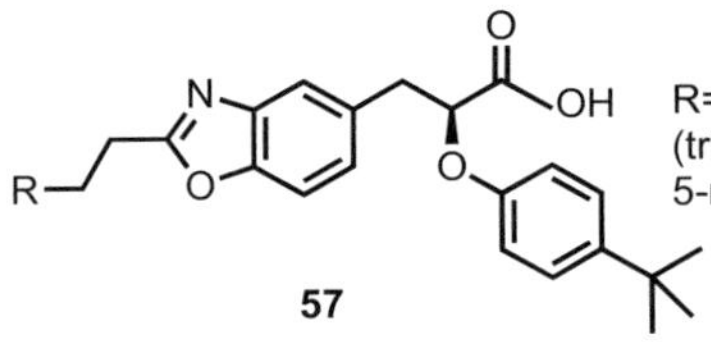

57

R= Phenyl, 4-isopropylphenyl, 4-fluorophenyl, 3,4,5-trimethoxyphenyl, (trifluoromethyl)imidazo[1,2-a]pyridin-2-yl, 1,3-oxazol-2-yl, benzofuran-2-yl, 5-methyl-2-oxazol-4-yl, isopropyl, *n*-pentyl, tetrahydro-2*H*-pyran-4-yl

Sweidan *et al.* have synthesized a series of novel butyrolactone analogues based on the known lichen antibacterial compounds and they have also evaluated their *in vitro* antibacterial activity against *Streptococcus gordonii*. Among the derivatives, where R = $C_{15}H_{31}$ and $C_{16}H_{33}$ (compound **58**) had the lowest MIC of 9.38 µg/mL where they have shown to be stronger bactericidal, by 2–3 times, than the reference antibiotic, doxycycline [171].

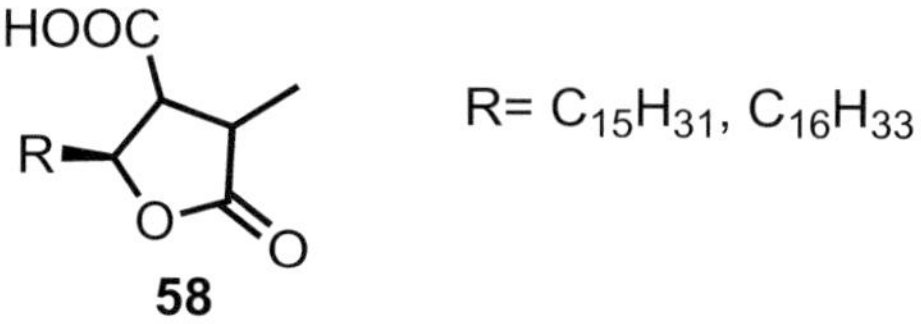

58

Kumar *et al.* have synthesized some novel imidazo[1,2-a]pyridine based organoselenium compounds (compounds **59-61**) and evaluated their antibacterial activity. Among the compounds, 3-nitro-2-(phenylselanyl)imidazo[1,2-a]pyridine (compound **59**) and 3-nitro-2-(*o*-tolylselanyl)imidazo[1,2-a]pyridine (compound **60**) were found active against gram negative bacterium *Escherichia coli* whereas compound 3-nitro-2-(pyridin-2-ylselanyl)imidazo[1,2-a]pyridine (compound **61**) was active against different fungal strains. Synergistic effects of active compounds 2-(phenylselanyl)-3-nitro-imidazo[1,2-a]pyridine and 2-(pyridin-2-ylselanyl)-3-nitro-imidazo[1,2-a]pyridine were tested with existing antibiotic drugs and this test showed that the antibiotic combination with synthesized organoselenium compounds efficiently enhanced the antimicrobial activity [172].

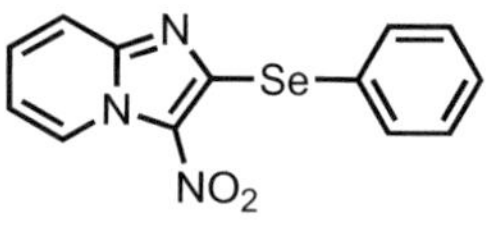

59

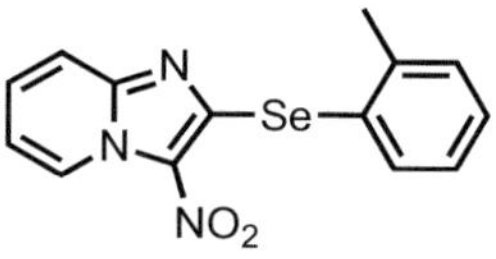

60

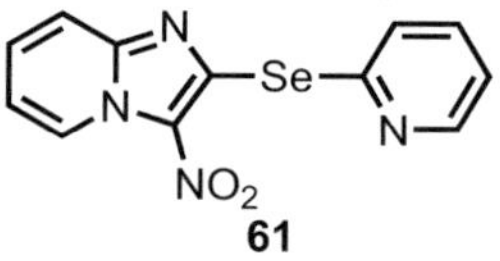

61

Alvarez-Elcoro and Enzler have compared stability and antimicrobial profile of azithromycin and clarithromycin macrolides now available in the United States with erythromycin. These two new macrolides are chemically more stable and more tolerated than erythromycin, and they have a broader antimicrobial spectrum than erythromycin against *Mycobacterium avium complex* (MAC), *Haemophilus influenzae*, *nontuberculous mycobacteria*, and *Chlamydia trachomatis*. Both azithromycin and clarithromycin are effective agents for MAC prophylaxis in patients with late-stage acquired immunedeficiency syndrome (AIDS), however azithromycin may be considered preferable compound due to less drug-drug interactions [173].

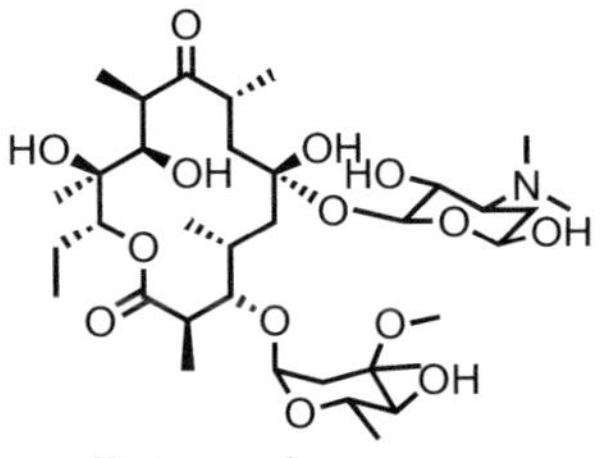

Erytromycin

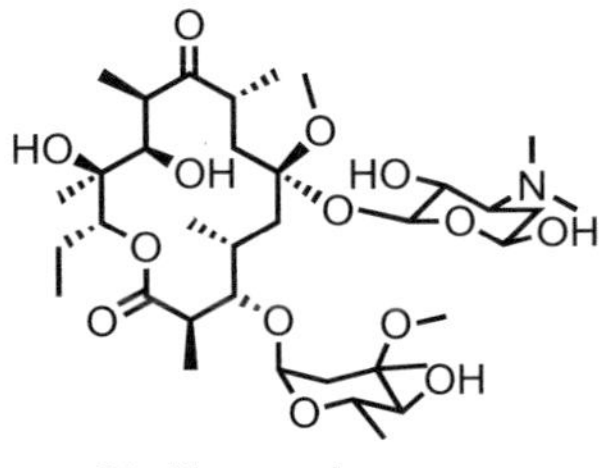

Clarithromycin

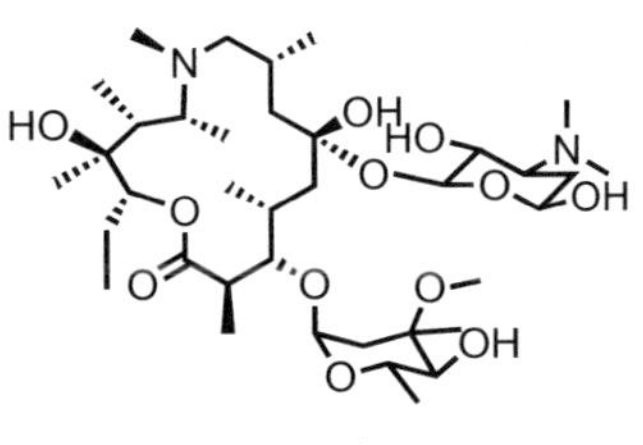

Azithromycin

Tuberculosis (TB) is the second leading lethal infective disease in the world after acquired immune deficiency (AIDs). Gandhi and his co-workers have synthesized and screened antimicobacterial properties of a number of nicotine analogues and one nicotine analogue [3-(5-(3-fluorophenyl)nicotinoyl)-1-methylpyrrol-din-2-one] (compound **62**) exhibited minimum inhibitory concentration of 1 μg/mL (2.86 nM) against *Mycobacterium tuberculosis* (H37Rv strain), a human pathogenic strain of clinically significant importance [174].

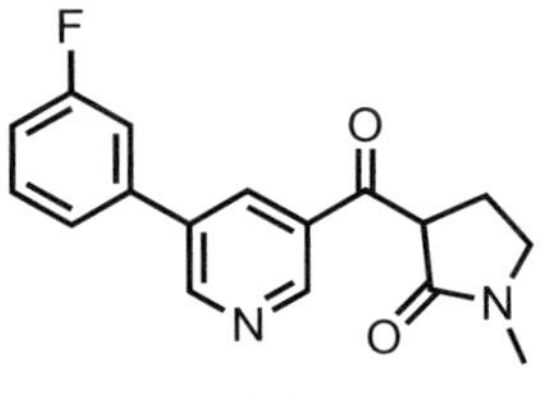

62

Nishimura *et al.* have described the effect of chitin and its derivatives on the activation of peritoneal macrophages *in vivo*, on the suppression of tumor growth in syngenetic mice and on the protection of the host against bacterial infection [175].

Kraljevic *et al.* have synthesized and explored a series of potentially active cytostatic and antibacterial agents based on coumarin–1,2,3-triazole pharmacophoric system. Among the coumarin derivatives compounds **63**, **64** and **65** exhibited high selectivity against *Enterococcus species*. These compounds were found to be superior in inhibiting the growth of clinically isolated vancomycin-resistant *Enterococcus faecium*, while the reference antibiotics exhibited the lack of activity [176].

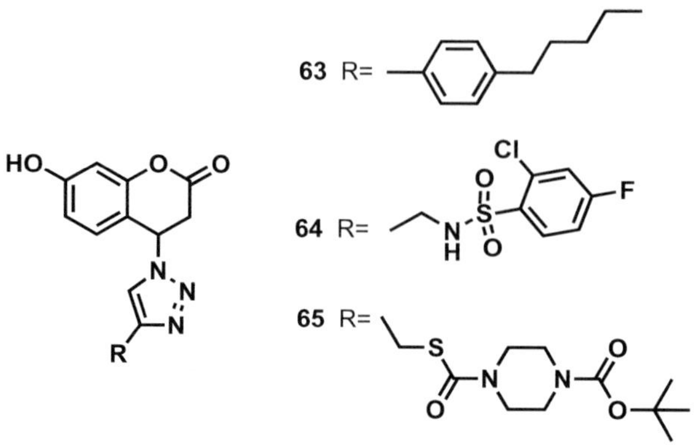

Ahn and his co-workers have synthesized the first, ultra-short pyrazole-arginin--based antimicrobial peptidomimetic derived from the newly synthesized *N*-alkyl/aryl pyrazole amino acids (compound **66**). According to their report, the shortest peptide exhibited greater antimicrobial activity against antibiotic-resistant bacteria, including MRSA, MDRPA, and VREF, which was approximately 2–4 times higher than that of melittin. It also exhibited higher anti-biofilm activity against MDRPA [177].

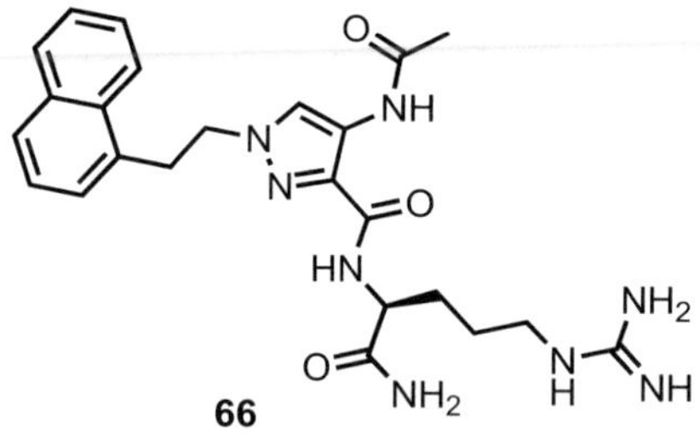

66

Pyrazole and triazole derivatives (compounds **67-72**) possess versatile biological activities such as anticancer, antibacterial, antifungal, and anti-diabetic. Some example of these type compounds are given in Fig. (**17**).

Chowdhury *et al.* have described 'green' silver nanoparticle synthesis using cacao (*Theobroma cacao*) extract and evaluated their toxic effects against microorganisms and human cells. The antimicrobial effects of the cacao AgNPs suspensions were then evaluated against *Staphylococcus aureus* ATCC 29213, *Staphylococcus epidermidis* ATCC 35984, *Escherichia coli* ATCC 25922 and *Pseudomonas aeruginosa* ATCC 27853. The cytotoxicity of the cacao AgNPs suspensions was also tested against primary human dermal fibroblast (HDFs) cells [178].

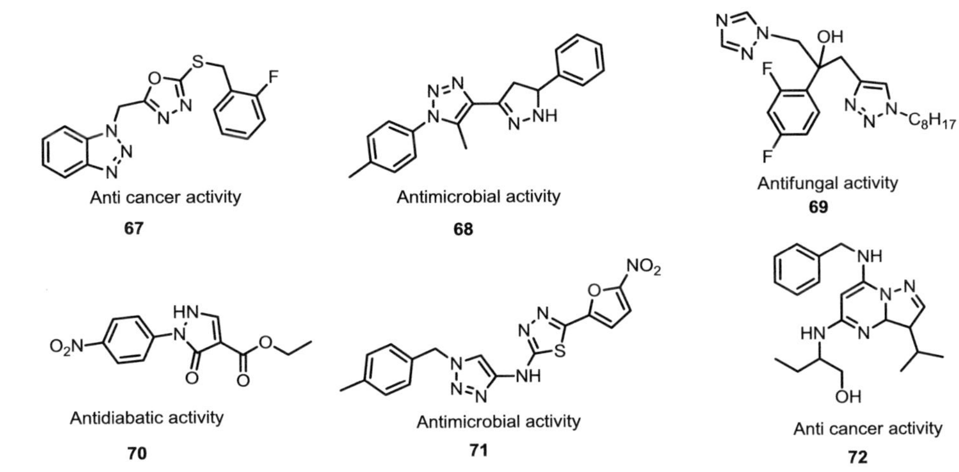

Fig. (17). Some biological active pyrazole and triazole derivatives.

Panda *et al.* have synthesized some amino acid and peptide conjugates of quinine using benzotriazole methodology. The *in vitro* antimalarial activity of these conjugates retain with IC_{50} values below 100 nm, similar to quinine [179].

Ibrahim *et al.* have synthesized a number of novel, cyclic peptidomimetics through benzotriazole methodology (Fig. **18**). Microbiological testing of some of the synthesized compounds revealed an exceptionally high activity against *Candida albicans* with a minimum inhibitory concentration (MIC) lower than the MIC of the antifungal reference drug amphotericin B (**73**) [180].

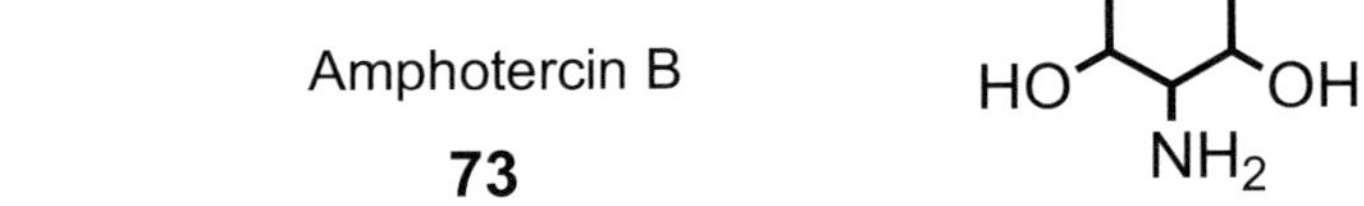

Amphotercin B

73

Chuang *et al.* have designed and synthesized two new series of pyrazole core structures conjugated with sulfonyl groups. One series of derivatives were pyridine-SCH_2-pyrazole (compound **75**) and pyridine-pyrazole (compound **76**) derivatives. According to their results one of the screened compound, namely, 5-(pyridin-2-yl)-1H-pyrazol-3-yl-2-nitrobenzenesulfonate exhibited potent activity against HBV in HepG2 2.2.15 cells with an IC50 value of 9.19 μM [181].

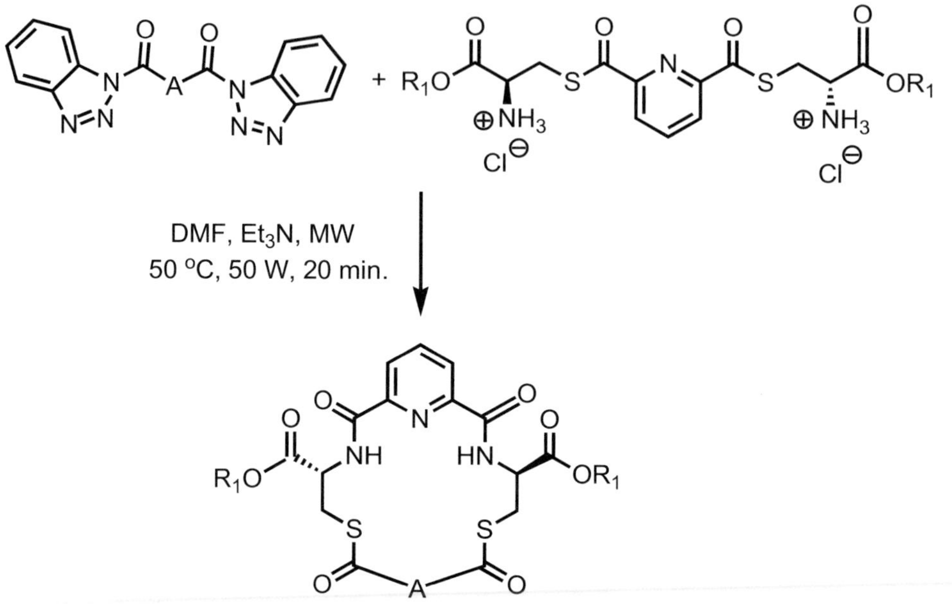

74

A= 2,6-pyridylene, 1,3-phenylene, isopropyl, O, S; R'= Methyl, Ethyl

Fig. (18). Synthesis method for the cyclic peptidomimetics through benzotriazole methodology.

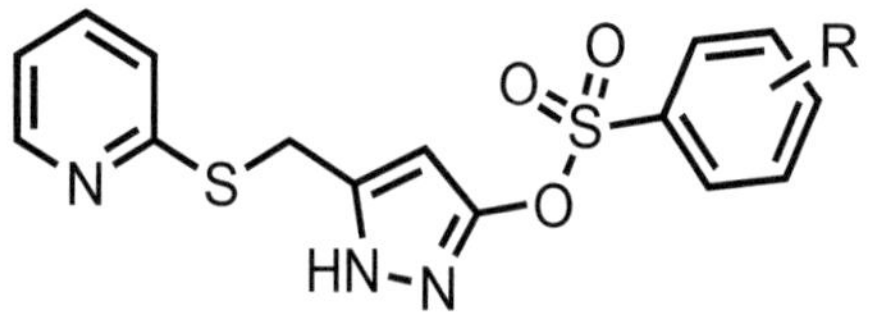

R: H, *p*-Me, *p*-NO_2, *o*-NO_2, *p*-F, *p*-Br, *p*-OMe, OSO_2Me

75

PyridineSCH2-pyrazole derivatives

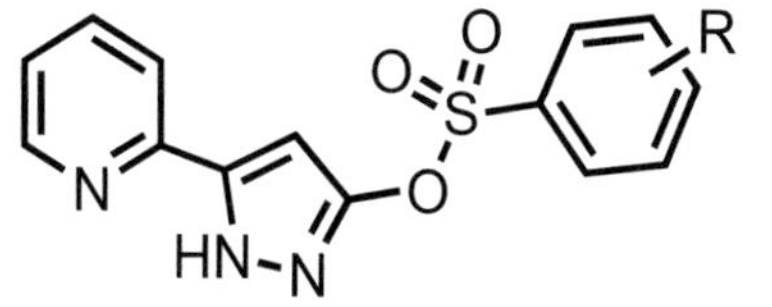

R: H, *p*-Me, *p*-NO_2, *o*-NO_2, *p*-F, *p*-Br, *p*-OMe, OSO_2Me

76

Pyridine-pyrazole derivatives

Apohan *et al.* have synthesized fourteen novel cobalt (II) or zinc (II) complexes of benzimidazoles from reacting of 1-(4-substitutedbenzyl)-1*H*-benzimidazoles (compound **77**) and $CoCl_2.6H_2O$ or $ZnCl_2$. Cytotoxic activities of novel complexes were investigated against A549 and BEAS-2B cell lines. Three of the examined compounds (compounds **78**, **81** and **82**) showed high cytotoxic activity against A549. While the IC_{50} of the cisplatin was 2.56 µg/mL for A549 cells at 72 h, the IC_{50} values of compounds **78**, **81** and **82** were 1.97, 1.87 and 1.9 µg/mL, respectively. IC_{50} values of these compounds for BEAS-2B cells were higher than the IC_{50} values for A549. While the IC_{50} values for BEAS-2B cells were 59.8, 24.5 and 32.67 µg/mL, respectively, the IC_{50} of the cisplatin was determined as 2.53 µg/mL in the present work [182].

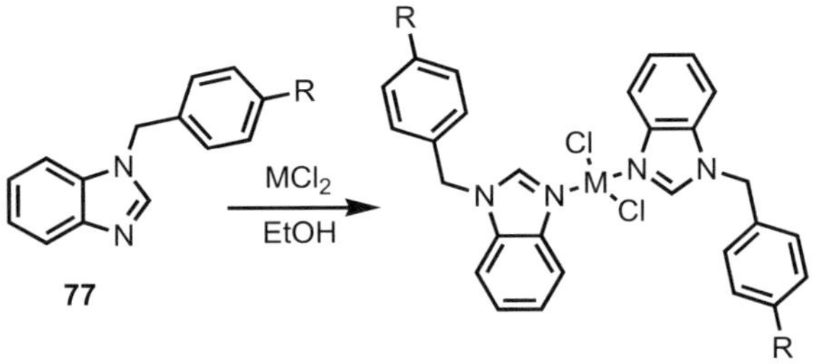

78 R = Cl, M = Zn **85** R = CN, M = Co
79 R = Cl, M = Co **86** R = OCH_3, M = Zn
80 R = Br, M = Zn **87** R = OCH_3, M = Co
81 R = Br, M = Co **88** R = NO_2, M = Zn
82 R = CH_3, M = Zn **89** R = NO_2, M = Co
83 R = CH3, M = Co **90** R = $CH{=}CH_2$, M = Zn
84 R = CN, M = Zn **91** R = $CH{=}CH_2$, M = Co

Tung *et al.* reported synthesis and antimicrobial properties of Fe_3O_4-Ag hybrid nanoparticles against methicilline-resistant *Staphylococcus aureus* (MRSA) pathogen. The characterization of dimer-like nanostructure of Fe_3O_4–Ag hybrid NPs has been identified using X-ray diffraction and High-resolution Transmission Electron Microscopy. According to their biological analysis, novel Fe_3O_4–Ag hybrid NPs exhibited better bactericidal activity than that of plain Fe_3O_4 NPs and Ag-NPs [183].

Thanna *et al.* have synthesized a library of 42 2AT (2-Aminothiophene) compounds. Among these, ethyl 6-ethyl-2-(perfluorobenzamido)-4,5,6,7-tetrahydrothieno[2,3-c]pyridine-3- carboxylate (compound **92**) showed remarkable potency against *Mycobacterium tuberculosis* (Mtb) H37RV (MIC = 0.23 µM) and showed an impressive potency (MIC = 0.20–0.44 µM) against Mtb strains resistant to isoniazid, rifampicin and fluoroquinolones [184].

Surresh *et al.* have synthesized copper nanoparticles (CuNPs) using two- stage chemical reduction method, where a separate reducing agent hydrazine hydrate and a separate stabilizing agent Gum Kondagogu extract are used. The anti-biofilm effect of Gum Kondagogu extract stabilized CuNPs tested against clinical isolate *Klebsiella Pneumoniae* (Gram negative, ATCC 27736) and they obtained promising results for the development of anti-bacterial coated medical devices against pathogenic microorganisms [185].

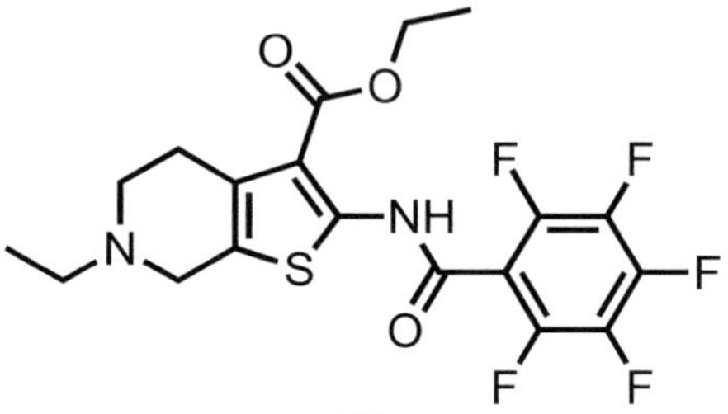

92

El-Sharkawy and Mahmoud reported that *L. mucronata* extract have various cytotoxic activities against HCT116, HepG2 and MCF-7. According to their report 6-isobutylcoumarin (compound **93**) and 6-isobutyl-4-methylcoumarin (compound **94**) showed high significant cytotoxic activity against different cell lines [186].

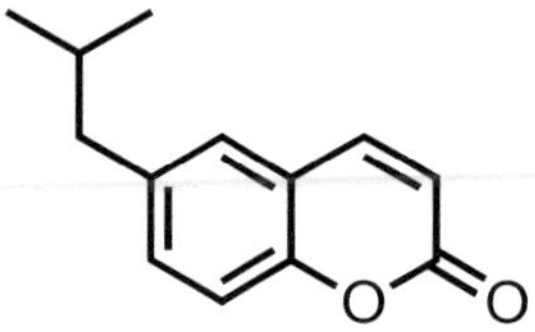

93

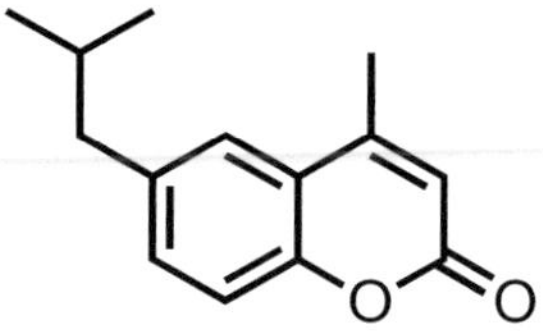

94

CONCLUDING REMARKS

An extensive review of literature survey on commonly used anti-infective drugs, recent development relating to the novel antibiotics and their classifications are provided briefly in this chapter. The classification focused on the main group antibiotics such as β-lactams, macrolides, fluroquinolones, tetracyclines and aminoglycosides. However, despite the remarkable progress in anti-infective therapy, infective diseases caused by bacteria and fungi remain a major worldwide health problem due to the rapid development of resistance to the existing anti-infective drugs. Hence, it is quite important to understand natural products structures and their action mechanism to synthesize semi and full synthetic anti-infective drugs. Therefore, it is realized that there is continuous need to design new drugs as microbes are expected to develop resistance mechanism against new drugs in future. Natural products will continue to act as reservoir of new class of novel anti-infective agents or template for new drug discovery. We hope, this chapter will be useful resource for pharmacy, medicine, biology and chemistry students and researchers.

ABBREVIATIONS

6-APA	6-Aminopenicillanic acid
7-ACA	7-Aminocephalosporanic acid
7-ADCA	Aminodesacetoxycephalosporanic acid
A2780	Ovarian cancer cell line
A549	Adenocarcinomic human alveolar basal epithelial cells
ABP	Acute bacterial prostatitis
AChE	Acetylcholinesterase
AG	Aminoglycoside
AgNPs	Silver nanoparticles
AIDS	Acquired immune deficiency syndrome
AMA	Aspergillomarasmine A
AME	Alternariol-9-methyl ether
Anti-MRSA	Anti-methicillin-resistant *Staphylococcus aureus*
AO/EtBr	Acridine orange/ethidium bromide
ATCC	American type culture c*ollection*
ATIs	Aza-tricyclic indolines
BEAS-2B	Non-tumorigenic human bronchial epithelial cells
BODIPY-FL	Boron-dipyrromethene based fluorescent dye
BTZ	Bisthiazolidine
CA	Clavulanic acid
CBP	Chronic bacterial prostatitis
CephC	Cephamycin C
CPNP	Calcium phosphate nanoparticle
CTB1	Cyclothiazomycin B1
DNA	Deoxyribonucleic acid
ESI	Electrospray ionization
FDA	Food and drug administration
GEM	Gemifloxacin
GNPs	Gold nanoparticles
GT	Gentamicin
hCA I	The human carbonic anhydrase I
hCA II	The human carbonic anhydrase II
HCT116	Human colon cancer cells
HEAC	Hydroethanol extract of *Annona coriacea*

HeLa	Cervical cancer cells
Hep G2	Human liver cancer cell line
HIV	Human immunodeficiency virus
HPLC	High-performance liquid chromatography
IC50	The half maximal inhibitory concentration
I-PSS	International prostate symptom score
LZH	Layered zinc hydroxide
MAC	*Mycobacterium avium complex*
MBC	Minimum bactericidal concentration
MBL	Metallo-β-lactamase
MCF-7	Breast cancer cells
MDR	Multiple drug resistance
MDRPA	Multidrug resistant Pseudomonas aeruginosa
MIC	Minimum inhibitory concentration
MI*milR*	A regulatory gene in the milbemycin
MRSA	Methicillin-resistant *Staphylococcus aureus*
MS	Mass Spectrometry
Mtb	*Mycobacterium tuberculosis*
MTT	3-(4,5-Dimethylthiazol-2-yl)-2,5-diphenyltetrazolium bromide
NBD	Nitrobenzoxadiazole
NDM	New Delhi metallo-β-lactamase
NIH	National institutes of health
NIH-CPSI	National institutes of health -chronic prostatitis symptom index
NPs	Nanoparticles
ODIPY FL	A bright, green-fluorescent dye with similar excitation
OEHHA Prop 65	The office of environmental health hazard assessment proposition 65
OEHHA	Office of environmental health hazard assessment
PC3	Prostate cancer cell lines
PVP	Poly(N-vinylpyrrolidone)
QSAR	Quantitative structure-activity relationship
QTOF-MS	Quadrupole time-of-flight mass spectrometry
TB	Tuberculosis
Tet-CPNPs	Tetracycline-loaded calcium phosphate nanoparticles
TR	Texas Red
UHPLC	Ultrahigh pressure liquid chromatography

VIM MBLs	Verona integron-encoded metallo-β-lactamase
VISA	Vancomycin-intermediate *Staphylococcus aureus*
VRE	Vancomycin-resistant *Enterococcus*
VRSA	Vancomycin-resistant *Staphylococcus aureus"*

CONFLICT OF INTEREST

The authors declare no conflict of interest, financial or otherwise.

ACKNOWLEDGEMENTS

Declared none.

REFERENCES

[1] Trudinger PA, Bubela B. Microorganisms and the natural environment. Miner Depos 1967; 2(3): 147-57.
[http://dx.doi.org/10.1007/BF00201911]

[2] Baker DD, Chu M, Oza U, Rajgarhia V, Oza U, Rajgarhia V. The value of natural products to future pharmaceutical discovery. Nat Prod Rep 2007; 24(6): 1225-44.
[http://dx.doi.org/10.1039/b602241n] [PMID: 18033577]

[3] Wright PM, Seiple IB, Myers AG. The evolving role of chemical synthesis in antibacterial drug discovery. Angew Chem Int Ed Engl 2014; 53(34): 8840-69.
[http://dx.doi.org/10.1002/anie.201310843] [PMID: 24990531]

[4] Bbosa GS, Mwebaza N, Odda J, Kyegombe DB, Ntale M. Antibiotics / antibacterial drug use, their marketing and promotion during the post-antibiotic golden age and their role in emergence of bacterial resistance. Health 2014; 6(5): 410-25.
[http://dx.doi.org/10.4236/health.2014.65059]

[5] Gowri M, Anonthalakshmi S, Therese P. In-Vitro antimicrobial screening of naphthalene acetic acid compounds. Int J Pharm Life Sci 2013; 4(7): 2780-4.

[6] Tan SY, Tatsumura Y. Alexander Fleming (1881-1955): Discoverer of penicillin. Singapore Med J 2015; 56(7): 366-7.
[http://dx.doi.org/10.11622/smedj.2015105] [PMID: 26243971]

[7] Wolfe DW. Tales from the Underground: A natural History of Subterranean Life. Cambridge, Massachusetts, USA: Persus Publishing 2001.

[8] Peláez F. The historical delivery of antibiotics from microbial natural products--can history repeat? Biochem Pharmacol 2006; 71(7): 981-90.
[http://dx.doi.org/10.1016/j.bcp.2005.10.010] [PMID: 16290171]

[9] Fair RJ, Tor Y. Antibiotics and bacterial resistance in the 21st century. Perspect Medicin Chem 2014; 6: 25-64.
[PMID: 25232278]

[10] Cragg GM, Newman DJ. A continuing source of novel drug leads. BBA - Gen Subj. Biochim Biophys Acta 2013; 1830(6): 3670-95.
[http://dx.doi.org/10.1016/j.bbagen.2013.02.008] [PMID: 23428572]

[11] Abad MJ, Bedoya LM, Bermejo P. Marine Compounds and their Antimicrobial Activities. In: Mendez-Vilas A, Ed. Science Against Microbial Pathogens: Communicating Current Research and Technological Advances. Formatex 2011; pp. 1293-306.

[12] Kanoh K, Matsuo Y, Adachi K, Imagawa H, Nishizawa M, Shizuri Y. Mechercharmycins A and B, cytotoxic substances from marine-derived Thermoactinomyces sp. YM3-251. J Antibiot 2005; 58(4): 289-92.
[http://dx.doi.org/10.1038/ja.2005.36] [PMID: 15981418]

[13] Feling RH, Buchanan GO, Mincer TJ, Kauffman CA, Jensen PR, Fenical W. Salinosporamide A: a highly cytotoxic proteasome inhibitor from a novel microbial source, a marine bacterium of the new genus salinospora. Angew Chem Int Ed Engl 2003; 42(3): 355-7.
[http://dx.doi.org/10.1002/anie.200390115] [PMID: 12548698]

[14] Li F, Maskey RP, Qin S, *et al.* Chinikomycins A and B: isolation, structure elucidation, and biological activity of novel antibiotics from a marine Streptomyces sp. isolate M045. J Nat Prod 2005; 68(3): 349-53.
[http://dx.doi.org/10.1021/np030518r] [PMID: 15787434]

[15] Maloney KN, Macmillan JB, Kauffman CA, Jensen R, Dipasquale AG, Rheingold AL. vd. Lodopyridone, a Structurally Actinomycete. Org Lett 2009; 11: 5422-4.
[http://dx.doi.org/10.1021/ol901997k] [PMID: 19883103]

[16] Macherla VR, Liu J, Bellows C, *et al.* Glaciapyrroles A, B, and C, pyrrolosesquiterpenes from a Streptomyces sp. isolated from an Alaskan marine sediment. J Nat Prod 2005; 68(5): 780-3.
[http://dx.doi.org/10.1021/np049597c] [PMID: 15921430]

[17] Bruntner C, Binder T, Pathom-aree W, *et al.* Frigocyclinone, a novel angucyclinone antibiotic produced by a Streptomyces griseus strain from Antarctica. J Antibiot 2005; 58(5): 346-9.
[http://dx.doi.org/10.1038/ja.2005.43] [PMID: 16060387]

[18] Oh DC, Gontang EA, Kauffman CA, Jensen PR, Fenical W. Salinipyrones and pacificanones, mixed-precursor polyketides from the marine actinomycete Salinispora pacifica. J Nat Prod 2008; 71(4): 570-5.
[http://dx.doi.org/10.1021/np0705155] [PMID: 18321059]

[19] Subramani R, Aalbersberg W. Marine actinomycetes: an ongoing source of novel bioactive metabolites. Microbiol Res 2012; 167(10): 571-80.
[http://dx.doi.org/10.1016/j.micres.2012.06.005] [PMID: 22796410]

[20] Harbarth S, Samore MH. Antimicrobial resistance determinants and future control. Emerg Infect Dis 2005; 11(6): 794-801.
[http://dx.doi.org/10.3201/eid1106.050167] [PMID: 15963271]

[21] Barbour PM, Wang W, Chang L, *et al.* Property-guided synthesis of aza-tricyclic indolines: Development of gold catalysis en route. Adv Synth Catal 2016; 358(9): 1482-90.
[http://dx.doi.org/10.1002/adsc.201501101] [PMID: 28360827]

[22] Neu HC. The crisis in antibiotic resistance. Science 1992; 257(5073): 1064-73.
[http://dx.doi.org/10.1126/science.257.5073.1064] [PMID: 1509257]

[23] Davies J, Davies D. Origins and evolution of antibiotic resistance. Microbiol Mol Biol Rev 2010; 74(3): 417-33.
[http://dx.doi.org/10.1128/MMBR.00016-10] [PMID: 20805405]

[24] Gottfried J. History Repeating ? Avoiding a Return to the Pre-Antibiotic Age. Third Year Paper, Harward University 2005. Available at: http://nrs.harvard.edu/urn-3:HUL.InstRepos:8889467

[25] Cragg GM, Newman DJ. Natural products: a continuing source of novel drug leads. Biochim Biophys Acta 2013; 1830(6): 3670-95.
[http://dx.doi.org/10.1016/j.bbagen.2013.02.008] [PMID: 23428572]

[26] von Nussbaum F, Brands M, Hinzen B, Weigand S, Häbich D. Antibacterial natural products in medicinal chemistry--exodus or revival? Angew Chem Int Ed Engl 2006; 45(31): 5072-129.
[http://dx.doi.org/10.1002/anie.200600350] [PMID: 16881035]

[27] Singh SB, Barrett JF. Empirical antibacterial drug discovery--foundation in natural products. Biochem Pharmacol 2006; 71(7): 1006-15.
[http://dx.doi.org/10.1016/j.bcp.2005.12.016] [PMID: 16412984]

[28] Aljamali NM, Jwad SM, Jawad AM. Survey on antibiotics and bacteria resistance. Int J Pharm Physiol 2015; 1(1): 1-16.

[29] Barzic AI, Ioan S. Antibacterial Drugs- From Basic Concepts to Complex Therapeutic Mechanisms of Polymer Systems. In: Bobbarala V, Ed. Immunology and Microbiology "Concepts, Compounds and the Alternatives of Antibacterials" World' s largest Science, Technology & Medicine Open Access book publisher. 2015; pp. 1-28.
[http://dx.doi.org/10.5772/60755]

[30] Kohanski MA, Dwyer DJ, Hayete B, Lawrence CA, Collins JJ. A common mechanism of cellular death induced by bactericidal antibiotics. Cell 2007; 130(5): 797-810.
[http://dx.doi.org/10.1016/j.cell.2007.06.049] [PMID: 17803904]

[31] Moore D. Antibiotic classification and mechanismm 2017. Available at: http://www.orthobullets.com/basic-science/9059/antibiotic-classification-and-mechanism

[32] Fedorenko V, Genilloud O, Horbal L, *et al.* Antibacterial Discovery and Development: From Gene to Product and Back. Biomed Res Int. 2015; pp. 1-16.

[33] Procópio RE, Silva IR, Martins MK, *et al.* Antibiotics produced by Streptomyces. Braz J Infect Dis 2012; 16(5): 466-71.
[http://dx.doi.org/10.1016/j.bjid.2012.08.014] [PMID: 22975171]

[34] Etebu E, Arikekpar I. Antibiotics : Classification and mechanisms of action with emphasis on molecular perspectives. Int J Appl Microbiol Biothech Res 2016; 4: 90-101.

[35] Neuhauser MM, Danziger LH. β -Lactam Antibiotics. In: Piscitelli SC, Rodvold KA, Eds. Drug Interactions in Infectious Diseases. New York: Humana Press 2001; pp. 151-84.

[36] Kotra LP, Mobashery S. Beta-Lactam antibiotics, beta-1actamases and bacterial resistance. Bull Inst Pasteur 1998; 96(3): 139-50.
[http://dx.doi.org/10.1016/S0020-2452(98)80009-2]

[37] Zaffiri L, Gardner J, Toledo-Pereyra LH. History of antibiotics. From salvarsan to cephalosporins. J Invest Surg 2012; 25(2): 67-77.
[http://dx.doi.org/10.3109/08941939.2012.664099] [PMID: 22439833]

[38] Hamilton-Miller JM. Development of the semi-synthetic penicillins and cephalosporins. Int J Antimicrob Agents 2008; 31(3): 189-92.
[http://dx.doi.org/10.1016/j.ijantimicag.2007.11.010] [PMID: 18248798]

[39] Silver R, Bostian K. Historically, "antibiotics" stood for natural products and their derivatives, whereas "antibacterials" meant synthetic compounds. Eur J Clin Microbiol Infect Dis 1990; 9(7): 455-61.
[http://dx.doi.org/10.1007/BF01964283] [PMID: 2226472]

[40] Lai JC. Their chemical history and legal disputes in New Zealand. Chem New Zealand 2009; pp. 116-24.

[41] Bentley R. Different roads to discovery; Prontosil (hence sulfa drugs) and penicillin (hence β-lactams). J Ind Microbiol Biotechnol 2009; 36(6): 775-86.
[http://dx.doi.org/10.1007/s10295-009-0553-8] [PMID: 19283418]

[42] Chain EB. The chemical structure of the penicillins. Nobel Lecture 1946; pp. 110-43.

[43] Elander RP. Industrial production of β-lactam antibiotics 2003; 61: 385-92.
[http://dx.doi.org/10.1007/s00253-003-1274-y]

[44] Batchelor FR, Doyle FP, Nayler JH, Rolinson GN. Synthesis of penicillin: 6-aminopenicillanic acid in

penicillin fermentations. Nature 1959; 183(4656): 257-8.
[http://dx.doi.org/10.1038/183257b0] [PMID: 13622762]

[45] Pur FN, Dilmaghani KA. Calixpenams : synthesis, characterization, and biological evaluation of penicillins V and X clustered by calixarene scaffold. Turk J Chem 2014; 38: 288-96.
[http://dx.doi.org/10.3906/kim-1307-32]

[46] Rolinson GN. Forty years of β-lactam research. J Antimicrob Chemother 1998; 41(6): 589-603.
[http://dx.doi.org/10.1093/jac/41.6.589] [PMID: 9687097]

[47] Kaur SP, Rao R, Nanda S. Amoxicillin: A broad spectrum antibiotic. Int J Pharm Pharm Sci 2011; 3(3): 30-7.

[48] Kennedy WP, Wallace AT, Murdoch JM. Ampicillin in treatment of certain gram-negative bacterial infections. BMJ 1963; 2(5363): 962-5.
[http://dx.doi.org/10.1136/bmj.2.5363.962] [PMID: 14056923]

[49] Raut MR, Kumari S, Vichare VV, Mane VS, Gangaware AK. Isolation and Purification of Cephalosporin ' s from cheese whey. Res J Pharm Biol Chem Sci 2013; 4(1): 1054-67.

[50] Wegman MA, Janssen MH, Van Rantwijk F, Sheldon RA. Towards Biocatalytic Synthesis of β-Lactam Antibiotics. Adv Synth Catal 2001; 343: 559-76.
[http://dx.doi.org/10.1002/1615-4169(200108)343:6/7<559::AID-ADSC559>3.0.CO;2-Z]

[51] Singh J, Arrieta AC. New Cephalosporins. Semin Pediatr Infect Dis 1999; 10(1): 14-22.
[http://dx.doi.org/10.1016/S1045-1870(99)80005-3]

[52] García-Rodríguez JA, Muñoz Bellido JL, García Sánchez JE. Oral cephalosporins: current perspectives. Int J Antimicrob Agents 1995; 5(4): 231-43.
[http://dx.doi.org/10.1016/0924-8579(95)00015-Z] [PMID: 18611674]

[53] Marshall WF, Blair JE. The cephalosporins. Mayo Clin Proc 1999; 74(2): 187-95.
[http://dx.doi.org/10.4065/74.2.187] [PMID: 10069359]

[54] Garaul J, Wilson W, Wood M, Carlefl J. Fourth-generation cephalosporins : A review of *in vitro* activity, pharmacokinetics, pharmacodynamics and clinical utility. Clin Microbiol Infect 1997; 3 (Suppl. 1): 87-101.
[http://dx.doi.org/10.1111/j.1469-0691.1997.tb00649.x]

[55] Greenwood D. Chronicle of a twentieth century medical triumph Oxford. Antimicrobial Drugs. Oxford University Press 2008; pp. 1-423.

[56] Mandell GL. Drugs Five Years Later. Ann Intern Med 1973; 79: 561-5.
[http://dx.doi.org/10.7326/0003-4819-79-4-561] [PMID: 4748274]

[57] Bonnet R. Growing group of extended-spectrum β-lactamases: the CTX-M enzymes. Antimicrob Agents Chemother 2004; 48(1): 1-14.
[http://dx.doi.org/10.1128/AAC.48.1.1-14.2004] [PMID: 14693512]

[58] Yahav D, Paul M, Fraser A, Sarid N, Leibovici L. Efficacy and safety of cefepime: a systematic review and meta-analysis. Lancet Infect Dis 2007; 7(5): 338-48.
[http://dx.doi.org/10.1016/S1473-3099(07)70109-3] [PMID: 17448937]

[59] Duplessis C, Crum-Cianflone NF. Ceftaroline: A new cephalosporin with activity against methicillin-resistant *Staphylococcus aureus* (MRSA). Clin Med Rev Ther 2011; 3(a2466): 1-25.
[PMID: 21785568]

[60] Kisgen J, Whitney D. Ceftobiprole , a broad-spectrum cephalosporin with activity against methicillin-resistant *Staphylococcus aureus* (MRSA). P&T 2008; 33(11): 631-41.
[PMID: 19750059]

[61] Jelić D, Antolović R. From erythromycin to azithromycin and new potential ribosome-binding antimicrobials. Antibiotics (Basel) 2016; 5(3): 1-13.
[http://dx.doi.org/10.3390/antibiotics5030029] [PMID: 27598215]

[62] Weisblum B. Macrolide resistance. Drug Resist Updat 1998; 1(1): 29-41. [http://dx.doi.org/10.1016/S1368-7646(98)80212-4] [PMID: 17092794]

[63] Davis S. Macrolides and ketolides : more than just antimicrobials. S Afr Pharm 2011; 78(5): 24-7.

[64] Gaillard T, Dormoi J, Madamet M, Pradines B. Macrolides and associated antibiotics based on similar mechanism of action like lincosamides in malaria. Malar J 2016; 15(85): 85. [http://dx.doi.org/10.1186/s12936-016-1114-z] [PMID: 26873741]

[65] Mutak S. Azalides from azithromycin to new azalide derivatives. J Antibiot 2007; 60(2): 85-122. [http://dx.doi.org/10.1038/ja.2007.10] [PMID: 17420561]

[66] Zuckerman JM. Macrolides and ketolides: azithromycin, clarithromycin, telithromycin. Infect Dis Clin North Am 2004; 18(3): 621-649, xi. [http://dx.doi.org/10.1016/j.idc.2004.04.010] [PMID: 15308279]

[67] Schlünzen F, Harms JM, Franceschi F, *et al.* Structural basis for the antibiotic activity of ketolides and azalides. Structure 2003; 11(3): 329-38. [http://dx.doi.org/10.1016/S0969-2126(03)00022-4] [PMID: 12623020]

[68] Song QL, Guo BQ, Zhang W, Lan P, Sun PH, Chen WM. Design, synthesis and antibacterial activity of novel ketolides bearing an aryltetrazolyl-substituted alkyl side chain. J Antibiot 2011; 64(8): 571-81. [http://dx.doi.org/10.1038/ja.2011.50] [PMID: 21772308]

[69] Wagh B, Paul T, Debrosse C, *et al.* Desmethyl Macrolides: Synthesis and Evaluation of 4,8,10-Tridesmethyl Cethromycin. ACS Med Chem Lett 2013; 4(11): 1114-8. [http://dx.doi.org/10.1021/ml400337t] [PMID: 24470840]

[70] Leclercq R, Courvalin P. Resistance to macrolides and related antibiotics in *Streptococcus pneumoniae.* Antimicrob Agents Chemother 2002; 46(9): 2727-34. [http://dx.doi.org/10.1128/AAC.46.9.2727-2734.2002] [PMID: 12183222]

[71] Yang B, Zöllner T, Gebhardt P, Möllmann U, Miller MJ. Preparation and biological evaluation of novel leucomycin analogs derived from nitroso Diels-Alder reactions. Org Biomol Chem 2010; 8(3): 691-7. [http://dx.doi.org/10.1039/B922450E] [PMID: 20090988]

[72] Grundy WE. Chemotherapy of bacterial infections part II chemotherapy of fungal infections. In: Schnitzer RJ, Hawking F, Eds. Experimental Chemotherapy. New York: Academic Press 1964; pp. 172-207.

[73] Furuuchi T, Miura T, Kurihara K, Yoshida T, Watanabe T, Ajito K. Design and synthesis of novel leucomycin analogues modified at the C-3 position. Part II: 3-O-(3-Aryl-2-propenyl)leucomycin analogues. Bioorg Med Chem 2008; 16(8): 4401-18. [http://dx.doi.org/10.1016/j.bmc.2008.02.064] [PMID: 18329276]

[74] Karray F, Darbon E, Oestreicher N, *et al.* Organization of the biosynthetic gene cluster for the macrolide antibiotic spiramycin in Streptomyces ambofaciens. Microbiology 2007; 153(Pt 12): 4111-22. [http://dx.doi.org/10.1099/mic.0.2007/009746-0] [PMID: 18048924]

[75] Jakopović IP, Kragol G, Forrest AK, *et al.* Synthesis and properties of macrolones characterized by two ether bonds in the linker. Bioorg Med Chem 2010; 18(17): 6578-88. [http://dx.doi.org/10.1016/j.bmc.2010.07.007] [PMID: 20688524]

[76] Kapić S, Cipcić Paljetak H, Alihodzić S, *et al.* 6-Alkylquinolone-3-carboxylic acid tethered to macrolides synthesis and antimicrobial profile. Bioorg Med Chem 2010; 18(17): 6569-77. [http://dx.doi.org/10.1016/j.bmc.2010.06.048] [PMID: 20673633]

[77] Pallo-Zimmerman LM, Byron JK, Graves TK. Fluoroquinolones: then and now. Compend Contin Educ Vet 2010; 32(7): E1-9.

[PMID: 20957609]

[78] Bisacchi GS. Origins of the quinolone class of antibacterials: An expanded "Discovery Story". J Med Chem 2015; 58(12): 4874-82.
[http://dx.doi.org/10.1021/jm501881c] [PMID: 25738967]

[79] Newman RL, Holt RJ, Frankcombe CH. Nalidixic Acid: microbiological and clinical studies on urinary infections in children. Arch Dis Child 1966; 41(218): 389-94.
[http://dx.doi.org/10.1136/adc.41.218.389] [PMID: 21032438]

[80] Misra GC, Willcox MC. A clinical trial with nalidixic acid on 22 acute and chronic urinary tract infections with follow-up for i-5 months. Postgrad Med J 1965; 41: 508-11.
[http://dx.doi.org/10.1136/pgmj.41.478.508] [PMID: 14325647]

[81] Goodman LS, Gilman A. The pharamcoclogical basis of therapeutics. 8th., New York: Macmillan 1992.

[82] Tillotson GS, Lesher G. Quinolones: structure-activity relationships and future predictions. J Med Microbiol 1996; 44(5): 320-4.
[http://dx.doi.org/10.1099/00222615-44-5-320] [PMID: 8636945]

[83] Chai Y, Liu M, Lv K, *et al.* Synthesis and *in vitro* antibacterial activity of a series of novel gati fl oxacin derivatives. Eur J Med Chem 2011; 46(9): 4267-73.
[http://dx.doi.org/10.1016/j.ejmech.2011.06.032] [PMID: 21764484]

[84] Mouton Y, Leroy O. Ofloxacin. Int J Antimicrob Agents 1991; 1(2-3): 57-74.
[http://dx.doi.org/10.1016/0924-8579(91)90001-T] [PMID: 18611493]

[85] Nightingale CH. Moxifloxacin, a new antibiotic designed to treat community-acquired respiratory tract infections: a review of microbiologic and pharmacokinetic-pharmacodynamic characteristics. Pharmacotherapy 2000; 20(3): 245-56.
[http://dx.doi.org/10.1592/phco.20.4.245.34880] [PMID: 10730681]

[86] Guay DR. Moxifloxacin in the treatment of skin and skin structure infections. Ther Clin Risk Manag 2006; 2(4): 417-34.
[http://dx.doi.org/10.2147/tcrm.2006.2.4.417] [PMID: 18360653]

[87] Naber KG, Adam D. Classification of fluoroquinolones. Int J Antimicrob Agents 1998; 10(4): 255-7.
[http://dx.doi.org/10.1016/S0924-8579(98)00059-4] [PMID: 9916897]

[88] Soni K. Fluoroquinolones : Chemistry & Action – A Review. Indo Glob J Pharam Sci 2012; 2(1): 43-53.

[89] National Toxicology program. California Office of Environmental Health Hazard Assessment (OEHHA) Available at: https://ntp.niehs.nih.gov/pubhealth/impact/1990s/1998

[90] Ambrose PG, Owens RC Jr, Quintiliani R, Nightingale CH. New generations of quinolones: with particular attention to levofloxacin. Conn Med 1997; 61(5): 269-72.
[PMID: 9197076]

[91] Hamzah J, Skinner-Adams T, Davis TM. *In vitro* antimalarial activity of trovafloxacin, a fourth-generation fluoroquinolone. Acta Trop 2000; 74(1): 39-42.
[http://dx.doi.org/10.1016/S0001-706X(99)00051-0] [PMID: 10643906]

[92] Brighty KE, Gootz TD. The chemistry and biological profile of trovafloxacin. J Antimicrob Chemother 1997; 39 (Suppl. B): 1-14.
[http://dx.doi.org/10.1093/jac/39.suppl_2.1] [PMID: 9222064]

[93] Oliphant CM, Green GM, Hershey MS. Quinolones: a comprehensive review. Am Fam Physician 2002; 65(3): 455-64.
[PMID: 11858629]

[94] Andersson MI, MacGowan AP. Development of the quinolones. J Antimicrob Chemother 2003; 51 (Suppl. 1): 1-11.

[http://dx.doi.org/10.1093/jac/dkg212] [PMID: 12702698]

[95] Thaker M, Spanogiannopoulos P, Wright GD. The tetracycline resistome. Cell Mol Life Sci 2010; 67(3): 419-31.
[http://dx.doi.org/10.1007/s00018-009-0172-6] [PMID: 19862477]

[96] Nelson ML, Levy SB. The history of the tetracyclines. Ann N Y Acad Sci 2011; 1241: 17-32.
[http://dx.doi.org/10.1111/j.1749-6632.2011.06354.x] [PMID: 22191524]

[97] Chopra I, Roberts M. Tetracycline antibiotics: mode of action, applications, molecular biology, and epidemiology of bacterial resistance. Microbiol Mol Biol Rev 2001; 65(2): 232-60.
[http://dx.doi.org/10.1128/MMBR.65.2.232-260.2001] [PMID: 11381101]

[98] Fluit AC, Visser MR, Schmitz FJ. Molecular detection of antimicrobial resistance. Clin Microbiol Rev 2001; 14(4): 836-71.
[http://dx.doi.org/10.1128/CMR.14.4.836-871.2001] [PMID: 11585788]

[99] Chopra I, Hawkey PM, Hinton M. Tetracyclines, molecular and clinical aspects. J Antimicrob Chemother 1992; 29(3): 245-77.
[http://dx.doi.org/10.1093/jac/29.3.245] [PMID: 1592696]

[100] Chopra I. Glycylcyclines: third-generation tetracycline antibiotics. Curr Opin Pharmacol 2001; 1(5): 464-9.
[http://dx.doi.org/10.1016/S1471-4892(01)00081-9] [PMID: 11764771]

[101] Fuoco D. Classification framework and chemical biology of tetracycline-structure-based drugs. Antibiotics (Basel) 2012; 1(1): 1-13.
[http://dx.doi.org/10.3390/antibiotics1010001] [PMID: 27029415]

[102] Chiwunze TE, Azumah R, Ramtahal M, *et al.* Organocatalyzed mannich reactions on minocycline : Towards novel tetracycline antibiotics. S Afr J Chem 2016; 9: 72-8.

[103] Zakeri B, Wright GD. Chemical biology of tetracycline antibiotics. Biochem Cell Biol 2008; 86(2): 124-36.
[http://dx.doi.org/10.1139/O08-002] [PMID: 18443626]

[104] Chopra I. Tetracycline analogs whose primary target is not the bacterial ribosome. Antimicrob Agents Chemother 1994; 38(4): 637-40.
[http://dx.doi.org/10.1128/AAC.38.4.637] [PMID: 8031024]

[105] Rasmussen B, Noller HF, Daubresse G, *et al.* Molecular basis of tetracycline action: identification of analogs whose primary target is not the bacterial ribosome. Antimicrob Agents Chemother 1991; 35(11): 2306-11.
[http://dx.doi.org/10.1128/AAC.35.11.2306] [PMID: 1725100]

[106] van Hoek AH, Mevius D, Guerra B, Mullany P, Roberts AP, Aarts HJ. Acquired antibiotic resistance genes: an overview. Front Microbiol 2011; 2: 203.
[http://dx.doi.org/10.3389/fmicb.2011.00203] [PMID: 22046172]

[107] Kudo F, Eguchi T. Biosynthetic genes for aminoglycoside antibiotics. J Antibiot 2009; 62(9): 471-81.
[http://dx.doi.org/10.1038/ja.2009.76] [PMID: 19644520]

[108] Mahmud T, Flatt PM, Wu X. Biosynthesis of unusual aminocyclitol-containing natural products. J Nat Prod 2007; 70(8): 1384-91.
[http://dx.doi.org/10.1021/np070210q] [PMID: 17661520]

[109] Ginbsberg J. Selman Waksman and antibiotics ASC national historic chemical landmarks 2005. Available at: http://www.acs.org/content/acs/en/education/whatischemistry/landmarks/selmanwaksman.html

[110] Woodruff HB, Selman A. Selman A. Waksman, winner of the 1952 Nobel Prize for physiology or medicine. Appl Environ Microbiol 2014; 80(1): 2-8.
[http://dx.doi.org/10.1128/AEM.01143-13] [PMID: 24162573]

[111] Caminero JA, Sotgiu G, Zumla A, Migliori GB. Best drug treatment for multidrug-resistant and extensively drug-resistant tuberculosis. Lancet Infect Dis 2010; 10(9): 621-9. [http://dx.doi.org/10.1016/S1473-3099(10)70139-0] [PMID: 20797644]

[112] Sandhu JS, Sehgal A, Gupta O, Singh A. Aminoglycoside nephrotoxicity revisited nephrotoxicity experimental nephroprotection treatment. J Indian Acad Clin Med 2007; 8(4): 331-3.

[113] Peck RL, Hoffhine CE, Paul KG, Folkers K. Streptomyces Antibiotics. XXIII. Isolation of neomycin A 1949; 71(7): 2590-1.

[114] Zembower TR, Noskin GA, Postelnick MJ, Nguyen C, Peterson LR. The utility of aminoglycosides in an era of emerging drug resistance. Int J Antimicrob Agents 1998; 10(2): 95-105. [http://dx.doi.org/10.1016/S0924-8579(98)00033-8] [PMID: 9716286]

[115] Waterworth PM. The in-vitro activity of tobramycin compared with that of other aminoglycosides. J Clin Pathol 1972; 25(11): 979-83. [http://dx.doi.org/10.1136/jcp.25.11.979] [PMID: 4648543]

[116] Fukami H, Ikeda S, Ahara KK, Nakajima M. Total synthesis of ribostamycin. Agric Biol Chem 1977; 41(9): 1689-94.

[117] Noone P. Sisomicin, netilmicin and dibekacin. A review of their antibacterial activity and therapeutic use. Drugs 1984; 27(6): 548-78. [http://dx.doi.org/10.2165/00003495-198427060-00003] [PMID: 6376062]

[118] Okba NM, Aboshanab KM, El-banna TS, Abd AA, Aziz E. Isolation, heterologous expression and gene duplication of certain ribostamycin biosynthetic genes from Streptomyces ribosidificus NRRL B-11466. Arch Clin Microbiol 2013; 4(5): 1-10.

[119] Willis B, Arya DP. An expanding view of aminoglycoside–nucleic acid recognition. Adv Carbohydr Chem Biochem 2006; 60: 251-302 s. [http://dx.doi.org/10.1016/S0065-2318(06)60006-1]

[120] Stead DA. Current methodologies for the analysis of aminoglycosides. J Chromatogr B Biomed Sci Appl 2000; 747(1-2): 69-93. [http://dx.doi.org/10.1016/S0378-4347(00)00133-X] [PMID: 11103900]

[121] Dionex Corporation. Analysis of the aminoglycoside antibiotics kanamycin and amikacin matches USP requirements. 2011; pp. 1-6. Application Note 267. Sunnyvale, CA

[122] Dion HW, Woo PW, Willmer NE, Kern DL, Onaga J, Fusari SA. Butirosin, a new aminoglycosidic antibiotic complex: isolation and characterization. Antimicrob Agents Chemother 1972; 2(2): 84-8. [http://dx.doi.org/10.1128/AAC.2.2.84] [PMID: 4670491]

[123] Young LS, Hindler J. Aminoglycoside resistance: a worldwide perspective. Am J Med 1986; 80(6B): 15-21. [http://dx.doi.org/10.1016/0002-9343(86)90474-2] [PMID: 3089000]

[124] Arjomandi OK, Hussein WM, Vella P, *et al.* Design, synthesis, and *in vitro* and biological evaluation of potent amino acid-derived thiol inhibitors of the metallo-β-lactamase IMP-1. Eur J Med Chem 2016; 114: 318-27. [http://dx.doi.org/10.1016/j.ejmech.2016.03.017] [PMID: 27017264]

[125] Bisht SP, Praveen B, Panda A, Mishra R, Dhillon HP. Isolation, purification and detection of antimicrobial activity of beta-lactam antibiotics from few fungal strains. Int J Pharm Sci Rev Res 2012; 12(1): 126-9.

[126] Deng H, McShan D, Zhang Y, *et al.* Mechanistic study of the synergistic antibacterial activity of combined silver nanoparticles and common antibiotics. Environ Sci Technol 2016; 50(16): 8840-8. [http://dx.doi.org/10.1021/acs.est.6b00998] [PMID: 27390928]

[127] Genç H, Kalin R, Köksal Z, *et al.* Discovery of potent carbonic anhydrase and acetylcholinesterase inhibitors: 2-aminoindan β-lactam derivatives. Int J Mol Sci 2016; 17(10): 1736.

[http://dx.doi.org/10.3390/ijms17101736] [PMID: 27775608]

[128] Turan B, Şendil K, Şengül E, *et al.* The synthesis of some β-lactams and investigation of their metal-chelating activity, carbonic anhydrase and acetylcholinesterase inhibition profiles. J Enzyme Inhib Med Chem 2016; 31(sup1) (Suppl. 1): 79-88. [http://dx.doi.org/10.3109/14756366.2016.1170014] [PMID: 27075164]

[129] González MM, Kosmopoulou M, Mojica MF, *et al.* Bisthiazolidines: A substrate-mimicking scaffold as an inhibitor of the NDM-1 carbapenemase. ACS Infect Dis 2015; 1(11): 544-54. [http://dx.doi.org/10.1021/acsinfecdis.5b00046] [PMID: 27623409]

[130] Kalita S, Kandimalla R, Sharma KK, Kataki AC, Deka M, Kotoky J. Amoxicillin functionalized gold nanoparticles reverts MRSA resistance. Mater Sci Eng C 2016; 61: 720-7. [http://dx.doi.org/10.1016/j.msec.2015.12.078] [PMID: 26838902]

[131] Koteva K, King AM, Capretta A, Wright GD. Total synthesis and activity of the metallo-β-lactamase inhibitor aspergillomarasmine A. Angew Chem Int Ed Engl 2016; 55(6): 2210-2. [http://dx.doi.org/10.1002/anie.201510057] [PMID: 26709849]

[132] Liao D, Yang S, Wang J, *et al.* Total synthesis and structural reassignment of aspergillomarasmine A. A Angew Chem Int Ed Engl 2016; 55(13): 4291-5. [http://dx.doi.org/10.1002/anie.201509960] [PMID: 26592805]

[133] Leite CA, Cavallieri AP, Baptista AS, Araujo ML. Dissociation of cephamycin C and clavulanic acid biosynthesis by 1,3-diaminopropane in Streptomyces clavuligerus. FEMS Microbiol Lett 2016; 363(1): fnv215. [http://dx.doi.org/10.1093/femsle/fnv215] [PMID: 26564965]

[134] Mikolasch A, Hildebrandt O, Schlüter R, Hammer E, Witt S, Lindequist U. Targeted synthesis of novel β-lactam antibiotics by laccase-catalyzed reaction of aromatic substrates selected by pre-testing for their antimicrobial and cytotoxic activity. Appl Microbiol Biotechnol 2016; 100(11): 4885-99. [http://dx.doi.org/10.1007/s00253-016-7288-z] [PMID: 26780358]

[135] Tufariello JJ, Lee GE, Senaratne PA, Al-Nuri M. Thienamycin. A solution of the stereochemical problem. Tetrahedron Lett 1979; 20(45): 4359-62. [http://dx.doi.org/10.1016/S0040-4039(01)86588-6]

[136] Pieczykolan M, Staszewska-Krajewska O, Furman B, Chmielewski M. 1,3-Dipolar cycloaddition of a cyclic nitrone derived from 2-deoxy-D-ribose to α,β-unsaturated lactones: An entry to carbapenem antibiotics. Carbohydr Res 2016; 433: 89-96. [http://dx.doi.org/10.1016/j.carres.2016.07.002] [PMID: 27471832]

[137] Vangala VB, Pati HN. Efficient synthesis of β -lactam containing α -hydroxy phosphonates using tartaric acid and fumaric acid as mild catalysts. Synth Commun 2016; 46(4): 374-8. [http://dx.doi.org/10.1080/00397911.2016.1139722]

[138] Seiple IB, Zhang Z, Jakubec P, *et al.* A platform for the discovery of new macrolide antibiotics. Nature 2016; 533(7603): 3-45.

[139] Domagalska J, Janas A, Pyta K, *et al.* 16-Membered macrolide lactone derivatives bearing a triazole-functionalized arm at the aglycone C13 position as antibacterial and anticancer agents. ChemMedChem 2016; 11(17): 1886-91. [http://dx.doi.org/10.1002/cmdc.201600250] [PMID: 27411730]

[140] Hirama M. Total synthesis and related studies of large, strained, and bioactive natural products. Proc Jpn Acad, Ser B, Phys Biol Sci 2016; 92(8): 290-329. [http://dx.doi.org/10.2183/pjab.92.290] [PMID: 27725470]

[141] Klich K, Pyta K, Kubicka MM, *et al.* Synthesis, antibacterial, and anticancer evaluation of novel spiramycin-like conjugates containing C(5) triazole arm. J Med Chem 2016; 59(17): 7963-73. [http://dx.doi.org/10.1021/acs.jmedchem.6b00764] [PMID: 27501415]

[142] Zhang Y, He H, Liu H, Wang H, Wang X, Xiang W. Characterization of a pathway-specific activator

of milbemycin biosynthesis and improved milbemycin production by its overexpression in Streptomyces bingchenggensis. Microb Cell Fact 2016; 15(1): 152. [http://dx.doi.org/10.1186/s12934-016-0552-1] [PMID: 27604457]

[143] Tereshchenkov AG, Shishkina AV, Karpenko VV, *et al.* New fluorescent macrolide derivatives for studying interactions of antibiotics and their analogs with the ribosomal exit tunnel. Biochemistry (Mosc) 2016; 81(10): 1163-72. [http://dx.doi.org/10.1134/S0006297916100138] [PMID: 27908240]

[144] Walmsley S, de Poire E, Rawlings B, Caffrey P. Engineered biosynthesis and characterisation of disaccharide-modified 8-deoxyamphoteronolides. Appl Microbiol Biotechnol 2016. [http://dx.doi.org/10.1007/s00253-016-7986-6] [PMID: 27858138]

[145] Ude Z, Romero-Canelón I, Twamley B, Fitzgerald Hughes D, Sadler PJ, Marmion CJ. A novel dual-functioning ruthenium(II)-arene complex of an anti-microbial ciprofloxacin derivative - Anti-proliferative and anti-microbial activity. J Inorg Biochem 2016; 160: 210-7. [http://dx.doi.org/10.1016/j.jinorgbio.2016.02.018] [PMID: 26993079]

[146] Chugunova E, Akylbekov N, Bulatova A, *et al.* Synthesis and biological evaluation of novel structural hybrids of benzofuroxan derivatives and fluoroquinolones. Eur J Med Chem 2016; 116: 165-72. [http://dx.doi.org/10.1016/j.ejmech.2016.03.086] [PMID: 27061980]

[147] Komarnicka UK, Starosta R, Kyzioł A, Płotek M, Puchalska M, Jeżowska-Bojczuk M. New copper(I) complexes bearing lomefloxacin motif: Spectroscopic properties, *in vitro* cytotoxicity and interactions with DNA and human serum albumin. J Inorg Biochem 2016; 165: 25-35. [http://dx.doi.org/10.1016/j.jinorgbio.2016.09.015] [PMID: 27764707]

[148] Komarnicka UK, Starosta R, Płotek M, de Almeida RF, Jeżowska-Bojczuk M, Kyzioł A. Copper(I) complexes with phosphine derived from sparfloxacin. Part II: a first insight into the cytotoxic action mode. Dalton Trans 2016; 45(12): 5052-63. [http://dx.doi.org/10.1039/C5DT04011F] [PMID: 26674970]

[149] Hiltensperger G, Hecht N, Kaiser M, *et al.* Quinolone amides as antitrypanosomal lead compounds with *In Vivo* activity. Antimicrob Agents Chemother 2016; 60(8): 4442-52. [http://dx.doi.org/10.1128/AAC.01757-15] [PMID: 27139467]

[150] Nabipour H, Hossaini Sadr M, Soltani B. Synthesis, identification and *in vitro* drug release of layered zinc hydroxide-gemifloxacin nanohybrids. J Incl Phenom Macrocycl Chem 2016; 85(3-4): 261-9. [http://dx.doi.org/10.1007/s10847-016-0625-0]

[151] Chopra I, Roberts M. Tetracycline antibiotics: Mode of action, applications, molecular biology, and epidemiology of bacterial resistance. Microbiol Mol Biol Rev 2001; 65(2): 232-60.

[152] Buszewski B, Rafińska K, Pomastowski P, Walczak J, Rogowska A. Novel aspects of silver nanoparticles functionalization. Colloids Surfaces A Physicochem Eng Asp 2016; 506: 170-8. [http://dx.doi.org/10.1016/j.colsurfa.2016.05.058]

[153] Railean-Plugaru V, Pomastowski P, Wypij M, *et al.* Study of silver nanoparticles synthesized by acidophilic strain of Actinobacteria isolated from the of Picea sitchensis forest soil. J Appl Microbiol 2016; 120(5): 1250-63. [http://dx.doi.org/10.1111/jam.13093] [PMID: 26864807]

[154] Devi J, Kumari S, Batra N, Kumar P, Narasimhan B, Malhotra R. Synthesis, antimicrobial activities and QSAR studies of heterocyclic Schiff base ligands with organosilicon(IV) halides. Med Chem Res 2016; 25(2): 235-46. [http://dx.doi.org/10.1007/s00044-015-1478-6]

[155] Mukherjee R, Patra M, Dutta D, Banik M, Basu T. Tetracycline-loaded calcium phosphate nanoparticle (Tet-CPNP): Rejuvenation of an obsolete antibiotic to further action. Biochim Biophys Acta 2016; 1860(9): 1929-41. [http://dx.doi.org/10.1016/j.bbagen.2016.06.006] [PMID: 27288585]

[156] Boucher HW, Talbot GH, Bradley JS, *et al.* Bad bugs, no drugs: no ESKAPE! An update from the Infectious Diseases Society of America. Clin Infect Dis 2009; 48(1): 1-12. [http://dx.doi.org/10.1086/595011] [PMID: 19035777]

[157] Chandra S, Chowdhuri AR, Mahto TK, Samui A. Sahu S kumar. One-step synthesis of amikacin modified fluorescent carbon dots for the detection of Gram-negative bacteria like Escherichia coli. RSC Advances 2016; 6(76): 72471-8. [http://dx.doi.org/10.1039/C6RA15778E]

[158] Júnior JG, Coutinho HD, Boris TC, *et al.* Chemical characterization and cytoprotective effect of the hydroethanol extract from Annona coriacea Mart. (Araticum). Pharmacognosy Res 2016; 8(4): 253-7. [http://dx.doi.org/10.4103/0974-8490.188882] [PMID: 27695264]

[159] Kato T, Yang G, Teo Y, *et al.* Synthesis and antiribosomal activities of 4′-O-, 6′-O-, 4″-O-, 4′,6′-O- and 4″,6″-O-derivatives in the kanamycin series indicate differing target selectivity patterns between the 4,5- and 4,6-Series of disubstituted 2-deoxystreptamine aminoglycoside antibiotics. ACS Infect Dis 2015; 1(10): 479-86. [http://dx.doi.org/10.1021/acsinfecdis.5b00069] [PMID: 27623314]

[160] Magri V, Montanari E, Marras E, Perletti G. Aminoglycoside antibiotics for NIH category II chronic bacterial prostatitis: A single-cohort study with one-year follow-up. Exp Ther Med 2016; 12(4): 2585-93. [PMID: 27698761]

[161] Ni X, Zong T, Zhang H, *et al.* Biosynthesis of 3″-demethyl-gentamicin C components by genN disruption strain of Micromonospora echinospora and test their antimicrobial activities *in vitro.* Microbiol Res 2016; 185: 36-44. [http://dx.doi.org/10.1016/j.micres.2016.01.005] [PMID: 26946376]

[162] Sganappa A, Bellucci MC, Nizet V, Tor Y, Volonterio A. Multicomponent domino synthesis and antibacterial activity of neomycin-sugar conjugates. Synthesis (Germany) 2016; 48: 4443-50. [http://dx.doi.org/10.1055/s-0035-1562727]

[163] Woiwode U, Sievers-Engler A, Lämmerhofer M. Preparation of fluorescent labeled gentamicin as biological tracer and its characterization by liquid chromatography and high resolution mass spectrometry. J Pharm Biomed Anal 2016; 121: 307-15. [http://dx.doi.org/10.1016/j.jpba.2015.12.053] [PMID: 26775580]

[164] Zimmermann L, Das I, Désiré J, *et al.* New broad-spectrum antibacterial amphiphilic aminoglycosides active against resistant bacteria: From neamine derivatives to smaller neosamine analogues. J Med Chem 2016; 59(20): 9350-69. [http://dx.doi.org/10.1021/acs.jmedchem.6b00818] [PMID: 27690420]

[165] Al-Khodir FAI, Refat MS. Synthesis, spectroscopic, and antimicrobial study of Ca(II), Fe(III), Pd(II), and Au(III) complexes of amoxicillin antibiotic drug. Russ J Gen Chem 2016; 86(3): 7-17.

[166] Reda FM, Shafi SA, Ismail M. Efficient inhibition of some multi-drug resistant pathogenic bacteria by bioactive metabolites from Bacillus amyloliquefaciens S5I4 isolated from archaeological soil in Egypt. Appl Biochem Microbiol 2016; 52(6): 593-601. [http://dx.doi.org/10.1134/S0003683816060144]

[167] Mizuhara N, Kuroda M, Ogita A, Tanaka T, Usuki Y, Fujita K. Antifungal thiopeptide cyclothiazomycin B1 exhibits growth inhibition accompanying morphological changes via binding to fungal cell wall chitin. Bioorg Med Chem 2011; 19(18): 5300-10. [http://dx.doi.org/10.1016/j.bmc.2011.08.010] [PMID: 21885289]

[168] Valle DL Jr, Cabrera EC, Puzon JJ, Rivera WL. Antimicrobial activities of methanol, ethanol and supercritical CO2 extracts of philippine Piper betle L. on clinical isolates of Gram positive and Gram negative bacteria with transferable multiple drug resistance. PLoS One 2016; 11(1): e0146349. [http://dx.doi.org/10.1371/journal.pone.0146349] [PMID: 26741962]

[169] Téllez MA, Téllez AN, Vélez F, Ulloa JC. *In vitro* antiviral activity against rotavirus and astrovirus infection exerted by substances obtained from Achyrocline bogotensis (Kunth) DC. (Compositae). BMC Complement Altern Med 2015; 15(1): 428.
[http://dx.doi.org/10.1186/s12906-015-0949-0] [PMID: 26630872]

[170] Zhang W, Liu J, Macho JM, *et al.* *In vitro* antiviral activity against rotavirus and astrovirus infection exerted by substances obtained from Achyrocline bogotensis (Kunth) DC. (Compositae). C. 126. Eur J Med Chem 2017; 27: 7-14.
[http://dx.doi.org/10.1016/j.ejmech.2016.10.010] [PMID: 27744188]

[171] Sweidan A, Chollet-Krugler M, van de Weghe P, *et al.* Design, synthesis and biological evaluation of potential antibacterial butyrolactones. Bioorg Med Chem 2016; 24(22): 5823-33.
[http://dx.doi.org/10.1016/j.bmc.2016.09.040] [PMID: 27687969]

[172] Kumar S, Sharma N, Maurya IK, *et al.* Facile synthesis, structural evaluation, antimicrobial activity and synergistic effects of novel imidazo[1,2-a]pyridine based organoselenium compounds. Eur J Med Chem 2016; 123: 916-24.
[http://dx.doi.org/10.1016/j.ejmech.2016.07.076] [PMID: 27565415]

[173] Alvarez-Elcoro S, Enzler MJ. The macrolides: erythromycin, clarithromycin, and azithromycin. Mayo Clin Proc 1999; 74(6): 613-34.
[http://dx.doi.org/10.4065/74.6.613] [PMID: 10377939]

[174] Gandhi PT, Athmaram TN, Arunkumar GR. Novel nicotine analogues with potential anti-mycobacterial activity. Bioorg Med Chem 2016; 24(8): 1637-47.
[http://dx.doi.org/10.1016/j.bmc.2016.02.035] [PMID: 26951892]

[175] Nishimura K, Nishimura S, Nishi N, Saiki I, Tokura S, Azuma I. Immunological activity of chitin and its derivatives. Vaccine 1984; 2(1): 93-9.
[http://dx.doi.org/10.1016/S0264-410X(98)90039-1] [PMID: 6397928]

[176] Kraljević TG, Harej A, Sedić M, *et al.* Synthesis, *in vitro* anticancer and antibacterial activities and in silico studies of new 4-substituted 1,2,3-triazole-coumarin hybrids. Eur J Med Chem 2016; 124: 794-808.
[http://dx.doi.org/10.1016/j.ejmech.2016.08.062] [PMID: 27639370]

[177] Ahn M, Gunasekaran P, Rajasekaran G, *et al.* Pyrazole derived ultra-short antimicrobial peptidomimetics with potent anti-biofilm activity. Eur J Med Chem 2017; 125: 551-64.
[http://dx.doi.org/10.1016/j.ejmech.2016.09.071] [PMID: 27718471]

[178] Chowdhury NR, MacGregor-Ramiasa M, Zilm P, Majewski P, Vasilev K. 'Chocolate' silver nanoparticles: Synthesis, antibacterial activity and cytotoxicity. J Colloid Interface Sci 2016; 482: 151-8.
[http://dx.doi.org/10.1016/j.jcis.2016.08.003] [PMID: 27501038]

[179] Panda SS, Ibrahim MA, Küçükbay H, *et al.* Synthesis and antimalarial bioassay of quinine - peptide conjugates. Chem Biol Drug Des 2013; 82(4): 361-6.
[http://dx.doi.org/10.1111/cbdd.12134] [PMID: 23497252]

[180] Ibrahim MA, Panda SS, Oliferenko AA, *et al.* Macrocyclic peptidomimetics with antimicrobial activity: synthesis, bioassay, and molecular modeling studies. Org Biomol Chem 2015; 13(36): 9492-503.
[http://dx.doi.org/10.1039/C5OB01400J] [PMID: 26256838]

[181] Chuang H, Huang L-C, Kapoor M, *et al.* Design and synthesis of pyridine-pyrazole-sulfonate derivatives as potential anti-HBV agents. MedChemComm 2016; 7(5): 832-6.
[http://dx.doi.org/10.1039/C6MD00008H]

[182] Apohan E, Yilmaz U, Yilmaz O, Serindag A, Küçükbay H. Synthesis, cytotoxic and antimicrobial activities of novel cobalt and zinc complexes of benzimidazole derivatives. J Organomet Chem 2017; 828: 52-8.

[http://dx.doi.org/10.1016/j.jorganchem.2016.11.020]

[183] Tung M, Cong NX, Huy T, *et al.* Synthesis, characterizations of superparamagnetic Fe_3O_4-Ag hybrid nanoparticles and their application for highly effective bacteria inactivation. J Nanosci Nanotechnol 2016; 16(6): 5902-12.
[http://dx.doi.org/10.1166/jnn.2016.11029] [PMID: 27427651]

[184] Thanna S, Knudson SE, Grzegorzewicz A, *et al.* Synthesis and evaluation of new 2-aminothiophenes against Mycobacterium tuberculosis. Org Biomol Chem 2016; 14(25): 6119-33.
[http://dx.doi.org/10.1039/C6OB00821F] [PMID: 27251120]

[185] Suresh Y, Annapurna S, Singh AK, Chetana A, Pasha C, Bhikshamaiah G. Characterization and evaluation of anti-biofilm effect of green synthesized copper nanoparticles. Materials Today: Proceedings 2016; 3(6): 1678-85.
[http://dx.doi.org/10.1016/j.matpr.2016.04.059]

[186] El-Sharkawy ER, Mahmoud K. Cytotoxity of two new coumarin derivatives isolated from Launaea mucronata. Nat Prod Res 2016; 30(4): 394-8.
[http://dx.doi.org/10.1080/14786419.2015.1017492] [PMID: 25751124]

CHAPTER 4

Antitubercular Agents and Tubercular Vaccines in Clinical Trials

Mohammed Jawed Ahsan*

Department of Pharmaceutical Chemistry, Maharishi Arvind College of Pharmacy, Ambabari Circle, Jaipur, Rajasthan 302 039, India

Abstract: In 2015, an estimated 10.4 million people were infected with and 1.8 million people were killed by tuberculosis (TB). Multi-drug resistant (MDR) and extensively drug resistant (XRD) TB were other reported complications in the treatment of TB. Almost 3.3% of new TB cases and 20% of previously treated cases have multi-drug resistance (MDR) TB while 9.7% of people with MDR-TB have XDR-TB. Recently, two chemical entities, namely bedaquiline and delamanid were granted conditional approval for the treatment of MDR-TB, and are recommended only to those patients for whom other treatments fail to cure. The diagnostic platform, including GeneXpert Omni® and Xpert Ultra® is in development. There are seven new compounds and eight approved or repurposed antitubercular drugs in advanced phases of clinical trials, while thirteen vaccine candidates are in clinical trials. New diagnostics, anti-tubercular drugs and tubercular vaccines will be needed to achieve the targets set in the End TB strategy. This chapter explores the medicinal chemistry of anti-tubercular agents in various phases of clinical trials. The present chapter also deals with various diagnostic technologies for early detection of tuberculosis, as well as the tubercular vaccines in various phases of clinical trials.

Keywords: Anti-tubercular agents, Delamanid, Diagnostics, TMC207, Tubercular, Tuberculosis vaccines.

INTRODUCTION

Tuberculosis, (TB) a dreadful disease, mainly caused by *Mycobacterium tuberculosis*, (MTB), is one of the major health problems worldwide. It primarily affects the lungs (pulmonary TB) and can also affect other sites as well (extra pulmonary TB). In 2015, there were an estimated 10.4 million new cases of TB and 1.8 million people died from TB, including almost 1.4 million deaths among HIV-negative individuals and 0.4 million among HIV-positive individuals.

* **Corresponding author Mohammed Jawed Ahsan:** Department of Pharmaceutical Chemistry, Maharishi Arvind College of Pharmacy, Ambabari Circle, Jaipur, Rajasthan 302 039, India; Tel: +91 9694087786; Fax: +91 141 2335120; Email: jawedpharma@gmail.com

Atta-ur-Rahman & M. Iqbal Choudhary (Eds.)

Globally, there were an estimated 580,000 people who have developed the multidrug resistant tuberculosis (MDR-TB) in 2015. An estimated 49 million lives have been saved through TB diagnostic and treatment between 2000 and 2015 [1]. Nearly 10 percent of infected people usually develop active TB in their lifetime [2]. A research led by the scientists at Stanford University revealed that the MTB can persist in the hostile intracellular microenvironment, evading immune cells and drug treatment. They isolated MTB from bone marrow, derived CD271+/CD45-mesenchymal stem cells [3]. Tubercular bacteria are spread through the air by active TB patients and most commonly affect the lungs. The directly observed treatment short-course (DOTS), and a multidrug therapy program developed by WHO, is one of the most efficient artilleries against the global plague with success rate of 85% among all new TB cases and 87% among new cases of sputum smear-positive pulmonary TB in 2010. Unfortunately, the first-line treatments can fail due to poor compliance and lead to the emergence of multi-drug resistant (MDR) strains of TB. The drug resistant TB is classified into two categories, such as multi drug resistant tuberculosis (MDR-TB) that is resistant to isoniazid and rifampicin, and extensively drug resistant tuberculosis (XDR-TB) that is resistant to isoniazid and rifampicin, plus the fluoroquinolones and any one of the three injectable second line drugs (kanamycin, capreomycin, or amikacin). In 2016, US$ 6.6 billion were available for TB care and prevention in low and medium-income countries [1].

Today we have comparatively sufficient number of antitubercular agents in preclinical, as well as, clinical stages of development. In this chapter, we emphasize the chemical entities currently in the clinical trials, the new tubercular vaccines in the developmental pipeline, and the new diagnostic tests either endorsed by WHO, or commercialized. After four decades since the discovery of rifampicin, two new chemical entities bedaquiline (Sirturo) and delamanid (Deltyba) were granted approval for the treatment of MDR-TB. However, both of the drugs induce arrhythmia, and are recommended only in patients for whom other treatments fail [4 - 7].

CURRENT THERAPY

Antitubercular agents are drugs used in the treatment of TB. WHO has recommended Directly Observed Treatment Short-course (DOTS) for the treatment of TB. DOTS, for the treatment of TB is nothing, but a combination of antitubercular drugs including isoniazid (INH), rifampin RIF, ethambutol (EB) and pyrazinamide (PZA) for a 6 months therapy. WHO has also recommended the use of second-line drugs, which include aminoglycosides (kanamycin, amikacin), capreomycin, cycloserin, *p*-aminosalicylic acid, thioamides (ethionamide (ETH), prothionamide), and fluoroquinolones (ciprofloxacin, ofloxacin, levofloxacin, *etc.*) for the treatment of MDR-TB. Bedaquiline (Sirturo) and delamanid (Deltyba) were also included in the treatment of MDR-TB. Both of the drugs induce arrhythmia and are recommended only when other treatments fail to cure the patients.

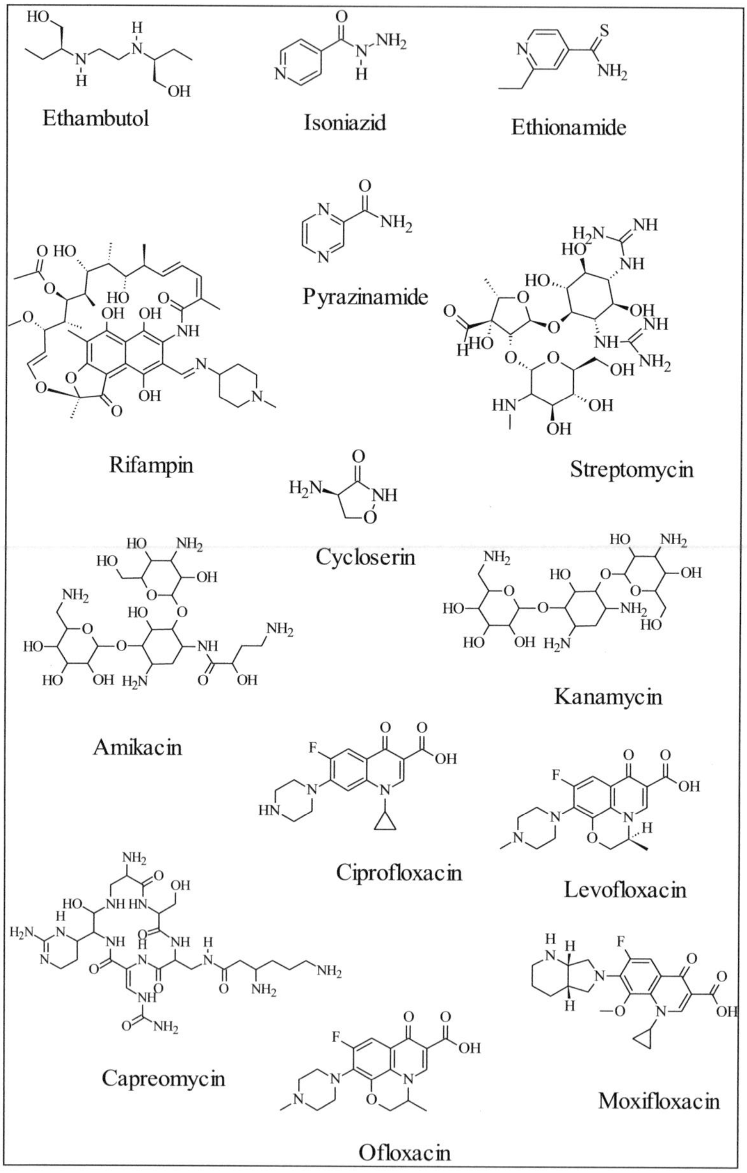

Fig. (1). Some of the anti-tubercular drugs in current therapy.

Some of the antitubercular drugs in current therapy are shown in Fig. (**1**). Rifampicin (RIF) is the drug of choice in the tubercular disease. RIF has been further modified as rifalazil, rifabutin and rifapentine to increase their half-lives, as well as *in vitro* potency, and hence recommended once or twice weekly, instead of daily RIF dosing [4]. The chemical analogues of RIF are shown in Fig. (**2**).

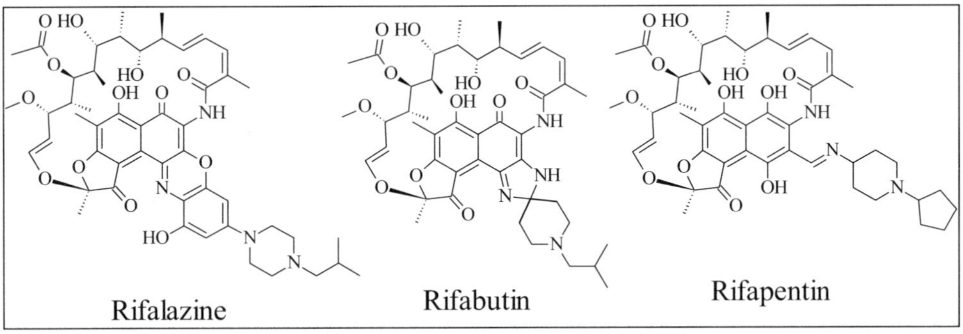

Fig. (2). Chemical structures of RIF analogues (rifalazine, rifabutin and rifapentin).

Classification of Antitubercular Drugs

Antitubercular agents are drugs used in the treatment of TB are classified as follows [8 - 12]:

First line drugs (high efficacy and low toxicity)

1. Ethambutol (EB)
2. Isoniazid (INH)
3. Pyrazinamide (PZA)
4. Rifampin (RIF)
5. Streptomycin
6. Ethionamide (ETH)

Second line drugs (low efficacy and high toxicity or both)

1. Aminoglycosides
   Amikacin (AMK), Kanamycin (KM)
2. Polypeptides
   Capreomycin, Viomycin, Enviomycin
3. Quinolones
   Ciprofloxacin (CIP), Levofloxacin, Moxifloxacin (MXF)
4. Thioamides
   Ethionamide (ETH), Prothionamide

5. Cycloserine
6. Para amino salicylic acid

Third line drugs (Other drugs that may be useful, but are not on the WHO list of SLDs)

1. Rifabutin
2. Clarithromycin
3. Linezolid
4. Thiacetazone
5. Thioridazine
6. Arginine
7. Vitamin D
8. R207910

WHO Grouping of Anti-Tubercular Drugs

According to the WHO guidelines, the programmatic management of drug resistant T, the anti-tubercular drugs are placed in five different groups. This grouping is given in Table **1**.

Table 1. WHO grouping of anti-tubercular drugs

Group	Description	Drugs
Group A	First-line oral agents	Ethambutol, Isoniazid, Pyrazinamide, Rifampicin, Rifabutin, Rifapentine
Group B	Injectable drugs	Amikacin, Capreomycin, Kanamycin, Streptomycin
Group C	Fluoroquinolones	Gatifloxacin, Levofloxacin, Moxifloxacin,
Group D	Oral bacteriostatic second-line drugs	Ethionamide, Cycloserine, Prothionamide, *p*-aminosalicylic acid, Terizidone
Group E	Drugs with limited data on efficacy and long-term safety	Amoxicillin/clavulanate, Bedaquiline, Clarithromycin, Clofazimine, Delamanid, Imipenem/cilastatin, Linezolid, Thioacetazone

Ethambutol

Ethambutol is an alkylenediamine discovered in 1961. It possesses bacteriostatic action on MTB and inhibits the mycobacterial cell wall synthesis, and acts by inhibiting the polymerization of arabinogalactane and lipoarabinomannan [13, 14]. Ocular toxicity is the most common side effect of ethambutol [15, 16]. It is prepared from 2-amino-1-butanol and dichloroethane. 2-Amino-1-butanol is synthesized by the catalytic reduction of 2-nitro-1-butanol [17].

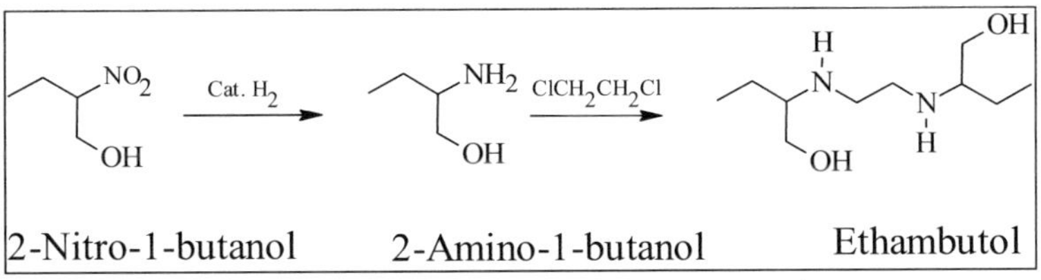

Isoniazid

Isoniazid, also known as isonicotinylhydrazide, was discovered in 1952. It exhibits a bactericidal action on MTB, and acts by inhibiting mycolic acid synthesis, one of the essential components of the mycobacterial cell wall [18 - 20]. It is synthesized from isonicotinic acid, which in turn is obtained by the oxidation of γ-picoline. Esterification of the resulting acid with ethanol in the presence of acid gives ethyl ester of isonicotinic acid, which on treatment with hydrazine, gives isoniazid [17]. Hepatotoxicity, peripheral neuropathy, and CNS toxicity are the most common adverse effects associated with isoniazid [15, 16].

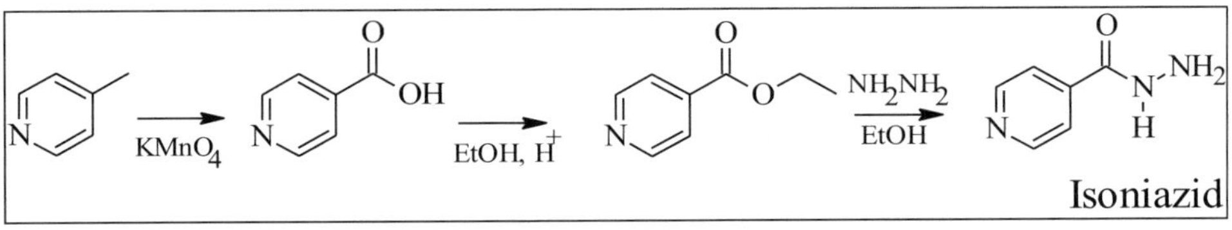

Pyrazinamide

Pyrazinamide or pyrazincarboxamide, a nicotinamide discovered in 1952. It possesses bactericidal action on intracellular mycobacteria. It acts by releasing pyrazinoic acid, which causes not only the pH imbalance of mycobacteria but also inhibits the ribosomal protein S1, by interfering trans-translation [21 - 24]. It is synthesized by catalytic oxidation (with sodium permanganate) of quinoxaline to pyrazin-2,3-dicarboxylic acid followed by decarboxylation to give pyrazin--carboxylic acid. This acid is esterified with methanol, in an acidic medium, and the ester further reacts with ammonia to give pyrazinamide. The quinoxaline is obtained from the reaction of *o*-phenylendiamine and glyoxal [17]. Hepatotoxicity and gout are the most common side effects of pyrazinamide [15, 16].

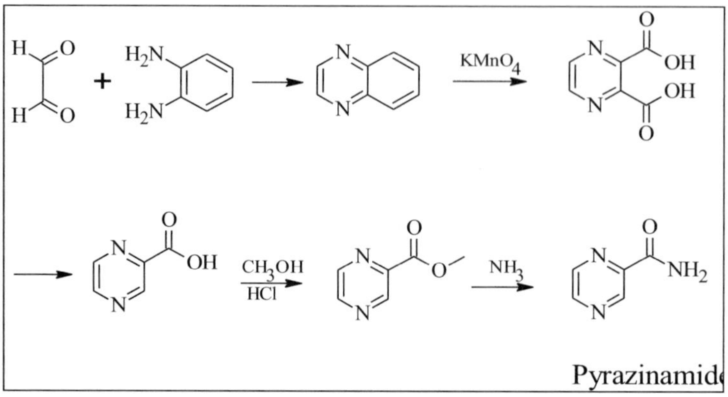

Rifamycins

The rifamycin complex is the mixture of five antibiotics (rifamicins A, B, C, D, and E) discovered in 1959 as metabolites of the microorganism *Streptomyces mediteranei (Nocardia mediteranei)*. Rifampicin is a semi-synthetic derivative of rifamycin B. It exhibits a bactericidal effect by inhibiting the mycobacterial RNA synthesis by binding to the β-subunit of the DNA-dependent polymerase [25]. Several hundred rifamycin derivatives were prepared and evaluated, and finally the most promising derivatives, rifampicin was introduced in 1968, rifapentine was introduced in 1978, rifabutin was introduced in 1983, and rifalazil was introduced in 1993 [15]. These derivatives are shown in Fig. (**2**). Clinical studies have suggested that a dose of 35 mg/kg of rifampicin was found to be safe [26]. Further rifapentine regimen was found to be safer, but not significantly more promising than rifampicin regime in patients, receiving either rifapentine or rifampicin (10 mg/kg/dose) along with isoniazid, ethambutol and pyrazinamide [27]. Cutaneous reactions and gastrointestinal disturbances are the common adverse effects of rifamycin [15].

Streptomycin

Streptomycin is an aminoglycoside antibiotics discovered in 1944 as a fermentation product of *Streptomyces griseus* [15]. Streptomycin is an *N*-methyl-L-glucosaminidostreptosidostreptidine composed of three components (streptidine, streptose, and *N*-methyl-L-glucosamine). It has both bacteriostatic and bactericidal activities and interferes with the biosynthesis of protein through interaction with the 30S subunit of the ribosome [28 - 30]. The most common side effects of streptomycin are nephrotoxicity, ototoxicity and electrolyte derangement [15, 16].

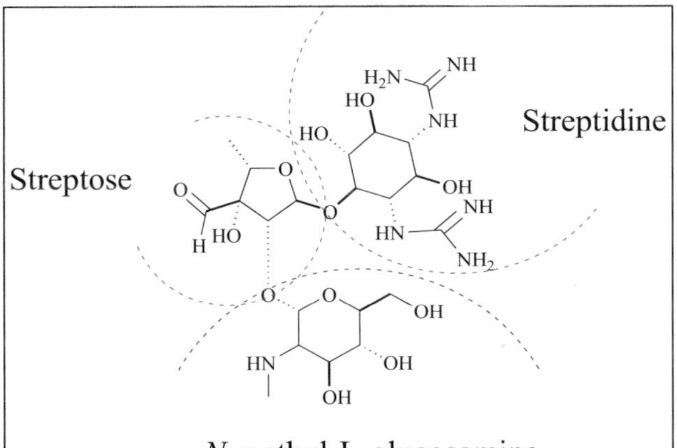

Streptomycin

Ethionamide

Ethionamide or 2-ethylpyridine-2-carbothioamide was discovered in 1956. It acts by inhibiting mycolic acid biosynthesis through *InhA* [20, 31]. It is synthesized by reacting 4-cyano-2-ethylpyridine with hydrogen sulphide under appropriate condition [32]. The most common side effects of ethionamide includes hypothyroidism, nausea and vomiting [15, 16].

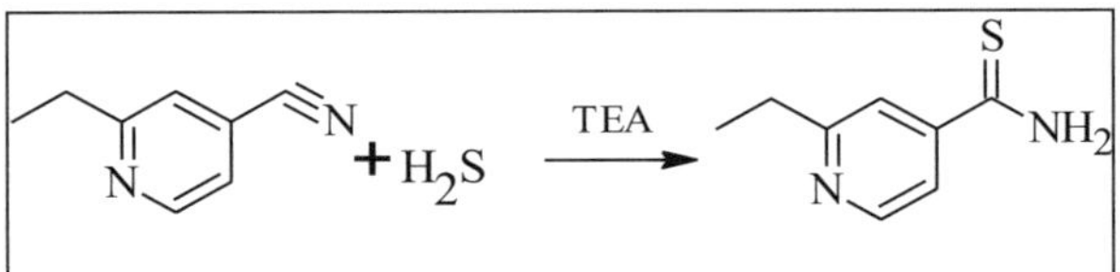

Ethionamide

Kanamycin

Kanamycin is an aminoglycoside, and was isolated as a fermentation product of *Stereptomyces kanamyceticus* in 1957. It is composed of deoxystreptamine, and two amino sugars kanosamine and 6-glucosamine. Its activity against MTB is comparatively weaker than the streptomycin and hence used in combination with other antitubercular drugs [15]. It has both bacteriostatic and bactericidal actions and interferes with the biosynthesis of protein through interaction with the 30S subunit of the ribosome [33]. Ototoxicity and nephrotoxicity are the most common adverse effects of kanamycin [15, 16].

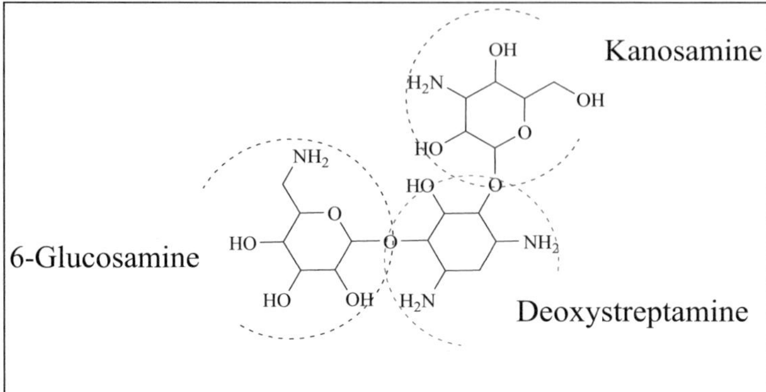

Kanamycin

Amikacin

Amikacin is a semi-synthetic analogue of kanamycin prepared by the amidation of the C-1 amino group with 2-hydroxy-4-aminobutyric acid. It is not activated by many of the R-factor mediated enzymes that attack kanamycin. It is used in the treatment of resistant MTB as well as non-tuberculous mycobacterial (NTM) infections. It acts by interfering with the biosynthesis of protein through interaction with the 30S subunit of the ribosome [33]. Ototoxicity and nephrotoxicity are the most common adverse effects of amikacin [15, 16].

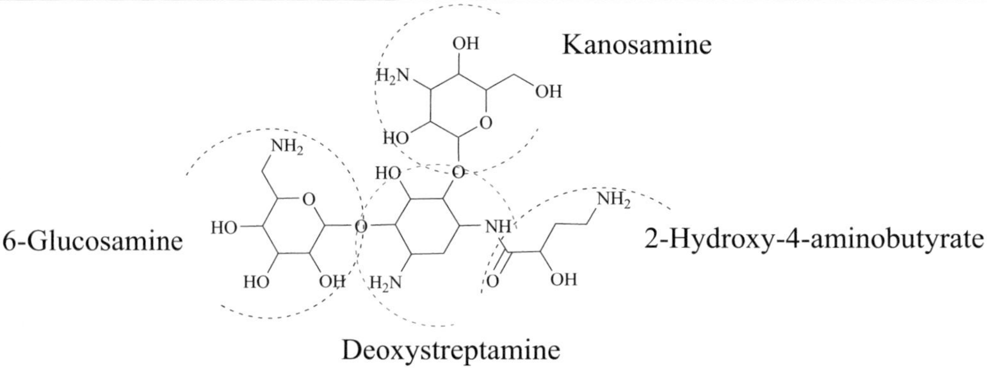

Amikacin

Viomycin

Viomycin is a polypeptide complex isolated by two individual groups of investigators from actinomyces, namely *Strptomyces puniceus* and *S. floridae* respectively in 1951. It has comparatively higher activity against mycobacteria than against other bacteria. It inhibits the protein synthesis and targets the small subunit, 30S of the ribosome [34]. Some of the severe and frequent side effects, include nephrotoxicity, ototoxicity, and electrolyte imbalance [15, 16].

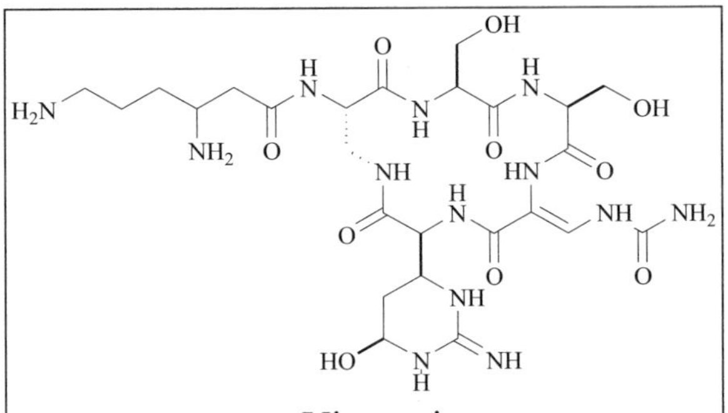

Viomycin

Capreomycin

Capreomycin is a polypeptide complex isolated from *Strptomyces capreolus* in 1960. It is active against MTB and *M. Kanassi*. It inhibits the protein synthesis by targeting the small subunit, 30S of the ribosome [35]. Nephrotoxicity is the most common side effect of capreomycin [15, 16].

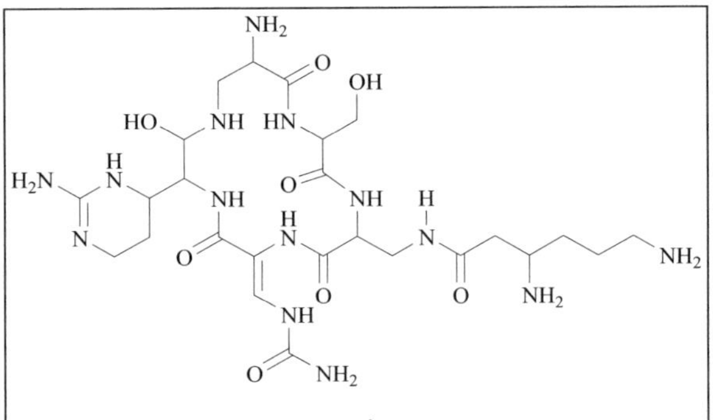

Capreomycin

Enviomycin

Enviomycin is a polypeptide antibiotics isolated from *S. griseoverticillatus* [36, 37]. It is used in the treatment of TB. Vestibular dysfunction is the main side effect of enviomycin [38].

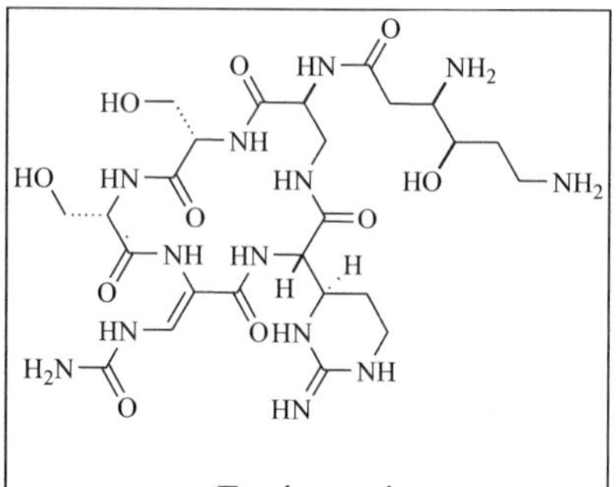

Enviomycin

Ciprofloxacin

Ciprofloxacin is a fluoroquinolone discovered in 1960. It has a bactericidal action targeting the DNA gyrase, which is the sole type II topoisomerase in the mycobacterium [39 - 41]. It is synthesized from 3-chloro-4-fluoroaniline and ethyl ethoxymethylenmalonate to an intermediate product, which upon heating gets converted to biphenyl esters, and further treatment with cyclopropyl bromide in triethyl amine followed by alkali hydrolysis afford the synthesis of 1-cyclopropy- -6-fluoro-7-chloro-1,4-dihydro-3-quinolin-4-on-carboxylic acid, which reacts with piperazine to produce ciprofloxacin [17]. Gastrointestinal reactions, central nervous disturbances, and hypersensitivity (mainly photosensitivity) are the most common side effects [15, 16].

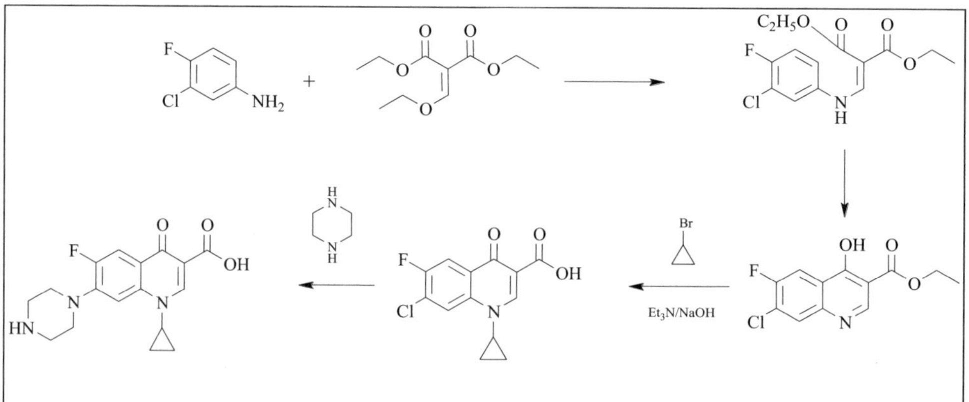

Ciprofloxacin

Levofloxacin

Levofloxacin is a fluoroquinolone discovered in 1992. It has a bactericidal action targeting the DNA gyrase, which is the sole type II topoisomerase in this mycobacterium [39 - 41]. It is synthesized from 2,3,4,5-tetrafluorobenzoic acid to an acid chloride, and further to diethyl-2,3,4,5-tetrafluoro benzoyl malonate. Decarboxylation and partial hydrolysis of the diethyl-2,3,4,5-tetrafluoro benzoyl malonate leads to ethyl-2,3,4,5-tetrafluorobenzoyl acetate. Ethyl-2,3,4,5-tetrafluorobenzoyl acetate is further converted to ethyl-2-(2,3,4,5-tetrafluorobenzol)-3-ethoxy acrylate. Condensing the ethyl-2-(2,3,4,5-tetrafluoro benzoyl)---ethoxy acrylate with (S)-2-aminopropanol and methylene chloride, gives ethyl---(2,3,4,5-tetrafluorobenzoyl)-3-[(l-hydroxyprop-2(S)-yl) amino]acrylate and further cyclises to give (S)-ethyl-9,10-difluoro-2,3-dihydro-3-methyl-7-oxo-7H-pyrido-[l,2,3-cfe]-l,4-benzoxazine-6-carboxylate, which is hydrolysed to (S)-ethyl-9,10-difluoro-2,3-dihydro-3-methyl-7-oxo-7H-pyrido-[l,2,3-cfe]-l,4-benzoxazine-6-carboxylic acid. Further treatment with methyl piperazine results in the synthesis of levofloxacin [42]. The main side effect includes QTc prolongation [16].

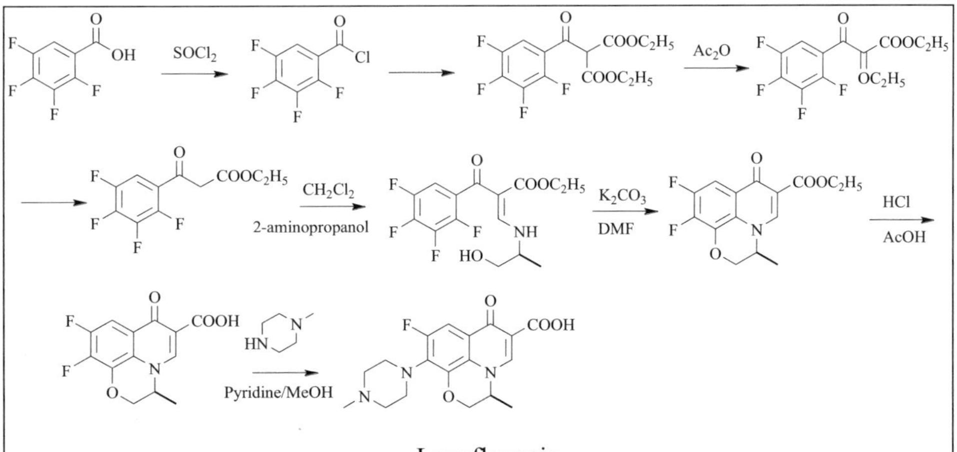

Levofloxacin

Moxifloxacin (MXF)

Moxifloxacin is a fluoroquinolone discovered in 1996. It has a bactericidal action and acts by targeting the DNA gyrase, which is the sole type II topoisomerase in the mycobacterium [39 - 41]. The quinolone ring (ethyl 1-cyclopropyl-6-7-difluoro-8-methoxy-4-oxo-1,4-dihydroquinoline-3-carboxylate) is obtained from 2,4,5-trifluoro-3-methoxybenzoyl chloride in a 4 step procedure. The substitution with appropriate secondary amine followed by the hydrolysis of the ethyl ester leads to the synthesis of moxifloxacin [43, 44]. The main side effect includes QTc prolongation [16].

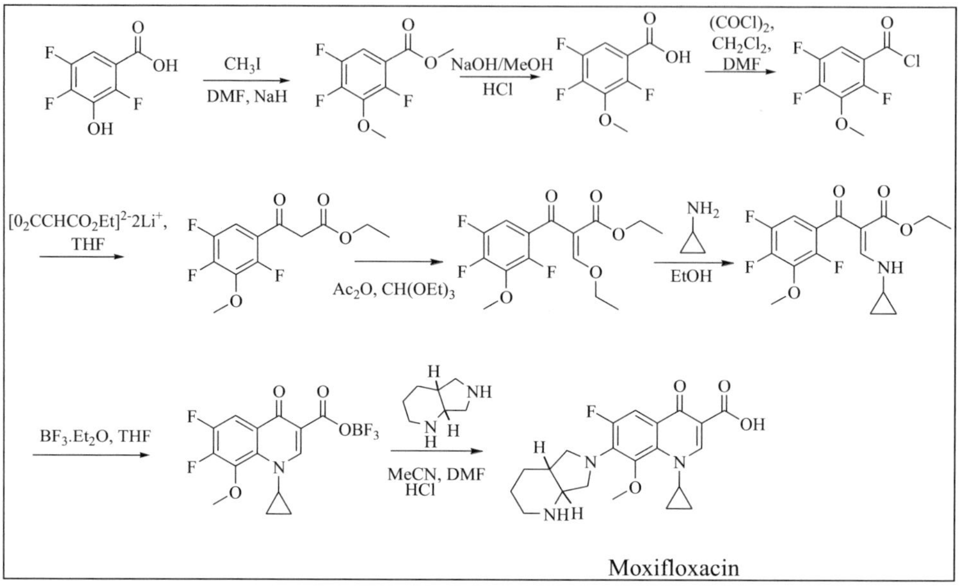

Cycloserine

D-Cycloserine was isolated in 1955 by several groups independently from the cultures of *Streptomyces garyphalus*, *S. orchidaceus*, and *S. lavenduale* respectively. D-Cycloserine is chemically 4-amino-3-isoxalidinone and can be obtained both biosynthetically from the actinomycetes as well as synthetically from the ethyl ester of D-serine. Ethyl ester of D-serine reacts with phosphorous pentachloride, to give an intermediate product which reacts with hydroxylamine to give the desired cycloserine by heterocyclization [17]. It causes severe side effects in the CNS including psychosis, confusion and depression [15, 16].

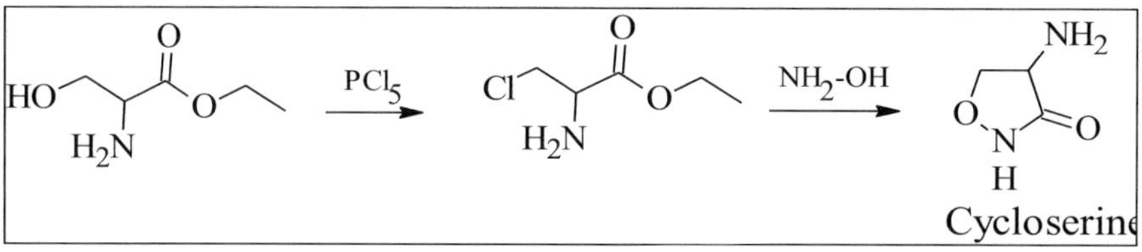

p-Amino-salicylic Acid

p-Aminosalicylic acid, 5-amino-2-hydoxybenzoic acid is an aminosalicylate discovered in 1946. It possesses a bacteriostatic action and the exact mechanism of action is still under investigation [45, 46]. It is synthesized by heating *m*-

aminophenol, potassium bicarbonate, and carbon dioxide at 5-10 atm pressure using Kolbe's reaction [17]. The most common side effects of *p*-aminosalicylic acid are gastrointestinal irritation and hypersensitivity reactions [15, 16].

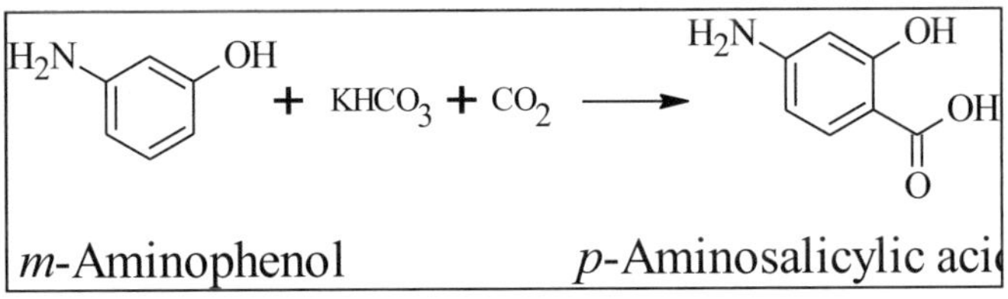

Thiacetazone

Thiacetazone, *p*-acetylaminobenzaldehyde is a thiosemicarbazone analogue discovered in 1940. It has a bacteriostatic action that targets the mycolic acid in mycobacteria by inhibiting cyclopropanation [47]. It is synthesized by heating *p*-acetylaminobenzaldehyde and thiosemicarbazide in an ethanolic solution [17]. The most common side effects of thiacetazone are gastrointestinal disorders, liver damage and anaemia. It also causes severe skin reactions in patients with HIV infection [15, 16].

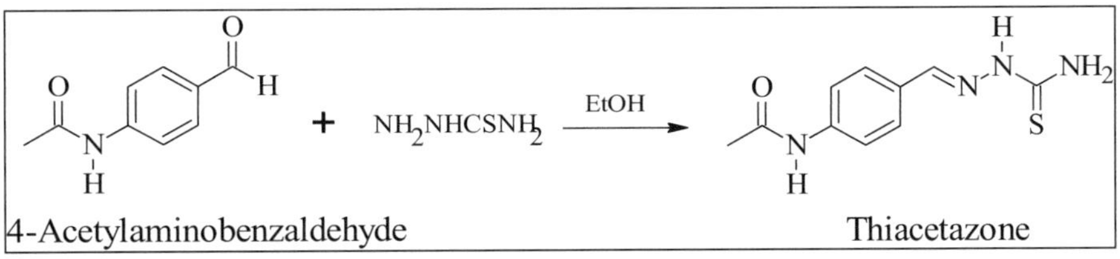

ANTITUBERCULAR DRUGS IN CLINICAL TRIALS

Currently, there are fifteen anti-TB drugs in advanced phases of clinical development for the treatment of drug-susceptible TB, multi drug resistant tuberculosis (MDR-TB), or latent tuberculosis infection (LTBI). Seven are new compounds (bedaquiline, delamanid, sutezolid, pretomanid, SQ109, PBTZ169, and Q203), while eight compounds (moxifloxacin, levofloxacin, linezolid, nitazoxanide, clofazimine, mepopenem/clavulanate, rifampicin and rifapentine) are approved or repurposed, and are undergoing further testing. The development of AZD5847 and TBA-354 was discontinued due to lack of demonstrated antitubercular activity and signs of toxicity respectively. There are seven compounds in preclinical developmental stage. Of these four compounds (TBI-166, CPZEN-45, SQ609 and 1599) are in early stage developments, while three compounds (BTZ-043, TBA-7371 and GSK-070) are in good laboratory practice toxicity stage [1, 48, 49]. The global tuberculosis drugs' pipeline is shown in Figs. (**3-4**).

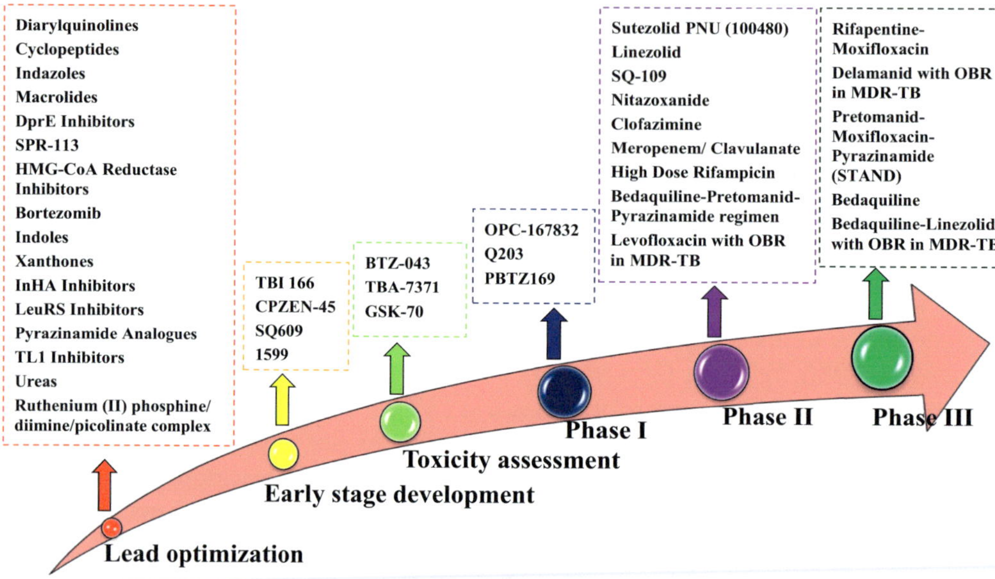

Fig. (3). The global tuberculosis drugs' pipeline. The pipeline is mainly based on data compiled by the New Drugs Working Group of the Stop TB Partnership and WHO Global tuberculosis report 2016 [1, 48, 49].

Discovery: Lead Optimization

There are several new classes and novel targets discovered for the treatment of TB. Currently, there are nearly seventeen compounds/ targets are under investigation [48]. HMG-CoA reductase inhibitor is the repurposed class of drug. Simvastatin (HMG-CoA reductase inhibitor) significantly increased the tuberculocidal activity of the standard oral regimen of isoniazid, rifampicin and pyrazinamide. Some of the new classes and targets are given in Table **2**.

Preclinical Development

Early Stage Development

There are four different classes of compounds in the early stage development, including riminophenazines antibiotics (TBI-166), nucleoside antibiotics (CPZEN-45), dipiperidines (SQ609) and spectinomycin analogs (1599). Their mechanisms of action and developers are given in Table **3**.

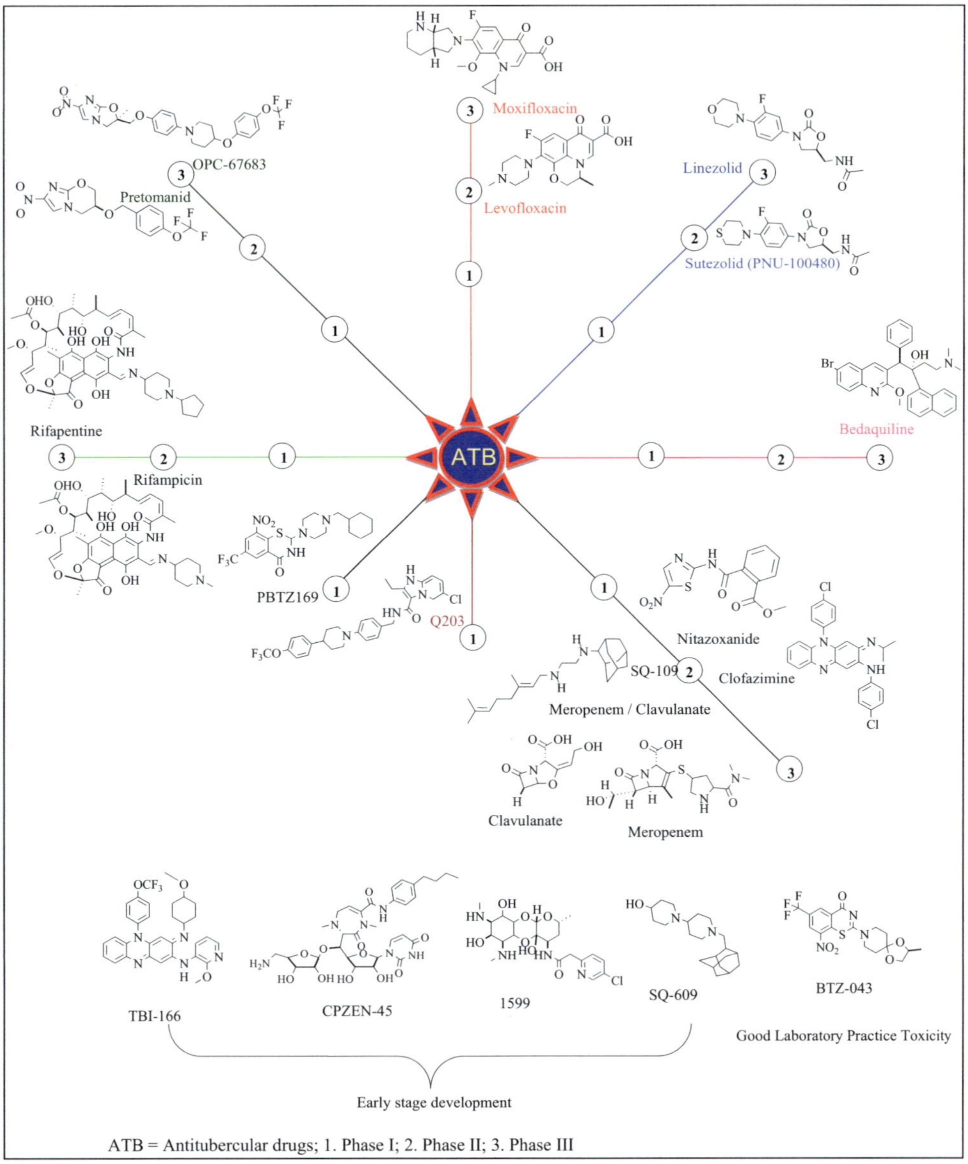

Fig. (4). The global portfolio of current tuberculosis drugs' pipeline in preclinical and clinical development.

Table 2. Some of the new class compounds and novel targets.

S. No.	Compound/ Target	Sponsor/ Developer	Description
1	Indazoles	GlaxoSmithKline Global Alliance for TB Drug Development	Identified to have an excellent *in vitro* and *in vivo* activity [48].
2	Macrolides	Sanofi Global Alliance for TB Drug Development	Identified to have an excellent activity against MTB. Its analogues are being synthesized to improve efficacy [48].
3	DprE1 Inhibitors	Caliber Global Alliance for TB Drug Development	DprE1 is a novel target identified by high throughput screening against mycobacterial whole cells [48].
4	SPR113	Kanury Rao, Sudeep Duggar	SPR113 showed an excellent *in vitro* anti-mycobacterial activity of MTB infected human macrophages with an EC_{50} of < 50 nM against MDR- and XDR-TB strains [48].
5	HMG-CoA reductase inhibitor	Generic	Simvastatin (25 mg/kg) significantly increased the tuberculocidal activity of the standard oral regimen of isoniazid (10 mg/kg), rifampicin (10 mg/kg) and pyrazinamide (150 mg/kg) [48, 50].
6	Bortezomib	SPRINT-TB (National University of Singapore)	The Bortezomib (human proteasome inhibitor) was identified as a potent inhibitor of mycobacterial *ClpP* in a target mechanism based whole cell screen [48].
7	Xanthone	SPRINT-TB (National University of Singapore)	Novel xanthone based leads were identified in a whole cell growth inhibition [48].
8	Indoles	SPRINT-TB (National University of Singapore)	Novel indoles based leads were identified in a whole cell growth inhibition [48].
9	*InhA* Inhibitors	GlaxoSmithKline	Isoniazid is supposed to be activated within the MTB by the KatG catalase and inhibits the biosynthesis of mycolic acid through *inhA* enzyme. Mutation in KatG leads to isoniazid resistance. The goal is to identify compounds having similar efficacy to that of the isoniazid and avoid much of the current resistance to isoniazid by bypassing the requirement for KatG activation and directly inhibiting *inhA* [48].
10	LeuRS Inhibitors	Anacor Pharmaceuticals GlaxoSmithKline	Development of leucyl-tRNA synthetase (LeuRS) inhibitor is ongoing [48].

(Table 2) contd.....

S. No.	Compound/ Target	Sponsor/ Developer	Description
11	TL1 Inhibitors	Sequella	Translocase 1 (TL1), is a very attractive target for the development of new drugs that inhibit biosynthesis of the peptidoglycan layer of the bacterial cell wall, that is absent in the eukaryotes. Capuramycins a semi-synthetic nucleoside is TL1 inhibitor [48].
12	Ruthenium (II) phosphine/diimine/ picolinate complexes	UNESP/ School of Pharmaceutical Sciences	Ruthenium complexes (SCAR) showed up to 150 time higher activity against MTB than its organic molecule, without the metal (free ligand), with low cytotoxicity and high selectivity [48].
13	Diarylquinolines	TB Alliance, University of Auckland, Janssen	Bedaquiline, a diarylquinoline, is used in MDR-TB, which inhibits the MTB's ATP synthase. The development of next-generation diarylquinolines is in progress [48].
14	Cyclopeptides	Sanofi TB Alliance	New optimized derivatives from Streptomyces-derived griselimycin (natural cyclic peptide) are highly active against MTB, both *in vitro* and *in vivo* studies [48]. It acts by inhibiting the DNA polymerase sliding clamp DnaN [51].

Table 3. The antitubercular drugs in early stage development.

S. No.	Compound/ Structure	Family and Sponsor/Developer	Description
1	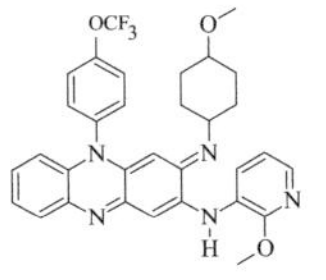 TBI-166	Riminophenazines antibiotics Institute of Materia Medica	Targeting the outer membrane and possibly the bacterial respiratory chain and the ion transporters [52]
2	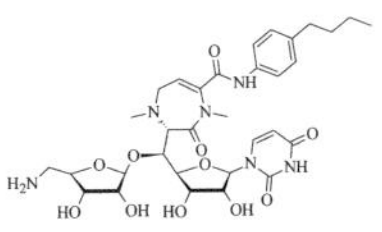 CPZEN-45	Nucleoside antibiotics Institute of Microbial Chemistry (BIKAKEN), Japan, Lilly TB Drug Discovery Initiative, NIAID, IDRI, Lilly, YourEncore	Inhibits a novel target WecA [53]
3	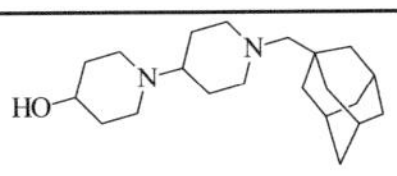 SQ609	Dipiperidines	Cell wall synthesis inhibitor [54]
4	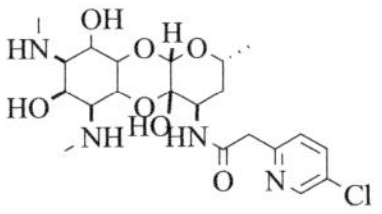 1599	Spectinomycin analogs St. Jude Chidren's Research Hospital, University of Tennessee Health Science Centre, Colorado State University, University of Zurich, Microbiotix	Selective ribosomal inhibitor and an excellent narrow-spectrum antitubercular activity [55].

TBI166

TBI166 belongs to the riminophenazine class of drugs discovered through lead optimization of clofazimine, in order to obtain similar compounds with less adverse effects (accumulation in fat tissues, long half-life and skin discoloration) [56]. TBI166 has an improved physiochemical and pharmacokinetic profile. Clofazimine was reported by Barry *et al.* in 1957, is "Group 5" drug not recommended for routine use for drug resistant TB due to ambiguous efficacy [57]. The SAR study of clofazimine suggested the para substitution on phenyl ring enhances activity, but is not essential, while the imine group should be substituted with alkyl or cycloalkyl groups in order to increase the activity [57]. In order to improve the physiochemical and pharmacokinetic property, chemical modification of **clofazimine**, leads in the discovery of TBI166. The SAR analysis shows that, N5 substitution with electron withdrawing groups is important for antimycobacterial activity, 4-methoxycyclohexyl substituent is preferred at imine nitrogen to improve pharmacokinetic property, while 2-methoxypyridyl group C2 nitrogen demonstrated reduced skin pigmentation [58]. The SAR of clofazimine and TBI166 are given in Fig. (**5**).

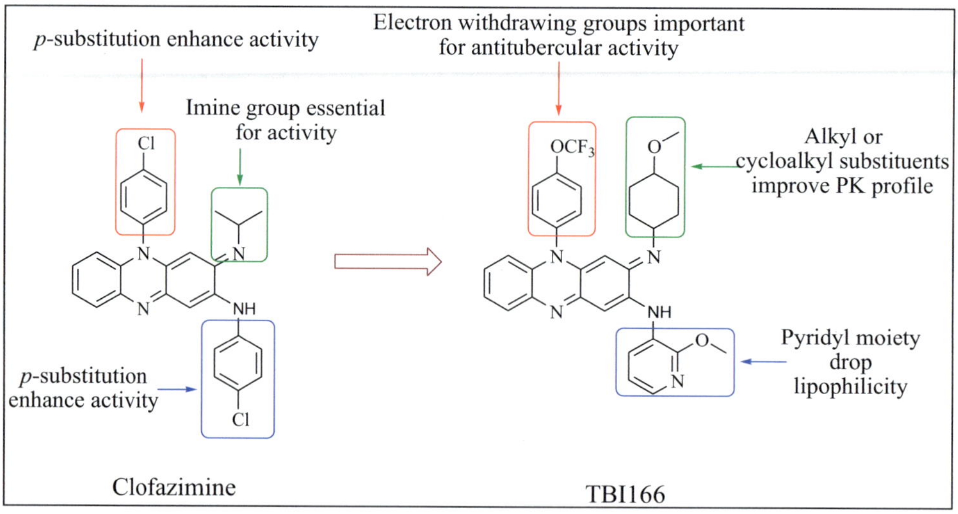

Fig. (5). The SAR analysis of clofazimine and TBI166.

TBI166 is synthesized with the stirring of a mixture of 2-fluronitobenzene, *p*-anisidine and KF at 160 °C to afford the synthesis of *N*-(4-methoxyphenyl--2-nitroaniline which is reduced to *N*-(4-methoxyphenyl)benzene-1,2-diamine with 10% Pd/C and further treated with 1,5-difluoro-2,4-dinitrobenzene (DFDNB) in ethanol and triethylamine (TEA) to obtain *N*-(5-fluoro-2,4-dinitrophenyl)-*N'*-

(4-methoxyphenyl)benzene-1,2-diamine which is treated with 3-amino-2-methoxypyridine and further reduced, and the reduced product is finally treated with 4-methoxycyclohexanamine in dioxane and glacial acetic acid followed by cyclization leads to the synthesis of TBI166. The outline for its synthesis is given in Fig. (**6**) [58]. The mechanism of action of TBI166 is still ambiguous. It possibly acts by targeting the outer membrane and possibly the bacterial respiratory chain and the ion transporters [52, 59].

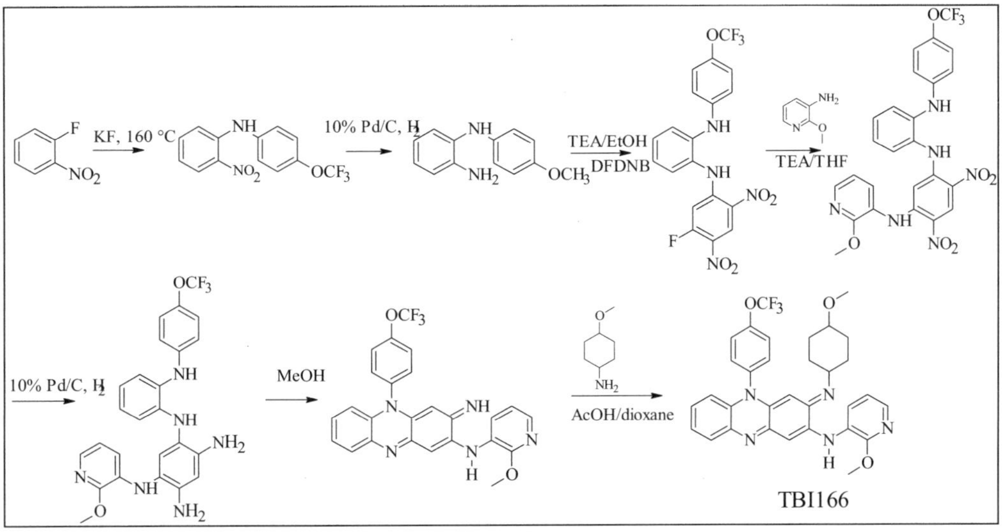

Fig. (6). The synthetic pathway for TBI166.

SQ609

SQ609 is a new dipiperidine analogue, that demonstrated activity against MTB, and discovered through the solid phase combinatorial synthesis, and screening of 10,358 diamines analogues. The SAR studies suggests that the (piperidin---ylmethyl)piperidine scaffold is an essential structural element required for antibacterial activity. *In vitro*, SQ609 inhibited more than 90% of intracellular bacterial growth of MTB-infected macrophages at 4 μg/ml and completely prevented the weight loss in MTB infected mice and prolonged the therapeutic effect by 10-15 days after therapy cessation. The synthetic protocol of SQ609 is given in Fig. (7) [60, 61].

Toxicity Assessment

Currently there are three new classes of anti-tubercular drugs in the preclinical stage of development, with toxicity assessment profile (Good Laboratory Practice toxicity). A brief description of these drugs is given in Table **4**.

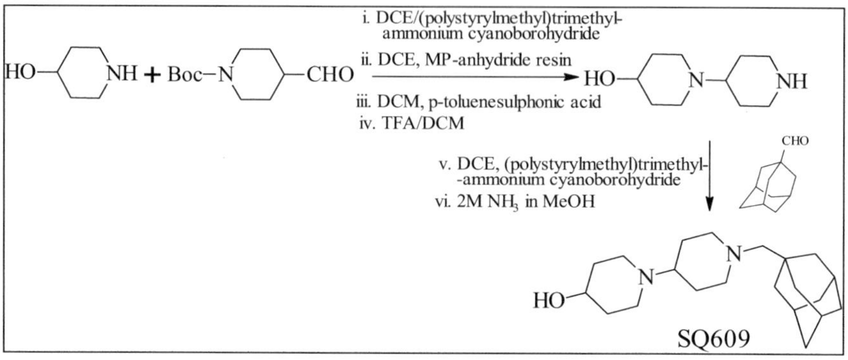

Fig. (7). The synthetic pathway for SQ609.

Table 4. List of drugs in preclinical GLP toxicity evaluation

S. No.	Anti-tubercular Agent	Family and Sponsor/Developer	Description
1	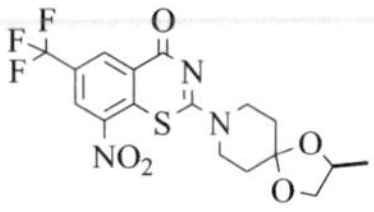 BTZ-043	Benzthiazinone Medical Centre of the University of Munich (LMU), Hans-Knöll-Institut (HKI), German Center for Infection Research (DZIF)	It acts by inhibiting the synthesis of cell wall arabinans by targeting the enzyme decaprenylphosphoryl-β-d-ribose 2'-epimerase (DprE) [62].
2	TBA-7371	DprE1 Inhibitor Eli Lilly	TBA-7371 inhibits the arabinan synthesis by targeting the enzyme DprE1 [62].
3	GSK-070	Leucyl-tRNA synthetase inhibitor Anacor Pharmaceuticals; GlaxoSmithKline; Global Alliance for TB Drug Development	GSK070 has an excellent activity against a set of 98 strains of MTB, including drug-sensitive, multidrug and extremely drug-resistant strains. It acts by inhibiting the leucyl-tRNA synthetase [63].

BTZ043

BTZ043 belongs to benzthiazinone class of antitubercular drugs. The protocol for the synthesis of BTZ043 is given in Fig. (**8**). 2-Chloro-3-nitro-5-trifluoromethylbenzoyl chloride on treatment with ammonia solution in acetonitrile, gives 2-chloro-3-nitro-5-(trifluoromethyl)benzamide, which reacts with 1,4-dioxa-8-azaspiro[4.5]decane-8-carbodithioic acid sodium salt, to form an intermediate, which further cyclises to obtain BTZ043 [64, 65]. The SAR analysis shows the crucial role of 8-nitro group of BTZ043 in inhibiting decaprenylphosphoryl-β-D-ribose 2'-oxidase (DprE1) for bactericidal activity against MTB [66].

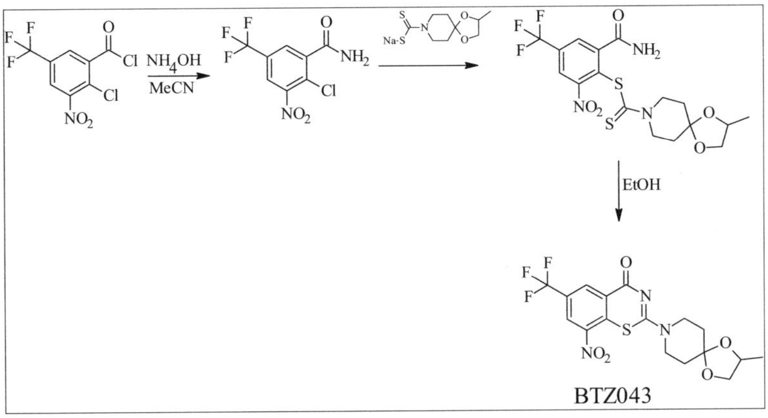

Fig. (8). The synthetic pathway for BTZ043.

Clinical Development

There are fourteen antitubercular drugs entered the various phases of clinical trials, including 3,4-carbostyril derivatives (OPC-167832), imidazopyridine amide (Q203), benzthiazinone (PTBZ169), oxazolidinone (sutezolid and linezolid), rifamycin (rifampicin and rifapentin), diarylquinoline (bedaquiline), nitro-imidazole (pretomanid and delmanid), nitrothiazole (nitazoxanide), fluoro-quinolone (levofloxacin, and moxifloxacin), and mepropenem/ clavulanate (carbapenem antibiotics).

OPC-167832

OPC-167832 is a 3,4-carbostyril derivative developed by Otsuka Pharmaceutical, Japan and is currently undergoing Phase I clinical trial.

Q203

Q203 is a new chemical class (imidazopyridine) of antitubercular drug currently in Phase I clinical trials, developed by Qurient Co. Ltd./LLC "Infectex", a portfolio firm of Maxwell Biotech Venture Fund. Q203 blocks the MTB growth by targeting the respiratory cytochrome *bc*1 complex. It also inhibited the growth of MDR and XDR MTB clinical isolates, both *in vitro* and *in vivo* studies [67, 68]. A dose escalation and study of safety evaluation, tolerability, and pharma-cokinetics of single doses Q203 in human volunteers, and Phase 1B of randomized, placebo-controlled, double-blind, multiple ascending dose study of safety evaluation, tolerability and pharmacokinetics of Q203 in healthy adults is undergoing [48]. The synthetic pathway of Q203 is given in Fig. (**9**). A solution of ethyl-2-bromo-3-oxopentanoate and 2-amino-5-chloropyridine in ethanol gives ethyl 6-chloro-2-ethylimidazo[1,2-*a*]pyridine-3-carboxylate, which coupled with

1-(4-{4-[4-(trifluoromethoxy)phenyl]piperidin-1-yl}phenyl)-methanamine, to give Q203 [67]. The structure activity relationship (SAR) of imidazopyridine amide is given in Fig. (**10**). The SAR analysis shows that (i) 6-chloro substituent is the best substitute, (ii) –CONH- is essential for antitubercular activity, and replacement of hydrogen of NH with alkyl/phenyl group decreases the activity, (iii) carboxamide moiety with *N*-benzylic group is critical for antimycobacterial activity, (iv) *para* substitution on *N*-benzylic group increases activity, while the substituent 4-[4-(trifluoromethoxy)phenyl]-piperidine is promising, and (v) trifluoromethoxy substituent is metabolically stable.

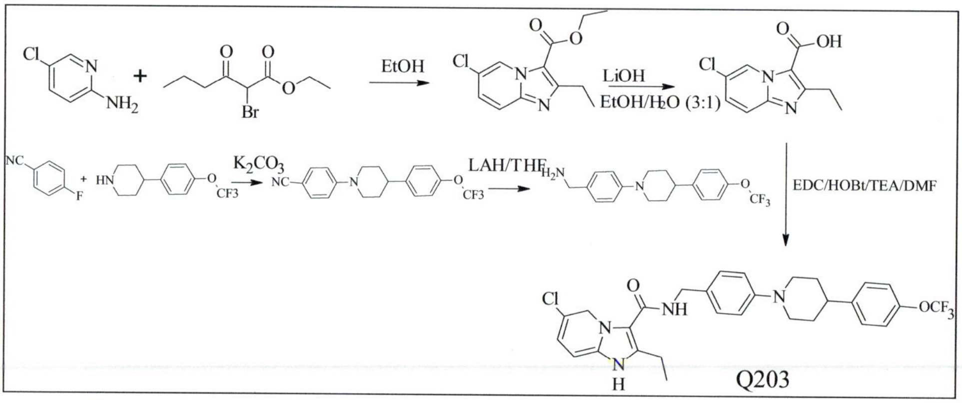

Fig. (9). The synthetic pathway for Q203.

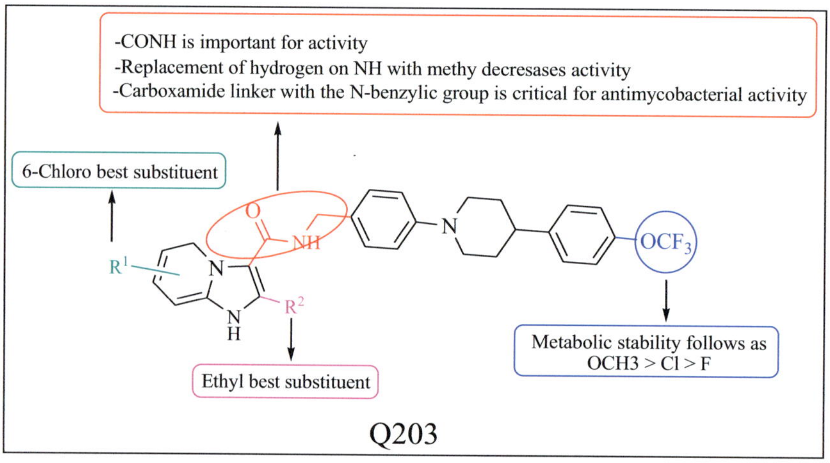

Fig. (10). SAR analysis of imidazopiridine amides.

PBTZ169

PBTZ169 belongs to the class benzthiazinone containing a piperazine ring. It was developed by Innovative Medicine for Tuberculosis (iM4TB) and now it is in Phase I clinical trials. It is not stereo-selective and comparatively easier to synthesize than BTZ043. It is 3-fold more active than BTZ043, against the MTB, and 10-time less cytotoxic for the HepG2 human cell lines. In a murine model of chronic TB infection, PBTZ169 showed better efficacy than BTZ043. In zebra fish model, PBTZ169 showed improved potency, safety, and efficacy profile compared to BTZ-043 [68]. Also in a murine model of chronic TB infection, PBTZ169 with PZA and BDQ showed a better efficacy than the standard triple therapy of INH, RIF and PZA. It acts by inhibiting the cell wall biosynthesis by inhibiting DprE1 [66, 69].

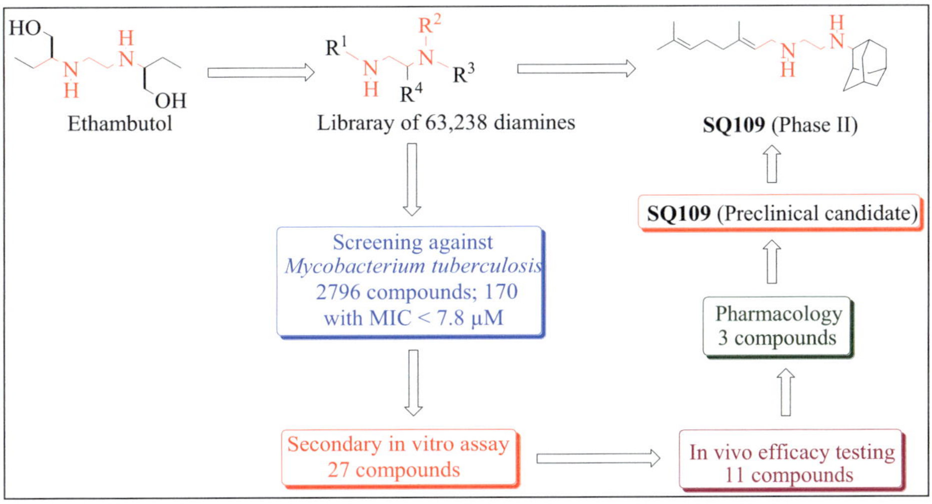

Fig. (11). Process to identify new drug candidate, SQ109, from a focused combinatorial library of 1,2-ethylenediamine small-molecule compounds [73].

SQ109

SQ109 is a 1,2-ethylenediamine based compound in Phase II clinical trials, developed by Sequela Incorporated. It was identified from a combinatorial library of 63,238 diamines (Fig. **11**) [70 - 72]. The SAR analysis shows that ethambutol pharmacophore is required for activity, and change in the basicity of either nitrogens, leads to the loss of antitubercular activity. Further, the long chain alkyl group (isoprenyl unit) and the bulky core 2-adamantyl moiety are favourable for activity (Fig. **12**). The outline for the synthesis of SQ109 is given in (Fig. **13**). Trans-trans farnesyl bromide is reacted with ethylenediamine to yield the corresponding mono-substituted amine, which on further reductive treatment with 2-adamantanone yields SQ109 [73]. SQ109 is active on all types of MTB, including MDR- and XDR-TB clinical strains. It possesses bactericidal action with an MIC range of 0.2–0.78 µg/ml. SQ109 demonstrated synergistic effect with INH and RIF, and additive effect when combined with EB or streptomycin. It also improves the efficacy of TMC207 by 4-8 folds [74]. SQ109 was found to be safe, and well tolerated with mild to moderate dose dependent, gastrointestinal discomfort [75]. SQ109 interferes with the cell wall synthesis targeting the MmpL3, a membrane transporter of trehalose monomycolate (TMM), the precursor of TDM and the cell wall mycolates [76, 77].

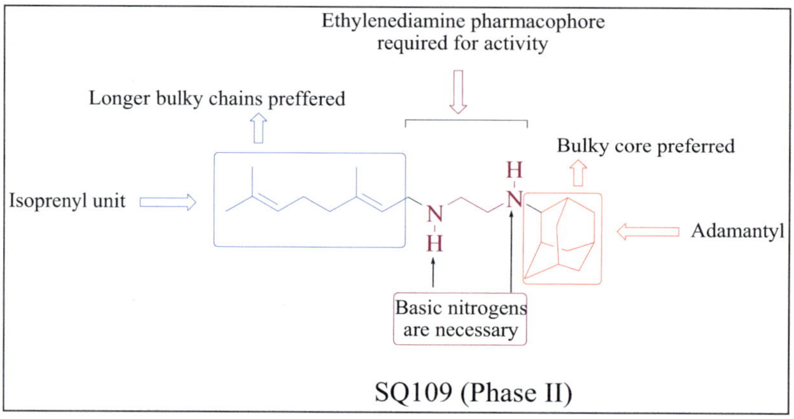

Fig. (12). SAR analysis of SQ109.

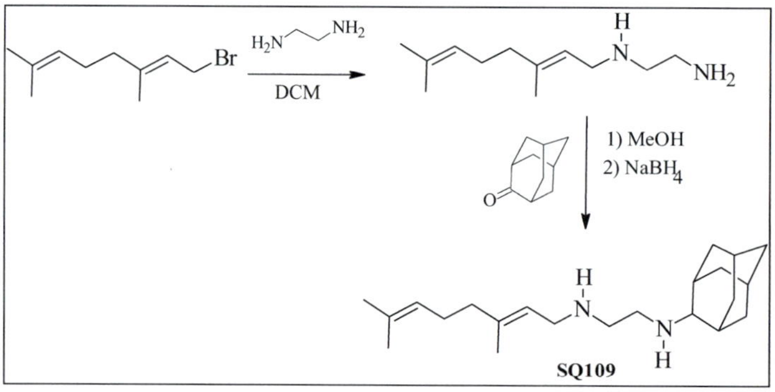

Fig. (13). The synthetic pathway for SQ109.

Nitazoxanide

Nitazoxanide (NTZ), nitro-thiazolyl antiparasitic drug is a repurposed antitubercular drug in Phase II clinical trials developed by Romark Laboratories. Nitazoxanide (NTZ) and its active metabolite kill replicating and non-replicating MTB [78]. It has a bactericidal activity against the *H37Rv* laboratory strain of MTB with an MIC of 16 µg/ml, while the MICs against 50 clinical isolates ranged from 12-28 μg/ml [79]. NTZ and its active metabolite tizoxanide strongly stimulate autophagy and inhibit signalling by mammalian target of rapamycin complex 1 (mTORC1), a major negative regulator of autophagy. It also targets the human quinone oxidoreductase (NQO1), which is partly responsible for mTORC1 inhibition [80]. The synthetic protocol of nitazoxanide is given in (Fig. **14**). 2-Amino-5-nitrothiazole reacts with the substituted benzoyl chloride (methyl 2-(chlorocarbonyl)benzoate) to give nitazoxanide [81].

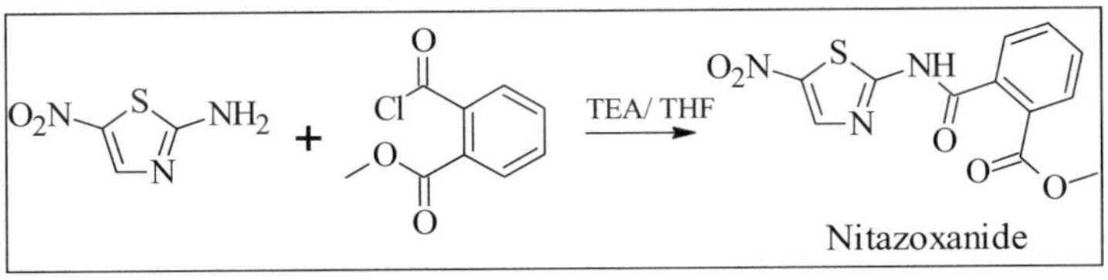

Fig. (14). The synthetic pathway for nitazoxanide.

Clofazimine

Clofazimine, a member of the riminophenazine class, was first introduced in 1960 for the treatment of leprosy. It is a repurposed antitubercular drug which showed an excellent activity against various drugs-resistant MTB strains and is currently in clinical trials as a component of new regimens for the treatment of MDR-TB [82, 83]. Randomized controlled study of clofazimine for the treatment of MDR-TB prompted cavity closure, accelerated sputum culture conversion, and improved treatment success rates; however it is found to be associated with skin discoloration and ichthyosis as the side effects [84]. Clofazimine is placed in "Group 5" of WHO grouping of antitubercular drug. It is being used for treatment of MDR/XDR TB when other choices are not available [82].

Mepropenem/ Clavulanate

Meropenem and clavulanate belong to carbapenem antibiotics, and are US FDA–approved drugs. They are the repurposed drugs for the treatment of TB, and were developed by TASK Foundation NPC, GlaxoSmithKline, and University Eduardo Mondlane. Phase II clinical a trial of early bactericidal activity, safety, and tolerability evaluation was ongoing for the drug combination. The combination of meropenem and clavulanate (β-lactamase inhibitor) showed potent activity against laboratory strains of MTB [85]. The MTB is resistant to β-lactams due to constitutive production of chromosomally encoded Ambler class A, β-lactamase (BlaC). The clavulanate inactivate BlaC to hydrolytically stable form, and could have potential to be used in combination with approved *β*-lactam antibiotics for the treatment of MDR/XDR TB [86]. The most common side effect of mepropenem/ clavulanate is seizure [16].

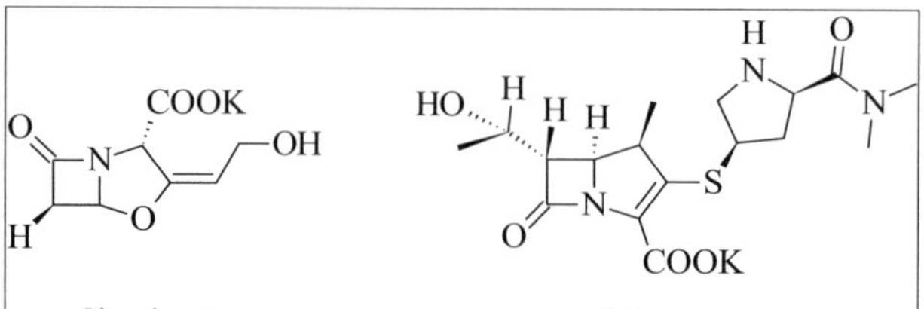

Clavulanate Meropenem

Fluoroquinolones

Fluoroquinolones class of drugs represent the major advancement over the original DNA gyrase inhibitor, nalidixic acid (Fig. **15**) [87, 88]. Various fluoroquinolones were discovered till date. Ciprofloxacin, levofloxacin, and moxifloxacin are used as second line antitubercular drugs. Phase II clinical trials of levofloxacin are undergoing. Similarly, Phase III clinical trials of moxifloxacin in combination with other antitubercular drug (rifapentin-moxifloxacin-delamanid and pretomanid-moxifloxacin-pyrazinamide) are also undergoing. The SAR was discussed elsewhere in detail and briefly summarized here [87, 88]. The best substituent at C2 (R^2) is hydrogen, to avoid steric hindrance; C5 substituent is hydrogen, for antitubercular activity, while presence of amino ($-NH_2$) and methyl ($-CH_3$) enhance activity against gram positive bacteria; C6 substituent should be small halogen (most probably fluorine) to confer greater potency to the target enzyme between 5 and 100 fold; C3 carboxylic group and C4 carbonyl functions are responsible and essential for the binding with the DNA gyrase; C7 substituent should be five or six member heterocyle containing nitrogen; R^1 should be a cyclopropyl or a fused cycle with R^5, and R^5 should be a methoxy group (OCH_3) or fused with 'O' containing ring with R^1; the substituents at C7 (R^4), C8 (R^5) and N1 (R^1) influence the pharmacokinetic profile of the drug candidates. A brief SAR analysis is given in Fig. (**16**).

Levofloxacin

Levofloxacin, a newer fluoroquinolone, and a repurposed antitubercular drug, has potent activity against TB both *in vitro* and *in vivo* studies and is currently in Phase II clinical trials for the study of an efficacy and safety for the treatment of MDR-TB. It acts by targeting specifically the mycobacterial topoisomerase II DNA gyrase [37 - 39]. The study led by group of researchers showed that, an optimized dose of 17-20 mg/kg, of levofloxacin, was required to improve its efficacy against TB and MDR-TB [89].

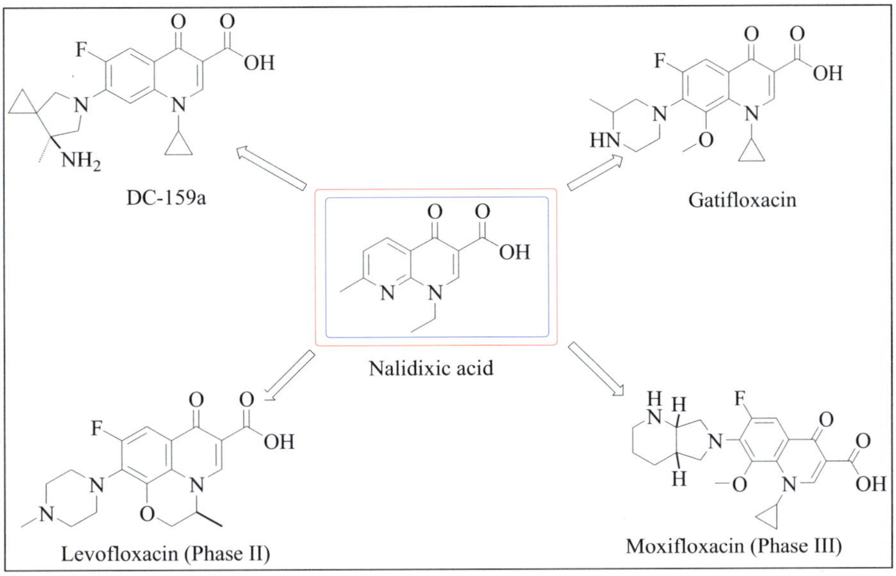

Fig. (15). Discovery of fluoroquinolone.

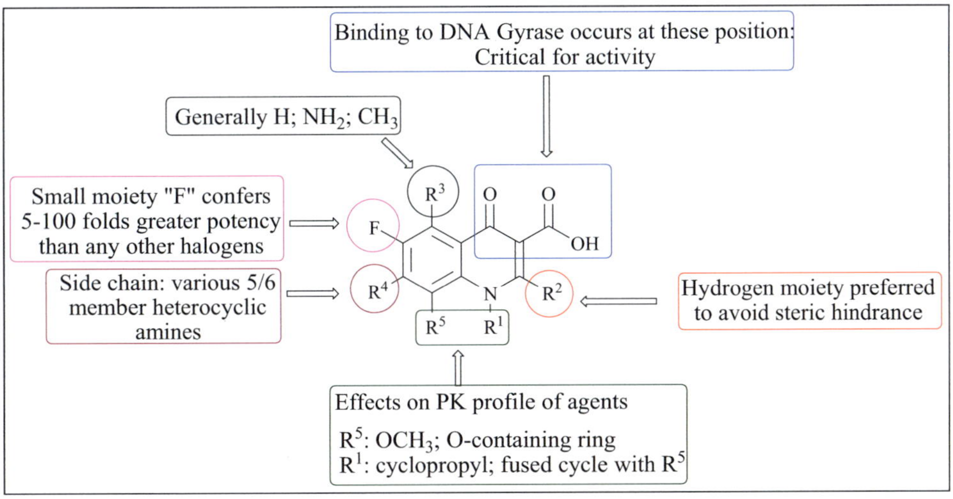

Fig. (16). SAR analysis of fluoroquinolone.

Moxifloxacin

Moxifloxacin, a drug belongs to fluoroquinolone class, is currently in Phase III clinical trials. The clinical trials of moxifloxacin in combination with pretomanid and pyrazinamide to evaluate the efficacy, safety, and tolerability as well as early bactericidal activity in pulmonary TB are being conducted. It is also being evaluated in combination with rifapentin. In a phase IIb study, the addition of moxifloxacin to the standard therapy regimen (RIF/INH/PZA/EMB) shortened the time to culture conversion, and substitution of the moxifloxacin with INH was not found to be very significant, however EMB can be substituted with moxifloxacin [90 - 93]. The main side effects of moxifloxain are headache and gastrointestinal disturbances [94].

Oxazolidinone (PNU-100480)

Oxazolidinones, a class of antibacterial compounds, are analogues of DuP105 and DuP721 having an MIC_{50} range of 4-16 and 2-8 μg/ml, respectively, but were discontinued due to Phase I toxicity issues [95]. Linezolid, an oxazolidinone, was introduced for Gram positive bacterial infections [96]. It acts by inhibiting protein synthesis targeting the 23S RNA in the 50S ribosomal subunit [97]. The most common side effects of linezolid include peripheral neuropathy, myelo-suppression, and ocular toxicity [16, 98]. The further development of linezolid is restricted due to its toxic profile and new analogue (PNU-100480), showing identical and better *in vivo* activity and with better therapeutic index was initiated by Upjohn. Two oxazolidinones that were structural analogue of linezolid include PNU-100480 (sutezolid) and AZD-5847. The development of AZD-5847 by Astra-Zeneca was discontinued (due to lack of demonstrated antimycobacterial activity). The development of oxazolidinones is given in (Fig. **17**).

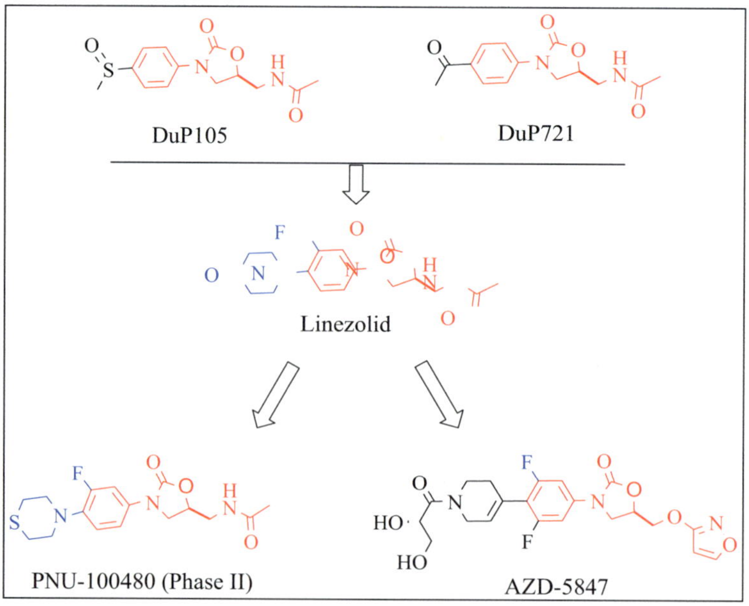

Fig. (17). Development of oxazolidinones from DuP105 and DuP721 by structural modifications.

PNU-100480 exhibits an MIC range of 0.03-0.50 μg/ml against sensitive and drug resistant strains of MTB, and it is more potent than linezolid in the mouse model. Single doses of PNU-100480 (up to 1000 mg) were well tolerated in healthy volunteers. It also demonstrated superior antitubercular activity to linezolid (300 mg) at steady state [99]. Phase I study of PNU-100480 is completed and now the drug enters into the Phase II study. The SAR analysis shows that *N*-aryl group is required for activity; electron withdrawing group (fluoro) in the aromatic ring improve activity; 5-S-configuration is necessary; the morpholine or thiomorpholino enhances pharmacokinetics; 5-acylamino methyl is essential for activity (Fig. **18**) [100, 101]. The synthetic pathway of PNU-100480 is similar to that of the synthesis of linezolid. The PNU-100480 is synthesized by the treatment of 3,4-difluoronitrobenzene with thiomorpholine, followed by the reduction of nitro intermediate to the corresponding amine, which reacts with benzyloxy-carbonyl chloride to obtain benzyl[3-fluoro-4-(thiomorpholin-4-yl)phenyl]-carbamate, which reacts with lithium *t*-amylate and potassium salt of tertiary butanol to form 3-[3-fluoro-4-(thiomorpholin-4-yl)phenyl]-5-(hydroxymethyl)-1, 3-oxazolidin-2-one, and further reacts with 3-nitrobenzenesulfonyl chloride followed by treatment with ammonium chloride and acetic anhydride leads to the synthesis of PNU-100480 (Fig. **19**) [102, 103].

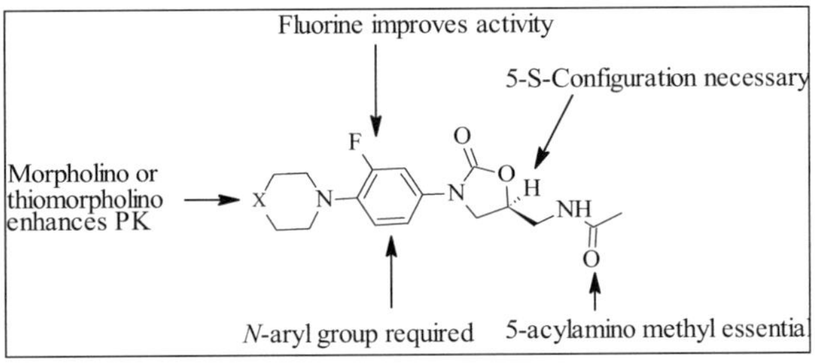

Fig. (18). SAR analysis of oxazolidinones.

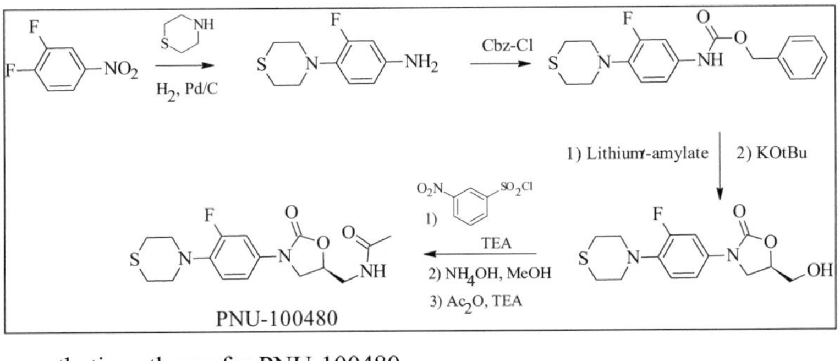

Fig. (19). The synthetic pathway for PNU-100480.

Nitroimidazole (Delamanid and Pretomanid)

Metronidazole was developed in the 1960s, and is currently used to treat protozoal and anaerobic bacterial infections. It exhibited modest antitubercular activity *in vitro* and *in vivo* studies [104]. Since metronidazole was found to have therapeutic potential in the treatment of bacterial infections, 5-nitroimidazole (CGI 17341) was developed and initially promising results were obtained against MTB. Its activity was found to be comparable to isoniazid and rifampin and superior to streptomycin, ciprofloxacin or norfloxacin, and oxazolidinone, but it was found to be associated with mutagenicity [105, 106]. However, the lead of CGI 17341 was considered in the synthesis of a library of 328 bicyclic nitroimidazolepyran analogues, and finally PA-824 was identified as promising antitubercular agent [107]. Similarly, OPC-67683 and TBA-354 were also designed from CGI 17341. PA-824 and OPC-67683 are now in Phase III clinical trials, but the further development of TBA-354 was discontinued due to the presence of toxicity in Phase I clinical trials [1]. Some of the nitroimidazoles are given in Fig. (**20**).

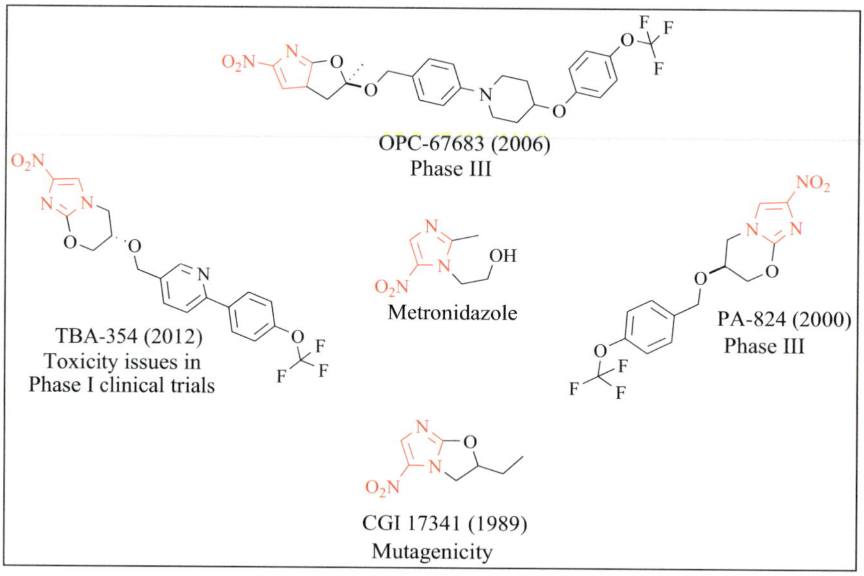

Fig. (20). Some of the nitroimidazole analogues.

Pretomanid (PA-824)

The activity of PA-824 against MTB complex was found to be promising, devoid of any cross resistant with other antitubercular drugs. Its activity was found to be comparable to rifampin and moxifloxacin under anaerobic conditions [108, 109]. The Phase IIa early bactericidal activity was completed for PaMZ, (PA-824, moxifloxacin and pyrazinamide), in which they killed TB bacteria faster when compared with the current TB regimen. PaMZ has the potential to cure both TB and some forms of MDR-TB in 4 months, drastically improving the treatment. The shortening treatment by advancing novel drug (STAND) is being planned for the drug combination (PaMZ). The Phase II trials to evaluate the efficacy, safety and tolerability of PaMZ in drug sensitive and multi-drug resistant patients are ongoing. PA-824 is a prodrug, that requires bioreductive activation of the aromatic nitro group by the deazaflavin F_{420} dependent glucose-6-phosphate dehydrogenase (FGD1) and deazaflavin-dependent nitroreducatase Rv3547 (Ddn) to its major metabolite des-nitroimidazole to generate reactive nitrogen species (NO) and inhibits cytochrome c oxidase, that exerts anaerobic killing of MTB [110 - 112].

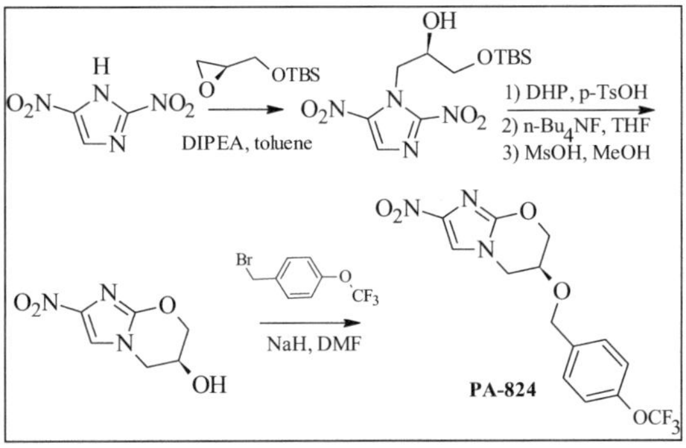

Fig. (21). The synthetic pathway for PA-824.

The synthesis of PA-824 requires the following steps, alkylated on *N*-1 of 2,4-dinitroimidazole, followed by cyclization to affords the synthesis of nitroimidazopyran, and then finally alkylated with 1-(bromomethyl)-4-(trifluoromethoxy)benzene to form PA-824 [113, 114]. The synthetic pathway of PA-824 is given in Fig. (**21**). The SAR analysis of nitroimidazo[2,1-b]oxazine series shows that nitro group is essential for antitubercular activity; bicyclic system is essential and opening of ring abolishes the activity, replacement of O atom with CH_2 decreases activity, while N and S atoms were well tolerated; ether linkage can be replaced with urea, carbamate or carbonate *etc*; *p*-substitution is favourable, but the *o* and *m*-substitution on the benzyl group is detrimental for activity (Fig. **22**) [8, 101, 115 - 118].

Delamanid (OPC-67683)

The development of CGI 17341 was discontinued due to its mutagenicity. It was speculated that the antitubercular activity can be increased and mutagenicity of

CGI 17341 can be eliminate by modification at 2-position of 6-nitro-2-3-dihydroimidazo[2,1-*b*]oxazoles, and finally OPC-67683 was discovered [117]. It has an MIC of 0.006-0.024 µg/ml against MTB and MDR-TB. OPC-67683 in combination with rifampicin and pyrazinamide quickly eradicated the viable TB bacilli in the lung than in the comparison to the standard regimen of rifampicin, isoniazid, ethambutol, and pyrazinamide (REF-INH-EB-PZA) [118, 119]. The 6 month treatment of OPC-67683 in combination with an optimized background regimen can improve outcomes and reduce mortality among patients with both MDR and XDR-TB [120]. OPC-67683 acts by inhibiting the mycolic acid synthesis (methoxy- and keto-mycolic acid) [119].

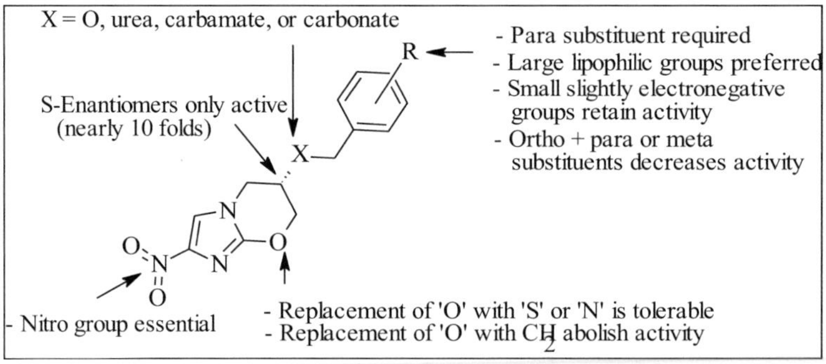

Fig (22). SAR analysis of nitroimidazo[2,1-b]oxazine series (related to PA-824).

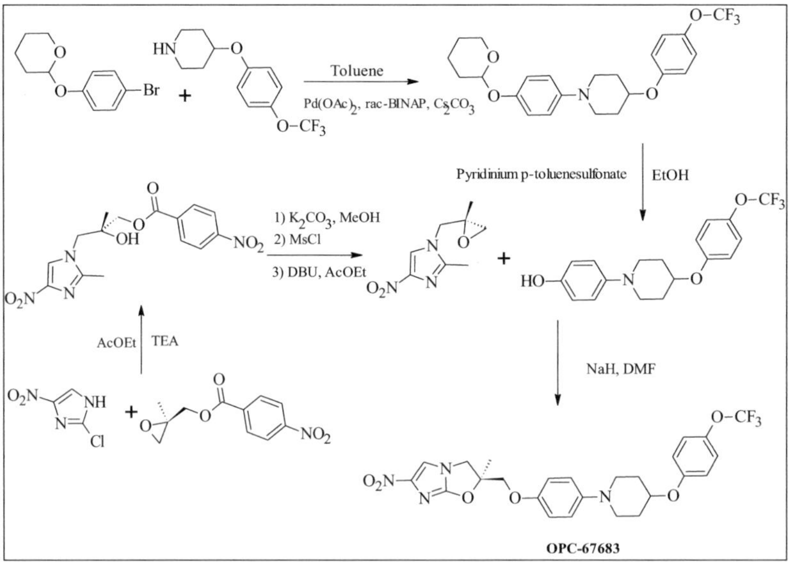

Fig. (23). The synthetic pathway for OPC-67683.

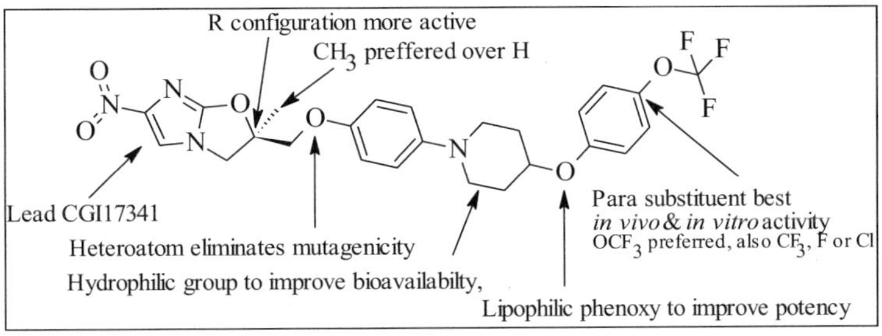

Fig. (24). Summary of the SAR in the nitroimidazo[2,1-b]oxazole series (related to OPC-67683).

The synthetic pathway of OPC-67683 is given in Fig. (**23**). The SAR analysis of nitroimidazo[2,1-b]oxazole series is given in Fig. (**24**). Methyl group preferred at position 2, and R configuration is active; phenoxymethyl group at position 2 linked to piperidino confers the best *in vivo* activity; lipophilic phenoxy terminal having *p*-trifluoromethoxy group (*p*-OCF_3) confers the best activity than the CF_3, F or Cl [118]. The most common side effects of OPC-67683 include nausea, vomiting, dizziness and QTc prolongation [16].

Diarylquinoline (Bedaquiline)

Bedaquiline, TMC207 is a novel diarylquinoline class of antitubercular drug. It is a potent agent against MTB and MTB clinical isolate with an MIC_{99} of 0.030-0.120 µg/ml [121]. It has a bactericidal action on both growing and dormant TB bacilli [122]. In combination with first and second line drugs TMC207 significantly shortens the duration of treatment in mice. It was well tolerated, as no serious adverse effects occurred [123]. TMC207 inhibits the proton pump of the mycobacterial ATP synthase [121, 122]. It is synthesized in the following steps, starting with the reaction of *p*-bromoaniline and 3-phenylpropanoic acid. The quinoline ring is obtained by Vilsmeir-Haack reaction and the final condensation leads to a mixture of four stereoisomers which are separated by column chromatography and the desired R,S compound is obtained (Fig. **25**) [122, 124].

The SAR analysis of TMC207 series compounds is shown in Fig. (**26**). The SAR analysis shows that the presence of bromo substituent at C6 and alkyloxy preferably methoxy at C2 are optimal to retain activity; the presence of two lipophilic groups enhances steric hindrance and promotes the active conformation; the most active conformations are RS and SR; methyl is the best substituent (in tertiary amine). The most common side effects of TMC207 include arthralgia, hepatitis, headache and QTc prolongation [16].

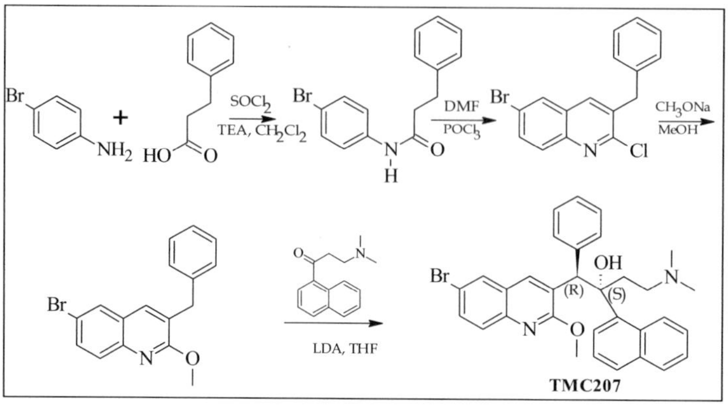

Fig. (25). The synthetic pathway for TMC207 (bedaquiline).

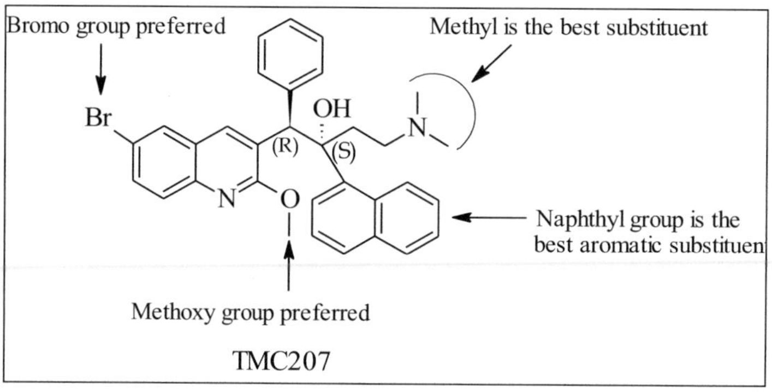

Fig. (26). The SAR analysis of TMC207 series.

MODE OF ACTION OF ANTITUBERCULAR DRUGS

A simplified version of MTB and MTB cell envelop and cytoplasmic membrane and mode of actions of antitubercular drugs are shown in Fig. (**27**). The drug diarylquinoline (TMC207), primarily targets the c-ring portion of the F_0 subunits of ATP synthase and inhibits them leading to the energy depletion and finally kill the MTB. Interestingly 10,000 fold higher concentration of drug is required to inhibit eukaryotic ATP synthase. The nitroimidazoles (PA-824 and OPC-67683) act through F_{420}-deazaflavin dependent nitroreductase (Ddn) release of nitric oxide, which is thought to inhibit cytochrome oxidase and as well as some other targets [109 - 111]. OPC-67683 also inhibits the mycolic acid synthesis (methoxy- and keto-mycolic acid) [119]. The oxazolidinones (PNU-100480 and linezolid) inhibit the synthesis of protein by targeting 23S RNA in the 50S ribosomal subunit [97]. The fluoroquinolones (ciprofloxacin, levofloxacin, moxifloxacin, *etc.,*) primarily target the DNA gyrase, which is the sole type II topoisomerase in the mycobacterium, and inhibit the DNA super-coiling [37 - 39].

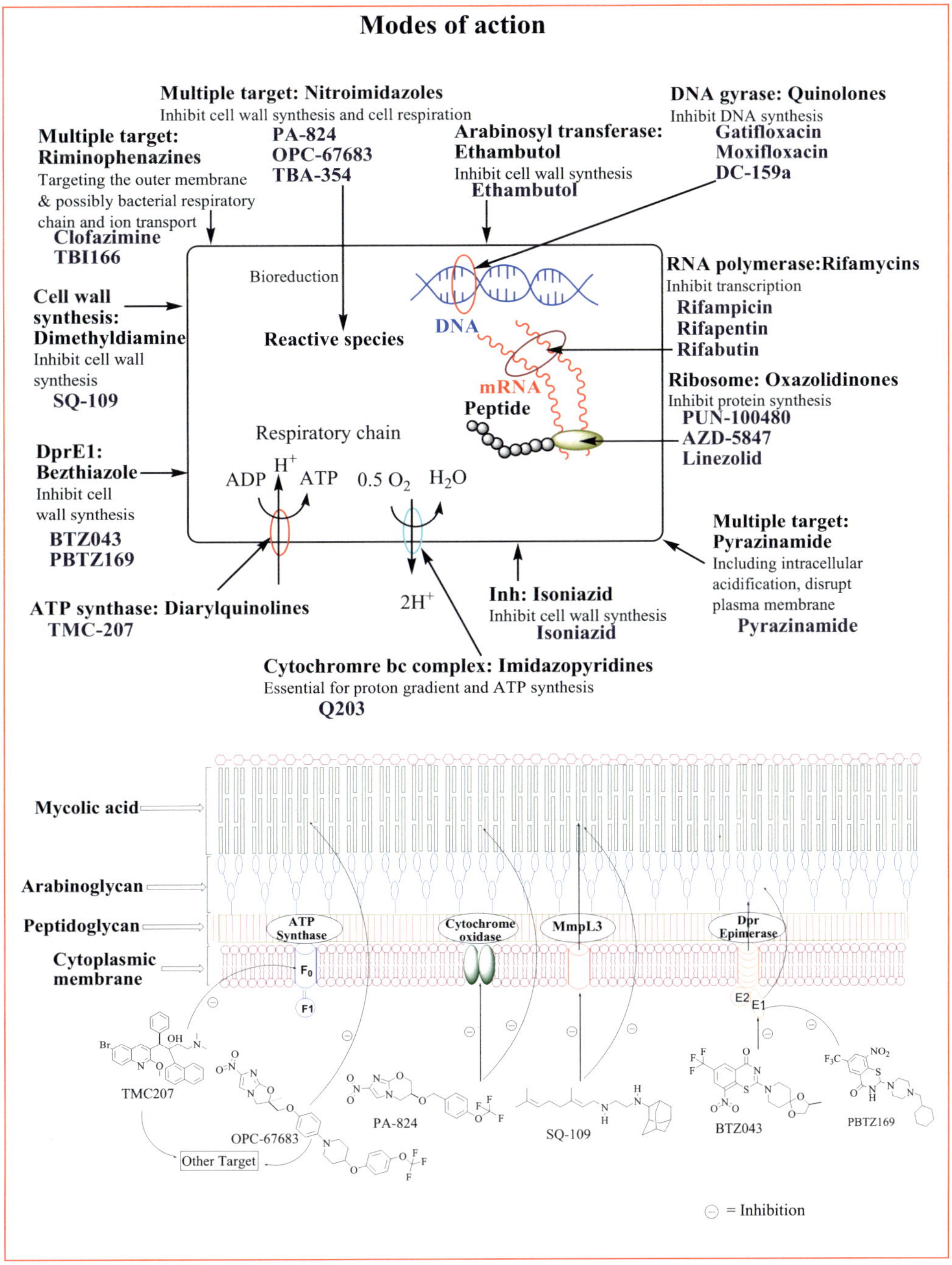

Fig. (27). The mode of action of antitubercular drugs in clinical trials.

The benzthiazinones (BTZ043 and PBTZ169) class of antitubercular drugs inhibit the cell wall biosynthesis by targeting the enzyme decaprenylphosphoryl---dribose2'-epi- merase (DprE1) that catalyses the conversion of decaprenyl-phosphoryl-d ribose (DPR) to decaprenyl-phosphoryl-d arabinose (DPA) the arabinan donor for arab-inogalactan [62, 69]. Similarly, TBA-7371 an antitubercular drug in GLP toxicity evaluation phase also targets the DprE1 and inhibits arabinan synthesis [62].

The riminophenazines class of antitubercular drugs (clofazimine and TBI166) target the outer mycobacterium membrane and possibly inhibit the bacterial respiratory chain and the ion transport system [52, 59]. The imidazopyridine (Q203) class of antitubercular drug inhibits the growth of MTB, by targeting the respiratory cytochrome bc1 complex [67, 68]. The ethylenediamine (SQ109) class of antitubercular drug interferes with the cell wall synthesis, targeting the MmpL3, a membrane transporter of trehalose monomycolate (TMM), which is the precursor of TDM and cell wall mycolate [77]. The translocase 1 (TL1), leucyl-tRNA synthase (LeuRS) and HMG Co reductase are some of the new and attractive targets, which are in developmental phase. The antitubercular drug in good laboratory practice toxicity stage, GSK-070 inhibits the LeuRS [48].

TUBERCULAR VACCINES IN CLINICAL TRIALS

Bacille Calmette Guerin (BCG) is the only vaccine used in practice for the last one century. The progress of genetic manipulation techniques of the genome sequence of MTB invigorates the development of TB vaccines [125]. Nowadays, vaccine development is an active area of Research & Development (R & D) to limit TB infection and to tackle the spread of MDR/XDR-TB. The Millennium Development Goal of eliminating TB by 2050 would not be possible without the introduction of new and effective vaccines. Today we have enough number of vaccines in clinical developmental phase. There are three types of TB vaccines, which include mycobacterial whole cell or extract, protein/adjuvant, and viral vector. Tubercular vaccines are mainly used as prime, boost, immunotherapy, and post infection. There are five mycobacterial whole cell or extract vaccines, which include Vaccae, VPM 1002, DAR-901, MTBVAC, and RUTI, four viral vectored vaccines which include ChAdOx1.85A/MVA85A, Ad5Ag85A, MVA85A/MVA85A, and TB-FLU-04L, and four protein/adjuvant vaccines include M72+AS01$_E$, H1/H56: IC31, H4:IC31, and ID93+GLA-SE. All these thirteen vaccines are in various phases of clinical trials, eight vaccines are in Phase III and Phase II clinical trial and five vaccines are in Phase I clinical trials. MVA85A is an aerosolized vaccine that was developed at University of Oxford. The TB vaccines in the clinical, developmental phases are shown in Fig. (**28**). There are eight antigens that have been used in the preparation of TB vaccines.

These antigens are nothing but protein that are found on the cell surface of bacteria and evoke an immune response in an infected person. T-cells (CD4+, CD8+ and γ/δ T cells) and T-cell derived cytokines play a pivotal role in protection against the MTB [126, 127]. The various indications, antigens, immune responses, and target population of each TB vaccines in clinical trials are summarized in Table **5** [152, 153].

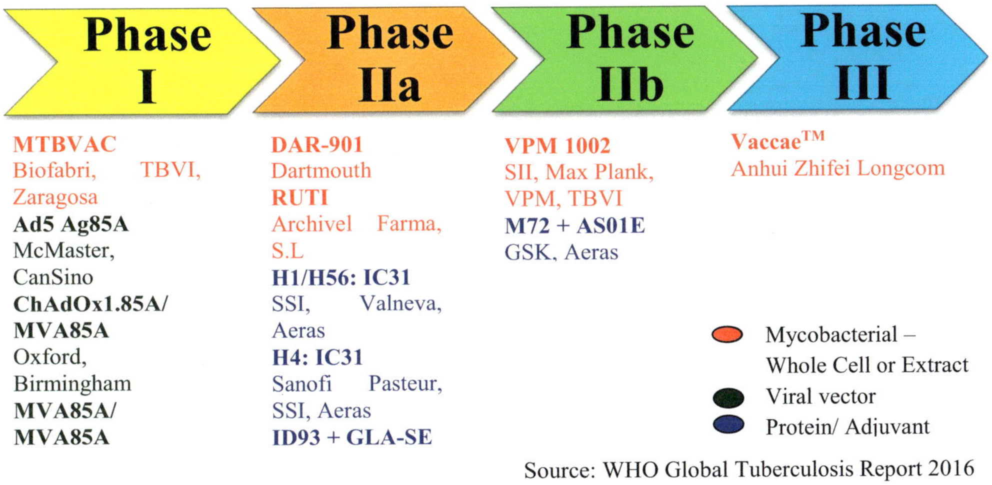

Fig. (28). The tubercular (TB) vaccines in clinical trials.

MOLECULAR TUBERCULOSIS DIAGNOSTICS

The diagnostic technology continues to look promising today. Three new commercial technologies are intended for use at the microscopic level include, Epistem Genedrive (Epistem, United Kingdom), EasyNAT (Ustar Biotechnologies, China), and Molbio True NAT, (Molbio, India) [1]. Cephoid is also developing new TB diagnostic platforms (GeneXpert Omni and Xpert Ultra). WHO reviewed three diagnostic technologies in 2016; loop-mediated isothermal amplification test for TB (TB-LAMP); line probe assays (LPAs) to test for resistance to first-line anti-TB drugs; and LPAs to test for resistance to second-line anti-TB drugs. QuantiFERON-TB Plus (QFT-Plus, Qiagen, Hilden, Germany), was developed to stimulate gamma interferon production by both CD4 and CD8 T-cells [151]. An overview of the progress in the development (not an exhaustive list of technologies) of the molecular TB diagnostics is given in Table **6** [1, 16, 152].

Table 5. Tubercular vaccines in clinical trials.

Phase	TB Vaccines	Type of Vaccines	Sponsor	Indication	Antigens	Immune response	Target population
Phase III	Vaccae	Mycobacterial – Whole cell or extract	Anhui Zhifei Longcom, China	Immunotherapy	-	$CD4^+$ T-cells (IFN-γ and IL-10) [128]	BCG-vaccinated HIV + adult
Phase IIb	VPM 1002	Mycobacterial – Whole cell or extract	Max Plank, VPM, TBVI, Serum Institute	Prime & Boost	-	$CD4^+$ and $CD8^+$ T-cell [129, 130]	Infants
	$M72+AS01_E$	Protein/ Adjuvant	GSK, Aeras	Boost & Post infection	Rv0125 (Mtb32A), Rv1196 (Mtb39A)	$CD4^+$ T-cell [131] $CD4^+$ and $CD8^+$ T-cell [132]	Adolescents/adult, infants
Phase IIa	DAR-901	Mycobacterial – Whole cell or extract	Darmouth, Aeras	Prime & Boost	-	IFN-γ [133]	BCG-vaccinated, HIV-infected adults
	RUTI	Mycobacterial – Whole cell or extract	Archivesl Farma, S.I.	Boost, Post infection & Immunotherapy	-	T_H1 (IFN-γ), T_H2, T_H3, $CD4^+$ and $CD8^+$ T-cells [134 - 136]	HIV+ adult, LTBI diagnosed
	H1/H56: IC31	Protein/ Adjuvant	SSI, Aeras, Intercell	Prime, Boost, Post infection	Rv0288 (TB10.4), Rv1886 (Ag85B), Rv2660, Rv3875 (ESAT6)	T_H1 (IFN-γ, IL-2) [137, 138] $CD4^+$ T-cell [139]	Adolescents, adult
	H4:IC31	Protein/ Adjuvant	SSI, Sanofi-Pasteur, Aeras, Intercell	Boost	Rv0288 (TB10.4), Rv1886 (Ag85B),	$CD4^+$ T-cell (IFN-γ, TNF-α and IL-2) [140]	Infants
	ID93+GLA-SE	Protein/ Adjuvant	Infectious Disease Research Institute (IDRI), Aeras	Boost	Rv1813, Rv2608, Rv3619, Rv3620	T_H1 (IFN-γ, TNF-α and IL-2); $CD4^+$ T-cell (IFN-γ and TNF-α) [141, 142]	Adolescents, adult
Phase I	MTBVAC	Mycobacterial – Whole cell or extract	TBVI, Zaragoza, Biofabri	Prime	-	$CD4^+$ T-cells [143]	HIV negative new born
	Ad5 Ag85A	Viral-vectored	McMaster CanSino	Prime, Boost, Post infection	Rv3804 (Ag85A)	IFN-γ [144] $CD4^+$ and $CD8^+$ T-cells [145]	Infants, adolescents, HIV+
	ChAdOx1.85A/ MVA85A	Viral-vectored	Oxford, Birmingham	Prime & Boost	Rv3804 (Ag85A)	-	BCG-vaccinated adults
	MVA85A/ MVA85A	Viral-vectored	Oxford, Aeras	Boost, Post infection & Immunotherapy	Rv3804 (Ag85A)	IFN-γ [146] $CD4^+$ T-cell [147] $CD4^+$ T-cell (IFN-γ and IL-2) [148] $CD4^+$ T-cell (IFN-γ, TNF-α, IL-2 and IL-17) [149]	BCG-vaccinated infants, children, and adults
	TB-FLU-04L	Viral-vectored	Research Institute for Biological Safety Problems, Research Institute of Influenza	Boost	Rv3804 (Ag85A), Rv3875 (ESAT6)	IFN- γ, IL-1β, TNFα and IL2 [150]	Infants, adolescents, adults

IFN-γ, antigen-specific interferon γ; IL, interleukin; TH1, T helper 1; TNF-α, tumour necrosis factor α.

Table 6. An overview of progress in the development of molecular TB diagnostics, August 2016.

Name of the Test	Sponsor	Assay Principle	Measurement	Estimated Year of WHO Review/ Recommend
Loop mediated isothermal amplification test for TB (TB-LAMP)	Eiken Chemical, Japan	NAAT (LAMP)	Pulmonary TB (not recommended for MDR-TB)	2016
Line probe assays (LPA) to test for resistance to first-line anti-TB drugs	Nipro Corporation, Japan Hain Lifesciences, Germany	NAAT (LPA)	Active TB disease diagnosis Drug resistance (isoniazid and rifampicin)	2016
Line probe assay to test for resistance to second-line anti-TB drugs	Hain Lifesciences, Germany	NAAT (LPA)	Drug resistance (fluoroquinolones and second-line injectable drugs)	2016
Mycobacterium tuberculosis complex assay	Eiken Chemical, Japan	NAAT (LAMP)	Active TB disease diagnosis	2016
Xpert Ultra	Cepheid	NAAT	Rapid and simultaneous detection of TB and rifampicin resistance	2017
Light-emitting diode (LED)	Carl Zeiss Micro Imaging GmbH, Germany	Use the sensitive fluorescent	TB bacteria	2009
Xpert MTB/RIF	Cepheid, Sunnyvale, USA	NAAT (qPCR)	Rapid and simultaneous detection of TB and rifampicin resistance	2010
Mycobacterium tuberculosis lipoarabinomannan (LAM)	Alere Inc., Waltham, MA, USA	Antigen detection	Moderate sensitivity and high specificity in a subgroup of TB patients living with HIV who had advanced immuno-suppression (CD4 cell-counts <50)	2015

FUTURE PROSPECT

Despite the availability of an effective treatment for TB for the last 40 years, TB is spreading globally and till date not completely eradicated. The current TB treatment is of longer duration, and the patient non-compliance and some other factors (cross resistant, *etc.*) leads to the emergence of MDR/ XDR-TB. Today there is an urgent need of shortening, and more effective regimens of TB. Over the last one decade an exhaustive effort by various groups make the TB drug pipeline healthy with an approval of two new antitubercular drugs (bedaquiline and delmanid) for the treatment of MDR-TB. The development of AZD5847 (oxazolidinone) and TBA-354 (nitroimidazole) was discontinued due to lack of demonstrated antitubercular activity and signs of toxicity respectively. Discontinuation of some of the preclinical and clinical phases TB drug is an apprehension that needs to be addressed by promoting more research, from basic to translational, and clinical. We need to understand the pathogenesis and immunology of MTB infection, which is still partly understood. Understanding of MTB's resistance development together with knowledge of genome sequencing, and molecular platforms need to be developed in the near future to support the introduction of new drug regimens. Some new targets (DprE1, HMG-Co reductase, LeuRS *etc.*) were identified, while some new target was identified and validated (mycobacterial ATP synthase; bedaquiline). Hopefully, we can say that some new antitubercular drugs with novel targets may be introduced in the preclinical and clinical developmental pipeline in near future. Lack of adequate funding is a big obstacle that needs to be overcome if we really want to eradicate TB globally, not in the development of TB drugs, but also in the development of TB vaccines as well as diagnostics technology of TB. BCG is the only licensed TB vaccine used since 1921. Although there are 13 TB vaccine candidates in the pipeline, a new TB vaccine is not expected to reach the market in near future. Similarly, we need to develop more effective diagnostic technology for identification of active TB in the near future.

CONCLUSION

TB is spreading globally even though an effective treatment was introduced 40 years ago. There is an urgent need to shorten the TB regimen to improve patients' compliance and affective treatment of MDR/XDR-TB. Two new TB drugs were granted accelerated approval for MDR-TB treatment when the other treatments fail to cure, however, both the drugs are associated with cardiac complications. There are fourteen new and repurposed antitubercular drugs in the developmental pipeline. Some of the newer anti-TB drugs and novel targets were identified today. Various anti-TB drugs in clinical development phases, their synthesis, structure activity relationship (SAR) and mode of action were discussed. There are 13 vaccine candidates in clinical trials: five in Phase I, seven in Phase II and one in Phase III trials. The diagnostic technologies continue to look promising with the review of the three more diagnostic technologies by WHO in 2016, and three new technology were commercialized at the microscopic level. Two new TB diagnostic platforms are in development.

CONFLICT OF INTEREST

The author (editor) declares no conflict of interest, financial or otherwise.

ACKNOWLEDGEMENTS

I acknowledge the constant support and encouragement of the Chairperson, Ms Bharti Prashar of the Maharishi Arvind Group, and the Director, Dr. Bharat Prashar, Maharishi Arvind College of Pharmacy (MACP), India. I am also indebted to many of my colleagues who were an ever ready source of inspiration and motivation, all through the project. Last but not the least, my colleague, Mr. Sadiq Umar, Maharishi Arvind Institute of Science and Management (MAISM) needs to be mentioned, and whose unflinching support in language editing has no parallel…

ABBREVIATIONS

AcOH	acetic acid
AMK	amikacin
BCG	Bacille Calmette Guerin
BDQ	bedaquiline
CIP	ciprofloxacin
CNS	central nervous system
Ddn	deazaflavin-dependent nitroreducatase
DMF	N,N-dimethylformamide
DFDNB	1,5-difluoro-2,4-dinitrobenzene
DNA	deoxyribonucleic acid
DOTS	directly observed treatment short-course
DprE1	decaprenylphosphoryl-β-D-ribose 2'-oxidase
EB	ethambutol
ETH	ethionamide
EtOH	ethanol
FGD1	deazaflavin F420 dependent glucose-6-phosphate dehydrogenase
HIV	human immuno deficiency virus
HMG-CoA	3-hydroxy-3-methyl-glutaryl-coenzyme A reductase
INH	isoniazid
KM	kanamycin
LeuRS	leucyl-tRNA synthase
LTBI	latent tuberculosis infection

MDR	multidrug resistant
MIC	minimum inhibitory concentration
MXF	moxifloxacin
MTB	Mycobacterium tuberculosis
NTM	nontuberculous mycobacterial
NTZ	Nitazoxanide
p-TsOH	p-toluenesulfonic acid
PZA	pyrazinamide
RIF	rifampin
RNA	ribonucleic acid
SAR	structure activity relationship
TB	Tuberculosis
TEA	triethylamine
THF	tetrahydrofuran
TDM	trehalose dimycolate
TMM	trehalose monomycolate
XDR	extensively drug resistant
WHO	World Health Organization

REFERENCES

[1] WHO. Global Tuberculosis Report 2016. ISBN 9 789241 565394

[2] Cox HS, Ford N, Reeder JC. Are we really that good at treating tuberculosis? Lancet Infect Dis 2009; 9(3): 138-9.
[http://dx.doi.org/10.1016/S1473-3099(09)70025-8] [PMID: 19246014]

[3] Das B, Kashino SS, Pulu I, *et al.* CD271(+) bone marrow mesenchymal stem cells may provide a niche for dormant Mycobacterium tuberculosis. Sci Trans Med 2013; 5: 170-3.

[4] Cohen J. Infectious disease. Approval of novel TB drug celebrated-with restraint. Sci 2013; 339: 130.
[http://dx.doi.org/10.1126/science.339.6116.130]

[5] Ryan NJ, Lo JH. Delamanid: first global approval. Drugs 2014; 74(9): 1041-5.
[http://dx.doi.org/10.1007/s40265-014-0241-5] [PMID: 24923253]

[6] European public assessment report (EPAR) for Sirturo , [December 02, 2014]; Available at: http://www.ema.europa.eu/docs/en_GB/document_library/EPAR_-_Summary_for_the_public/human/002614/WC500163211.pdf

[7] European public assessment report (EPAR) for Deltyba , [December 02, 2014]; Available at: http://www.ema.europa.eu/docs/en_GB/document_library/EPAR_-_Summary_for_the_public/human/002552/WC500166235.pdf

[8] Rivers EC, Mancera RL. New anti-tuberculosis drugs in clinical trials with novel mechanisms of action. Drug Discov Today 2008; 13(23-24): 1090-8.
[http://dx.doi.org/10.1016/j.drudis.2008.09.004] [PMID: 18840542]

[9] Sriram D, Yogeeswari P. Medicinal Chemistry. 2nd ed., Doerge: Dorling Kindersley (India) Pvt. Ltd.

2014.

[10] David AW, Thomas LL, Foye WO. Principal of Medicinal Chemistry. 4th ed. Philadelphia: Lippincott William and Wilkins 2002; pp. 384-407.

[11] Wolf ME. Burger's Medicinal Chemistry. 5th ed. New York: John Wiley and Sons 2005; pp. 264-319.

[12] Tripathi KD. The Text Book of Medical Pharmacology. 5th ed. New Delhi: JP Publication 2005; pp. 369-80.

[13] Thomas JP, Baughn CO, Wilkinson RG, Shepherd RG. A new synthetic compound with antituberculous activity in mice: ethambutol (dextro-2,2′-(ethylenediimino)-di-l-butanol). Am Rev Respir Dis 1961; 83: 891-3.
[PMID: 13776497]

[14] Belanger AE, Besra GS, Ford ME, *et al.* The embAB genes of Mycobacterium avium encode an arabinosyl transferase involved in cell wall arabinan biosynthesis that is the target for the antimycobacterial drug ethambutol. Proc Natl Acad Sci USA 1996; 93(21): 11919-24.
[http://dx.doi.org/10.1073/pnas.93.21.11919] [PMID: 8876238]

[15] Sensai P, Grassi GG. Antimycobacterial agents. In: Abraham Donald J, Ed. Burger's Medicinal Chemistry & Drug Discovery. 6th ed. 807-80.

[16] Pai M, Behr MA, Dowdy D, *et al.* Tuberculosis. Nat Rev Dis Primers 2016; 2: 16076.
[http://dx.doi.org/10.1038/nrdp.2016.76] [PMID: 27784885]

[17] Vardanyan RS, Hruby VJ. Synthesis of essential drugs. the Netherland: Elsevier 2006.

[18] Timmins GS, Deretic V. Mechanisms of action of isoniazid. Mol Microbiol 2006; 62(5): 1220-7.
[http://dx.doi.org/10.1111/j.1365-2958.2006.05467.x] [PMID: 17074073]

[19] Winder FG, Collins PB. Inhibition by isoniazid of synthesis of mycolic acids in Mycobacterium tuberculosis. J Gen Microbiol 1970; 63(1): 41-8.
[http://dx.doi.org/10.1099/00221287-63-1-41] [PMID: 5500025]

[20] Banerjee A, Dubnau E, Quemard A, *et al.* inhA, a gene encoding a target for isoniazid and ethionamide in Mycobacterium tuberculosis. Science 1994; 263(5144): 227-30.
[http://dx.doi.org/10.1126/science.8284673] [PMID: 8284673]

[21] Malone L, Schurr A, Lindh H, McKENZIE D, Kiser JS, Williams JH. The effect of pyrazinamide (aldinamide) on experimental tuberculosis in mice. Am Rev Tuberc 1952; 65(5): 511-8.
[PMID: 14924173]

[22] Zhang Y, Mitchison D. The curious characteristics of pyrazinamide: a review. Int J Tuberc Lung Dis 2003; 7(1): 6-21.
[PMID: 12701830]

[23] Zhang Y, Wade MM, Scorpio A, Zhang H, Sun Z. Mode of action of pyrazinamide: disruption of Mycobacterium tuberculosis membrane transport and energetics by pyrazinoic acid. J Antimicrob Chemother 2003; 52(5): 790-5.
[http://dx.doi.org/10.1093/jac/dkg446] [PMID: 14563891]

[24] Shi W, Zhang X, Jiang X, *et al.* Pyrazinamide inhibits trans-translation in Mycobacterium tuberculosis. Science 2011; 333(6049): 1630-2.
[http://dx.doi.org/10.1126/science.1208813] [PMID: 21835980]

[25] Zhang Y. The magic bullets and tuberculosis drug targets. Annu Rev Pharmacol Toxicol 2005; 45: 529-64.
[http://dx.doi.org/10.1146/annurev.pharmtox.45.120403.100120] [PMID: 15822188]

[26] Boeree MJ, Heinrich N, Aarnoutse R, *et al.* PanACEA consortium. High-dose rifampicin, moxifloxacin, and SQ109 for treating tuberculosis: a multi-arm, multi-stage randomised controlled trial. Lancet Infect Dis 2017; 17(1): 39-49.
[http://dx.doi.org/10.1016/S1473-3099(16)30274-2] [PMID: 28100438]

[27] Dorman SE, Goldberg S, Stout JE, *et al.* Tuberculosis Trials Consortium. Substitution of rifapentine for rifampin during intensive phase treatment of pulmonary tuberculosis: study 29 of the tuberculosis trials consortium. J Infect Dis 2012; 206(7): 1030-40.
[http://dx.doi.org/10.1093/infdis/jis461] [PMID: 22850121]

[28] Schatz A, Waksman SA. Effect of streptomycin and other antibiotic substances upon Mycobacterium tuberculosis and related organisms. Proc Soc Exp Biol Med 1944; 57: 244-8.
[http://dx.doi.org/10.3181/00379727-57-14769]

[29] Carter AP, Clemons WM, Bordersen DE, Morgan-Warren RJ, Wimberly BT, Ramakrishnan B. Functional insights from the structure of the 30S ribosomal subunit and its interactions with antibiotics. Nature 2000; 407(6802): 340-8.

[30] Garvin RT, Biswas DK, Gorini L. The effects of streptomycin or dihydrostreptomycin binding to 16S RNA or to 30S ribosomal subunits. Proc Natl Acad Sci USA 1974; 71(10): 3814-8.
[http://dx.doi.org/10.1073/pnas.71.10.3814] [PMID: 4139702]

[31] Quémard A, Lanéelle G, Lacave C. Mycolic acid synthesis: a target for ethionamide in mycobacteria? Antimicrob Agents Chemother 1992; 36(6): 1316-21.
[http://dx.doi.org/10.1128/AAC.36.6.1316] [PMID: 1416831]

[32] Singh H, Kapoor VK. Medicinal and Pharmaceutical Chemistry. 2nd ed., Delhi: Vallabh Prakashan 2010.

[33] David HL, Takayama K, Goldman DS. Susceptibility of mycobacterial D-alanyl-D-alanine synthetase to D-cycloserine. Am Rev Respir Dis 1969; 100(4): 579-81.
[PMID: 4981706]

[34] Akbergenov R, Shcherbakov D, Matt T, *et al.* Molecular basis for the selectivity of antituberculosis compounds capreomycin and viomycin. Antimicrob Agents Chemother 2011; 55(10): 4712-7.
[http://dx.doi.org/10.1128/AAC.00628-11] [PMID: 21768509]

[35] Johansen SK, Maus CE, Plikaytis BB, Douthwaite S. Capreomycin binds across the ribosomal subunit interface using tlyA-encoded 2′-O-methylations in 16S and 23S rRNAs. Mol Cell 2006; 23(2): 173-82.
[http://dx.doi.org/10.1016/j.molcel.2006.05.044] [PMID: 16857584]

[36] Yamori S, Ichiyama S, Shimokata K, Tsukamura M. Bacteriostatic and bactericidal activity of antituberculosis drugs against Mycobacterium tuberculosis, Mycobacterium avium-Mycobacterium intracellulare complex and Mycobacterium kansasii in different growth phases. Microbiol Immunol 1992; 36(4): 361-8.
[http://dx.doi.org/10.1111/j.1348-0421.1992.tb02035.x] [PMID: 1406364]

[37] Selvakumar N, Kumar V, Acharyulu GS, Rehman F, Paramasivan CN, Prabhakar R. Susceptibility of south Indian strains of Mycobacterium tuberculosis to tuberactinomycin. Indian J Med Res 1992; 95: 101-4.
[PMID: 1506058]

[38] Nakayama M, Miura H, Kamei T. Investigation of Vestibular Damage by Antituberculous Drugs. Acta Oto-Laryngologica 1991; 111(Sup481): 481-5.

[39] Mitscher LA. Bacterial topoisomerase inhibitors: quinolone and pyridone antibacterial agents. Chem Rev 2005; 105(2): 559-92.
[http://dx.doi.org/10.1021/cr030101q] [PMID: 15700957]

[40] Aubry A, Pan XS, Fisher LM, Jarlier V, Cambau E. Mycobacterium tuberculosis DNA gyrase: interaction with quinolones and correlation with antimycobacterial drug activity. Antimicrob Agents Chemother 2004; 48(4): 1281-8.
[http://dx.doi.org/10.1128/AAC.48.4.1281-1288.2004] [PMID: 15047530]

[41] Lounis N, Roscigno G. *In vitro* and *in vivo* activities of new rifamycin derivatives against mycobacterial infections. Curr Pharm Des 2004; 10(26): 3229-38.
[http://dx.doi.org/10.2174/1381612043383287] [PMID: 15544512]

[42] Rammohan RD, Dwivedi SD, Sreenivasulu P, Sahu A, Trinadhachari GN, Sasi KS. An improved process for the preparation of levofloxacin hemihydrate Available at: https://www.google.com/patents/WO2006048889A1?cl=en

[43] Sanchez JP, Gogliotti RD, Domagala JM, *et al.* The synthesis, structure-activity, and structure-side effect relationships of a series of 8-alkoxy- and 5-amino-8-alkoxyquinolone antibacterial agents. J Med Chem 1995; 38(22): 4478-87. [http://dx.doi.org/10.1021/jm00022a013] [PMID: 7473575]

[44] Petersen U, Schröck W, Habich D, *et al.* Quinolonecarboxylic acids 1996. US 5480879 A

[45] Bernstein J, Lott WA, Steinberg BA, Yale HL. Chemotherapy of experimental tuberculosis. V. Isonicotinic acid hydrazide (nydrazid) and related compounds. Am Rev Tuberc 1952; 65(4): 357-64. [PMID: 14903503]

[46] Rengarajan J, Sassetti CM, Naroditskaya V, Sloutsky A, Bloom BR, Rubin EJ. The folate pathway is a target for resistance to the drug para-aminosalicylic acid (PAS) in mycobacteria. Mol Microbiol 2004; 53(1): 275-82. [http://dx.doi.org/10.1111/j.1365-2958.2004.04120.x] [PMID: 15225321]

[47] Alahari A, Trivelli X, Guérardel Y, *et al.* Thiacetazone, an antitubercular drug that inhibits cyclopropanation of cell wall mycolic acids in mycobacteria. PLoS One 2007; 2(12): e1343. [http://dx.doi.org/10.1371/journal.pone.0001343] [PMID: 18094751]

[48] http://www.newtbdrugs.org [Access on: December 02, 2016]

[49] https://www.tballiance.org [Access on: December 02, 2016]

[50] Skerry C, Pinn ML, Bruiners N, Pine R, Gennaro ML, Karakousis PC. Simvastatin increases the in vivo activity of the first-line tuberculosis regimen. J Antimicrob Chemother 2014; 69(9): 2453-7. [http://dx.doi.org/10.1093/jac/dku166] [PMID: 24855121]

[51] Kling A, Lukat P, Almeida DV, *et al.* Antibiotics. Targeting DnaN for tuberculosis therapy using novel griselimycins. Sci 2015; 348(6239): 1106-12. [http://dx.doi.org/10.1126/science.aaa4690]

[52] http://www.uccz.nl/media/36718/new_drug_ treatment_in_era_of_mdr_tb.pdf [Access on: 15 July 2014]

[53] Ishizaki Y, Hayashi C, Inoue K, *et al.* Inhibition of the first step in synthesis of the mycobacterial cell wall core, catalyzed by the GlcNAc-1-phosphate transferase WecA, by the novel caprazaymicin derivative CPZEN-45. J Biochem 2013; 288: 303039-30319.

[54] http://www.newtbdrugs.org/project.php?id=145 [Access on: 26 September 2013]

[55] Lee RE, Hurdle JG, Liu J, *et al.* Spectinamides: a new class of semisynthetic antituberculosis agents that overcome native drug efflux. Nat Med 2014; 20(2): 152-8. [http://dx.doi.org/10.1038/nm.3458] [PMID: 24464186]

[56] Kasim NA, Whitehouse M, Ramachandran C, *et al.* Molecular properties of WHO essential drugs and provisional biopharmaceutical classification. Mol Pharm 2004; 1(1): 85-96. [http://dx.doi.org/10.1021/mp034006h] [PMID: 15832504]

[57] Barry VC, Belton JG, Conalty ML, *et al.* A new series of phenazines (rimino-compounds) with high antituberculosis activity. Nature 1957; 179(4568): 1013-5. [http://dx.doi.org/10.1038/1791013a0] [PMID: 13430770]

[58] Zhang D, Lu Y, Liu K, *et al.* Identification of less lipophilic riminophenazine derivatives for the treatment of drug-resistant tuberculosis. J Med Chem 2012; 55(19): 8409-17. [http://dx.doi.org/10.1021/jm300828h] [PMID: 22931472]

[59] Yano T, Kassovska-Bratinova S, Teh JS, *et al.* Reduction of clofazimine by mycobacterial type 2 NADH:quinone oxidoreductase: a pathway for the generation of bactericidal levels of reactive oxygen

species. J Biol Chem 2011; 286(12): 10276-87.
[http://dx.doi.org/10.1074/jbc.M110.200501] [PMID: 21193400]

[60] Bogatcheva E, Hanrahan C, Nikonenko B, *et al.* Identification of SQ609 as a lead compound from a library of dipiperidines. Bioorg Med Chem Lett 2011; 21(18): 5353-7.
[http://dx.doi.org/10.1016/j.bmcl.2011.07.015] [PMID: 21807506]

[61] Bogatcheva E, Hanrahan C, Chen P, *et al.* Discovery of dipiperidines as new antitubercular agents. Bioorg Med Chem Lett 2010; 20(1): 201-5.
[http://dx.doi.org/10.1016/j.bmcl.2009.10.135] [PMID: 19917527]

[62] Makarov V, Manina G, Mikusova K, *et al.* Benzothiazinones kill Mycobacterium tuberculosis by blocking arabinan synthesis. Science 2009; 324(5928): 801-4.
[http://dx.doi.org/10.1126/science.1171583] [PMID: 19299584]

[63] Antitubercular profile of GSK070 a Mycobacterium tuberculosis leucyl-tRNA synthetase inhibitor Available at: https://www.escmid.org/escmid_publications/escmid_elibrary/material/?mid=31146

[64] Makarov V, Möllmann U, Cole ST. New benzothiazinone derivatives and their use as antibacterial agents 2007. WO2007134625

[65] Makarov V, Lechartier B, Zhang M, *et al.* Towards a new combination therapy for tuberculosis with next generation benzothiazinones. EMBO Mol Med 2014; 6(3): 372-83.
[http://dx.doi.org/10.1002/emmm.201303575] [PMID: 24500695]

[66] Makarov V, Neres J, Hartkoorn RC, *et al.* The 8-pyrrole benzthiazinones are noncovalent inhibitors of DprE1 from *Mycobacterium tuberculosis.* Antimicrob Agents Chemother 2015; 59(8): 4446-52.
[http://dx.doi.org/10.1128/AAC.00778-15] [PMID: 25987616]

[67] Kang S, Kim RY, Seo MJ, *et al.* Lead optimization of a novel series of imidazo[1,2-*a*]pyridine amides leading to a clinical candidate (Q203) as a multi- and extensively-drug-resistant anti-tuberculosis agent. J Med Chem 2014; 57(12): 5293-305.
[http://dx.doi.org/10.1021/jm5003606] [PMID: 24870926]

[68] Pethe K, Bifani P, Jang J, *et al.* Discovery of Q203, a potent clinical candidate for the treatment of tuberculosis. Nat Med 2013; 19(9): 1157-60.
[http://dx.doi.org/10.1038/nm.3262] [PMID: 23913123]

[69] Zumla A, Nahid P, Cole ST. Advances in the development of new tuberculosis drugs and treatment regimens. Nat Rev Drug Discov 2013; 12(5): 388-404.
[http://dx.doi.org/10.1038/nrd4001] [PMID: 23629506]

[70] Ge Z, Li R, Cheng T. An efficient synthesis of formylmethyl piperidine-1-carbodithioate diethyl acetal and analogs. Synth Commun 1999; 29: 3191-6.
[http://dx.doi.org/10.1080/00397919908085943]

[71] Sacksteder KA, Protopopova M, Barry CE III, Andries K, Nacy CA. Discovery and development of SQ109: a new antitubercular drug with a novel mechanism of action. Future Microbiol 2012; 7(7): 823-37.
[http://dx.doi.org/10.2217/fmb.12.56] [PMID: 22827305]

[72] Lee RE, Protopopova M, Crooks E, Slayden RA, Terrot M, Barry CE III. Combinatorial lead optimization of [1,2]-diamines based on ethambutol as potential antituberculosis preclinical candidates. J Comb Chem 2003; 5(2): 172-87.
[http://dx.doi.org/10.1021/cc020071p] [PMID: 12625709]

[73] Protopopova M, Hanrahan C, Nikonenko B, *et al.* Identification of a new antitubercular drug candidate, SQ109, from a combinatorial library of 1,2-ethylenediamines. J Antimicrob Chemother 2005; 56(5): 968-74.
[http://dx.doi.org/10.1093/jac/dki319] [PMID: 16172107]

[74] Onajole OK, Govender P, van Helden PD, *et al.* Synthesis and evaluation of SQ109 analogues as potential anti-tuberculosis candidates. Eur J Med Chem 2010; 45(5): 2075-9.

[http://dx.doi.org/10.1016/j.ejmech.2010.01.046] [PMID: 20149497]

[75] Heinrich N, Dawson R, du Bois J, *et al.* Pan African Consortium for the Evaluation of Antituberculosis Antibiotics (PanACEA). Early phase evaluation of SQ109 alone and in combination with rifampicin in pulmonary TB patients. J Antimicrob Chemother 2015; 70(5): 1558-66. [http://dx.doi.org/10.1093/jac/dku553] [PMID: 25630641]

[76] Reddy VM, Einck L, Andries K, Nacy CA. *In vitro* interactions between new antitubercular drug candidates SQ109 and TMC207. Antimicrob Agents Chemother 2010; 54(7): 2840-6. [http://dx.doi.org/10.1128/AAC.01601-09] [PMID: 20385864]

[77] Tahlan K, Wilson R, Kastrinsky DB, *et al.* SQ109 targets MmpL3, a membrane transporter of trehalose monomycolate involved in mycolic acid donation to the cell wall core of Mycobacterium tuberculosis. Antimicrob Agents Chemother 2012; 56(4): 1797-809. [http://dx.doi.org/10.1128/AAC.05708-11] [PMID: 22252828]

[78] de Carvalho LP, Lin G, Jiang X, Nathan C. Nitazoxanide kills replicating and nonreplicating Mycobacterium tuberculosis and evades resistance. J Med Chem 2009; 52(19): 5789-92. [http://dx.doi.org/10.1021/jm9010719] [PMID: 19736929]

[79] Shigyo K, Ocheretina O, Merveille YM, *et al.* Efficacy of nitazoxanide against clinical isolates of *Mycobacterium tuberculosis.* Antimicrob Agents Chemother 2013; 57(6): 2834-7. [http://dx.doi.org/10.1128/AAC.02542-12] [PMID: 23507275]

[80] Lam KK, Zheng X, Forestieri R, *et al.* Nitazoxanide stimulates autophagy and inhibits mTORC1 signaling and intracellular proliferation of Mycobacterium tuberculosis. PLoS Pathog 2012; 8(5): e1002691. [http://dx.doi.org/10.1371/journal.ppat.1002691] [PMID: 22589723]

[81] New derivatives of 2-benzamido-5-nitro thiazoles Available at: https://www.google.ch/patents/US3950351

[82] Dooley KE, Obuku EA, Durakovic N, Belitsky V, Mitnick C, Nuermberger EL. Efficacy Subgroup, RESIST-TB. World Health Organization group 5 drugs for the treatment of drug-resistant tuberculosis: unclear efficacy or untapped potential? J Infect Dis 2013; 207(9): 1352-8. [http://dx.doi.org/10.1093/infdis/jis460] [PMID: 22807518]

[83] Dey T, Brigden G, Cox H, Shubber Z, Cooke G, Ford N. Outcomes of clofazimine for the treatment of drug-resistant tuberculosis: a systematic review and meta-analysis. J Antimicrob Chemother 2013; 68(2): 284-93. [http://dx.doi.org/10.1093/jac/dks389] [PMID: 23054996]

[84] Tang S, Yao L, Hao X, *et al.* Clofazimine for the treatment of multidrug-resistant tuberculosis: prospective, multicenter, randomized controlled study in China. Clin Infect Dis 2015; 60(9): 1361-7. [PMID: 25605283]

[85] Hugonnet JE, Tremblay LW, Boshoff HI, Barry CE III, Blanchard JS. Meropenem-clavulanate is effective against extensively drug-resistant *Mycobacterium tuberculosis.* Science 2009; 323(5918): 1215-8. [http://dx.doi.org/10.1126/science.1167498] [PMID: 19251630]

[86] Hugonnet JE, Blanchard JS. Irreversible inhibition of the Mycobacterium tuberculosis beta-lactamase by clavulanate. Biochemistry 2007; 46(43): 11998-2004. [http://dx.doi.org/10.1021/bi701506h] [PMID: 17915954]

[87] Gootz TD, Brighty KE. Fluoroquinolone antibacterials: SAR mechanism of action, resistance, and clinical aspects. Med Res Rev 1996; 16(5): 433-86. [http://dx.doi.org/10.1002/(SICI)1098-1128(199609)16:5<433::AID-MED3>3.0.CO;2-W] [PMID: 8865150]

[88] Tillotson GS. Quinolones: structure-activity relationships and future predictions. J Med Microbiol 1996; 44(5): 320-4.

[http://dx.doi.org/10.1099/00222615-44-5-320] [PMID: 8636945]

[89] Alsultan A, An G, Peloquin CA. Limited sampling strategy and target attainment analysis for levofloxacin in patients with tuberculosis. Antimicrob Agents Chemother 2015; 59(7): 3800-7. [http://dx.doi.org/10.1128/AAC.00341-15] [PMID: 25870068]

[90] Wang JY, Wang JT, Tsai TH, *et al.* Adding moxifloxacin is associated with a shorter time to culture conversion in pulmonary tuberculosis. Int J Tuberc Lung Dis 2010; 14(1): 65-71. [PMID: 20003697]

[91] Dorman SE, Johnson JL, Goldberg S, *et al.* Tuberculosis Trials Consortium. Substitution of moxifloxacin for isoniazid during intensive phase treatment of pulmonary tuberculosis. Am J Respir Crit Care Med 2009; 180(3): 273-80. [http://dx.doi.org/10.1164/rccm.200901-0078OC] [PMID: 19406981]

[92] Conde MB, Efron A, Loredo C, *et al.* Moxifloxacin *versus* ethambutol in the initial treatment of tuberculosis: a double-blind, randomised, controlled phase II trial. Lancet 2009; 373(9670): 1183-9. [http://dx.doi.org/10.1016/S0140-6736(09)60333-0] [PMID: 19345831]

[93] Rustomjee R, Lienhardt C, Kanyok T, *et al.* Gatifloxacin for TB (OFLOTUB) study team. A Phase II study of the sterilising activities of ofloxacin, gatifloxacin and moxifloxacin in pulmonary tuberculosis. Int J Tuberc Lung Dis 2008; 12(2): 128-38. [PMID: 18230244]

[94] Moxifloxacin. Tuberculosis (Edinb) 2008; 88(2): 127-31. [http://dx.doi.org/10.1016/S1472-9792(08)70016-7] [PMID: 18486050]

[95] Barry AL. *In vitro* evaluation of DuP 105 and DuP 721, two new oxazolidinone antimicrobial agents. Antimicrob Agents Chemother 1988; 32(1): 150-2. [http://dx.doi.org/10.1128/AAC.32.1.150] [PMID: 3348606]

[96] Brickner SJ, Hutchinson DK, Barbachyn MR, *et al.* Synthesis and antibacterial activity of U-100592 and U-100766, two oxazolidinone antibacterial agents for the potential treatment of multidrug-resistant gram-positive bacterial infections. J Med Chem 1996; 39(3): 673-9. [http://dx.doi.org/10.1021/jm9509556] [PMID: 8576909]

[97] Zhang Y, Post-Martens K, Denkin S. New drug candidates and therapeutic targets for tuberculosis therapy. Drug Discov Today 2006; 11(1-2): 21-7. [http://dx.doi.org/10.1016/S1359-6446(05)03626-3] [PMID: 16478687]

[98] Schecter GF, Scott C, True L, Raftery A, Flood J, Mase S. Linezolid in the treatment of multidrug-resistant tuberculosis. Clin Infect Dis 2010; 50(1): 49-55. [http://dx.doi.org/10.1086/648675] [PMID: 19947856]

[99] Wallis RS, Jakubiec WM, Kumar V, *et al.* Pharmacokinetics and whole-blood bactericidal activity against Mycobacterium tuberculosis of single doses of PNU-100480 in healthy volunteers. J Infect Dis 2010; 202(5): 745-51. [http://dx.doi.org/10.1086/655471] [PMID: 20629533]

[100] Biava M, Porretta GC, Deidda D, Pompei R. New trends in development of antimycobacterial compounds. Infect Disord Drug Targets 2006; 6(2): 159-72. [http://dx.doi.org/10.2174/187152606784112173] [PMID: 16789877]

[101] Poce G, Cocozza M, Consalvi S, Biava M. SAR analysis of new anti-TB drugs currently in pre-clinical and clinical development. Eur J Med Chem 2014; 86: 335-51. [http://dx.doi.org/10.1016/j.ejmech.2014.08.066] [PMID: 25173852]

[102] Barbachyn MR, Ford CW. Oxazolidinone structure-activity relationships leading to linezolid. Angew Chem Int Ed Engl 2003; 42(18): 2010-23. [http://dx.doi.org/10.1002/anie.200200528] [PMID: 12746812]

[103] Pearlman B, Perrault AW, Barbachyn RM, *et al.* Process to prepare oxazolidinones 1997. WO/1997/037980

[104] Brooks JV, Furney SK, Orme IM. Metronidazole therapy in mice infected with tuberculosis. Antimicrob Agents Chemother 1999; 43(5): 1285-8.
[PMID: 10223954]

[105] Ashtekar DR, Costa-Perira R, Nagrajan K, Vishvanathan N, Bhatt AD, Rittel W. *In vitro* and *in vivo* activities of the nitroimidazole CGI 17341 against Mycobacterium tuberculosis. Antimicrob Agents Chemother 1993; 37(2): 183-6.
[http://dx.doi.org/10.1128/AAC.37.2.183] [PMID: 8452346]

[106] Ma Z, Ginsberg AM, Spigelman M. Antimycobacterial Agents. In: Taylor JB, Triggle DJ, Eds. Comprehensive Medicinal Chemistry II. Amsterdam: Elsevier Science B. V 2007; Vol. 7: pp. 699-730.
[http://dx.doi.org/10.1016/B0-08-045044-X/00224-8]

[107] Stover CK, Warrener P, VanDevanter DR, *et al.* A small-molecule nitroimidazopyran drug candidate for the treatment of tuberculosis. Nature 2000; 405(6789): 962-6.
[http://dx.doi.org/10.1038/35016103] [PMID: 10879539]

[108] Lenaerts AJ, Gruppo V, Marietta KS, *et al.* Preclinical testing of the nitroimidazopyran PA-824 for activity against Mycobacterium tuberculosis in a series of *in vitro* and *in vivo* models. Antimicrob Agents Chemother 2005; 49(6): 2294-301.
[http://dx.doi.org/10.1128/AAC.49.6.2294-2301.2005] [PMID: 15917524]

[109] Manjunatha UH, Boshoff H, Dowd CS, *et al.* Identification of a nitroimidazo-oxazine-specific protein involved in PA-824 resistance in Mycobacterium tuberculosis. Proc Natl Acad Sci USA 2006; 103(2): 431-6.
[http://dx.doi.org/10.1073/pnas.0508392103] [PMID: 16387854]

[110] Singh R, Manjunatha U, Boshoff HI, *et al.* PA-824 kills nonreplicating Mycobacterium tuberculosis by intracellular NO release. Science 2008; 322(5906): 1392-5.
[http://dx.doi.org/10.1126/science.1164571] [PMID: 19039139]

[111] Manjunatha U, Boshoff HI, Barry CE. The mechanism of action of PA-824: Novel insights from transcriptional profiling. Commun Integr Biol 2009; 2(3): 215-8.
[http://dx.doi.org/10.4161/cib.2.3.7926] [PMID: 19641733]

[112] Villemagne B, Crauste C, Flipo M, Baulard AR, Déprez B, Willand N. Tuberculosis: the drug development pipeline at a glance. Eur J Med Chem 2012; 51: 1-16.
[http://dx.doi.org/10.1016/j.ejmech.2012.02.033] [PMID: 22421275]

[113] Baker WR, Shaopei C, Keeler EL. Nitroimidazole antibacterial compounds and methods of use thereof 1997.WO/1997/001562

[114] Kim P, Zhang L, Manjunatha UH, *et al.* Structure-activity relationships of antitubercular nitroimidazoles. 1. Structural features associated with aerobic and anaerobic activities of 4- and 5-nitroimidazoles. J Med Chem 2009; 52(5): 1317-28.
[http://dx.doi.org/10.1021/jm801246z] [PMID: 19209889]

[115] Kim P, Kang S, Boshoff HI, *et al.* Structure-activity relationships of antitubercular nitroimidazoles. 2. Determinants of aerobic activity and quantitative structure-activity relationships. J Med Chem 2009; 52(5): 1329-44.
[http://dx.doi.org/10.1021/jm801374t] [PMID: 19209893]

[116] Blaser A, Palmer BD, Sutherland HS, *et al.* Structure-activity relationships for amide-, carbamate-, and urea-linked analogues of the tuberculosis drug (6S)-2-nitro-6-[4-(trifluoromethoxy)benzy-]oxy-6,7-dihydro-5H-imidazo[2,1-b][1,3]oxazine (PA-824). J Med Chem 2012; 55(1): 312-26.
[http://dx.doi.org/10.1021/jm2012276] [PMID: 22148391]

[117] Barry CE III, Boshoff HI, Dowd CS. Prospects for clinical introduction of nitroimidazole antibiotics for the treatment of tuberculosis. Curr Pharm Des 2004; 10(26): 3239-62.
[http://dx.doi.org/10.2174/1381612043383214] [PMID: 15544513]

[118] Sasaki H, Haraguchi Y, Itotani M, *et al.* Synthesis and antituberculosis activity of a novel series of

optically active 6-nitro-2,3-dihydroimidazo[2,1-b]oxazoles. J Med Chem 2006; 49(26): 7854-60. [http://dx.doi.org/10.1021/jm060957y] [PMID: 17181168]

[119] Matsumoto M, Hashizume H, Tomishige T, *et al.* OPC-67683, a nitro-dihydro-imidazooxazole derivative with promising action against tuberculosis *in vitro* and in mice. PLoS Med 2006; 3(11): e466.
[http://dx.doi.org/10.1371/journal.pmed.0030466] [PMID: 17132069]

[120] Skripconoka V, Danilovits M, Pehme L, *et al.* Delamanid improves outcomes and reduces mortality in multidrug-resistant tuberculosis. Eur Respir J 2013; 41(6): 1393-400.
[http://dx.doi.org/10.1183/09031936.00125812] [PMID: 23018916]

[121] Andries K, Verhasselt P, Guillemont J, *et al.* A diarylquinoline drug active on the ATP synthase of Mycobacterium tuberculosis. Science 2005; 307(5707): 223-7.
[http://dx.doi.org/10.1126/science.1106753] [PMID: 15591164]

[122] Guillemont J, Meyer C, Poncelet A, Bourdrez X, Andries K. Diarylquinolines, synthesis pathways and quantitative structure--activity relationship studies leading to the discovery of TMC207. Future Med Chem 2011; 3(11): 1345-60.
[http://dx.doi.org/10.4155/fmc.11.79] [PMID: 21879841]

[123] Rustomjee R, Diacon AH, Allen J, *et al.* Early bactericidal activity and pharmacokinetics of the diarylquinoline TMC207 in treatment of pulmonary tuberculosis. Antimicrob Agents Chemother 2008; 52(8): 2831-5.
[http://dx.doi.org/10.1128/AAC.01204-07] [PMID: 18505852]

[124] Guillemont JEG, Van Gestel JFE, Venet MG, Poignet HJJ, Decrane LFB, Vernier D. Quinoline derivatives and their use as mycobacterial inhibitors 2004.WO2004/011436 A1

[125] Cole ST, Brosch R, Parkhill J, *et al.* Deciphering the biology of Mycobacterium tuberculosis from the complete genome sequence. Nature 1998; 393(6685): 537-44.
[http://dx.doi.org/10.1038/31159] [PMID: 9634230]

[126] Flynn JL. Immunology of tuberculosis and implications in vaccine development. Tuberculosis (Edinb) 2004; 84(1-2): 93-101.
[http://dx.doi.org/10.1016/j.tube.2003.08.010] [PMID: 14670350]

[127] Flynn JL, Chan J, Triebold KJ, Dalton DK, Stewart TA, Bloom BR. An essential role for interferon gamma in resistance to Mycobacterium tuberculosis infection. J Exp Med 1993; 178(6): 2249-54.
[http://dx.doi.org/10.1084/jem.178.6.2249] [PMID: 7504064]

[128] Rodríguez-Güell E, Agustí G, Corominas M, Cardona PJ, Luquin M, Julián E. Mice with pulmonary tuberculosis treated with *Mycobacterium vaccae* develop strikingly enhanced recall gamma interferon responses to *M. vaccae* cell wall skeleton. Clin Vaccine Immunol 2008; 15(5): 893-6.
[http://dx.doi.org/10.1128/CVI.00477-07] [PMID: 18337379]

[129] Grode L, Ganoza CA, Brohm C, Weiner J III, Eisele B, Kaufmann SH. Safety and immunogenicity of the recombinant BCG vaccine VPM1002 in a phase 1 open-label randomized clinical trial. Vaccine 2013; 31(9): 1340-8.
[http://dx.doi.org/10.1016/j.vaccine.2012.12.053] [PMID: 23290835]

[130] http://www.vakzine-manager.de/en/resources/ Produkte/VPM1002_en.pdf

[131] Montoya J, Solon JA, Cunanan SR, *et al.* A randomized, controlled dose-finding Phase II study of the M72/AS01 candidate tuberculosis vaccine in healthy PPD-positive adults. J Clin Immunol 2013; 33(8): 1360-75.
[http://dx.doi.org/10.1007/s10875-013-9949-3] [PMID: 24142232]

[132] Day CL, Tameris M, Mansoor N, *et al.* Induction and regulation of T-cell immunity by the novel tuberculosis vaccine M72/AS01 in South African adults. Am J Respir Crit Care Med 2013; 188(4): 492-502.
[http://dx.doi.org/10.1164/rccm.201208-1385OC] [PMID: 23306546]

[133] http://www.tbvaccines2013.org/wp

[134] Vilaplana C, Montané E, Pinto S, *et al.* Double-blind, randomized, placebo-controlled Phase I Clinical Trial of the therapeutical antituberculous vaccine RUTI. Vaccine 2010; 28(4): 1106-16. [http://dx.doi.org/10.1016/j.vaccine.2009.09.134] [PMID: 19853680]

[135] Guirado E, Gil O, Cáceres N, Singh M, Vilaplana C, Cardona PJ. Induction of a specific strong polyantigenic cellular immune response after short-term chemotherapy controls bacillary reactivation in murine and guinea pig experimental models of tuberculosis. Clin Vaccine Immunol 2008; 15(8): 1229-37. [http://dx.doi.org/10.1128/CVI.00094-08] [PMID: 18524883]

[136] Cardona PJ, Amat I. [Origin and development of RUTI, a new therapeutic vaccine against *Mycobacterium tuberculosis* infection]. Arch Bronconeumol 2006; 42(1): 25-32. [PMID: 16426520]

[137] Reither K, Katsoulis L, Beattie T, *et al.* Safety and immunogenicity of H1/IC31®, an adjuvanted TB subunit vaccine, in HIV-infected adults with CD4+ lymphocyte counts greater than 350 cells/mm3: a phase II, multi-centre, double-blind, randomized, placebo-controlled trial. PLoS One 2014; 9(12): e114602. [http://dx.doi.org/10.1371/journal.pone.0114602] [PMID: 25490675]

[138] Mearns H, Geldenhuys HD, Kagina BM, *et al.* THYB04 study group. H1:IC31 vaccination is safe and induces long-lived TNF-α$^{(+)}$IL-2$^{(+)}$CD4 T cell responses in *M. tuberculosis* infected and uninfected adolescents: A randomized trial. Vaccine 2017; 35(1): 132-41. [http://dx.doi.org/10.1016/j.vaccine.2016.11.023] [PMID: 27866772]

[139] Hoang T, Aagaard C, Dietrich J, *et al.* ESAT-6 (EsxA) and TB10.4 (EsxH) based vaccines for pre- and post-exposure tuberculosis vaccination. PLoS One 2013; 8(12): e80579. [http://dx.doi.org/10.1371/journal.pone.0080579] [PMID: 24349004]

[140] Billeskov R, Elvang TT, Andersen PL, Dietrich J. The HyVac4 subunit vaccine efficiently boosts BCG-primed anti-mycobacterial protective immunity. PLoS One 2012; 7(6): e39909. [http://dx.doi.org/10.1371/journal.pone.0039909] [PMID: 22768165]

[141] Orr MT, Beebe EA, Hudson TE, *et al.* A dual TLR agonist adjuvant enhances the immunogenicity and protective efficacy of the tuberculosis vaccine antigen ID93. PLoS One 2014; 9(1): e83884. [http://dx.doi.org/10.1371/journal.pone.0083884] [PMID: 24404140]

[142] Orr MT, Duthie MS, Windish HP, *et al.* MyD88 and TRIF synergistic interaction is required for TH1-cell polarization with a synthetic TLR4 agonist adjuvant. Eur J Immunol 2013; 43(9): 2398-408. [http://dx.doi.org/10.1002/eji.201243124] [PMID: 23716300]

[143] Spertini F, Audran R, Chakour R, *et al.* Safety of human immunisation with a live-attenuated Mycobacterium tuberculosis vaccine: a randomised, double-blind, controlled phase I trial. Lancet Respir Med 2015; 3(12): 953-62. [http://dx.doi.org/10.1016/S2213-2600(15)00435-X] [PMID: 26598141]

[144] Pérez de Val B, Villarreal-Ramos B, Nofrarías M, *et al.* Goats primed with *Mycobacterium bovis* BCG and boosted with a recombinant adenovirus expressing Ag85A show enhanced protection against tuberculosis. Clin Vaccine Immunol 2012; 19(9): 1339-47. [http://dx.doi.org/10.1128/CVI.00275-12] [PMID: 22761299]

[145] Santosuosso M, Zhang X, McCormick S, Wang J, Hitt M, Xing Z. Mechanisms of mucosal and parenteral tuberculosis vaccinations: adenoviral-based mucosal immunization preferentially elicits sustained accumulation of immune protective CD4 and CD8 T cells within the airway lumen. J Immunol 2005; 174(12): 7986-94. [http://dx.doi.org/10.4049/jimmunol.174.12.7986] [PMID: 15944305]

[146] Minassian AM, Rowland R, Beveridge NE, *et al.* A Phase I study evaluating the safety and immunogenicity of MVA85A, a candidate TB vaccine, in HIV-infected adults. BMJ Open 2011; 1(2):

e000223.
[http://dx.doi.org/10.1136/bmjopen-2011-000223] [PMID: 22102640]

[147] Satti I, Meyer J, Harris SA, *et al.* Safety and immunogenicity of a candidate tuberculosis vaccine MVA85A delivered by aerosol in BCG-vaccinated healthy adults: a phase 1, double-blind, randomised controlled trial. Lancet Infect Dis 2014; 14(10): 939-46.
[http://dx.doi.org/10.1016/S1473-3099(14)70845-X] [PMID: 25151225]

[148] Dintwe OB, Day CL, Smit E, *et al.* Heterologous vaccination against human tuberculosis modulates antigen-specific CD4+ T-cell function. Eur J Immunol 2013; 43(9): 2409-20.
[http://dx.doi.org/10.1002/eji.201343454] [PMID: 23737382]

[149] Scriba TJ, Tameris M, Mansoor N, *et al.* Modified vaccinia Ankara-expressing Ag85A, a novel tuberculosis vaccine, is safe in adolescents and children, and induces polyfunctional CD4+ T cells. Eur J Immunol 2010; 40(1): 279-90.
[http://dx.doi.org/10.1002/eji.200939754] [PMID: 20017188]

[150] Walker KB, Guo M, Guo Y, Poecheim J, Velmurugan K, Schrager LK. Novel approaches to preclinical research and TB vaccine development. Tuberculosis (Edinb) 2016; 99 (Suppl. 1): S12-5.
[http://dx.doi.org/10.1016/j.tube.2016.05.012] [PMID: 27452413]

[151] Barcellini L, Borroni E, Brown J, *et al.* First evaluation of QuantiFERON-TB Gold Plus performance in contact screening. Eur Respir J 2016; 48(5): 1411-9.
[http://dx.doi.org/10.1183/13993003.00510-2016] [PMID: 27390280]

[152] Ahsan MJ, Garg SK, Vashistha B, Sharma P. Tuberculosis vaccines: hopes and hurdles. Infect Disord Drug Targets 2013; 13(5): 318-21.
[http://dx.doi.org/10.2174/18715265113666131201125513] [PMID: 24304353]

[153] Ahsan MJ. Recent advances in the development of vaccines for tuberculosis. Ther Adv Vaccines 2015; 3(3): 66-75.
[http://dx.doi.org/10.1177/2051013615593891] [PMID: 26288734]

CHAPTER 5

Recent Advances in Molecular Scaffolds towards the Identification of Novel Receptors in the Treatment of Hepatitis Diseases

Naseem Ahmed*

Department of Chemistry, Indian Institute of Technology Roorkee, Roorkee-247 667, Uttarakhand, India

Abstract: Widespread outbreak of numerous infectious diseases across the globe has created awareness in chemists for the novel design and synthesis of lead molecules. Like hepatitis is one of the viral infectious disease, damages the liver function and therefore causes major complications, even leads to death in many cases. More than one third population of the world is affected by hepatitis. Different viral hepatitis are Hepatitis A (HAV), B(HBV), C(HCV), D(HDV) and E(HEV), depending upon the infecting virus type. Hepatitis A and E viruses are usually contacted after eating and drinking contaminated food and water. While, HBV, HCV and HDV are transmitted through contaminated blood. Hepatitis B and C are typically chronic, but HDV may be acute or chronic in nature. Non-viral hepatitis are also reported either due to alcohol consumption or metabolic disorder medications, which causes the liver stress or inflammation.

The treatment options of hepatitis vary depending upon what form you have and what caused the infection. Until recently, the treatment of hepatitis B has been reported with interferons alone or pegylated interferons while hepatitis C with interferons only or pegylated interferon (PEG-IFN) and ribavirin in combination, both are less successful (35-40%) and have side effects. Thus, a virus-specific, efficient and drug resistant free, anti-HBV and anti-HCV therapeutics are needed. Since 2011, the use of new drugs in targeting NS3/4A protease, NS5B polymerase and NS5A enzymes have enhanced treatment rates (70-90%) but still showed some side effects. Furthermore, inhibitors are at diverse stages of clinical development for NS5B and NS5A polymerase targets. Future design and synthesis of novel drugs must address genetic difference in HBV and HCV with least drug resistance. Also, for the genetic over-expression in HCV, a number of investigational techniques have developed which led to the comprehensive analysis of different aspects of viral life-cycle and interactions between virus and host (human). Thus, a rising list of targets for therapeutic involvement has been revealed. The directly acting anti-virals (DAAs) is another therapy method which helps in exploring novel and highly developed combinations of drugs.

* **Corresponding Author Naseem Ahmed:** Department of Chemistry, Indian Institute of Technology Roorkee, Roorkee-247667, Uttarakhand, India; Tel/Fax: +91-1332 285745; E-mail: nasemfcy@iitr.ac.in

Atta-ur-Rahman & M. Iqbal Choudhary (Eds.)

In this chapter, we discuss the synthetic advances of receptor based anti-viral scaffolds in hepatitis, which afforded significant numbers of agents such as drugs or drug leads, their mechanisms of action (MOAs), structure-activity relationships (SARs) and future structural perspectives as drug candidates.

Keywords: Antiviral agents, Combination therapy, Direct acting anti-virals (DAAs), Drug resistance, Hepatitis, Receptor inhibitors, Structure-activity relationships (SARs).

1. GENERAL INTRODUCTION

More than one third of the world's population is affected by hepatitis diseases. It damages the liver and causes major complications, even leading to death in many cases. The viral hepatitis has been sub-divided into Hepatitis A (HAV), B(HBV), C(HCV), D(HDV) and E(HEV), depending upon the infecting virus. HAV and HEV are usually transmitted after eating and drinking contaminated food and water. While, HBV, HCV and HDV are transmitted through contaminated blood. Hepatitis B and C are chronic in nature, but HDV may be acute or chronic in nature. The non-viral hepatitis has also been reported either due to alcohol consumption or metabolic disorder medications that causes the liver stress or inflammation [1].

A number of anti-viral hepatitis inhibitors are obtained from plants or prepared by synthetic and semi-synthetic methods. Many of them have the drug-resistance because of different reasons and are used in combinations. In future, the design and the development of new molecules need greater attentions. This chapter reports research, recent development of drugs and directional trends in the past, present and near future for the hepatitis infections [2].

2. HEPATITIS A

Annually, about 1.4 million hepatitis A (HAV) infection arises worldwide either periodically or epidemically. In the developing and tropical countries, the virus is generally spread *via* the fecal-oral route due to low hygienic conditions [3] and in the industrialized countries may be due to travel to countries endemic of HAV infection or linked to frozen berries or imported pomegranate arils [4]. The infection is restricted to humans only which shows initial symptoms fever, vomiting, nausea, anorexia, weakness, abdominal discomfort and right upper quadrant pain. In advance stages, patients develop jaundice, darkened urine and uncolored stool and approximately 8% cases are associated with acute kidney injury [5].

This virus belongs to the hepadnavirus genus of *Picornaviridae* family. Genetically, HAV resembles typical picornavirus and insect picorna-like viruses which have a 27 nm long single-stranded, non-enveloped and icosahedral RNA, shown by immune electron microscopy in 1973. A rodent origin HAV is also suggested based on more than 200 small mammal species screening for hepatoviruses [6]. The host cell exosome membranes are used by virus as an envelope to protect itself from antibody mediated effects and facilitates detection of HAV by plasma cytoid dendritic cells for type-I interferon in infection [7]. Out of seven pathogenic HAV genotypes, four are able to infect humans. A limited type I interferon response is found in acute hepatitis A cases due to break down of vital adaptor proteins by HAV protease and polymerase precursor. The CD4+T cells play a major role in terminating HAV infection, has been shown in HAV-infected chimpanzees. Similarly, HAV-specific CD8+T cells have been reported a potential contributor to the infection in humans [8]. Anti-HAV IgM antibodies and/or HAV RNA is detected in acute HAV infection after vaccination and IgM antibodies persisting for at least 2-3 decades [9]. For the treatment of hepatitis A, drugs are not available. Recently, it was found that cyclosporine A and silibinin products inhibit HAV replication *in vitro* [10].

3. HEPATITIS B

3.1. Introduction

About 350-400 million people are surfacing HBV antigen (HBsAg) carriers and around one million people die annually due to HBV infections. The high mortality rate is found in HBsAg-positive patients due to chronic liver disease, non-Hodgkin lymphoma and hepatocellular carcinoma [11]. Since the discovery of HBV in 1965 by Blumberg, much development has been made in the vaccines and the advancement of potent anti-viral agents. However, the global burden of disease is still substantial. In chronic HBV therapy, the aim is either to inhibit the viral replication or to enhance immunological responses against virus or both. R-Interferon (R-IFN, Intron A) has been used effectively in 30-40% cases of chronic HBV infections. Thymosin-R1 (Zadaxin), interleukin-12 and therapeutic vaccines have been also used as immunotherapy regimens with limited success. Interferon-α and pegylated interferon-α-2a are used as immunomodulatory agents with poor response and adverse side effects [12].

Many Ape and African old world monkey species have been detected with HBV infection in the polymerase chain reaction (PCR) and pattern recognition receptors (PRR) screening [13]. Genetically, it is a lipid enveloped DNA virus with icosahedral core called Dane particles (the organizing framework of the virion) [14]. The lipid envelope is studded with surface protein (HBsAg) and loosely interact with cores. The mass spectrometry has further led to important insights into its structure [15] which showed virus compactness and adapts to its host to use full advantage of host systems [16]. The molecular mechanisms discovered that interferons and other inflammatory cytokines suppressed HBV replication and modulate HBV cccDNA metabolism and function. The activation and maturation of the HBV-specific adaptive immune response and the degree of HBV infection depend upon the intrahepatic innate immunity development and function status. Along with TLR7/8/9 or STING showed agonists pharmacological activation to control HBV infection [17], mediated by germline-encoded receptors to recognize the common structural and functional features of microbes or pathogen-associated molecular patterns (PAMPs). Thus far, many types of PRRs have been discovered like toll-like receptors (TLRs), leucine-rich repeat-containing receptors (NLRs), nucleotide-binding oligomerization domain (Nod), RIG-I-like receptors (RLRs), C-type lectin receptors (CLRs) and diversified DNA receptors [18]. Both type I and type II IFNs are required for a coordinated action of innate and adaptive immune responses in HBV clearance. However, T-cell appeared to be critical for the success of TLR3-mediated anti-viral action. Thus, the intrahepatic delivery of TLR3 agonists have a good potential for the treatment of chronic hepatitis B. Stimulator of interferon genes (STING) is the adaptor protein of multiple cytoplasmic DNA receptors and PRR recognizes bacterial 2°-messengers, cyclic di-adenosine monophosphate (c-di-AMP) and cyclic di-guanosine monophosphate (c-di-GMP). It was observed that cytoplasmic DNA activates cyclic guanosine monophosphate-adenosine monophosphate synthase (cGAS) to bind STING and induces IFNs and other cytokines for cGAMP production [19]. The STING can also be activated by cyclic di-nucleotides, TLR7 and TLR8 and other small molecules. It might be another potential target for pharmacological activation of innate immune responses and priming of an adaptive immune response [20]. The PRRs in microbial infections has physiological role for the curative therapeutic approaches of chronic hepatitis B [21] which led to prompt recognition of viral components by host cellular PRRs, induction of type I interferon (IFN) and IFN-stimulated genes of viral infections. In some other viruses, IFN and other inflammatory cytokine responses are impossible to detect in the early phase of humans HBV infection [22]. A recent report showed that HBV replication initiated by either HBV DNA transfection or virus infection elicited a type III not type I IFN response in HepG2 cells [23]. But, the treatment with lamivudine appreciably reduced the IFN response in HBV infected primary human hepatocytes and NTCP-expressing HepG2 cells. It is unclear that how RIG-I distinguish pgRNA has similar structural features of host cellular mRNA and why the type III IFN response was impossible to detect in HBV-infected chimpanzees and humans.

FDA approved drugs are immunomodulators (IFN-α, pegylated-IFN-α) and nucleoside analogues (lamivudine, adefovir dipivoxil, entecavir, telbivudine and tenofovir disoproxil fumarate) in HBV therapy [24]. Nucleosi/tide analogues (NA) and related compounds have also been approved for HBV infections like lamivudine (Epivir1), a reverse transcriptase (RT) inhibitor which inhibits HBV replication by lowering the HBV DNA level. A potent and orally available TLR7 agonist, GS-9620 is used as PRR agonists for the treatment of chronic hepatitis B [25, 26]. Mechanism of action by the activation of TLR-7 suggested that the anti-viral responses induced by GS-9620 is mediated by both the cytolytic activity of CD8+T cells and/or NK cells and type I/II IFN-mediated non-cytolytic activity with activation of B-cells in the liver micro-environment. It was also found that TLR8 is more important PRR than TLR7 in human liver, where TLR8 agonist, ssRNA40 selectively activates liver-resident and some extent the blood-derived NKT mucosal-associated invariant T and CD56 NK cells to produce IFN-c in both healthy and HBV- or HCV-infected livers [27]; adefovir dipivoxil (Hepsera1)- a purine nucleoside pro-drug can replace for dATP (adenosine). After integrated in the viral DNA chain, stopped the elongation of viral DNA synthesis. It also induces α-IFN production, boost NK cell activity, inspire the hosts' immune response and enhance efficacy in inhibiting HBV replication with low resistance rate [28]; drug entecavir (Baraclude1) is a guanine nucleoside for potent and selective inhibition of HBV polymerase [29]. The mechanism of action of nucleoside analogues revealed that the interaction of triphosphate derivatives (obtained from cellular metabolic transformation) with HBV DNA polymerase or RT as substrates and/or inhibitors are possible. Like Lamivudine inhibits all three functions of viral polymerase: (1) initiation of HBV polymerase; (2) synthesis of minus strand DNA from pregenomic RNA template and (3) synthesis of HBV DNA chain. HBV generates easily drug-resistance to lamivudine and the rate of resistance increases with the elongation of the therapeutic duration. Entecavir has 300 times more inhibitive efficacy than lamivudine or adefovir, even the resistance mutation frequency is very low [30], telbivudine (Tyzeka1, Sebivo1) showed advantages in inhibition of the synthesis for both strands of HBV DNA and only appropriate drug available in pregnant female patients. The antiviral efficacy of telbivudine is more than that of lamivudine [31] and tenofovir disoproxil fumarate (TDF) (Viread1)-an acyclic adenine nucleotide analogue has approved for the treatment of chronic hepatitis B in 2008 after it had been approved for the treatment of AIDS in 2001. It also inhibits HBV and HIV replication at RT step (tenofovir pro-drug is converted to tenofovir diphosphate *via* catalysis by a cellular kinase) (Fig. **1**) [32]. It was found that tenofovir disoproxil fumarate is significantly more effective than entecavir for complete viral suppression in HBeAg-positive hepatitis B patients. For HBeAg-negative patients, no significant difference in rates of viral suppression was observed [24].

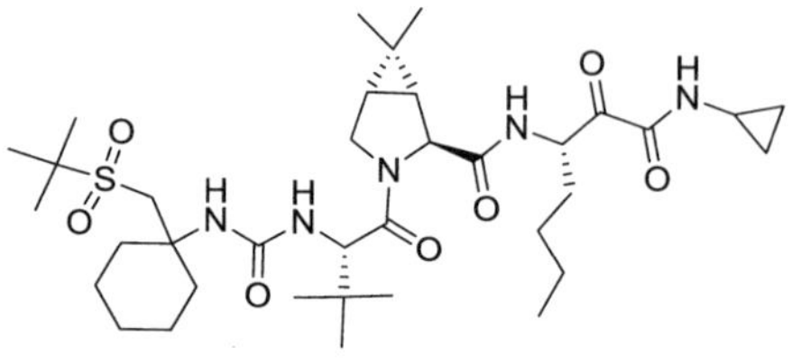

1
Narlaprevir (SCH900518)

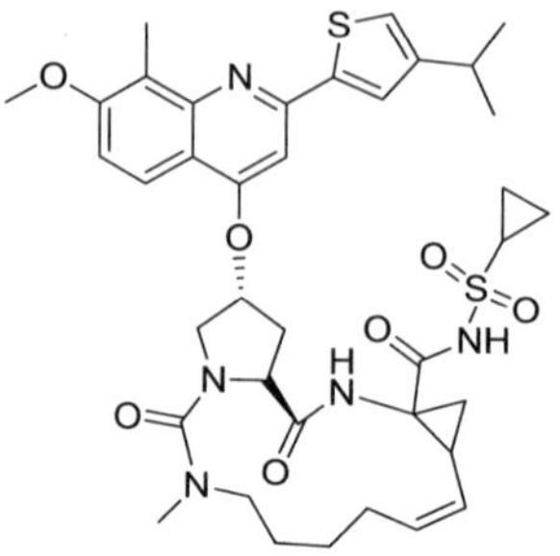

2
Simeprevir (TMC435)

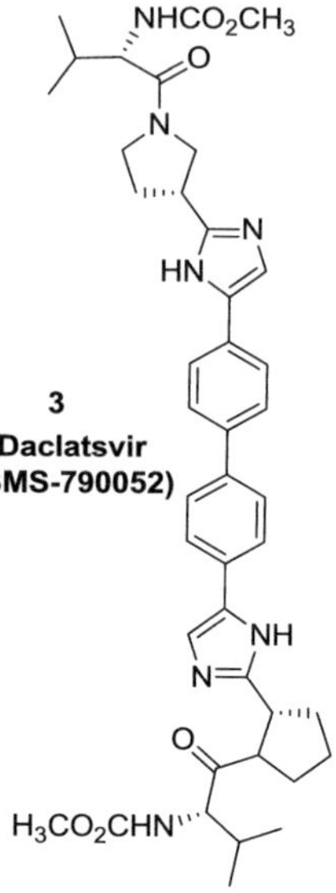

3
Daclatsvir
(BMS-790052)

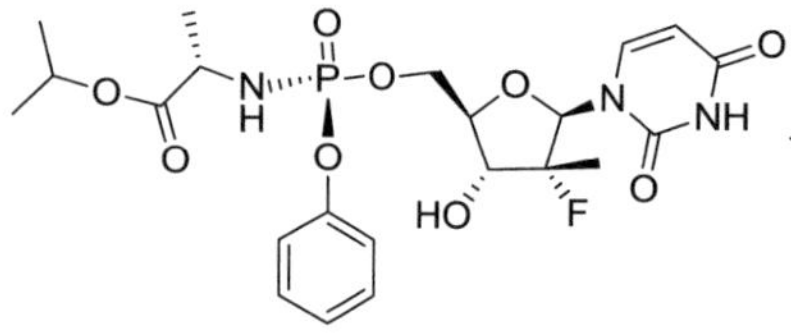

4
Sofosbuvir (GS-7977)

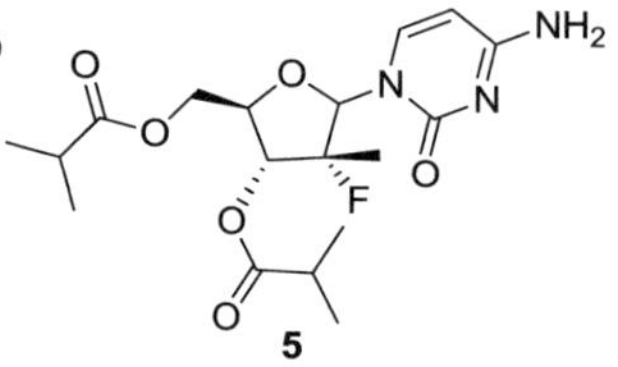

5
Mericitabine (RG7128; RO5024048)

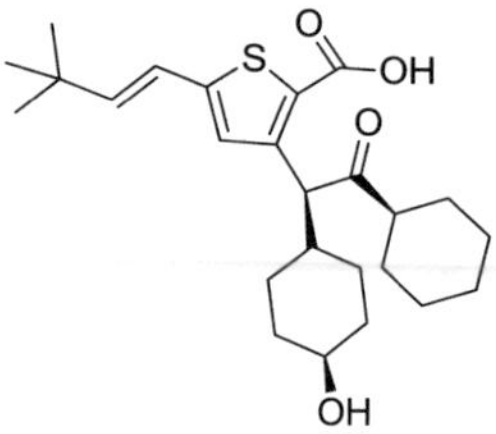

6
VX-222

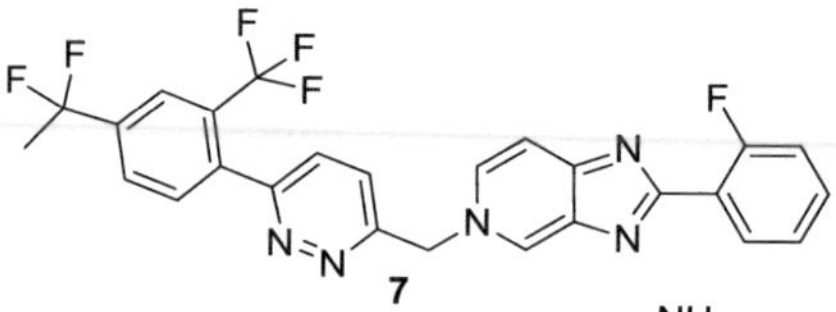

7
Tegobuvir (GS-9190)

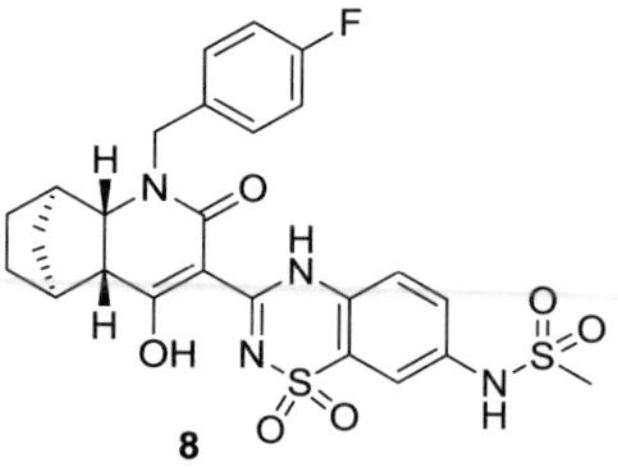

8
Setrobuvir

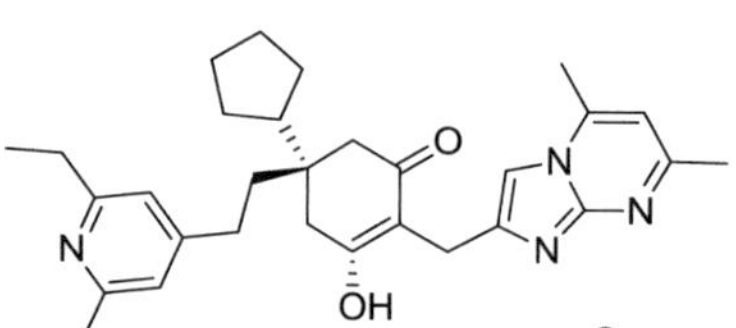

9
Filibuvir

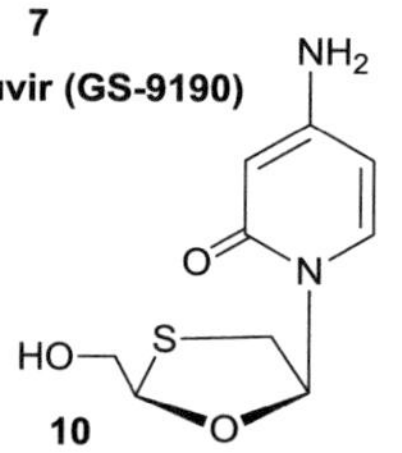

10
Lamivudine
2,3-Dideoxy-3-thiacytidine
3TC, Epivir

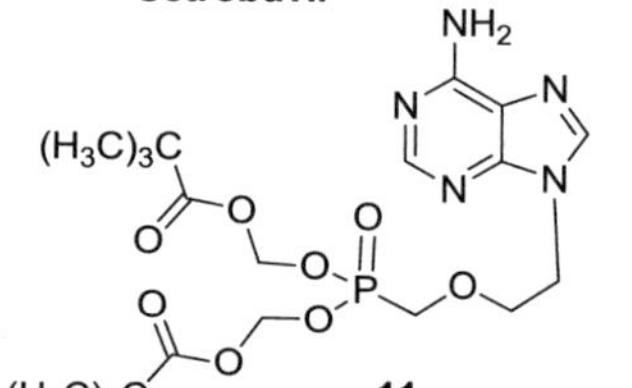

11
Adefovir dipivoxil
Hepsera

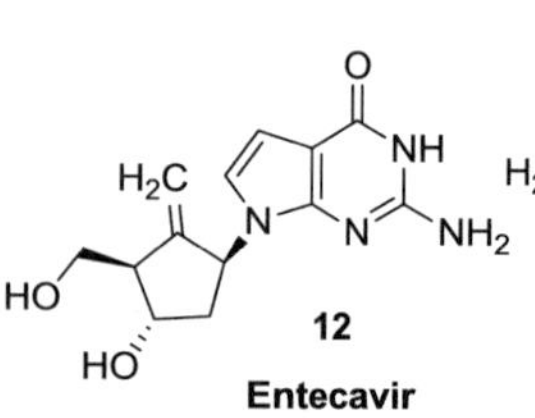

12
Entecavir
Baraclude

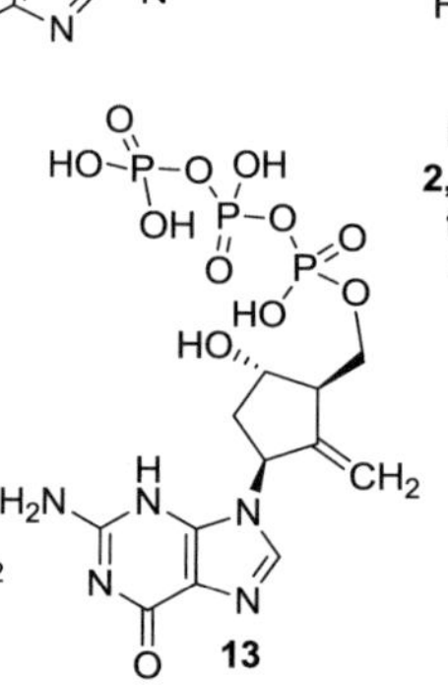

13
EC_{50} = 0.010-0.059 µM
Active form of Entacavir

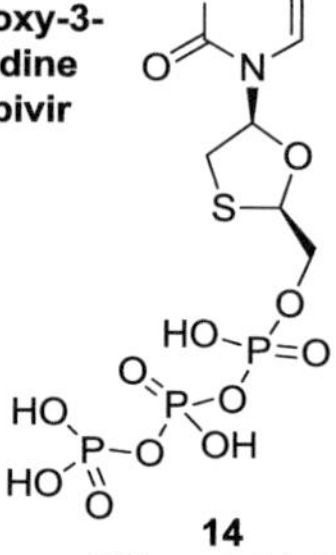

14
EC_{50} = 0.01-5.6 µM
Active form of lamivudine (EPIVIR-HBV)

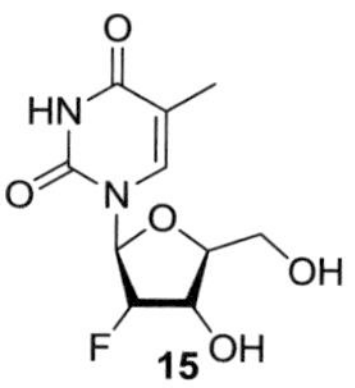

15
Clevudine

Fig. 1 contd.....

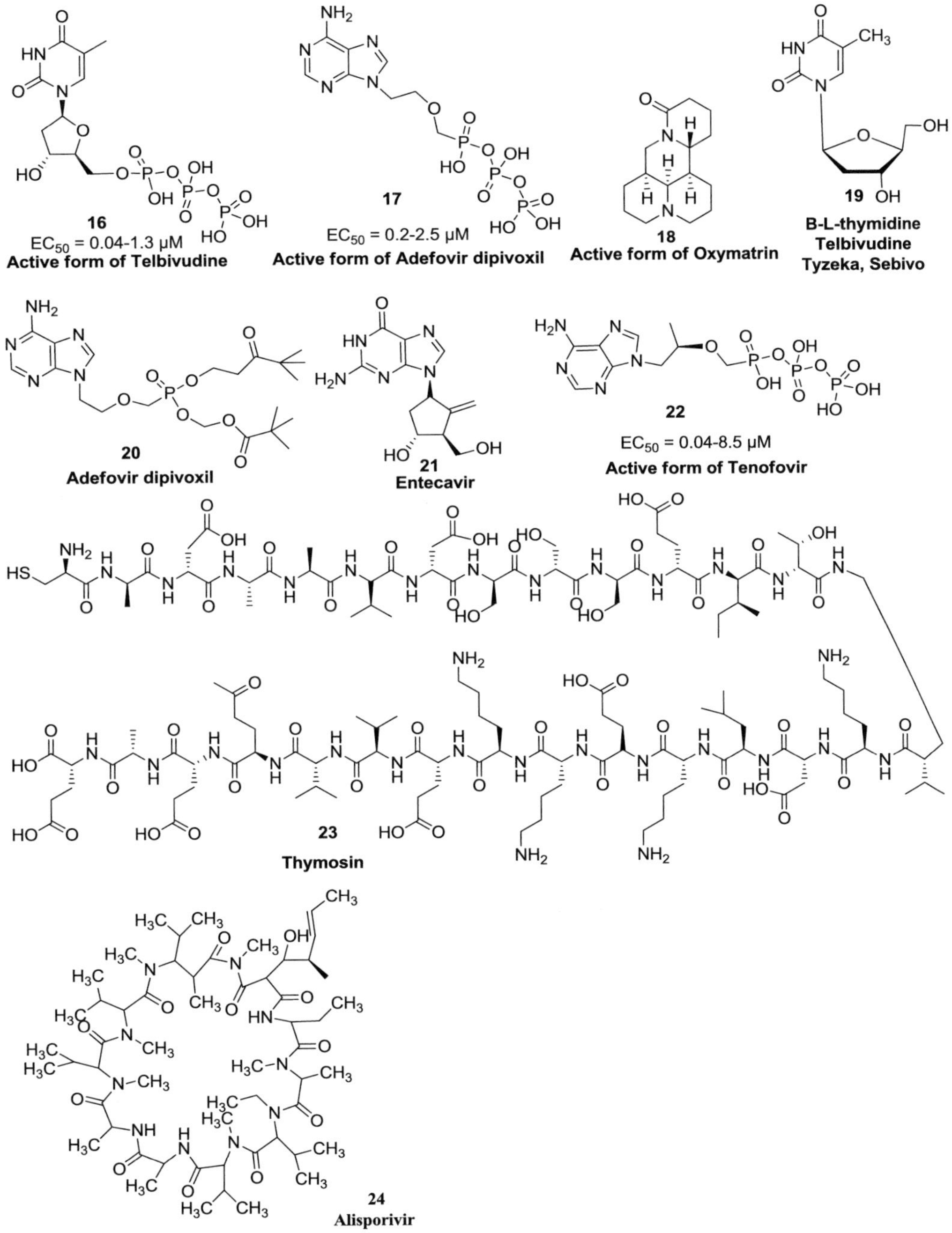

Fig. (1). HBV drugs.

3.2. HBV Life Cycle

The DNA of virus is circular and partially double-stranded of 3.2 kb. After entering the human hepatocyte, the relaxed circle DNA (rcDNA) is released from virus and transported to the nucleus. Inside the nucleus, converted to a cccDNA and then HBV replication started from the reverse transcription of pgRNA and sub-genomic mRNAs on the cccDNA template. Back to the cytoplasm, HBV polymerase recognizes RNA coded signal of pgRNA and binds to it and further packaged into the viral capsid having HBcAg. The process involves the reverse transcription of pgRNA to minus DNA, the incomplete plus DNA synthesis and RNase degradation is carried out in the nucleocapsid. Again, nucleocapsid containing minus-and plus-DNA re-entered in the nucleus or bud into the endoplasmic reticulum after enveloped and secreted outside the cells. It was observed that four different mRNAs are transcripted on the cccDNA template of 3.5 kb, 2.4 kb, 2.1 kb and 0.7 kb mRNA. The 3.5 kb mRNA serves as the reverse transcription substrate (pre-genomic mRNA, pgRNA) and the template for the HBV core antigen (HBcAg) and E antigen (HBeAg) polymerase proteins; the 2.4 kb and 2.1 kb mRNAs encode three surface proteins as the large (LHBs), middle (MHBs) and small (SHBs or HBsAg) surface proteins and 0.7 kb mRNA encodes the X antigen (HBxAg). Among these viral proteins, HBcAg is the main structure protein in HBV capsid and is very important for the packaging, RT and assembly. Three surface proteins are the envelope proteins associated with the attachment and invasion, the maturation and secretion of viruses and its immunogenicity. The polymerase protein is the key protein for HBV replication which contains three functional domains called terminal protein (TP), reverse transcriptase (RT) and RNase H which play an important role in HBV replication. HBeAg is processed in the endoplasmic reticulum and secreted out of the hepatocytes, possessing the function of immunoregulation and associated with the host immune tolerance and HBxAg is related to the virus replication, hepatocarcinogenesis and activation of some signal pathway [33].

3.3. Different Routes of HBV Transmission

Sexual (mainly in Western Europe) [34].

- Percutaneous (intravenous drug use)
- Perinatal (sub-Saharan Africa region) [35].
- Horizontal (in childhood) [36].
- Blood Transfusion [37].
- Nosocomial (due to patients, patient-health care workers and reverse contacts. The most common transmitted blood-borne virus in the health care setting including needle-stick injury) [38].

• Organ transplantation (*e.g.*, kidney, cornea) [39].

3.3.1. Acute Hepatitis

After HBV infection, the incubation period is 1-4 months. Then, a prodromal phase appears before acute hepatitis condition with prominent clinical symptoms of hepatitis [40].

3.3.2. Chronic Hepatitis

Mostly such patients have no symptom of acute hepatitis but chronic hepatitis B (CHB). Some have non-specific symptom as fatigue. However, significant clinical symptoms developed only after liver disease progresses to decompensated cirrhosis [41].

3.4. Drugs Targets/Receptors in Cellular Factors

Recent, an effective development of anti-virals across all genotypes of hepatitis C virus has enhanced interest for similar cure in chronic HBV infection. Therefore, new drug targets, novel small molecules and experimental strategies are under clinical evaluation. At least 38 new investigational agents are under development for the chronic hepatitis B of which 19 have reached human trials. 21 designated as DAAs and 17 as HTAs which are further sub-categorized as either immunomodulators (HTA-i) or targeting other host functions (HTA-hf) important for the virus [42]. Many other transcriptional regulatory elements are present in which four act as promoters (Cp, S1p, S2p, and Xp) and two enhancers (EnhI and EnhII). The transcription factors interact in these regions as activator protein 1 (Sp1), CAAT enhancer-binding protein (C/EBP) and hepatocyte nuclear factor-4α (HNF-4α) regulate HBV replication and transcription [43]. Oppositely, other host factors also involved directly or indirectly in the HBV life-cycle and impact on HBV replication and antigen expression. HBV RT catalyses the first step reaction of HBV genome replication and becomes an important target of anti-HBV drugs [44]. Nucleos(t)ide analogues have inhibitory effects due to the competition with natural dNTPs which inhibit HBV RT. They have strong anti-viral effects but all have same mechanism of action. They generate easily drug resistance or cross-resistance to cause moderate to serious side effects. In recent years, different class of compounds have been reported as anti-HBV activities such as natural agents, synthesized small molecules, peptide and proteins, nucleic acid, *etc.,* (Figs. **4-8**). Plants are an attractive source of finding new anti-HBV drugs and discover novel compounds with unique mode of action for controlling viral replication, preventing drug resistance and its long term complications.

3.5. HBV Receptors

Hepatitis B virus is covered with envelope proteins. It helps in protection of virus and also make it infectious and helped in viral entry inside the cells. The viral entry is further facilitated by specific interactions between viral envelope proteins and hepatocytes receptors. For example, the myristoylated preS1 domain of HBV L-protein played important role in viral infectivity by attachment to a hepatocyte-specific receptor [45].

3.5.1. Cp and cccDNA as Targets

Longer period of treatment with nucleoside analogs prevent formation of new virions but hardly results in loss of virus. Therefore, cccDNA remains throughout the cycle of infectivity. The virus has usual proteins of euchromatin along with two other proteins: X and Cp [46] where Cp is present as a dimer. The ends of dimer, distal to the four helix bundle are responsible for inter-dimer contacts. Cysteine placed in the middle of the four helix bundle which form a disulfide cross-linking [47]. The interaction of Cp with cccDNA is poorly understood. However, chromatin Immuno-Precipitation (ChIP) showed that Cp is preferentially associated with CpG islands. The association of Cp on CpG island 2 increased cccDNA activity (*i.e.* viral load) while methylation of DNA in CpG islands 2 and 3 decrease cccDNA activity [48]. Small molecules that drive Cp assembly, presumably deplete the concentration of free Cp which led to depletion in cccDNA-bound Cp and decrease production of viral RNA and proteins. It was also believed that the E3 ubiquitin ligase NIRF1 leads to suppression of cccDNA activity and so deplete cccDNA-bound Cp [49]. Cp-directed molecules (inhibitors) have their mechanism of action based on allostery called Cp Allosteric Modulators (CpAMs) (Fig. **2**) which can mis-direct assembly in two ways: (i) alter the subunit structure to stabilize an assembly-incompetent state or (ii) alter inter-subunit interactions. Either way, it will affects the assembled product formed due to the interactions with an intersubunit contact surface or indirectly by allostery. These effects have been demonstrated in Cp mutants. In the mis-direction of HBV capsid assembly, small molecules were first identified in *in vitro* assembly studies with a fluorescent dye 5,50-bis[8-(phenylamino--1-naphthalenesulfonate] (BisANS).

Sodium taurocholate co-transporting polypeptide (NTCP) is other important HBV receptor which mediates HBV and HDV entry and hence represents a new target for therapeutics in the blocking of HBV entry [50]. Myrcludex-B, a synthetic lipopeptide derivatized from HBV preS1 domain sequence showed specific binding to NTCP, and efficiently block *de novo* HBV infection. Thus, it prevents intrahepatic viral spreading *in vitro* and *in vivo* [51].

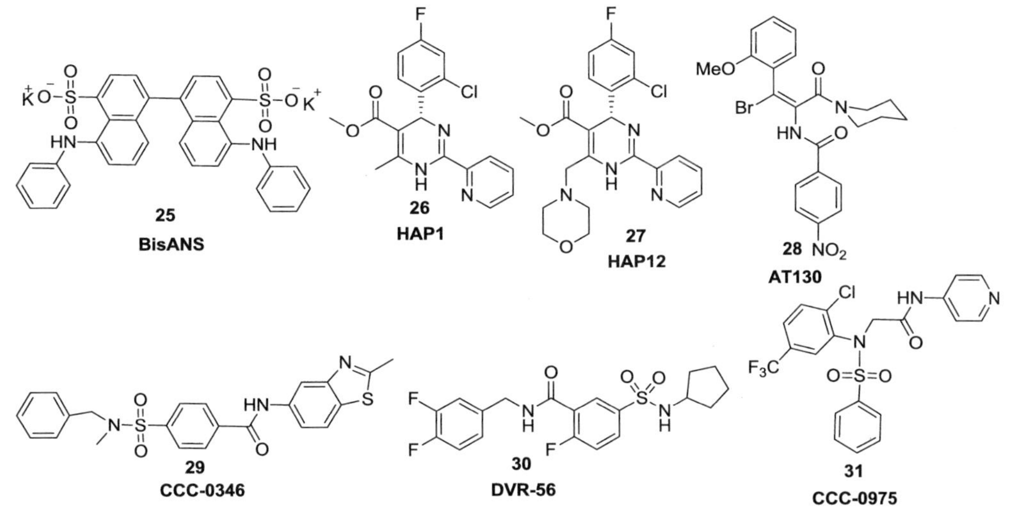

Fig. (2). Non-nucleoside and selected CpAM antivirals.

In addition, NTCP functions as a hepatic bile acid transporter for the uptake of most sodium-dependent bile salts into hepatocytes. Tsukuda *et al.* [52] demonstrated that RAR-selective antagonist, Ro41-5253 inhibits hNTCP promoter activity by decreasing cellular susceptibility to HBV infection. The IL-6 regulates NTCP expression and so effect HBV entry. Also, Bouezzedine *et al.* [53] found that NTCP mRNA expression, NTCP-mediated taurocholate uptake and HBV entry reduced 98%, 80% and 90% respectively upon pre-treatment of HepaRG cells with IL-6. Other important cellular factors include Toll-like receptors (TLRs) that involved in the HBV life-cycle [54]. The TLR-ligand interaction results in production and discharge of IFNs, pro-inflammatory cytokines and chemokines anti-viral molecules. However, virus can disrupt TLR expression and hinder intracellular signaling for evading the innate immune response. Thus, other treatment strategy involves as combination of anti-viral treatment with adjuvant therapy with TLR agonist to restore the innate immune response. TLR activated the TLR-mediated innate immune response for promising adjuvant drug candidates [55]. Like GS-9620 agonist of TLR7 was investigated for better safety, tolerability, pharmacokinetics and pharmaco-dynamics in HCV- and HBV-infected patients [56]. It is absorbed and tolerated at oral doses. The majority of patients serum has IFN-α at detectable levels in 16.7% and 12% respectively in HCV and HBV patients. However, no significant change was observed of HCV RNA in HCV-infected patients or reductions of the HBsAg or HBV DNA level in HBV-infected patients. Zhang *et al.* [57] reported a sub-group TLR family TLR3 and TLR2/4 to mediate innate immune responses to stop

HBV infection. Similarly, Kapoor *et al.* [58] gave the roles of TLR7 and TLR9 in chronic HBV infection.

3.6. Concerns about Receptor-Based Therapeutic Strategies

The main concern for the use of NTCP inhibitors are interference of NTCP physiological function during the treatment. Recently, it was found that the uptake of conjugated bile acids was impaired in NTCP knockout mice, even the serum level of bile acids in mice was normal [59]. No serious conditions associated with NTCP variants have been reported in humans. Similarly, no relationship between NTCP inhibition and drug-induced liver injury has been shown [60]. Humans may tolerate at least partial loss of NTCP function might be due to other transporters could compensate for NTCP function. Many drugs are transported by NTCP in the liver. Thus, more information on drug-drug interactions (DDIs) is needed to establish in the setting of NTCP blockage either by virus or by a HBV entry inhibitor. NTCP blockage will be a feasible option for anti-HBV therapy in chronically infected patients who may take other medications [61].

3.6.1. NTCP-Blocking Agents (Viral Entry Inhibitors)

The viral entry inhibition *via* NTCP is a promising option in the prevention and treatment of HBV/HDV infection to protect naive hepatocytes against primary infection and spread of vertical virus transmission, post-exposure prophylaxis and HBV recurrence after liver transplantation. It can also stopped viral spread and hinder amplification of cccDNA pools in the initial infected hepatocytes. For example, myr-preS1 lipopeptide binds to NTCP and inhibits viral infection *in vitro* and *in vivo*. Cyclosporine A (CsA), a cyclic peptide inhibits the transport activity of NTCP in the HBV life-cycle inside liver cells may be a good drug target [62]. The development of bile acid derivatives as blockers in the HBV and HDV infections with much higher efficiency than natural bile acids will be also a good target [63].

3.6.2. Immunoregulators

Immunoregulator drugs have been used in the treatment of severe pneumonia, immune-deficiency and chronic hepatitis B. They enhanced the patients immune response in the specific immunity to HBV and helped the immune cells to recognize and destroy HBV-infected cells and thus clearance of destructed HBV cells [64].

3.6.3. Interferon (IFN)

The host cells triggered the secretory glycoprotein, IFN which function as antiviral, anti-proliferation and various stimuli of immune regulatory cytokine. IFN on the basis of producing cells called white blood cells, fibroblasts and lymphocytes. IFNs used to treat chronic HBV infection is bound to the specific receptors on the cell surface and activate a series of signal transduction events which resulting in the production of anti-viral protein (AVP), degrade viral mRNA and inhibit viral replication. It also supported the activity of natural killer (NK) cells, macrophages and T lymphocytes. Chemical modification can extended the half-life of IFN [65]. For example, peg-IFN acquires a longer half-life (40 hours) and remains effective in inhibiting HBV replication for 168 hours with adverse effects like fever, hair loss and reduction of white blood cells.

3.6.4. Thymosin-α1

The main function of thymosin-α1, an immunoregulator is to promote differentiation of T-cells to the mature stage and enhance the response to antigens and other excitants. The boosting action in the host immune system helps host defense against chronic HBV infection. This can be combined with IFN to treat chronic hepatitis B [66].

3.6.5. Cytokines

Cytokines are secreted upon stimulation of multiple types of immune cells (monocytes, macrophages, T-, B- and NK-cells) and non-immune cells (endothelial cells, epidermal cells and fibroblasts). They are characterized as small molecules with extensive biological functions and strong anti-viral activity. Like interleukin (IL)-12 can induce TO cells into T1 cells leading to IFN production [67].

3.6.6. La Protein Inhibitor (HBSC11)

La protein is a phosphoprotein that has multi-functional RNA-binding protein which involved in HBV RNA metabolism. It showed that the La protein has protective effects against HBV where protein kinase CK2 (tyrosine kinase II) enables it to be phosphorylated at serine-366 and activates the La protein functions [68].

3.6.7. Anti-HBV Agents Derived from Natural Products

Several nucleoside and non-nucleoside analogues have been obtained from natural sources and synthesis or semi-synthesis methods. They are used as HBV inhibitors in the treatment of chronic HBV infections. Many of them exhibited good anti-HBV activity with novel mechanism of action which infer useful informations for the medicinal chemists to synthesize novel compounds [69].

These analogues inhibit HBV replication *via* unique interaction with HBV DNA polymerase. However, HBV variants resistant emerge to anti-viral therapy in these analogues that is almost inevitable and represents a clinical challenge. Therefore, further researches are needed to identify new anti-viral compounds as anti-HBV targets with unique mode of action for controlling viral replication and preventing drug resistance. Pro-drugs are used as chemical and molecular precursors of active drugs in the direct-acting antivirals (DAAs) and HBV polymerase inhibitors. They enhanced the performance of the active drug substance by decreasing toxicity, improving solubility, enhancing tissue absorption and increasing the half-life so that the agents can be dosed not more than once daily. As long as the prodrug can be efficiently and safely converted to the active agent, it may have better efficacy and safety profile [70]. Since current polymerase inhibitors are associated with the loss of HBsAg and the appearance of HBsAb in about 10% patients of those treated over 5 years, it is possible that a pro-drug that inhibits intrahepatic DNA replication could significantly increase seroconversion. About 34% approved drugs by FDA during the last 30 years consist of compounds from natural sources or derivatized from natural products. A fungal derived new tricyclic polyketide called "viral and NTCP inhibitor from *Talaromycesac* in A" (vanitaracin A) strongly inhibited HBV and HDV infections. Vanitaracin A **32** interaction with NTCP inhibited its bile acid uptake activity (IC_{50} 0.23 μM) without affecting the HBV replication process. It directly interacts with the HBV entry receptor NTCP and impairs its bile acid transport activity in all HBV genotypes tested (genotypes A to D except HCV). Thus, vanitaracin A and its related analogs could be part of an anti-viral strategy for preventing HBV reinfection [71].

3.6.8. Phyllanthus Extract and Related Active Compounds (Lignans and Phenols)

The phyllanthus (*Euphorbiaceae*) plants are extensively used in oriental countries as traditional medicines for the treatment of jaundice and hepatitis. The *P. amarus* extract was used as anti-HBV activity for the first time in 1982 which inhibits HBV polymerase, mRNA transcription and HBV replication activity. It also inhibits the interaction between HBV EnhI and transcript factor C/EBP α and β which suppresses HBV transcription. Huang *et al.* [72] isolated 25 compounds from four phyllanthus plants and explored their anti-HBV activities in HBV cell line MS-G2 which showed that amentoflavone **34**, niranthin, nirtetralin, hinokinin and geraniin significantly suppressed the secretion of HBsAg and HBeAg. Among these compounds, niranthin gave the best anti-HBsAg activity (EC_{50} 33.6 μM) and effectively inhibit HBsAg secretion (74.3% inhibition) at the non-cytotoxic concentration of 50 μM. Thus, the inhibitory effect is higher than IFN-α (EC_{50} 960 IU/ml); hinokinin showed the most potent anti-HBeAg activity at 50 μM (46.5%

inhibition). Phyltetralin and brevifolin at the non-cytotoxic concentrations of 120 and 200 μM suppressed both HBsAg and HBeAg about 42.6%, 29.5% and 54.0%, 61.8% respectively. Shin *et al.* [73] isolated a molecule ellagic acid from *P. urinaria* which showed inhibitory activity on HBeAg (IC_{50} 0.07 μg/ml) but have no impact on HBV polymerase, HBV replication and HBsAg secretion activity [74]. Robustaflavone **33**, a naturally occurring compound inhibited HBV replication *in vitro*. It is a biflavanoid composed of two units of apigenin (5,7,4'-trihydroxyflavone) joined *via* a biaryl linkage between the 6-position of one unit and the 3'-position of the other (I6,II3'-biapigenin). The natural material was isolated from the seed-kernels of *Rhus succedanea* and also synthesized under Suzuki coupling reaction to form the sterically congested 6-3'''-biaryl bond of robustaflavone, provided access to the desired biflavanoid system (Fig. **3**) [75].

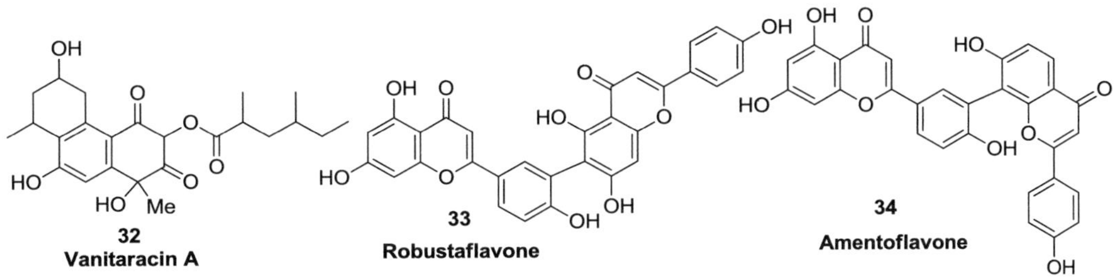

Fig. (3). Natural products as anti-HBV.

3.6.9. Curcumin

Phenolic curcumin **41** has shown anti-inflammatory, anti-oxidant and anti-viral effects in HBV and HCV with diverse mechanisms in different viruses by suppressing the AKT-SREBP-1 pathway which is essential for viral replication of HCV. It was also reported that curcumin effectively inhibits HBV expression in dose-dependent manner for the combination therapy with 3TC and exerts synergistical inhibition on HBV transcription [76]. Further, the study revealed that PGC-1α, a co-activator of key gluconeogenesis genes by interacting with the nuclear receptor, HNF4α and forkhead transcription factor (FOXO1) activates HBV transcription. Curcumin effectively decreased the PGC-1α protein levels by accelerating its degradation and shortening its half-life, hence inhibited HBV expression. Although, curcumin has favorable anti-HBV effect and specific action mechanism but need more study. It is insoluble in water and have short half-life and low bioavailability following oral administration, need to be improved.

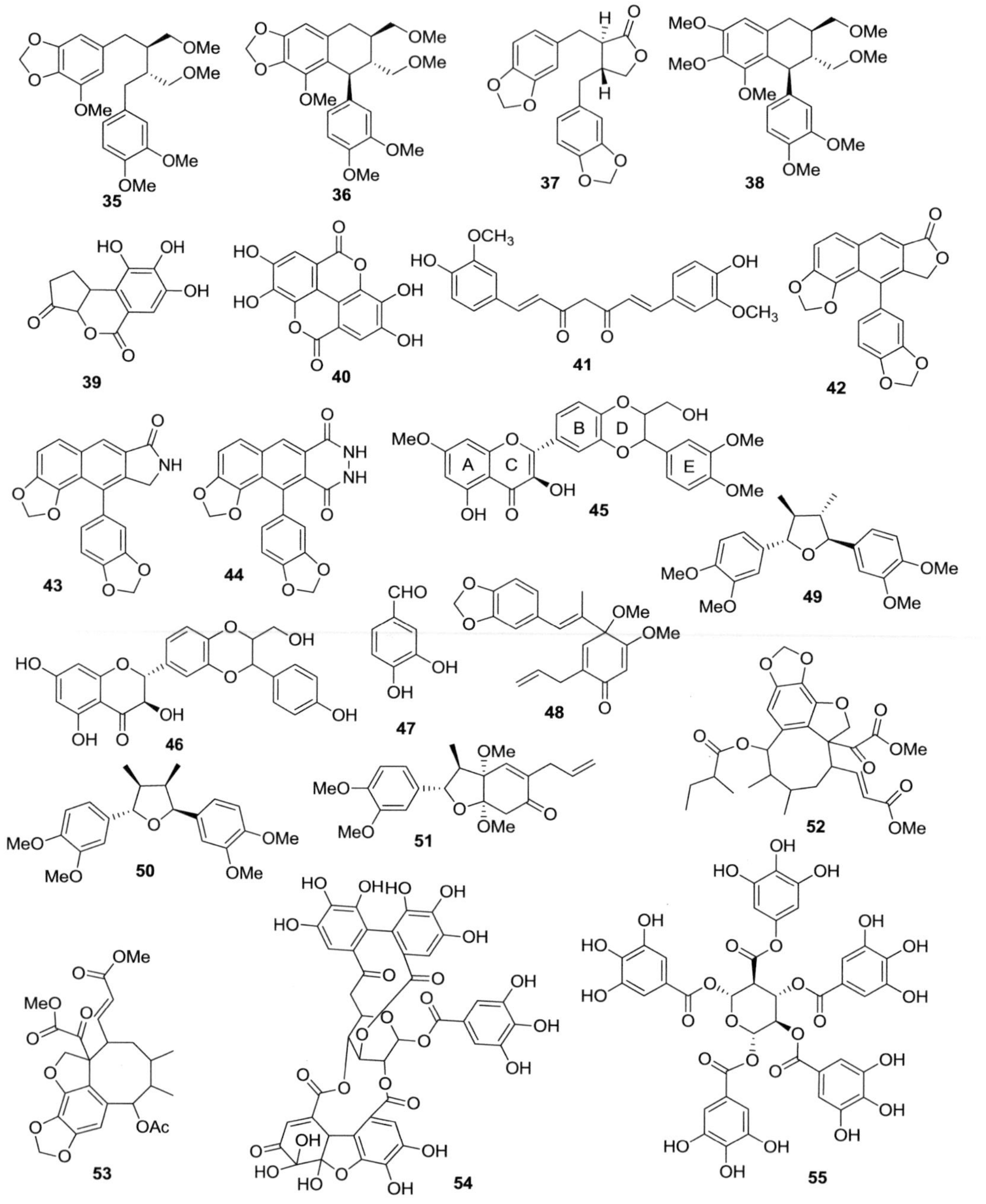

Fig. (4). Structure of active lignans and phenols.

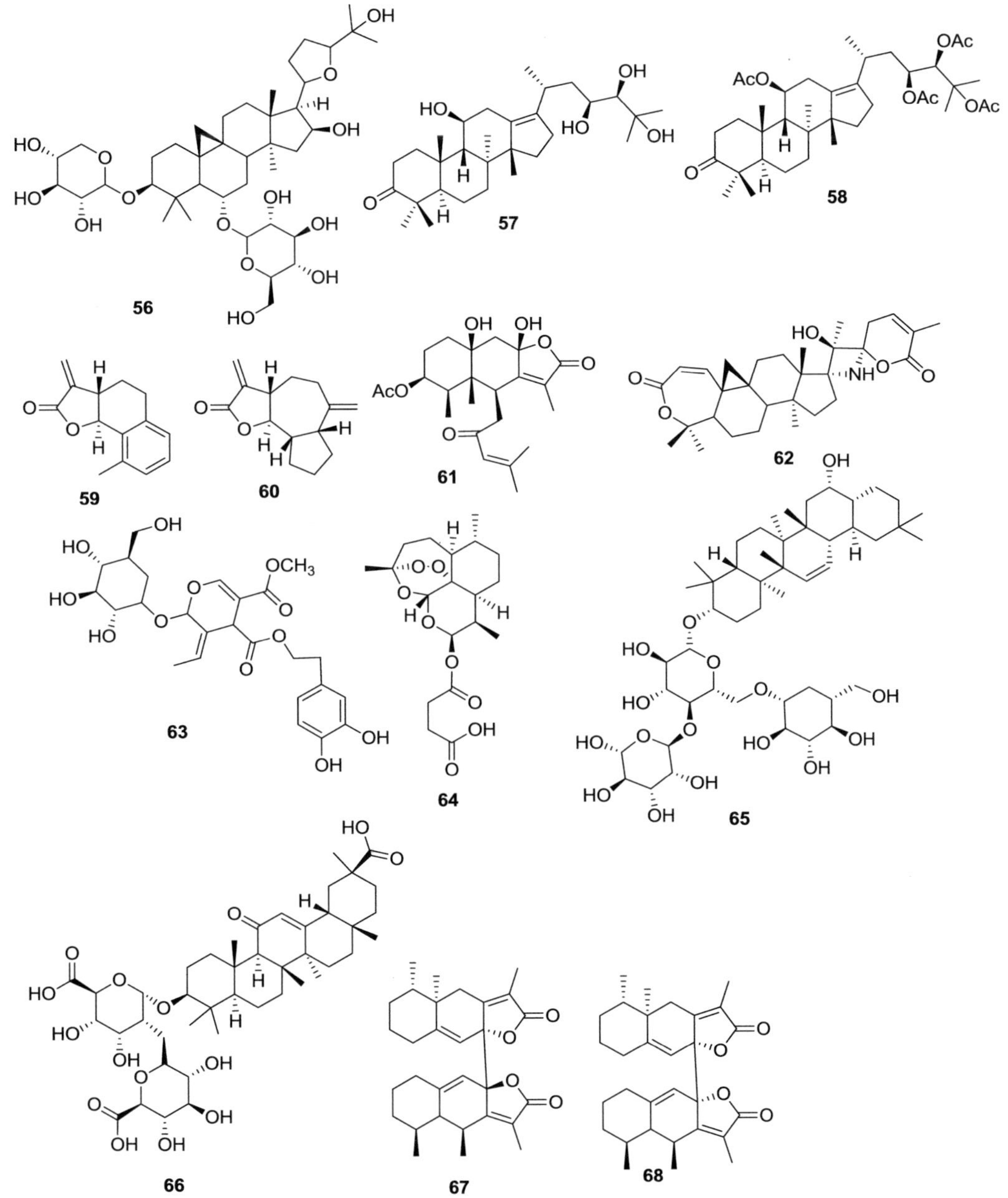

Fig. (5). Structure of active terpenoids.

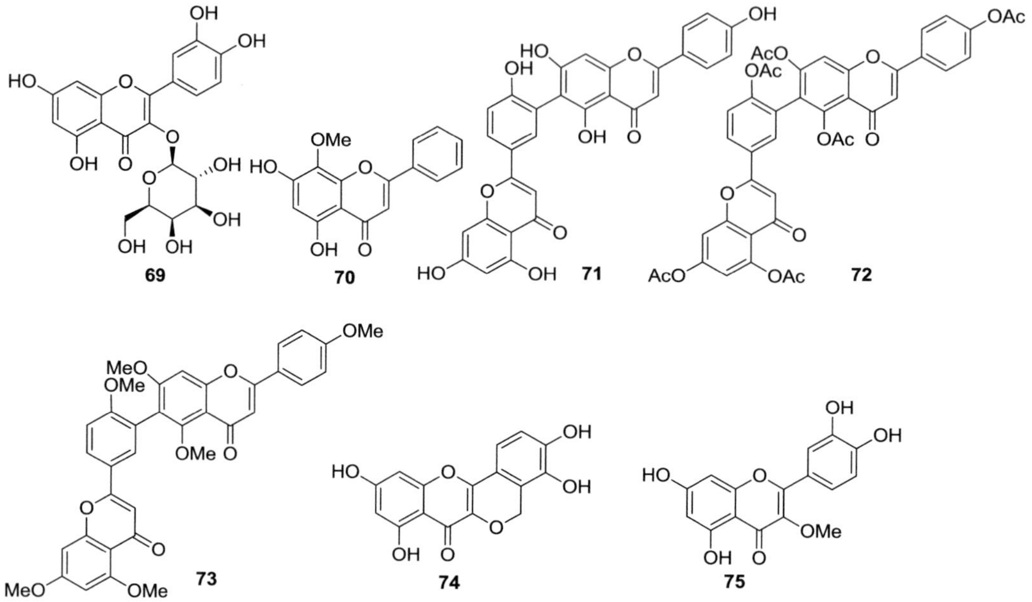

Fig. (6). Structure of active flavonoids.

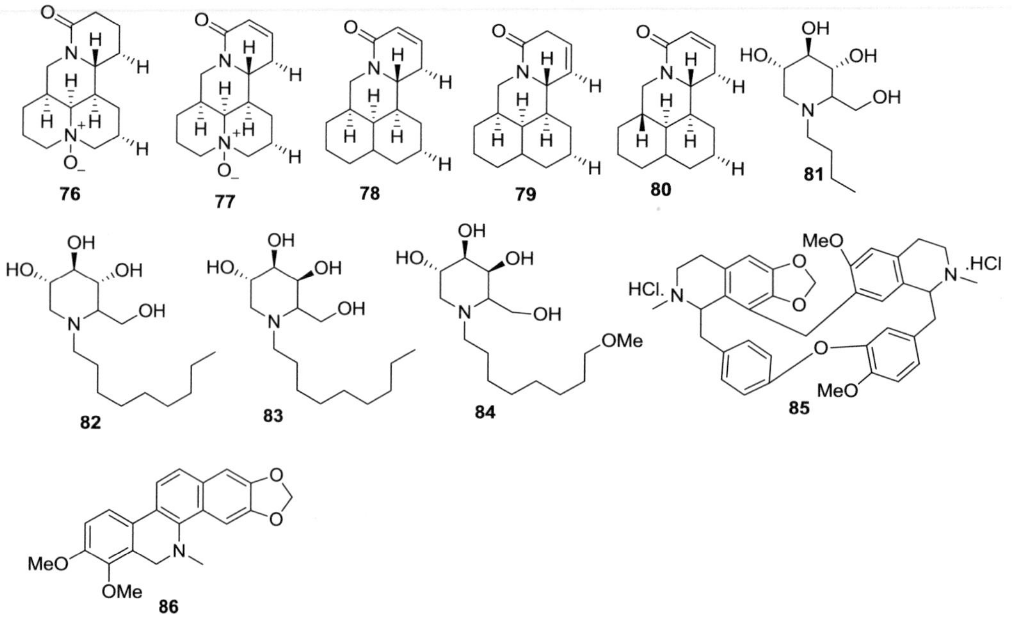

Fig. (7). Structure of active alkaloids.

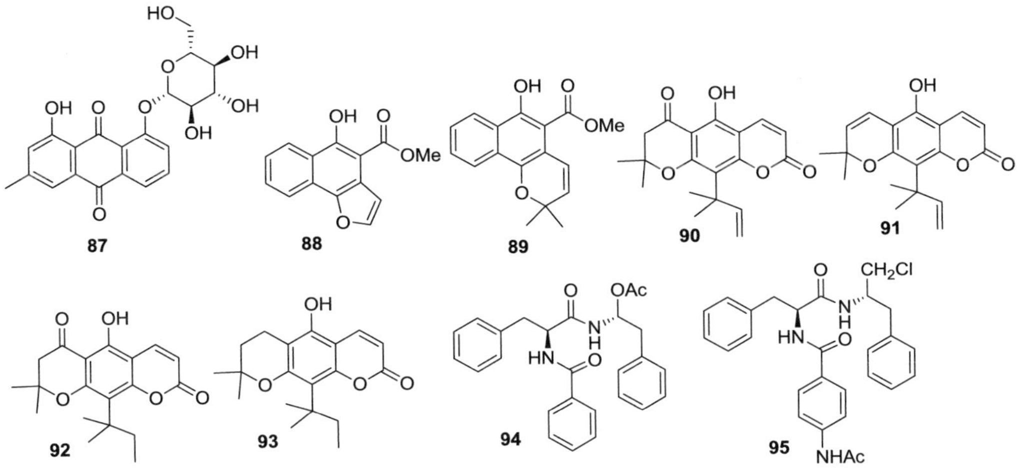

Fig. (8). Structure of other plants active compounds.

3.6.10. Oxymatrine

The herb *Sophora alopecuraides L*, extract isolated oxymatrine alkaloid which exhibited anti-HBV effect in HBV transgenic mice [77] and patients with chronic HBV infection by suppressing the levels of HBsAg and HBcAg in liver and HBV DNA in serum of transgenic mice, resulted in disrupting the packaging of pgRNA into the nucleocapsid or viral DNA polymerase [78]. Oxymatrine along with lamivudine prevent the resistance development in lamivudine in the chronic cases. The oxymatrine mechanisms against HBV is unclear [79] but it is reported in the Chinese Guideline for prevention and treatment of chronic HBV infection [80].

3.6.11. Wogonin and Its Analogues

Wogonin **96** (dose 20 mg/mL) isolated from *Scutellaria baicalensis* showed 45-48% inhibition by blocking anti-hepatitis B surface antigen (anti-HBsAg) activity. Both the linear and the relaxed circular form of HBV DNA were notably reduced in wogonin treatment. Similarly, significant reduction of secretion was observed in hepatitis B e antigen (HBeAg) in human hepatoblastoma-derived liver Hep-G2 cells (IC_{50} 4 mg/mL). Oppositely, wogonin's related analogue, baicalein **97** has minimal effects on HBsAg secretion. *In vitro* study of polyphenolic extract obtained from *Geranium carolinianum L.* also reduces the secretion of the HBV antigens and HBV DNA level. Similarly, the plasma and the liver DNA level was reduced in the DHBV infected ducks. The extract compounds, hyperin **98** showed significant inhibitory effect on HBsAg and HBeAg secretion but quercetin **99** had no activity against HBeAg (Fig. **9**) [81]. These results indicated that a galactose group at 3-position of quercetin skeleton enhanced the anti-HBV potency.

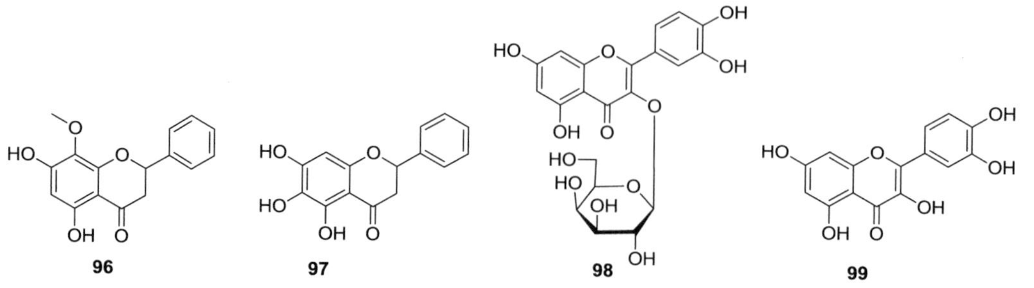

Fig. (9). Structure of wogonin, baicalin, hyperin, quercetine.

3.6.12. Helioxanthin and Its Analogues

Helioxanthin **100** isolated from the root of *Taiwania cryptomerioides* showed anti-HBV activity (EC_{50} 1.0 mmol/L). Derivatization of helioxanthin, an arylnaphthalene lignan lactone gave many products of improved activity. Structure-activity relationship (SAR) study found that the acid-hydrolysed derivative **101**, the lactam derivative **102** and the cyclic hydrazide derivative **103** have enhanced anti-HBV activity (EC_{50} 0.8, 0.08 and 0.03 mmol/L) respectively. However, halogens substitution at 5-position reduced the anti-viral activity. The carboxylic acid and amide groups modifications of compound **101** into dicarboxylic acid or diamide groups also resulted in a significant loss of activity. The methylenedioxy group replacement with two methoxy groups in A-ring exhibited reduced activity. The anti-viral mechanism was completely different from nucleoside analogues at the viral RNA transcription step [82]. The interaction of compound **108** with hepatocyte nuclear factors (HNF) and HBV promoters modified down-regulated HNF expression in HBV-harbouring cells [83]. The lactone ring and methylenedioxy unit modification of helioxanthin modulated the anti-viral activity. Among them, **108** was found the most effective anti-HBV agent which suppressed the secretion of viral surface antigen and e antigen in HepA2 cells (EC_{50} -0.06 and 0.14 mmol/L) respectively. Compound **108** also inhibited HBV DNA wild-type, lamivudine-resistant strain, HBV mRNA core protein and viral promoters (Fig. **10**).

3.6.13. Artemisinin and Its Analogues

Artemisia annua extract isolate Artemisinin **115** had been widely used as antimalarial, anticancer, antiangiogenesis, antiviral, immunosuppressive and antifungal agent. It was also found that artemisinin and its semi-synthetic derivative, artesunate **116** exhibited strong inhibition of HBsAg secretion (IC_{50} 55 and 2.3 mmol/L) respectively well below the host cell viability concentrations. Artesunate in combination with lamivudine gave synergic anti-HBV effects (Fig. **10**) [84].

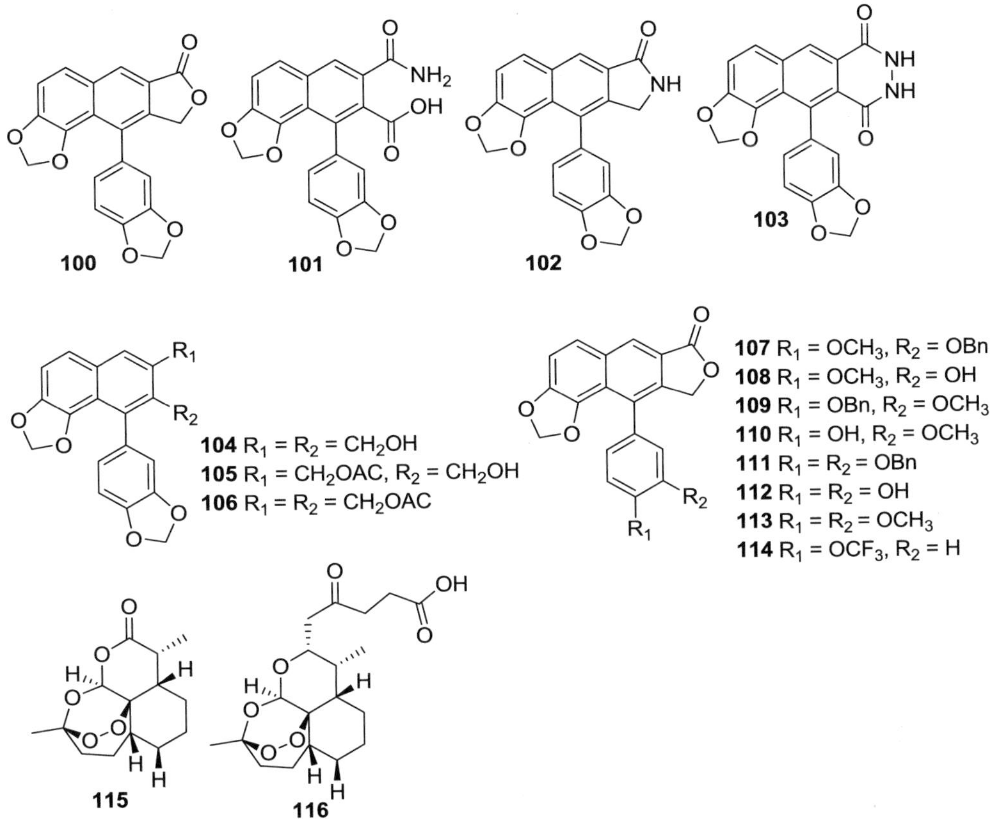

Fig. (10). Structure of helioxanthine and its analogues **100-103**, helioxanthin derivatives **104-114** and artemisinin **115** and artesunate **116**.

3.6.14. Alisol Analogues

The rhizome of *Alisma orientalis* extract afforded six triterpenes, alisol A 24-acetate **117**, 25-anhydroalisol A **118**, 13β,17β-epoxyalisol A **119**, alisol B 23-acetate **120**, alisol F **121**, and alisol F 24-acetate **122**. All compounds exhibited inhibitory activity against HBsAg (IC_{50} 0.6-15.4 mmol/L). Alisol F 24-acetate also displayed significant activity against HBeAg (IC_{50} 5.1 mmol/L). Alisol ester derivatives were synthesized [85] and its SAR study showed that acetylation at 25-position hydroxyl group enhanced potentially anti-HBV activity of alisol A derivatives. Similarly, acyloxy substituents at 11, 23, 24-positions are essential for anti-HBV activity. However, epoxide at 13(17)-position decreased suppressant property for the secretion of HBsAg and HBeAg. Thus, compound **120** showed better suppressant activity against secretion of HBsAg and HBeAg (IC_{50} 0.0048 and 0.011 mmol/L) respectively. Astragaloside IV **123** isolated from *Radix astragali* was also reported for anti-HBV activity (Fig. **11**) [86].

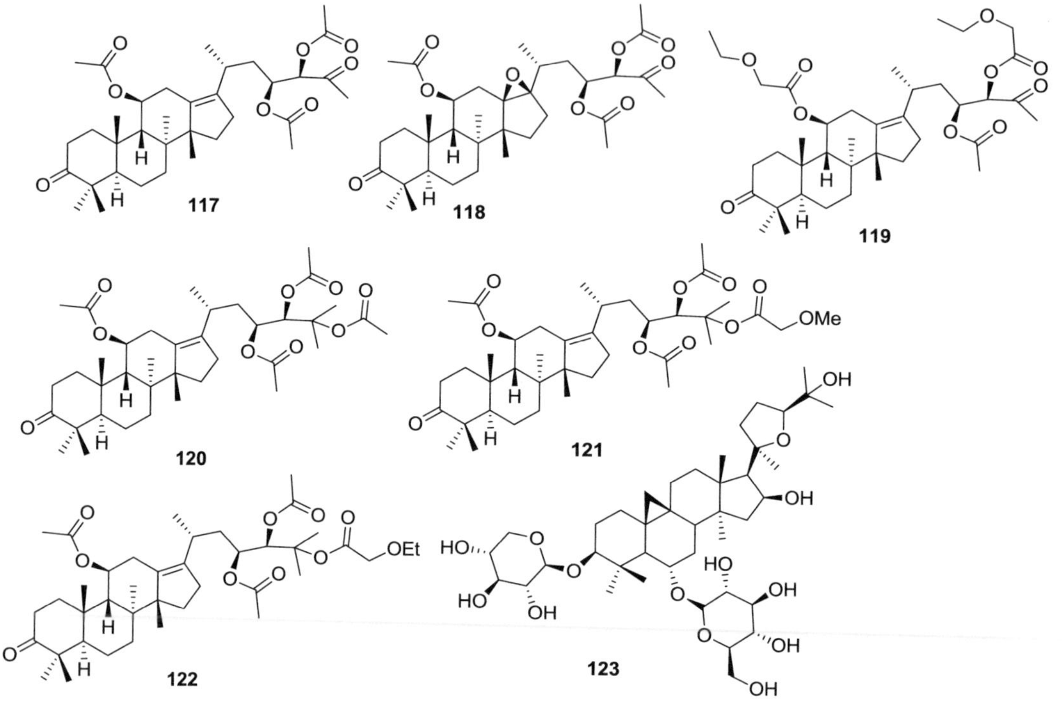

Fig. (11). Structures of ester derivatives of alisol and astragaloside IV **123**.

3.6.15. Matrine and Its Analogues

Matrine analogues isolated from the roots of *Sophora flavescens* and *Sophora tonkinensis* and their semi-synthetic products were investigated for anti-HBV activity *in vitro* [87]. Compounds **126, 128, 130** and **131** exhibited potential anti-HBV activity with low toxicity in HepG2.2.15 cells. Further, SAR study revealed that the N/O group compounds **129, 130** is less important for the activity. However, compounds with double bond in D ring and without hydroxyl group were more potent than other analogues. Introduction of a N/O group compound **130** or α-hydroxyl group compounds **132, 133** into compound **131** (unsaturated D ring) negatively influenced the anti-HBV activity and so the HBeAg inhibitory potency while compounds with saturated D ring showed dramatically opposite activity. The N/O group compound **129** and α-substituted hydroxyl group compound **125** in matrine **124** markedly enhanced the potency. While, proper substituents at 13- and/or 14-position(s) **126, 127, 128**, especially with electron-withdrawing groups might enhance the activity. Matrinic acid **134** and oxymatrinic acid **135** with D ring opening still retained moderate anti-HBV activity. Thus, D ring might not be required for activity. Twenty-six N-substituted matrinic acid analogues were synthesized [88]. Among these, compound **136** is host heat-stress cognate 70 (Hsc70) down-regulator has also exhibited a broad spectrum anti-HBV and anti-HCV effects with different mechanism than the nucleosides (Fig. **12**). SAR study showed that the carboxyl group at 11-position required for better activity and so introduction of a substituent on nitrogen atom at 12-position, especially with substituted benzyl might significantly improved the anti-HBV activity.

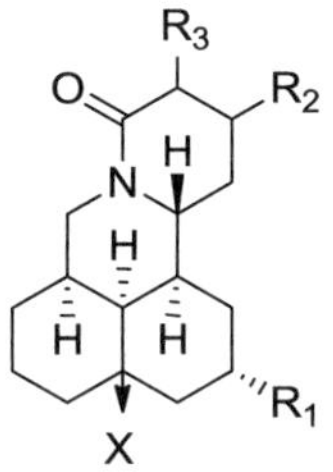

124 $R_1 = R_2 = R_3 = H$
125 $R_1 = OH, R_2 = R_3 = H$
126 $R_1 = R_3 = H, R_2 = OCH_3$
127 $R_1 = H, R_2 = R_3 = OCH_2C_6H_5$
128 $R_1 = H, R_2 = OCOCH_2Cl, R_3 = OH$
129 $R_1 = R_2 = R_3 = H, X = O$

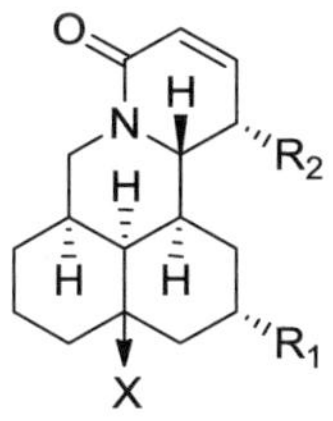

130 $R_1 = R_2 = H, X = O$
131 $R_1 = R_2 = H$
132 $R_1 = OH, R_2 = H$
133 $R_1 = H, R_2 = OH$

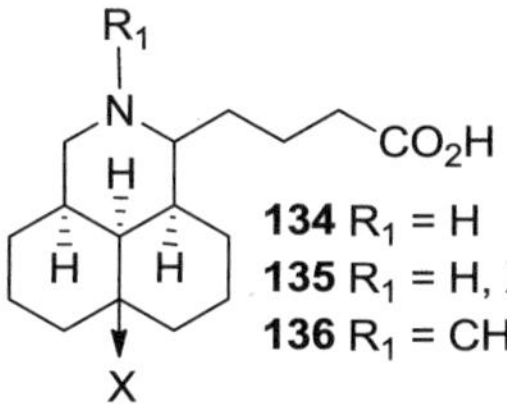

134 $R_1 = H$
135 $R_1 = H, X = O$
136 $R_1 = CH_2PhOCH_3$-P

Fig. (12). Structures of matrine and its analogues.

3.6.16. Acutumidine and Its Analogues

Hypserpa nitida Miers ethanol extract showed inhibitory effect against the secretion of HBsAg and HBeAg. Among the isolated alkaloids in ethanol extract, acutumidine **137** and its analogues **138-140** showed moderate activity against HBsAg secretion (IC_{50} 0.45-2.02 mmol/L) (Fig. **13**) [89]. While, N-methyl substituted derivatives were less potent than the corresponding non-substituted derivatives as anti-viral activities.

3.6.17. Chrysophanol and Its Analogues

Ethanol extract of *Rheum palmatum L.* afforded chrysophanol and its analogues and evaluated for anti-HBV activity (Fig. **14**). Among them, chrysophanol **141**, physcion **142**, aloe-emodin **143** and 8-O-β-D-glucoside **144** gave similar inhibitory activity against HBV DNA, HBsAg and HBeAg (IC_{50} 300 mg/mL) while **144** exhibited less toxicity than others. Therefore, a galactose group at 8-position of chrysophanol might be good to reduce the toxicity.

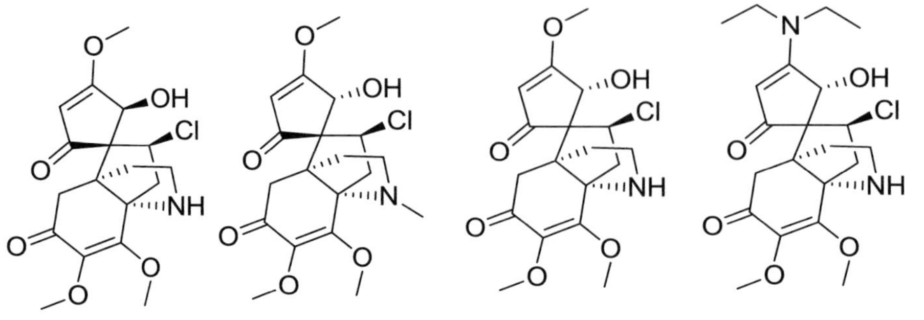

137 **138** **139** **140**

Fig. (13). Structures of acutumidine and its analogues.

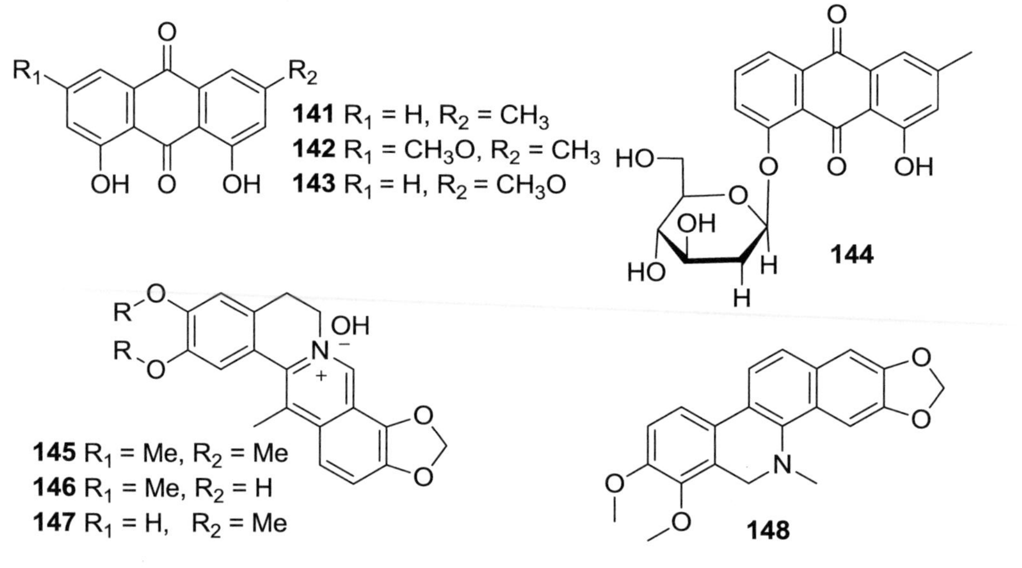

Fig. (14). Structures of chrysophanol and analogues **141-144** and dehydrocavidine and analogues **145-148**.

3.6.18. Dehydrocavidine and Its Analogues

Dehydrocavidine **145**, dehydeoapocavidine **146** and dehydroisoapocavidine **147** were isolated from *Corydalis saxicola* which demonstrated anti-HBsAg and anti-HBeAg effects with inhibition about 50% and 40% respectively. These compounds showed inhibitory effect on dose-dependent manner within the 16.5-250 mg/mL concentration range. Alkaloid dihydrochelerythrine **148** was also found to be a potent inhibitor for HBV secretion of both HBsAg and HBeAg (IC_{50} < 0.05 mmol/L) (Fig. **14**) [90].

3.6.19. Triterpenoid Saponin

Triterpenoid saponin **149** isolated from *Potentilla anserina L.* and used as

Traditional Chinese Medicine (TCM) in hepatitis B treatment. Compound **149** exhibited anti-HBV activity against secretion of HBsAg (IC_{50} 57.67 mg/mL), HBeAg (IC_{50} 30.05 mg/mL) and HBV DNA (IC_{50} 19.45 mg/mL) in HepG2.2.15 cells (Fig. **15**).

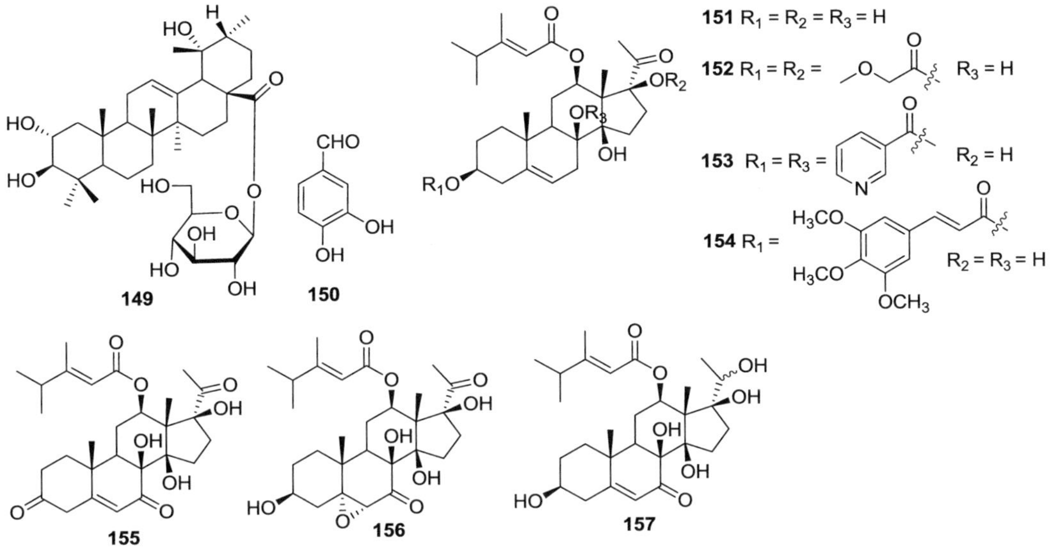

Fig. (15). Structures of tritepenoid saponin **149**, protocatechuic aldehyde **150**, caudatin and analogues **151-157**.

3.6.20. Protocatechuic Aldehyde

Salvia miltiorrhiza is the highly recommended and widely accepted medicines for hepatitis B treatment in China. The main active component, protocatechuic aldehyde **150** inhibits the production of HBV DNA (IC_{50} 4.17 mg/mL), HBsAg (EC_{50} 3.94 mg/mL) and HBeAg (EC_{50} 2.46 mg/mL). There might be at least two targets of protocatechuic aldehyde. It also reduces the level of DHBV DNA in DHBV-infected ducks at dosage of 50 mg/kg.

3.6.21. Caudatin and Its Analogues

Caudatin **151** isolated from *Cynanchum auriculatum* (Bai-Shou-Wu in Chinese) inhibited cell proliferation and induces cell apoptosis [91]. It has anti-HBV activity against the secretion of HBsAg and HBV DNA replication (IC_{50} 142.67 and 40.62 mmol/L) respectively in HepG2.2.15 cells. Several caudatin derivatives were synthesized. Among them, the 3-O-substituted derivatives showed effective anti-HBV activity by inhibiting the HBV DNA replication (IC_{50} 2.44-22.89 mmol/L) [92]. While, the 3,8-O-di and 3,17-O-diacyl derivatives **152**, **153** lost suppressant properties in the HBV and cytotoxicity. This suggested the importance of free hydroxyl groups for the activity and the cytotoxicity. Compound **155**, epoxide **156** and reduction product **157** exhibited decreased anti-HBV activity compared to caudatin. Among derivatives, compound **154** along with cinnamic acid displayed the most significant inhibitory effects on the secretion of HBsAg, HBeAg and HBV DNA replication (IC_{50} 5.52, 5.52, 2.44 mmol/L) respectively. The compound **154** mechanism exerted antiviral effects *via* interfering HBV promoters and enhancers to HBV transcriptions (Fig. **15**).

3.6.22. Hemslecin A and Its Analogues

Hemslecin A **158**, cucurbitane-type terpene is widely used to cure inflammatory diseases. Its derivatives were further evaluated for their anti-HBV activity in HepG2.2.15 cells [93]. Compound **158** showed moderate activity against HBV DNA replication (IC_{50} 11.4 mmol/L) with toxicity (CC_{50} 66.2 mmol/L) (Fig. **16**). However, their derivatives displayed enhanced anti-HBV activity. Compounds **159-164** exhibited significant activity against HBV DNA replication (IC_{50} 2.8-11.6 mmol/ L). SAR study also indicated that (i) mono- or di-acylation of hydroxyl group(s) at 2-position and/or 3-position resulted in enhancement of anti-viral activity. (ii) acylation of hydroxyls at 2-, 3- and 16-position decreased cytotoxicity. (iii) epoxide of double bond at 5(6)-position decreased the cytotoxicity and maintained activity against HBV DNA replication. (iv) presence of acetyl at 25-position was an important feature in conferring anti-HBV activity.

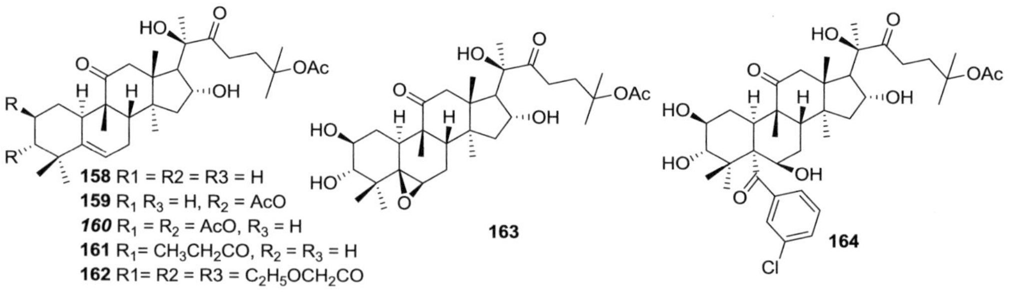

Fig. (16). Structures of hemslecin and analogues

Platycladus orientalis L. leaves extraction in water and alcohol precipitation afforded polysaccharide fraction, POP1 which constitutes of rhamnose 5.74%, arabinose 12.58%, mannose 10.97%, glucose 64.96% and galactose 6.55%. The periodate oxidation, Smith degradation and methylation gave main linkage types of POP1 consisted of (1→5)-linked α-L-Ara, (1→3)-linked α-L-Man, (1→6)-linked β-L-Rha, (1→4)-linked α-D-Glc, (1→6)-linked α-D-Glc, (1→6)-linked β-

D-Gal, (1→3,6)-linked β-D-Gal, and termination with α-L-Man and α-D-Glc residues. It gave excellent immune-stimulating activity by enhancing macrophage NO, TNF-α, IL-6 and IL-12 secretion and activating related mRNA expression. It also showed significant anti-HBV activity through inhibiting the expression of HBsAg (IC_{50} 1.33 mg/mL) and HBeAg (IC_{50} 1.67 mg/mL) by interfering with the HBV DNA replication (IC_{50} 0.80 mg/mL). The anti-viral screening in HepG2.2.15 cells identified three analogs **165-168** with good anti-HBV activity and low cytotoxicty (Fig. **17**) [94].

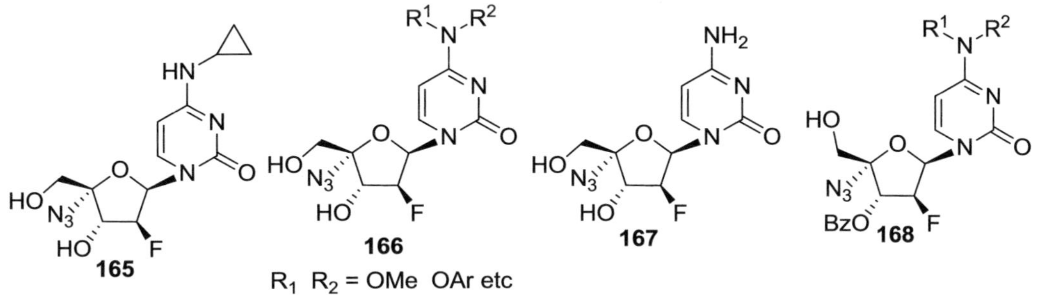

Fig. (17). Structure of the N^4-alkylated FNC derivatives.

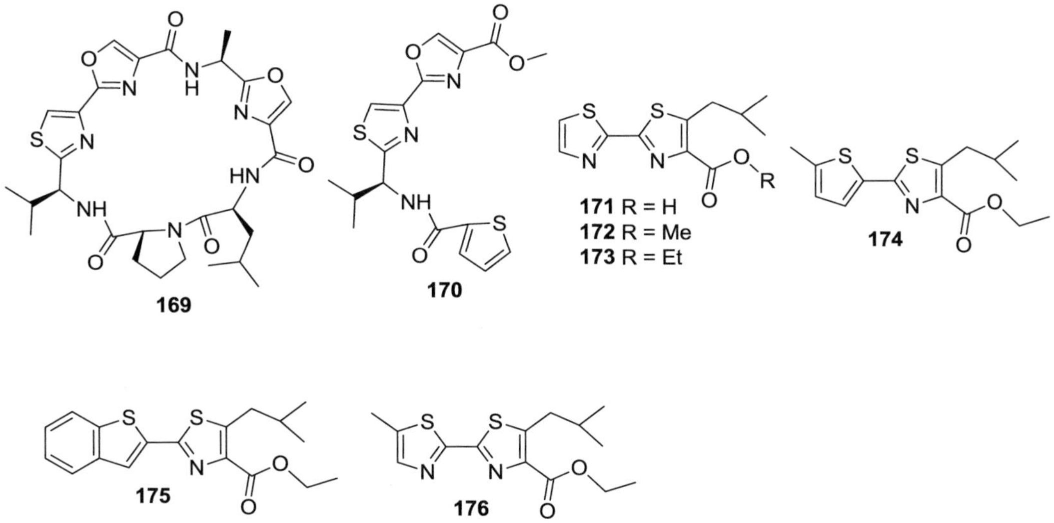

Fig. (18). Structure of leucamide **169** and 2,2-bishetrocycle tandems **170-176**.

3.7. Synthetic Compounds

3.7.1. 2,2-Bisheterocycles

In *in vitro* assays, molecular library of leucamide A **169**, a bioactive cydicheptapeptide were screened to determine their anti-viral activity. Compound **170** showed moderate activity against HBV DNA (IC_{50} 76.4 mmol/L) (Fig. **18**). Many 2,2-bisheterocycle compounds were synthesized and evaluated for their SAR and anti-HBV activity. It was found that a bulky aliphatic group at 5-positon of heterocycle B ring had an advantageous effect on the activity against HBV DNA replication. The inhibitory activity of acid analogue **171** (IC_{50} 60 mmol/L) was substantially diminished compared to its ester analogue **172** (IC_{50} 2.4 mmol/L) and **173** (IC_{50} 1.1 mmol/L). When A ring is replaced with thiophene ring **81** or the benzo[b]thiophene ring **175**, compound **176** showed significant potency (IC_{50} 0.14 mmol/L) against HBV DNA replication and about 500-fold more potent than the lead compound **169** (IC_{50} 76.4 mmol/L) and even more potent than lamivudine (IC_{50} 0.26 mmol/L) (Fig. **18**).

3.7.2. Acrylamide Derivatives

Phenylpropenamide derivatives **177-183** displayed potent anti-HBV activity (IC_{50} <4 mmol/L) without toxicity in the HepAD38 cellular assay [95]. The E-isomers showed weak activity or no activity against HBV. SAR study revealed that the vinyl bromides were slightly more active and less toxic than the corresponding vinyl chlorides. In general, substitution at 4-position of A ring had little effects on the activity. However, substitution at 4-position on B ring resulted in improved inhibitory activity but unsubstituted piperidine and pyrrolidine amides are much preferred. Additionally, AT-61 **177** and AT-130 **183** also showed anti-viral activity against YVDD lamivudine resistant variant in *in vitro*. AT-61 was highly selective and inhibits only the replication of human HBV but not the replication of other viruses. The mechanism of action indicated that the phenylpropenamide derivatives inhibit HBV replication in the packaging of pre-genomic RNA into immature core particles not in the HBV polymerase [96]. The replacement of the phenyl in phenylpropenamide with 1,2,3-thiadiazolyl gave a new class of acrylamide analogues which possess a similar SAR with the phenylpropenamides. Compounds **184-186** that replaced A or B ring by 1,2,3-thiadiazole had anti-HBV DNA activity (IC_{50} 10.4, 3.59 and 9.00 mg/mL) respectively. However, when A and B rings were simultaneously replaced by 1,2,3-thiadiazole **187**, the anti-HBV activity was eliminated and the cytotoxicity was higher than the mono-substituted analogues (Fig. **19**) [97].

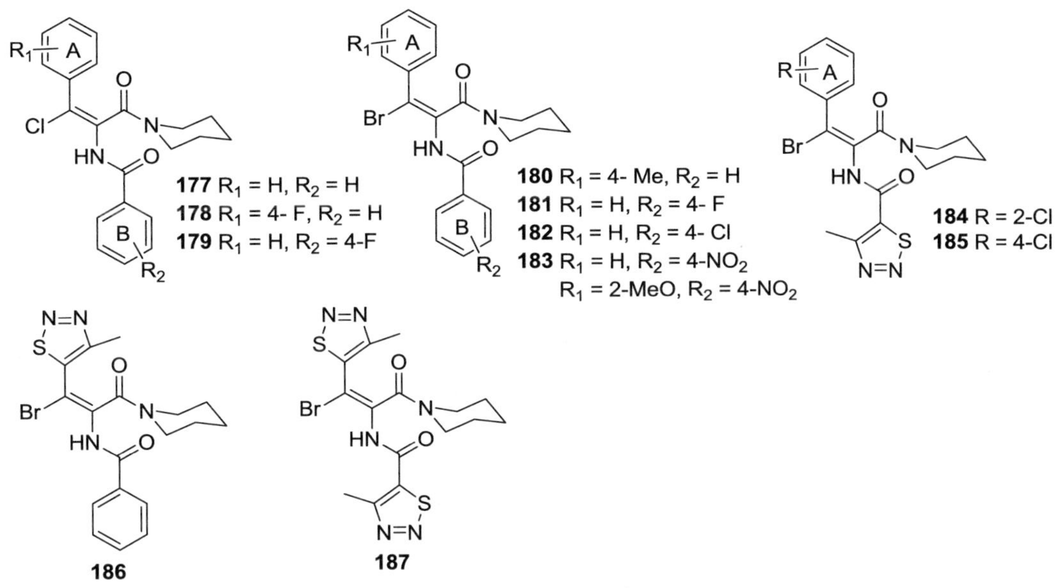

Fig. (19). Structure of phenylpropenamides **177-183** and 1,2,3 thiadiazole subsitituted acrylamides **184-187**.

3.7.3. Imino Sugars

N-butyl-deoxy-nojirimycin (N-Bu-DNJ, **188**) and N-nonyl-deoxy-nojirimycin (NN-DNJ, **189**), imino sugars had shown to be effective against HBV infection. For SAR study, many imino sugar derivatives were synthesized and classified into two groups: an imino sugar head group and an alkyl tail. It indicated that the head group played a critical role in anti-viral activity. Variation of the head group was allowed to maintain a large extent anti-viral activity. For alkyl tail, the side chain length appeared important for anti-viral activity and decreased sharply with side chains less than eight carbons. Also, pause of the side chain with oxygenation (N-7-oxa-decyl- DGJ, **192**) reduces anti-viral activity. NN-DGJ **190** was effective against the lamivudine resistant virus but not inhibit DNA polymerase or envelop antigen production by either prevented the maturation of HBV nucleocapsids or destabilized the formed nucleocapsids (Fig. **20**) [98].

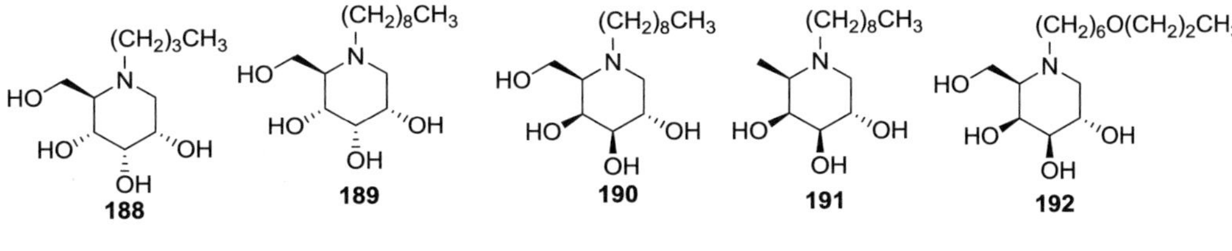

Fig. (20). Structures of imino sugars.

3.7.4. 2,5-Pyridine Dicarboxylic Acid Derivatives

Pyridine based dicarboxylic acid derivatives were synthesized and evaluated for their anti-HBV activity. Compounds **193-203** showed potent inhibitory effect against HBV polymerase (TC_{50} <10 mg/L) with low cytotoxicity (CC_{50} >100 mmol/L) which indicated their excellent anti-HBV property. SAR study also showed that isopropyl, tert-butyl and 3-imidazolylpropyl groups were preferred substitutents for better activity. For example, amino substituted with isobutyl group, resulted in compounds **195** and **196** with improved activity (Fig. **21**).

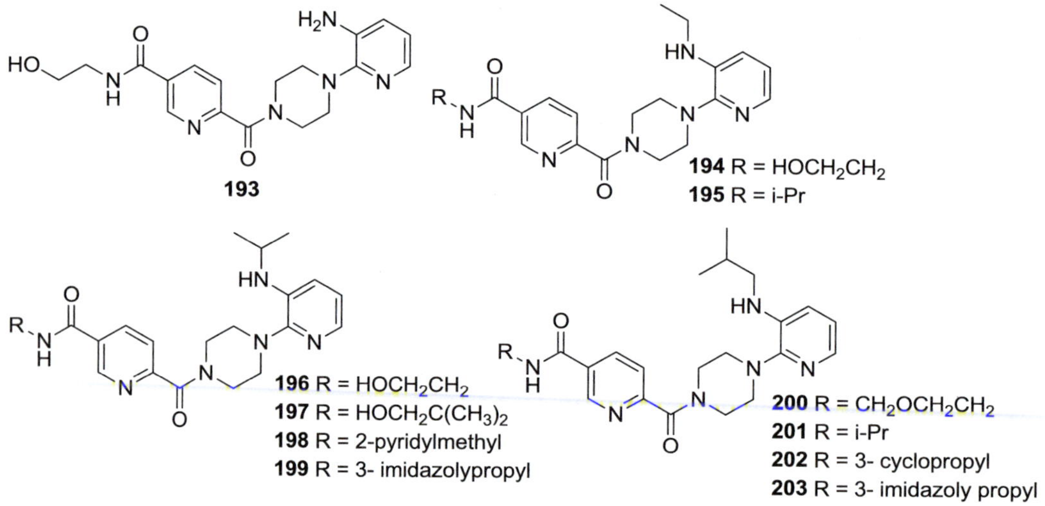

Fig. (21). Structures of 2,5 dipyridinedicarboxylic acids.

3.7.5. Triazoles

Triazoles have significant anti-fungal and anti-bacterial properties. Therefore, triazole derivatives were synthesized and evaluated for anti-HBV activity. Compounds **204-206** showed moderate activity against HBV (IC_{50} 35, 63 and 40 mmol/L) respectively [99]. Oxadiazole compound **207** was also exhibited anti-HBV activity (EC_{50} 1.63 mmol/L) for HBsAg and HBeAg in a concentration-dependent manner without affecting the transcription and HBV cytotoxic effects and not found that compound **207** affects downstream of transcription in the viral replication. 1,2,3-Thiadiazole derivatives, compound **208** was identified as a HBV inhibitor at 0.6 mmol/mL which reduces the secretion of HBsAg and HBeAg by 88.6% and 15.5% respectively and inhibits HBV DNA (IC_{50} 400 mmol/L) [100]. Screening of a chemical library of 5600 compounds in an enzyme-linked immunosorbent assay, showed the interaction between the core protein and PreS region in the surface protein. Among them, compound KKJ00626 **209** inhibited the production of HBV particles from transiently HBV-producing HuH7 cells (IC_{50} 0.12 mmol/L) (Fig. **22**) [101].

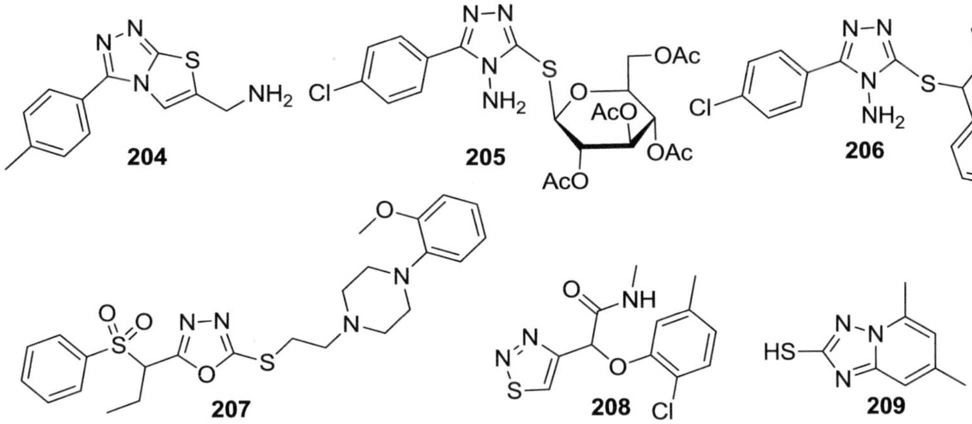

Fig. (22). Structure of 1,2,4-triazoles 1,2,3-oxadiazoles and 1,2,3-thiadiazole acetamides.

3.7.6. Benzimidazoles

Compound **210** was identified as an inhibitor of HBV (IC_{50} 14.2 mmol/L) against HBV DNA in a random screening. SAR study also revealed that the substituents such as methyl, isopropyl, methoxy and nitro group were tolerated at the benzenesulfonyl group at N-1 position of benzimidazole core. The N-1 substituent removal resulted in a tremendous loss of activity while introducing 4-methylbenzoyl to N-1 position of the benzimidazole core decreased the cytotoxicity. Replacement of the phthalimide group with maleimide yielded in compound **212** with improved anti-activity. Alkyl linkers are important for potent anti-viral activity but methylene and propylene analogues were more toxic. Contrarily, the replacement of sulfonyl group with alkyl substituents at N-1 position dramatically increased anti-viral activity and selectivity. The most promising compounds **213** and **214** showed potent anti-HBV activity (IC_{50} 0.9 and 0.7 mmol/L) respectively [102]. To improve the water-solubility and oral bioavailability, eighteen novel derivatives of compound **213** were synthesized and evaluated for anti-HBV activity and cytotoxicity in the HepG2.2.15 cell line [103]. Among them, compound **215** (IC_{50} <0.41 mmol/L) was the most promising compound (nearly three times higher selectivity than lamivudine). Large substituents at 5- or 6-position of the benzoimidazole ring resulted in a new series of benzimidazole derivatives **216-223** with better anti-HBV activity. SAR study showed that the substituent on the benzoyl ring is important at 6-position. The halide substituted analogues **217-220** demonstrated more inhibition activity than the methyl substituted analogue **221**. However, 5-position substituted derivative

222 without a substituent on the benzoyl ring was found to be more potent than the fluoro substituted derivative **223**. Thus, compounds **219** and **224** are better anti-viral agents (IC_{50} 0.70 mmol/L). Similarly, 1-methyl-1H-benzimidazol-5-ol analogues with different Mannich side chains at 4-position of the benzimidazole core were synthesized and evaluated for anti-HBV activity in HepG2.2.15 cells (Fig. **23**) [104].

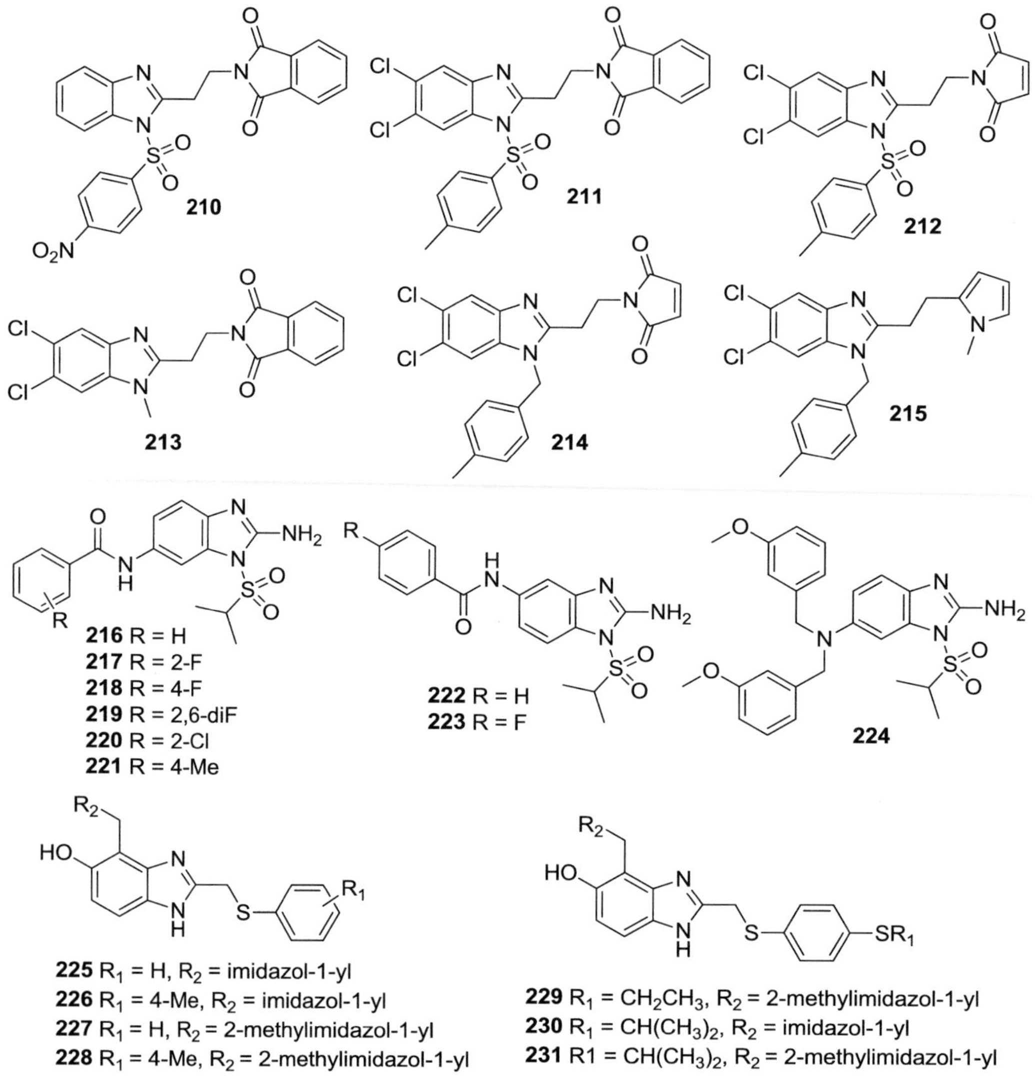

Fig. (23). Structures of benzimidazoles and 1*H*-benzimidazol-5-OH **225-231**.

3.7.8. Indoles

Compound arbidol **232** used for influenza A and B infections treatment in Russia, was reported to possess inhibitory activity of several viruses such as respiratory syncytial virus, para-influenza virus, rhinovirus and hepatitis C virus [105]. Recently, HBV inhibitory activity is also reported against HBV DNA (IC_{50} 22.85 mg/mL) and HBsAg 47.45 mg/mL. Derivatives **233-237** also exhibited significant anti-HBV activity (IC_{50} < 60 mg/mL). SAR study revealed that fluoro or chloro group on the phenyl ring could improve the anti-HBV activity and oxidation of sulfide into sulfinyl also resulted in increased activity. Bromo group at 6-position has small influence on activity and cytotoxicity. Arbidol was found to inhibit membrane fusion during influenza virus or HCV infection and suppress these viruses entry into target cells (Fig. **24**) [106].

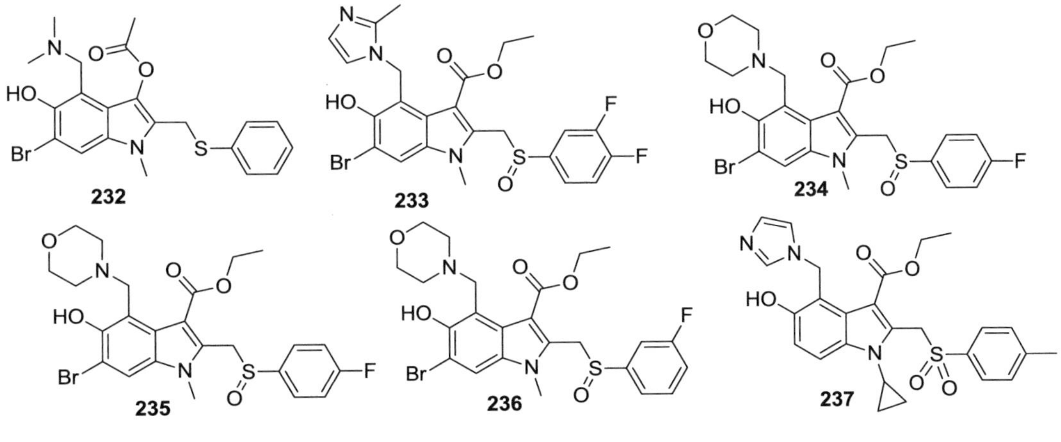

Fig. (24). Structure of ethyl 5 hydroxy 1-*H*-indole-3-carboxylates.

3.7.9. Quinolin-2-ones and Benzodiazepine-2-ones

4-Arylquinolin-2-one and 5-aryl-1,4-benzodizaepin-2-one derivatives were synthesized where compounds **238-252** inhibited the secretion of HBsAg (IC_{50} 0.01-2.84 mmol/L). SAR study revealed that compounds **241-243** are less active than corresponding hydroxyl ethyl derivatives **252-255** while introduction of hydroxyethyl to 3-position of 4-aryl-6-chloroquinoline-2-one confers enhanced anti-HBV activity. In addition, ester derivatives **256-259** displayed optimal profile inhibiting not only HBsAg and HBeAg secretion but also HBV DNA replication. 3-Amino derivatives **244-247** exhibited increased cytotoxicity and activity. A preliminary mechanism study suggested that compound **245** promoted the transcription activity of HBV enhancers ENI and ENII to exert anti-HBV action. The ring-expanded derivatives **251-252** were also active against HBsAg secretion (IC_{50} 67 and 56 mmol/L) and thiazolides have similar activity (Fig. **25**) [107].

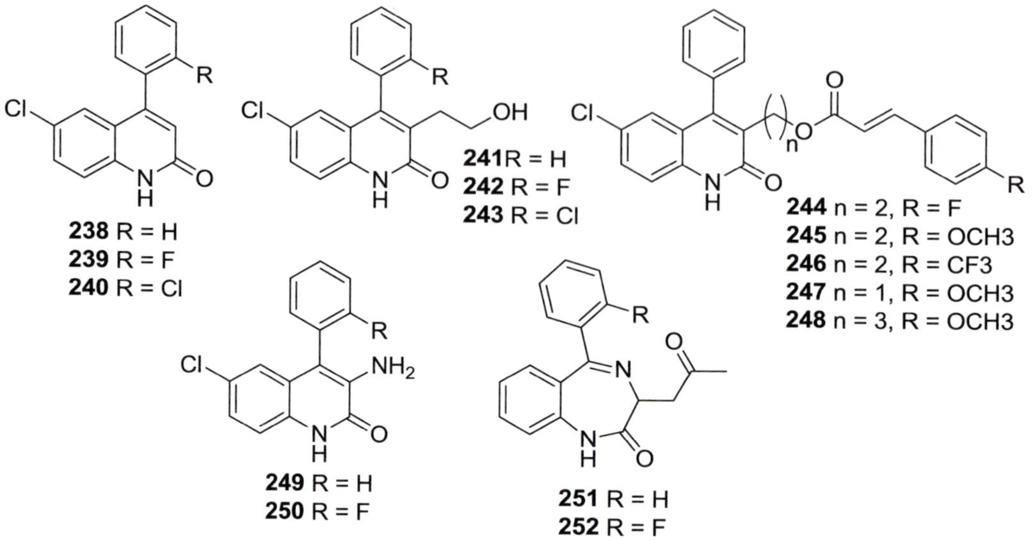

Fig. (25). Structure of 4-aryl-6-chloro-quinoline-2-one and benzodiaze-pine-2-one.

3.7.10. Quinolines

Several quinoline derivatives were reported with potent anti-HBV activity. 7-Hydroxyquinolines, compounds **253** (IC_{50} 3.5 mmol/L,) and **254** (IC_{50} 2.6 mmol/L) were found more potent than the lamivudine (IC_{50} 343.2 mmol/L) against HBV DNA [108]. Substitution of imidazolyl group by 2-methylimidazolyl group has little effect on anti-HBV activity. Electron-withdrawing fluoro atom on the phenyl at 2-postion was superior to the electron-donating methoxy, methyl or no substitution. In 6-hydroxyquinolines, compounds **255** and **256** inhibited the secretion of both HBsAg and HBeAg. They also demonstrated potent inhibition of HBV DNA replication (IC_{50} 10.7 and 4.7 mmol/L) respectively [109]. SAR study also revealed that fluoride could enhanced the activity while oxidation of the sulfide into the sulfinyl group had little influence on HBV activity and cytotoxicity. As for Mannich groups, pyrrolidinyl, piperidyl and imidazolyl were preferred at 5-position while morpholinyl and 4-methyl piperazinyl were not. A series of 4-aryl-6-chloro-quinoline derivatives were synthesized and assayed for anti-HBV activity and cytotoxicities in HepG2.2.15 cells [110]. Compounds **257-265** displayed significant inhibition against HBV DNA replication (IC_{50} 4.4-9.8 mmol/L) while compounds **261**, **263-264** had low cytotoxicities. SAR study indicated that TBDPS substitution at 3-position is an important feature in the conferring relatively low cytotoxicity. But in 2-N-substituted analogues, TBDPS substitution reduces the suppressant property on the secretion of HBsAg and HBeAg. A novel 6H-benzothiopyrano[4,3-b]quinoline skeleton was also found to be an inhibitor of HBV (Fig. **26**) [111].

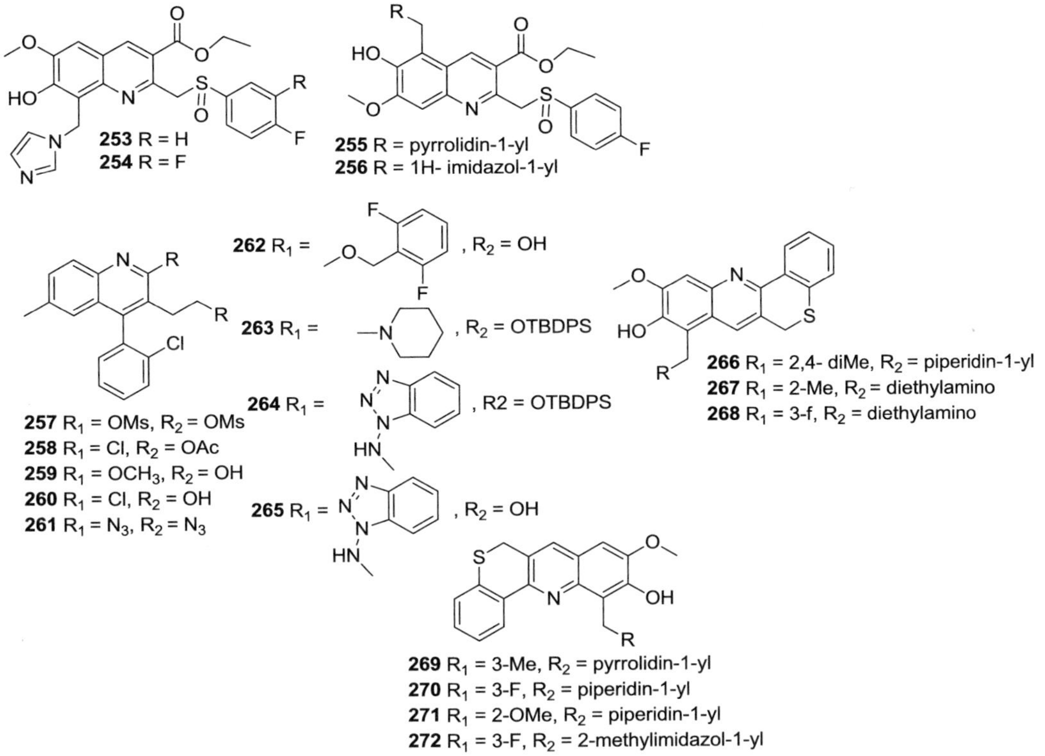

Fig. (26). Ethyl 6(7)-hydroxyquinoline-3-carboxylate, 4-aryl-6-chloroquinolines **257-265** and 6*H*- [1] benzothiopyrano[4,3-b]quinoline-9(10)-ols **266-272**.

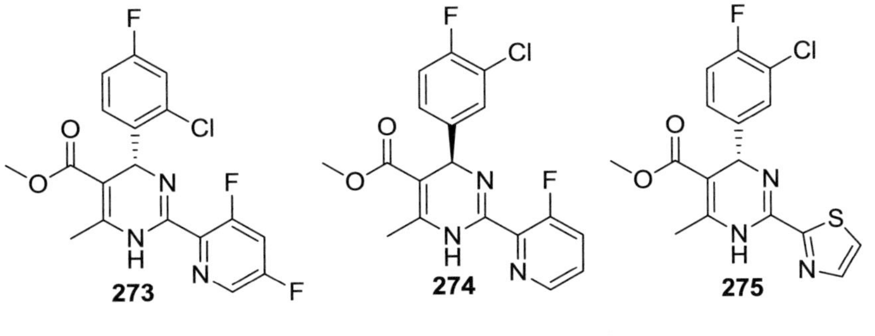

Fig. (27). Structures of Bay 41-4109, Bay 38-7690, Bay 39-5493.

3.7.11. Dihydropyrimidines

Bay 41-4109 **273**, Bay 38-7690 **274** and Bay 39-5493 **275** were revealed as highly potent inhibitors of HBV replication (IC_{50} 50, 150 and 30 nmol/L) respectively. SAR study showed that there was little tolerance for changes in the 2-chloro-4-fluoroaryl moiety at 4-position but have no effects for 2-position of the pyridyl nitrogen (Fig. **27**) [112]. Oppositely, larger aryl groups at 2-position could reduce the anti-HBV activity. The presence of phenyl, chloro or substituted amino groups in the β-position to 6-position was well tolerated and inhibited virus production by targeting viral capsid [113].

3.7.12. Qaphthoquinones

Naphthoquinone trimers act as potential HIV inhibitors. Compound **276** showed good inhibition of HBV DNA replication in *in vitro* assay (EC_{50} 0.009 mmol/L) [114]. The pyran/dihydropyan ring(s) of compound **276** were replaced by methoxy groups or deleted for inhibitor of HBV but not found as active as compound **276**. During re-synthesis of compound **276** for a proof of concept studies, a small molecule **277** was discovered as potent HBV inhibitor as active as against lamivudine resistant HBV in HepG2 B1 and HepG2 D88 cell assays having different mode of inhibition from nucleosides. SAR study of 2-hydroxyaroyl-N-(thiazol-2-yl)-amides (thiazolides) and related salicyloyl anilides against HBV showed excellent activities for intracellular virions led to the identification of 2-hydroxybenzoyl-N-(5-chlorothiazol-2-yl)amide **278** and O-glucuronide of **278** as a potent and selective anti-HBV agent (Fig. **28**) [115]. Irbesartan **281** weakly reduced HBV uptake but efficiently inhibits HBV covalently closed circular DNA (cccDNA) formation at physiological temperature. Thus, irbesartan targets HBV infection at post-uptake prior to cccDNA formation step like the cell membrane fusion [116].

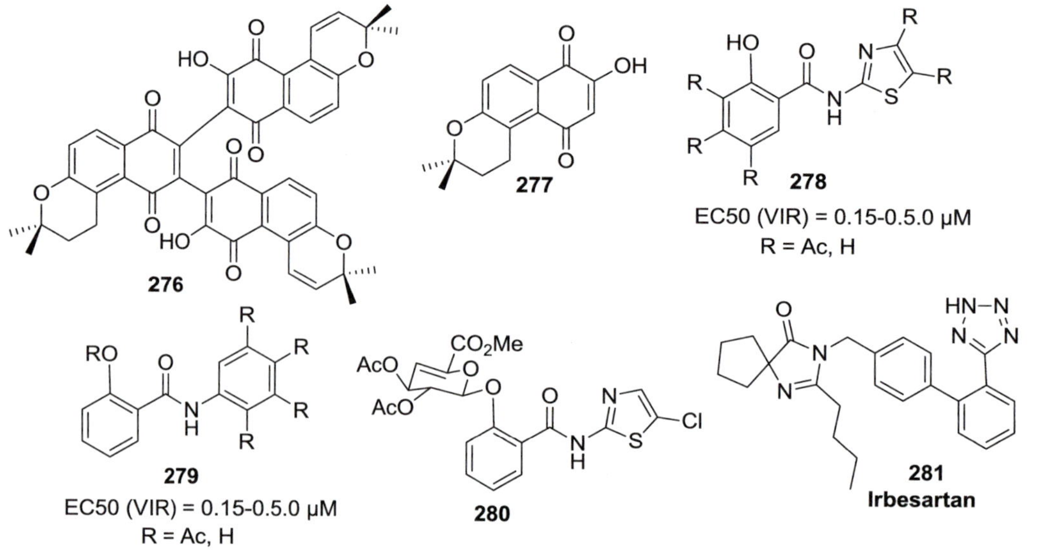

Fig. (28). Structure of naphthoquinone trimers, thiazolides **278-279**, *O*-glucuronide **280** and irbesartan **281**.

In neurotoxicity study, it was found that unnatural L-nucleosides are more potent antiviral agents than the corresponding D-nucleosides such as 2'-fluoro-5-metyl-β-D-arabino furanosyl uracil (D-FMAU). Also, the L-analogues of FMAU (L-FMAU) **282-284** were found to be potent anti-HBV agent (EC_{50} 0.1 μM in 2.2.15 cells). The thymine derivatives and the only 2'-deoxy nucleoside with a 3'-OH group have anti-HBV activity. The mode of action in L-FMAU differs from other cytosine derivatives acting as chain terminators. In *in vitro* study, 2.2.15 and HepG2 cells showed that L-FMAU is metabolized to its mono-, di- and tri-phosphates. It was also found that the 5'-triphosphate of L-FMAU is the active compound acting as a potent inhibitor of HBV DNA polymerase (*Ki* =0.12 μM) and a substrate for thymidine kinase and deoxycytidine kinase (Fig. **29**) [117].

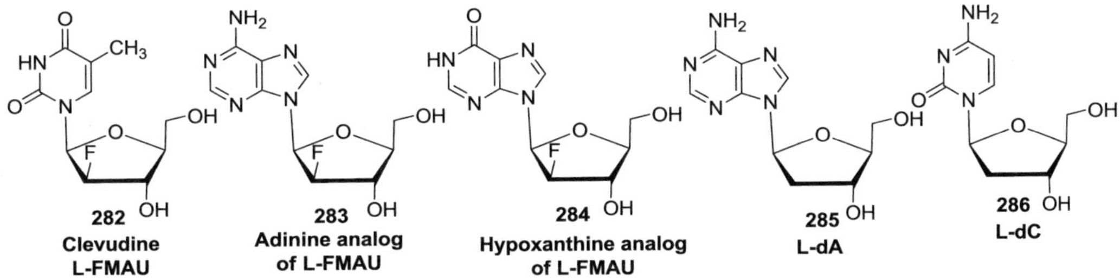

Fig. (29). Anti-HBV active 2'-fluoro-L-arabinofuranosyl nucleosides and β-L-2'-Deoxynucleosides **285-286**.

Different purine nucleosides containing the same 2-deoxy-2-fluor--β-L-arabinosyl moiety as in L-FMAU possessed potent anti-HBV activities (Fig. **30**). The adenine and hypoxanthine derivatives exhibited good *in vitro* anti-HBV activity (EC_{50} 1.5 and 8 μM) respectively in 2.2.15 cells compared to clevudine. Recently, compound **290** also showed strong and selective inhibition of replication of HBV and HTV.

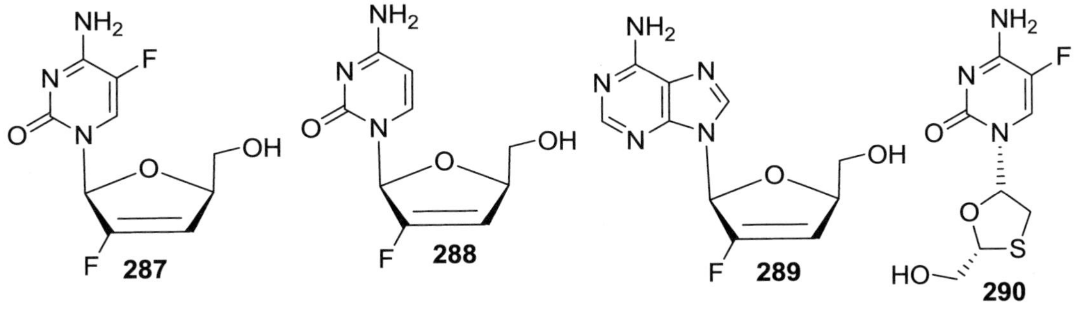

Fig. (30). Anti-HBV active 2'-Fluoro-2',3'-unsaturated L-nucleosides.

Pyrimidine nucleosides with variety of substituents at C-5 position and a 1-[(--hydroxy-1-(hydroxymethyl)ethoxy)methyl] showed flexible acyclic glycosyl moiety, possessing mimic property of natural 2'-deoxyribosyl moiety. They have shown potential anti-viral activity with variations at both C-5 and C-6 positions of the uracil base. Uracil other derivatives like 6-aza congeners and 4-amino and 4-methoxy pyrimidines were synthesized in which the base moiety was substituted by 5-chloro-(**296**), 5-(2-bromovinyl)-(**303**), or 5-bromo-6-methyl-(**308**) groups possess significant activity against duck-HBV, wild-type human HBV (2.2.15 cells) and lamivudine-resistant HBV containing single and double mutations. The anti-HBV activity of compounds **296**, **303** and **308** was found superior for human HBV and comparable for DHBV than the corresponding purine nucleoside, ganciclovir. Other derivatives in the series were moderately inhibitory against DHBV and wild-type human HBV. The size and electronegativity of halogen substituents at the 5- and 6-positions are important for anti-viral HBV activity. Generally, it was found inactive in these anti-viral assay (conc. upto 100 µg/mL). However, 1-[(2-hydroxy-1-(hydroxymethyl) ethoxy)methyl]-5-fluorocytosine **305** showed some inhibitory activity against hepatitis C virus [118].

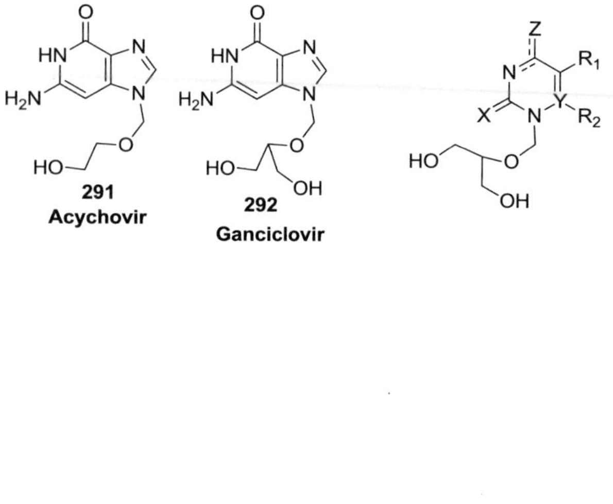

293 R_1 = H, R_2 = H, X = O, Y = C, Z = O
294 R_1 = F, R_2 = H, X = O, Y = C, Z = O
295 R_1 = Br, R_2 = H, X = O, Y = C, Z = O
296 R_1 = Cl, R_2 = H, X = O, Y = C, Z = O
297 R_1 = NO_2, R_2 = H, X = O, Y = C, Z = O
298 R_1 = NH_2, R_2 = H, X = S, Y = C, Z = O
299 R_1 = CH_3, R_2 = H, X =S, Y = C, Z = O
300 R_1 = C_2H_5, R_2 = H, X = O, Y = C, Z = O
301 R_1 = CH_2OH, R_2 = H, X = O, Y = C, Z = O
302 R_1 = CH_2CH_2OH, R_2 = H, X = S, Y = C, Z = O
303 R_1 = CH=CHBr, R_2 = H, X = O, Y = C, Z = O
304 R_1 = H, R_2 = H, X = O, Y = C, Z = NH_2
305 R_1 = F, R_2 = H, X = O, Y = C, Z = NH_2
306 R_1 = Br, R_2 = H, X = O, Y = C, Z = OCH_3
307 R_1 = H, R_2 = CH_3, X = O, Y = C, Z = O
308 R_1 = Br, R_2 = CH_3, X = O, Y = C, Z = O
309 R_1 = I, R_2 = CH_3, X = O, Y = C, Z = O
310 R_1 = H, X = O, Y = N, Z = O
311 R_1 = CH_3, X = O, Y = N, Z = O
312 R_1 = CH_3, X = S, Y = N, Z = O

Fig. (31). Anti-HBV active pyrimidines L-nucleosides.

The molecular modeling studies showed that acyclic nucleosides and a short chain connecting the base-sugar moiety provide torsional flexibility compared to the oxathiolane ring in lamivudine as confirmed in the HBV polymerase inhibition assays. Thus, among acyclic purine nucleosides, acyclovir 9-[(2-hydroxyethoxy) methyl]guanine **291** showed the modest inhibitor of HBV DNA polymerase in triphosphate form. Acyclovir exhibited both *in vitro* and *in vivo* activity in animal models, but not in HBV during human clinical trials. Ganciclovir, 9-[(2-hydro-y-1-(hydroxymethyl) ethoxy) methyl] guanine **292**, structurally similar to acyclovir with difference in the functional equivalent of a 3'-OH group is a potent inhibitor of HBV. SAR studies further supported the synthesis and enhanced anti-viral activities with 5-substituted pyrimidines of 1-[(2-hydroxy-1-(hydroxy-methyl) ethoxy)methyl] acyclic chain. Modifications at 4-, 5-, and 6-positions in these new series of promising anti-virals are also reported for their anti-HBV activity (Fig. **31**). Percent inhibition of viral replication by compounds **296** and **308** for resistant mutant HBV was close to that of wild-type HBV in contrast to lamivudine where single and double mutants of HBV were significantly less sensitive than wild-type HBV.

Nucleos(t)ides of reverse transcriptase and interferons inhibitors were resulted in low rate functional cure for HBV, called sustained off-therapy seroclearance of hepatitis B surface antigen (HBsAg) due to inability of therapies to reduce the levels of viral antigen production. This led to the high serum levels of HBsAg and exhaustion of the host immune system which unable to give effective anti-viral responses required for HBsAg clearance. A new mechanistic approaches are required to produce high rate of HBsAg seroclearance in order to greatly reduce off-treatment disease progression [119]. Clinically viable means of reducing gene expression, therapies based on RNA interference (RNAi) can directly target HBV transcripts with high specificity and awesome reduction of viral proteins. New methods effectively deliver the trigger to liver hepatocytes and cytoplasmic compartment resulted in increased efficacy and tolerability. RNAi-based drug, ARC-520 is currently in clinical trials showed dynamic polyconjugate where RNAi trigger conjugation to cholesterol and coinjected with a hepatocyte-targeted and membrane-active peptide. ARC-520 trial was well tolerated and resulted in significant dose-dependent reduction in HBsAg (up to 57 days in chronic HBV). The RNAi-based therapies may play an important role in future therapeutic regimes aimed at improving HBsAg seroclearance and eliminate the need for life-long therapy [120]. HBsAg in particular may directly suppress monocytes, dendritic cells and natural killer cells which leads to exhaustion of CD8+ and CD4+T cells.

3.8. Future Perspectives

Worldwide, chronic hepatitis B disease is 10 times more than HIV infection. A combination treatment gave better results in HIV infections, but less adopted in the HBV infections. Currently, immunomodulators and nucleos(t)ide analogues are used with limitations. In complete removal and rapid HBV replication, lower drug resistance nucleos(t)ide analogues (*e.g.*, TDF and ETV) are used as first-line therapy. The combination therapies are also attemped in different HBV mutant sites and/or different action mechanisms may display additive or synergistic effects. Similarly, nucleos(t)ides with modifications based on old ones are synthesized and screened for better inhibitory effects which lower drug resistance, cytotoxicities and side effects. Also, new anti-HBV agents based on peptides and proteins have been synthesized and screened *in vitro* and *in vivo* along with natural agents and nucleic acids for potent anti-HBV activities which are expected to be effective in drug-resistant strains and more suitable for the treatment of the patients.

Many plant agents have displayed recently inhibitory effects against HBV. Furthermore modifications based on active compounds may also be carried out for the better inhibitory effects and oral bioavailability with reduction of their toxicities and side effects. They have different mechanisms of action than the parent molecules in various stages of HBV life-cycle and function on host factors which are required for HBV replication and expression. They are also useful biomarkers for the clinical diagnosis and detection indicators for screening new anti-HBV agents. The proteomics technology, computational modeling and virtual screening methodology may facilitate current studies in the identification of novel and effective inhibitors against viral diseases in drug targets. The authenticated targets may be used as effective targets in new anti-HBV drug screening and also new biomarkers for clinical diagnosis and prognosis. Using x-ray crystallographic data and computational modeling for a structure-based virtual screening, molecules targeting viral proteins or host proteins impacting on virus replication and expression can be selected for evaluation of drug inhibitory effects. Due to the lack of anti-HBV drugs, new drugs with diverse skeleton types and various action mechanisms are urgently needed.

4. HEPATITIS C

4.1. Introduction

The World Health Organization (WHO) report shows 130–150 million people (2-2.5% of the world's population) are chronically infected with the hepatitis C virus (HCV) with slightly regional differences. First time in the late 1980s, HCV discovered which has significant global impacts as human pathogen. The first small-molecule inhibitors were tested in humans after 15 years. Still, the therapeutic intervention of anti-virals remains a challenge due to the diverse HCV genotypes and their ability to quickly evolve resistance [121]. Structurally, it is a small enveloped virus of Hepacivirus genus of *Flaviviridae* family. The infection is very complex process which requires many host entry factors [122]. The envelope glycoproteins E1-E2 present on viral surface play major role during entry. Initially, they bind to glycosaminoglycans (GAG) on the surface of the host cell. It was thought that the interactions between the LDL-receptor (LDL-R) and apolipoproteins of the viral particle might also participate in the initial binding of cell surface [123]. No vaccine is available for HCV because of the viral high diversity [124]. The treatment involves weekly injections of pegylated interferon-α with ribavirin as protease enzyme inhibitor with serious side effects. The protease enzyme has many binding sites which requires for HCV reproduction. Among these binding sites, NS3/4A and NS5B have garnered the most attention as drug targets [125]. However, *in vitro* and *in vivo* testing illustrated a rapid and error-prone mutations of HCV which causes the drug resistance and diminish susceptibility of compounds. For NS5A, enzymatic activity and its mechanisms of action during the HCV life-cycle are unclear. The crystal structures of NS5A showed dimer forms which may come together into large oligomeric arrays that channel RNA substrates within the cell [126].

The biology of hepatitis C virus is extremely complex nature for the development of anti-viral agents [127]. It has six major genotypes of the >50 subtypes of which genotype 1a/b accounts are responsible for approx. 70% of all infections. Their polyprotein processes both co- and post-translationally to produce structural (C, E1, E2, p7) and non-structural (NS2, NS3, NS4A, NS4B, NS5A, NS5B) proteins. The major non-structural proteins are the protease enzymes (NS2 and the N-terminal domain of the NS3), the helicase/ATPase (C-terminal domain of the NS3) and RNA-dependent RNA polymerase enzyme (NS5B) [128]. Initial studies designated that each of these enzymes is confirmed as a target for drug discovery by abrogating its catalytic function. In 2005, the production of infectious hepatitis C viral particles in tissue culture was finally achieved. On the other hand, inhibitors of the NS3 serine protease and the NS5B polymerase had entered clinical development (Fig. **32**) [129].

The direct anti-viral agent are targeted on HCV NS3/4A protein (protease), NS5B protein (polymerase) and NS5A protein. The use of interferon alone and PEG-IFN + ribavirin gave the patients cure for genotype 1 upto 30 and 45% respectively. Since 2011, the use of DAAs drugs, boceprevir and telaprevir improved the cure upto 70%. Furthermore, the DAAs drugs, sofosbuvir (Sovaldi), simeprevir (Olysio) and combination medicines like Harvoni and Viekira Pak are approved in 2013 for the more effective and less toxic in nature. They increased the cure rates upto 90% without interferon, effective for all HCV genotypes. Further, new HCV drugs is investigated and progressing rapidly, many combination medicines are in phase III clinical trials that include Viekirax, asunaprevir, daclatasvir. beclabuvir, grazoprevir, elbasvir and others (Fig. **33**) [130].

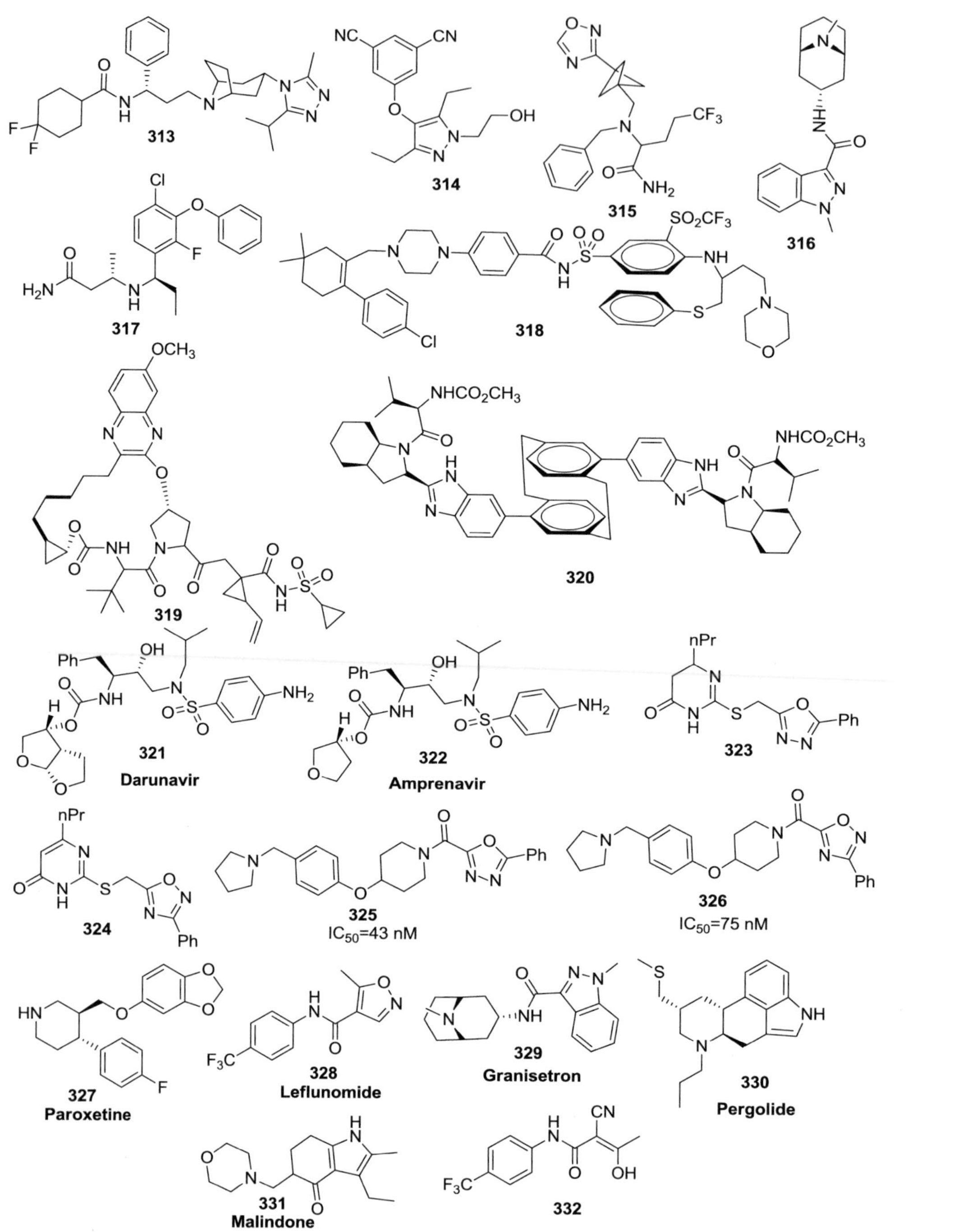

Fig. (32). Top scoring drugs ranked by the QED analysis.

Also, consensus interferon (CIFN, interferon alfacon-1, Infergen), a recombinant non-naturally occurring type-I IFN agent binds with high affinity with type-I IFN receptors and showed more portent biological activity than IFN-α. The CIFN utility in the clinic has yet to be proven and a limited number of Peg-interferon/ribavirin non-responders have been shown to achieve a sustained virological response with the use of high dose CIFN [131]. New drugs other than viral proteins are in clinical trials and will probably helpful in improving response to HCV therapy [132].

4.2. HCV Life Cycle

Heterogeneous viral particles with diameter between 50-80 nm were observed in a highly purified HCV protein and also found in the bloods sample of infected individuals. The virions bound to very low density lipoproteins (VLDL), low density lipoproteins (LDL), complexed with immunoglobulins and free circulating virions. The reasons for these association of a major portion of circulating virions with LDL and VLDL remain unknown. It might be due to that the HCV enters hepatocytes *via* the LDL receptor. These associations might be due to involvement of the LDL receptor led to non-productive HCV infection. First time the design and optimization study of sub-genomic and genomic HCV replicons in human hepatoma cell line, Huh7 offered to examine HCV RNA replication.

4.3. Different Routes of HCV Transmission

Hepatocellular carcinoma depends on region and environmental factors therefore observed more often in the Japan than the United States. However, the reasons are not clear. The different routes of its transmission are:

- Parenteral exposure to the hepatitis C virus: The most efficient means of transmission. Besides, European and US patients acquired the disease through intravenous drug use or blood transfusion [133].
- Sex with an intravenous drug user.
- Immunoglobulin injection.
- Organ transplantation: Transplant recipients who receive organs from HCV-positive donors have high risk for HCV infection (30 to 80% changes) [134].
- Sexual or household contact: Unprotected anal sex, fisting, having many sex partners in a short time period, a concomitant sexually transmitted disease including HIV and use of recreational drugs were identified as risk factors. Also, mucosal damage is a pre-requisite for HCV transmission [135]. The seroprevalence of HCV in MSM ranges from 4-8% is higher than the HCV prevalence reported for general European populations.
- Having been struck or cut with a bloody object.
- Piercing.

- Use of steroids: Steroids intake increase the HCV viral load but the effect on aminotransferases vary. It decreases in the most patients but increases in high transaminases and bilirubin cases. Reducing dosage of corticosteroids returns HCV viral load to baseline [136].
- Needle stick injury [137]:

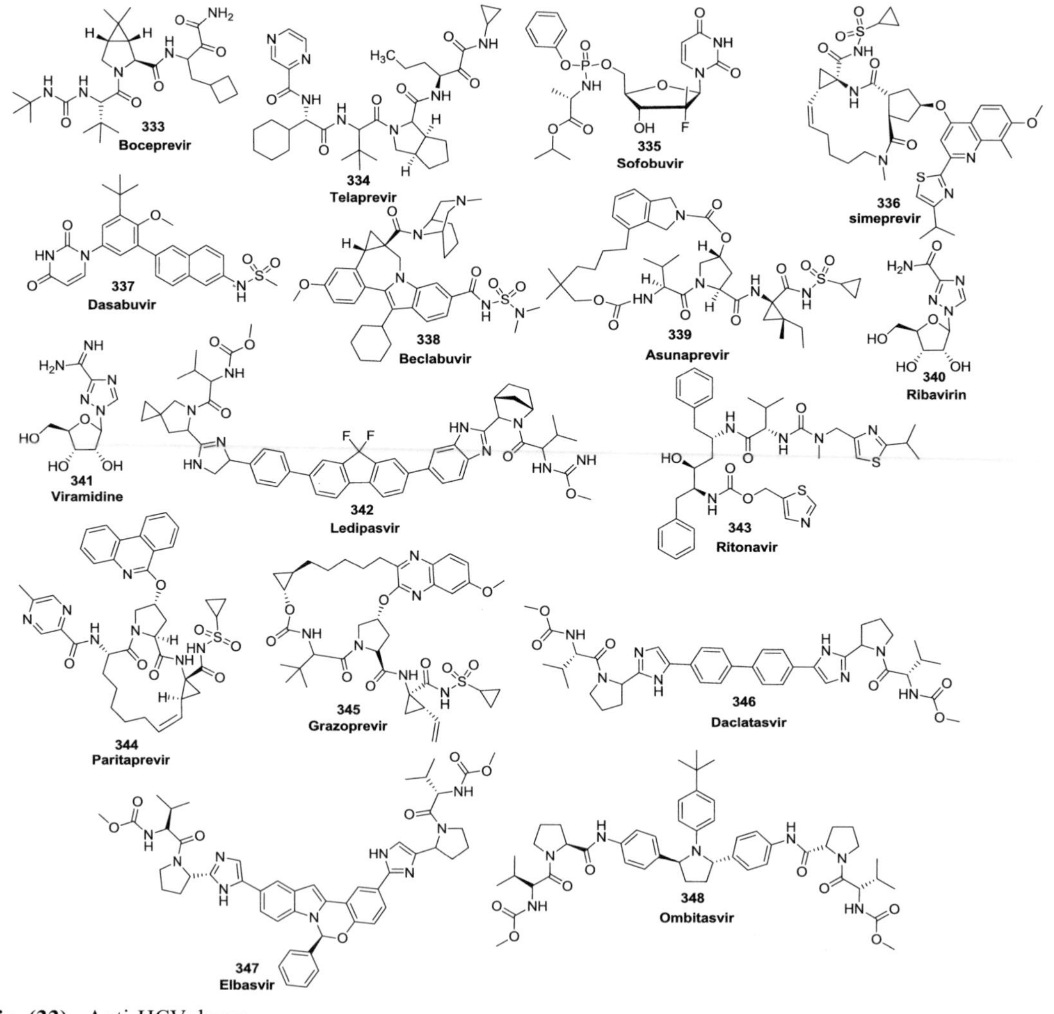

Fig. (33). Anti-HCV drugs.

4.3.1. Acute Hepatitis

Inoculation study showed aminotransferases become elevated approx. 6-12 weeks after exposure range 1-26 weeks in HCV. The elevation varies from individual to individual, more than 10-30 times the upper limit of normal (typically around 800 U/l) [138].

4.3.2. Chronic Hepatitis C

After acute hepatitis C, 75-100% of patients remained HCV RNA positive known as chronic hepatitis C [139].

4.4. Drugs Targets/Receptors in Cellular Factors

Hepatitis C virus has a single-stranded RNA genome, encodes with a large polyprotein of 3010 amino acids. The co- and post translational process of polyprotein gave cellular and viral encoded proteases to produce the mature structural and non-structural (NS) proteins. The NS3 serine-like protease and the RNA-dependent RNA polymerase (RdRp) are essential for the viral maturation and replication. Thus, the ideal targets for the development of small molecule anti-HCV agents [140]. Also, the HCV internal ribozyme entry site (IRES) possesses a unique functional structure which required for the viral translation and replication will be another specific target for drug developments [141].

4.5. Anti-HCV Agents Derived from Natural and Synthetic Products

A more efficacious and better tolerated treatment regimens are needed for all patients. The medicinal plants can be explored as a vital source for the novel drugs. Many plants were used in the treatment of liver problems and HCV infections [142]. In the laboratory synthesis, some novel compounds have shown promising results but the drug-resistant viruses emerged rapidly after the use of drugs, is a major concern for successful anti-HCV therapy. A fast turnover rate and the intrinsic low fidelity of the HCV replication machinery endows the virus with ability to fully explore its genome space and quickly come up with mutations that turn into a drug-resistant. Each newly generated HCV genome exhibited on average one nucleotide change per replication cycle.

4.6. HCV NS3/4A Protease Inhibitors

Hepatitis C protease enzyme cleaves the polyprotein at four junctions: NS3/NS4A, NS4A/NS4B, NS4B/NS5A and NS5A/NS5B. The cleavage at NS3/NS4A site is intramolecular (cis-cleavage), and other three junctions occurs intermolecular (trans-cleavage) [143]. The NS3 is a multi-functional protein in which the N-terminal third of the protein, contains a serine-like protease and the C-terminus possesses helicase and NTPase activities. Together NTPase and helicase unwinds duplex RNA structures and performs a crucial role in the replication. Thus, the NS3 protease is an attractive target for anti-viral involvement. The substrate-binding cleft of NS3/4A protease appeared flat and featureless, without cavities and flaps which may be exploited as anchor points to design selective inhibitors of other proteases [144].

Telaprevir, boceprevir, simeprevir and paritaprevir drugs used in the treatment of chronic HCV genotypes 1 and 4 infections (Fig. **33**) [145]. Asunaprevir drug is well tolerated but led to a moderate increase of amino transferases. Therefore, it is used in combination with daclatasvir as the NS5A inhibitor. Grazoprevir is used as NS3/4A inhibitor for all genotypes, has a distinct resistance profile compared to other NS3/4A inhibitors. Thus, it is developed as a fixed combination with elbasvir a NS5A inhibitor. ABT-493 is another 2nd generation NS3 protease inhibitor (PI), is currently in phase III development in combination with ABT-530 a NS5A inhibitor. Other NS3 PI are in earlier stages of clinical development include ACH-1625 (effective against all HCV genotypes), IDX320, GS-9256 and GS-9451.

4.6.1. Natural Products

A macrocyclic mimic of peptide product, BILN 2061 (Ciluprevir; Boehringer Ingelheim) was the first potent NS3 protease inhibitor for patients infected with genotype-1 but less effective on genotypes-2 and -3 [146]. In optimization of side chains and conversion of the linear peptides, derivatives of macrocyclic inhibitors were synthesized based on BILN 2061 skeleton with enhanced potencies and improved biopharmaceuticals properties (Fig. **34**) [147].

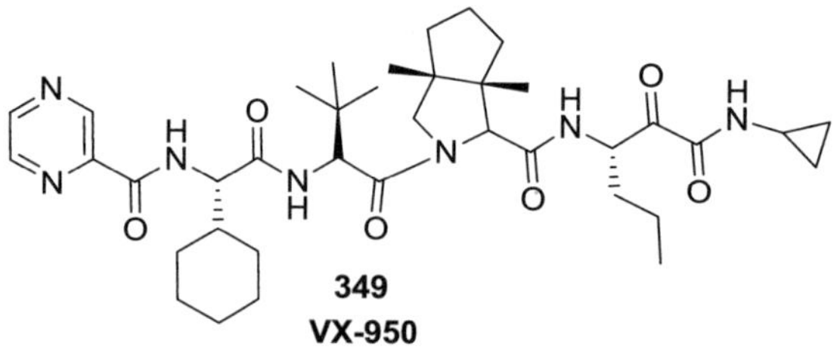

349
VX-950

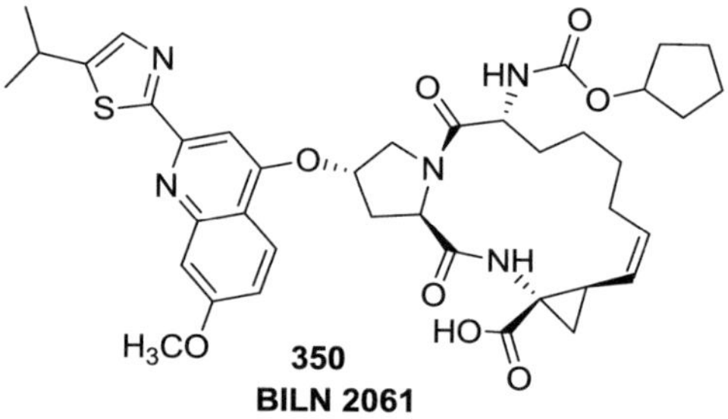

350
BILN 2061

Fig. (34). Structure of NS3-protease inhibitors BILN 2061 and VX-950.

The hexapeptide N-terminal products **351** and **352** derivatives have been used as NS3-protease cysteine residues as the P1 anchor, derived from the structure of the S1 specificity pocket. The small and lipophilic pocket lined by the hydrophobic residues of Val132, Leu135 and Phe154 is complementary to the small and lipophilic cysteine side-chain. The sulfhydryl group can also interact in a specific way with the aromatic ring of Phe154 (Figs. **35-37**) [148].

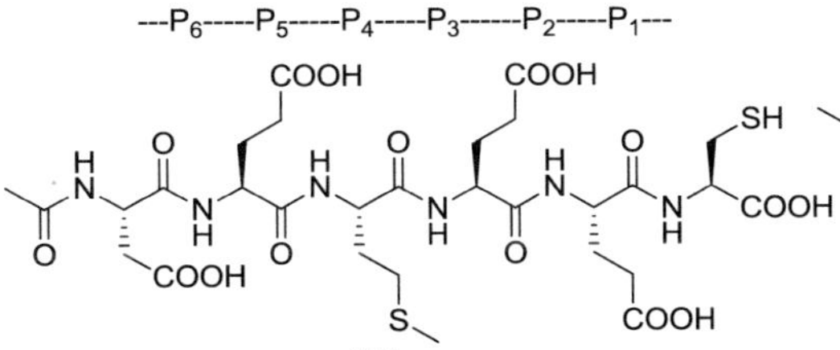

351
***k*$_i$ 0.60 μM**
NS4A/NS4B product

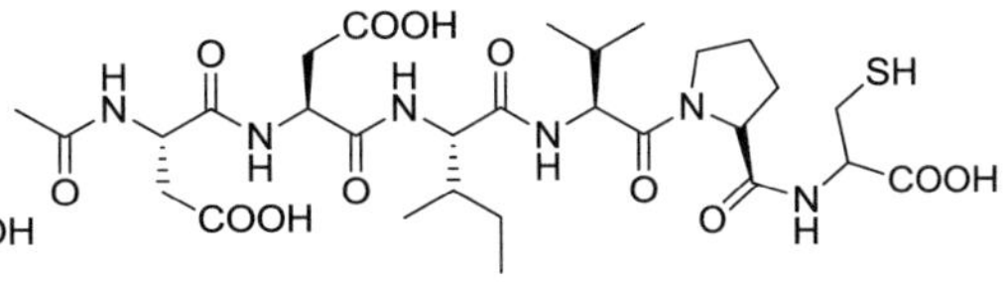

352
IC$_{50}$ 71 μM
NS5A/NS5B product

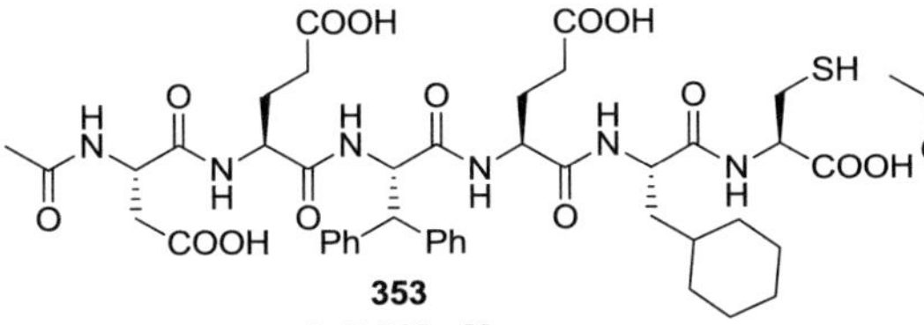

353
***k*$_i$ 0.040 μM**
NS4A/NS4B product mimic

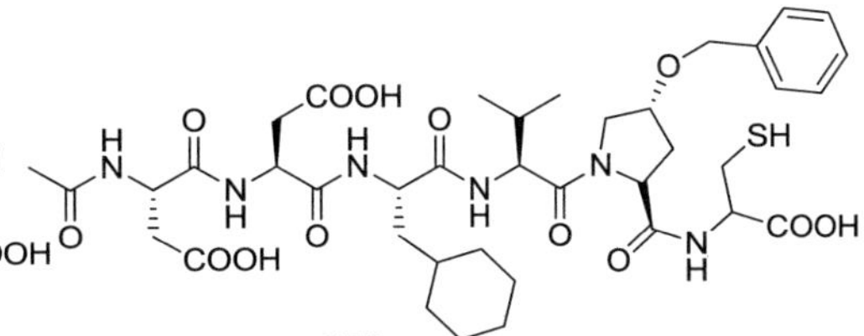

354
IC$_{50}$ 0.033 μM
NS5A/NS5B product mimic

Fig. (35). N-Terminal cleavage products of the peptide substrates **351** and **352**, hexapeptide **353** and **354** for protease inhibitors.

Further improvements in activity were obtained through traditional and combinatorial methods to optimize the P2-P6 amino acids which produce a number of highly active hexapeptides compounds [149].

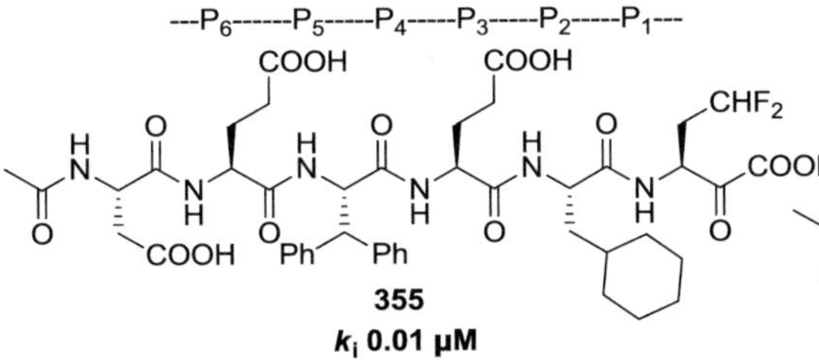

355
***k*$_i$ 0.01 μM**
NS4A/NS4B product

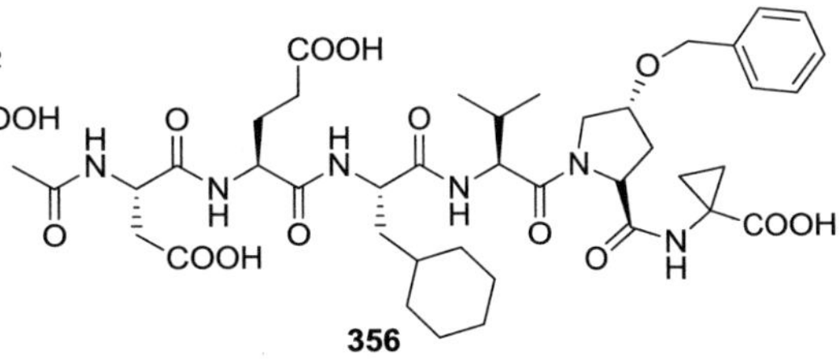

356
IC$_{50}$ 0.051 μM
NS5A/NS5B product

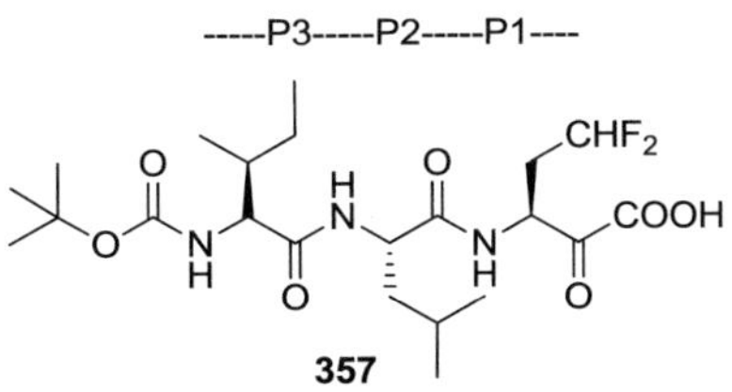

357
Boc-Ile-Leu-L-(difluoro)aminobutyric acid
IC$_{50}$ 1.0 μM

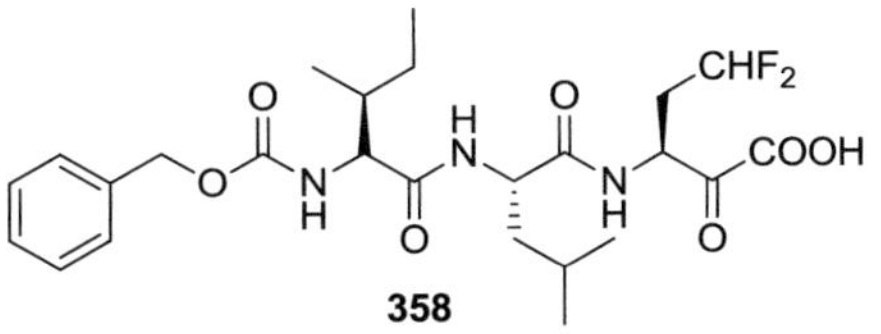

358
Cbz-Ile-Leu-L-(difluoro)aminobutyric acid
IC$_{50}$ 1.7 μM

Fig. 36 contd.....

----P_4-----P_3-----P_2-----P_1---

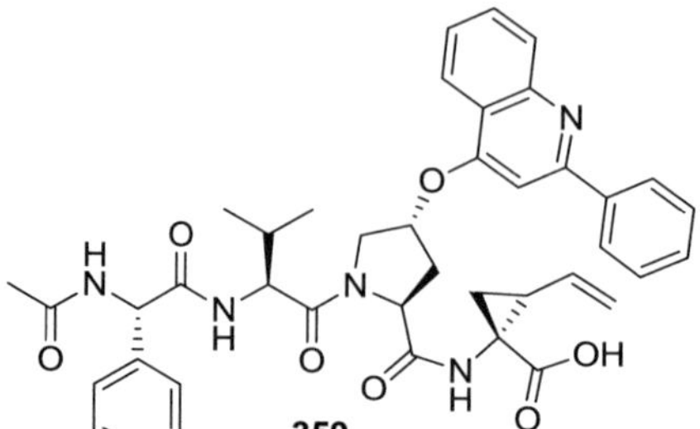

359

IC_{50} 0.013 µM

Fig. (36). Structure of peptidomimetic **355-56**, tripeptide **357-58** and tripeptide **359** of NS3 protease activity inhibitors.

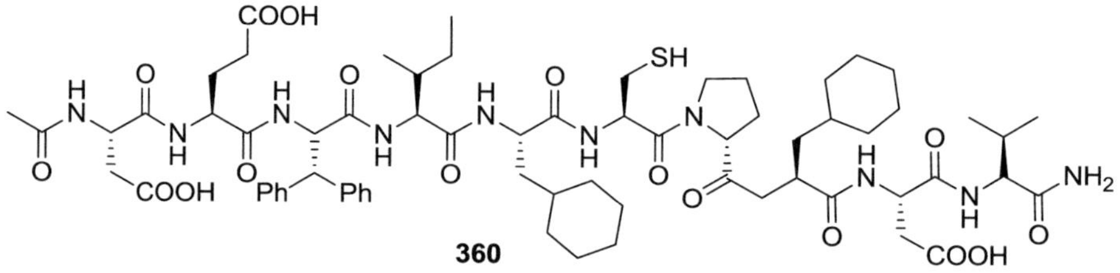

360

IC_{50} 1.3nM

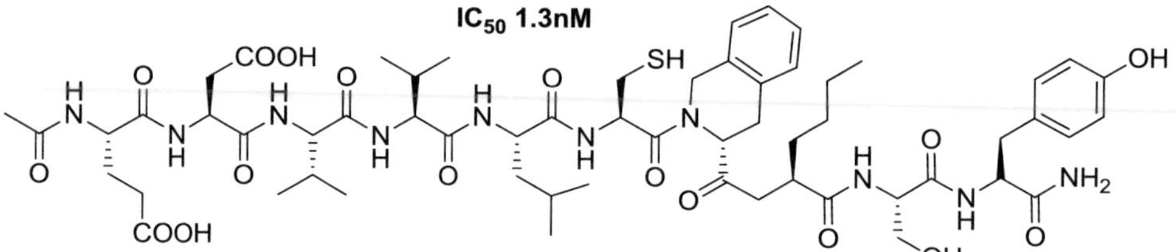

361

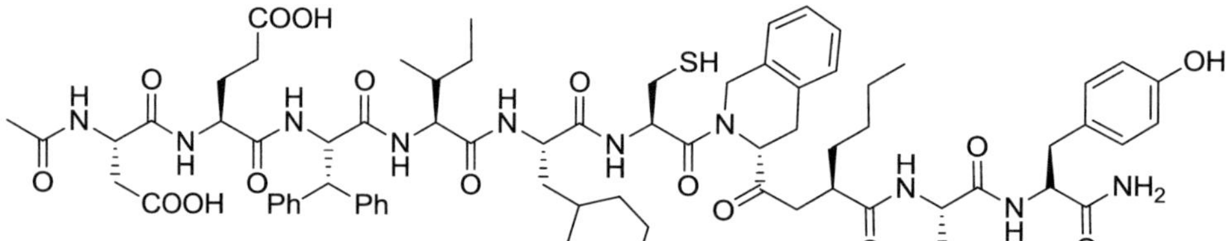

362

IC_{50} 0.1µM

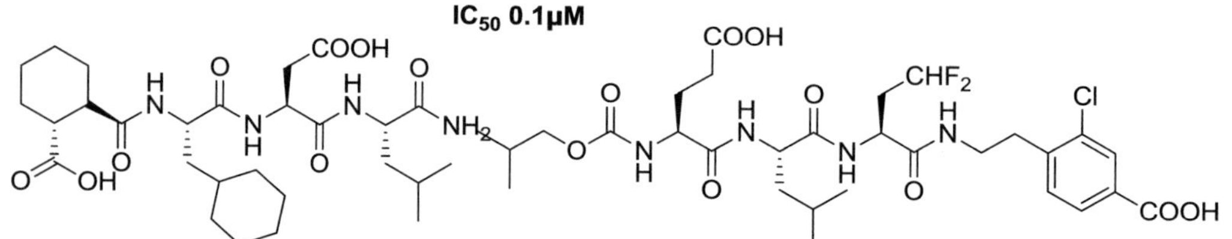

363

IC 15 µM

364

***k* 0 60 M**

Fig. (37). Structure of decapeptide **360-362**, a capped tripeptide and a tripeptide phenethyl amide **363-364** that simultaneously bind to the S and S'-regions of the NS3 protease active site.

Murayaquinone (Sch68631) **368** isolated from *Streptomyces* and so Sch351633 **369** along with derivatives **370** and **371** from *Penicllium griseofulvum* fungus. The major constituent is 2,4,6-trihydroxy-3-nitrobenzamides (THNBs) which showed NS3 protease inhibitor property on random screening (Fig. **38**) [150].

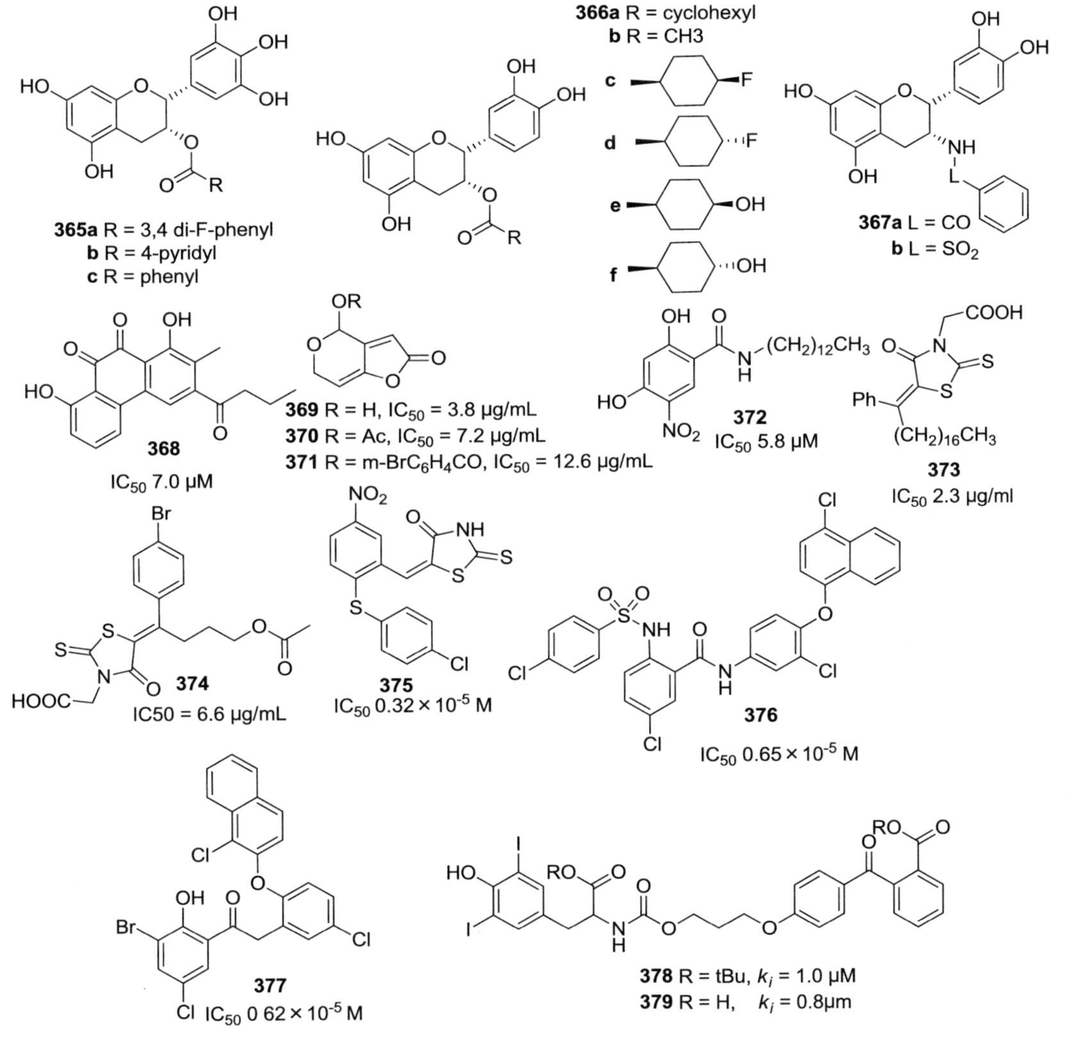

Fig. (38). Structure of murayaquinone **368**, **369** and derivatives **370-371**, the most potent NS3 protease inhibitor from the 2,4,6-trihydroxy-3-nitrobenzamides series **372** and structures of the NS3 protease inhibitors **373-374**. Structure of three potent NS3 protease inhibitors isolated from the screening of a 2000-compound library and structure of two non peptidic small-molecule inhibitors of NS3 protease **375-377** and the competitive inhibitors **378** and **379.**.

More than 4,500 flavonoids and bioflavonoids have been characterized and screened for potential anti-HCV agents (Fig. **39**).

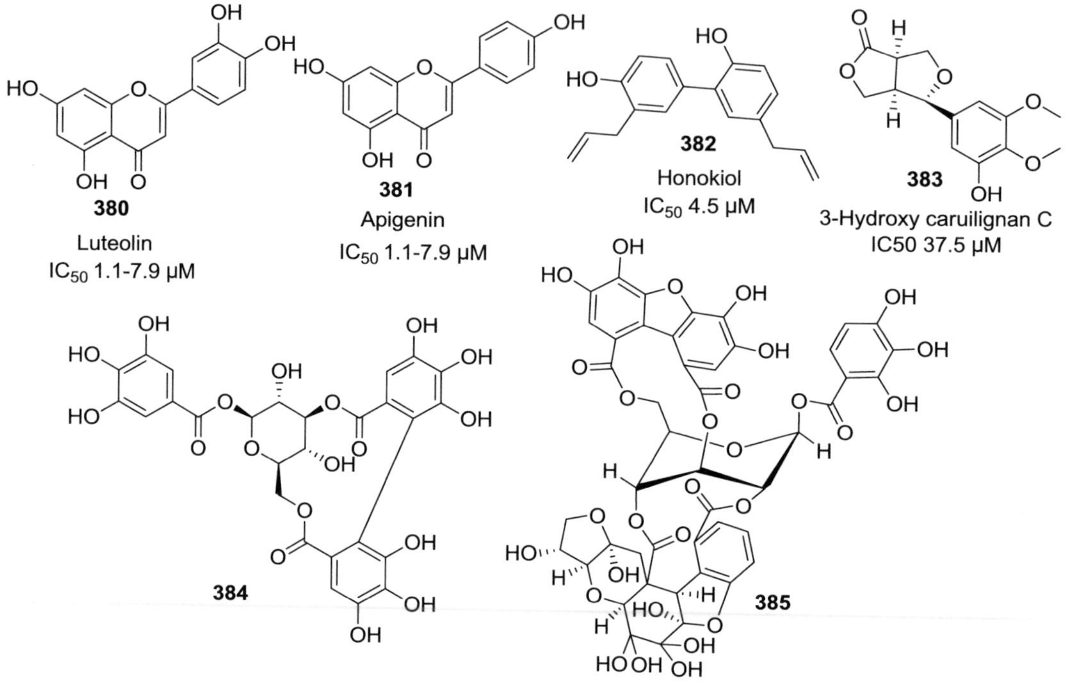

Fig. (39). Flavonoids or bioflavonoids anti-HCV molecules.

4.6.2. Silymarin/Silibinin

The seeds of milk thistle *Silybum marianum* extract are used in liver disease and as hepatoprotectant. Extract contains seven flavonolignans (silybin A, silybin B, isosilybin A, isosilybin B, silychristin, isosilychristin, silydianin) and taxifolin. Flavonolignans are polyphenols having flavonoid and lignan moieties. These compounds present are silymarin and silibinin (a mixture of silybin A and silybin B) which have anti-HCV activity [151] by inhibiting HCV replication and NS5B RNA-dependent RNA polymerase [152].

4.6.3. (−)-Epigallocatechin-3-gallate (EGCG)

EGCG is present in green tea extract (a single cup of tea contains up to 150 mg), a flavonoid of catechin sub-class [153]. It inhibits HCV entry in dose-dependent manner of infection (IC_{50} 2.5-9.7 I1/4g/mL corresponding to 5 I1/4M and 21 I1/4M) against the NS3 and NS5B in *in vitro* Huh-7 cells assays (Fig. **40**) [154].

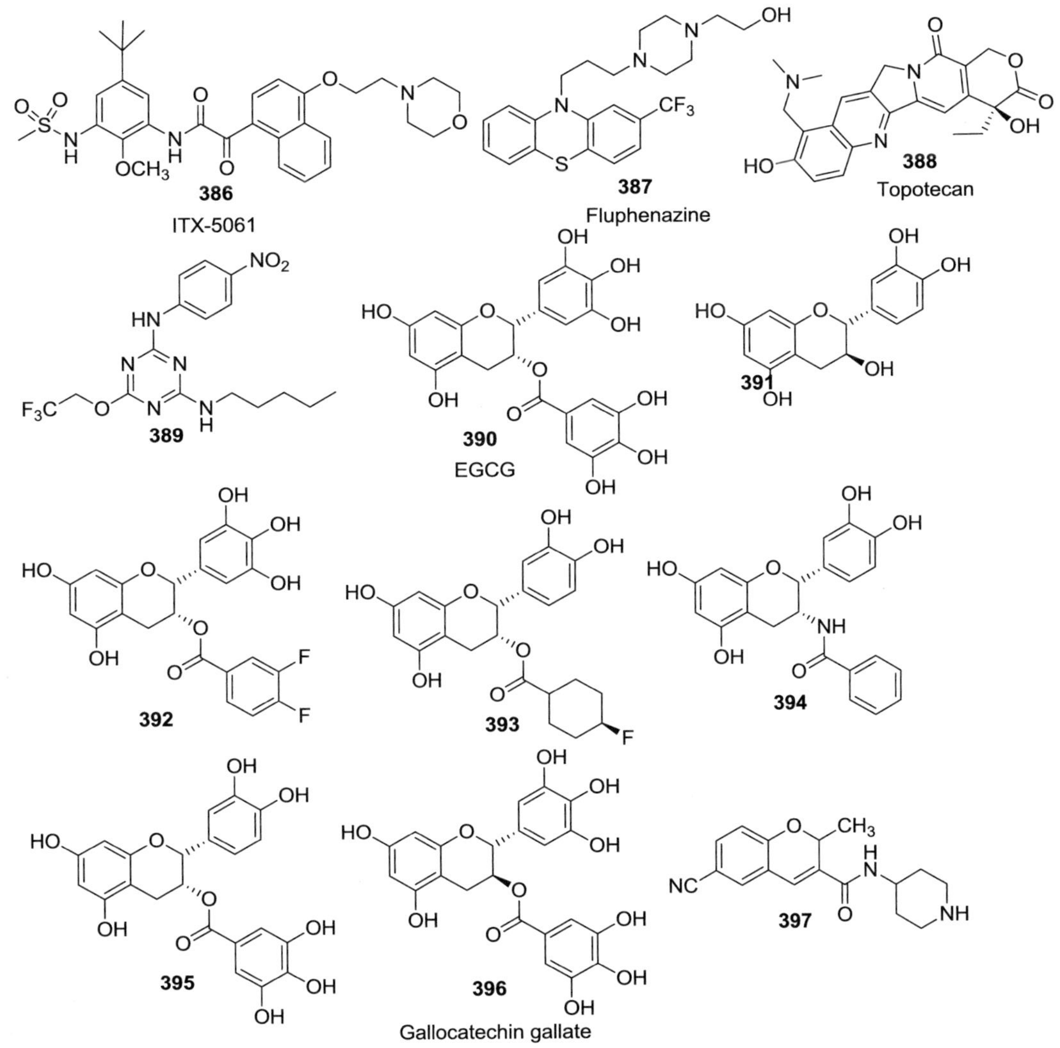

Fig. (40). EGCG derivatives.

4.6.7. Ladanein

Isolated from plant *Marrubium peregrinum* L. (*Lamiaceae*) extract, contains major flavones which inhibit HCV entry (IC_{50} 2.5 I1/4M) in a genotype-independent manner [155].

4.6.8. Naringenin

Used as dietary supplement and showed a dose-dependent manner decrease in core protein and HCV-positive strand RNA infectious particles in the supernatant of infected Huh-7 cells [156].

4.6.9. Quercetin

It is a plant-derived flavonol molecule present in fruits, vegetables, leaves and grains, also showed anti-HCV activity in NS3 and NS5A H77 strain, a genotype-1a [157].

4.6.10. Luteolin and Apigenin

Luteolin and apigenin are natural flavone molecules have anti-HCV activity against NS5B polymerase [158].

4.6.11. Honokiol

A lignan class compound present in the cones, the bark and the leaves of *Magnolia officinalis*. The plant is used in the traditional Japanese medicine Saiboku-to. In 2011, it was tested as an inhibitor for HCV infection [159] by HCV entry, translation and replication in Huh-7 cells using HCVcc, HCVpp and sub-genomic replicons.

4.6.12. 3-Hydroxy Caruilignan C

3-Hydroxy caruilignan C (3-HCL-C) isolated from *Swietenia macrophylla* stems was used for anti-HCV activity [160].

4.6.13. Polyphenols

Polyphenols have shown potential anti-HCV activity in *in vitro* assays. For example, 3',4',5,6,7,8-hexamethoxyflavone (nobiletin) obtained from citrus unshiu peel (*Aurantii nobilis* pericarpium) extract, an ingredient of traditional Japanese Kampo medicine is responsible for the anti-HCV activity (10 μg/mL) in MOLT-4 cells infection assay [161]. Similarly, SCH 644343 and SCH 644342 (oligophenolic compounds) obtained from Peruvian plant *Stylogne cauliflora* and 1,2,3,4,6-penta-*O*-galloyl-β-D-glucoside from plant *Saxifraga melanocentra* Franch have potent inhibitory activity against NS3 protease [162]. Polyphenols, 1,2,6-tri-*O*-galloyl-β-D-glucose, 1,2,3,6-tetra-*O*-galloyl-β-D-glucose and 1,2,3,4, 6-penta-*O*-galloyl-β-D-glucose were obtained from traditional Chinese medicine *Galla Chinese* have shown inhibition against NS3 protease *in vitro* (IC_{50} 1.89, 0.75 and 1.60 μM) respectively [163]. Four polyphenolic compounds were identified from Chinese mangrove plant *Excoecaria agallocha* L. (*Euphorbiaceae*) as inhibiting NS3 protease. However, excoecariphenol D and corilagin had a significant inhibitory action in the replicon assay (IC_{50} 12.6 and 13.5 μM) respectively.

A related compound series of a basic amine at the N-terminus of the P3-amino acid residue, P2-P4 macrocyclic inhibitors is reported for anti-NS3 protease (Fig. **41**) [164]. Substitution of the electroneutral P3-amino acid capping group is a feature of almost all tripeptide-like inhibitors of NS3 protease, which is not only tolerated but can result in advantageous cell based potency. Optimization gave the new class of P3-amine based inhibitors as compounds **400** and **401** that combine cell based activity with pharmacokinetic properties (Fig. **42**) [165]. Thus, the basic alkylamine functionality at N-terminus of active-site P1-P3 peptidomimetic inhibitors in NS3 is not only tolerated but can be beneficial in terms of enhanced cell based potency or improved pharmacokinetic properties (Fig. **43**).

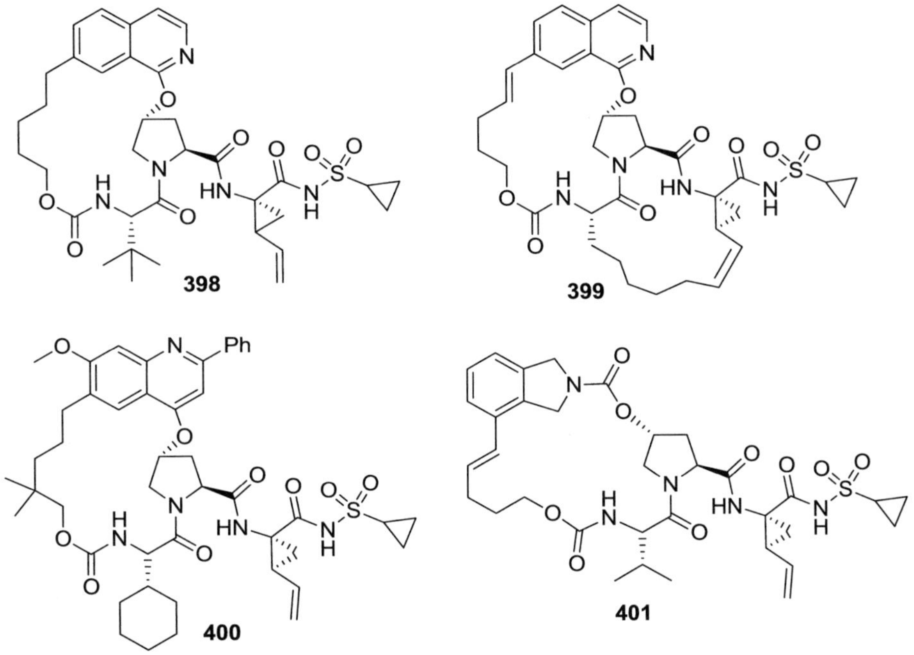

Fig. (41). P2-P4 Macrocyclic inhibitors of the HCV NS3 protease enzyme.

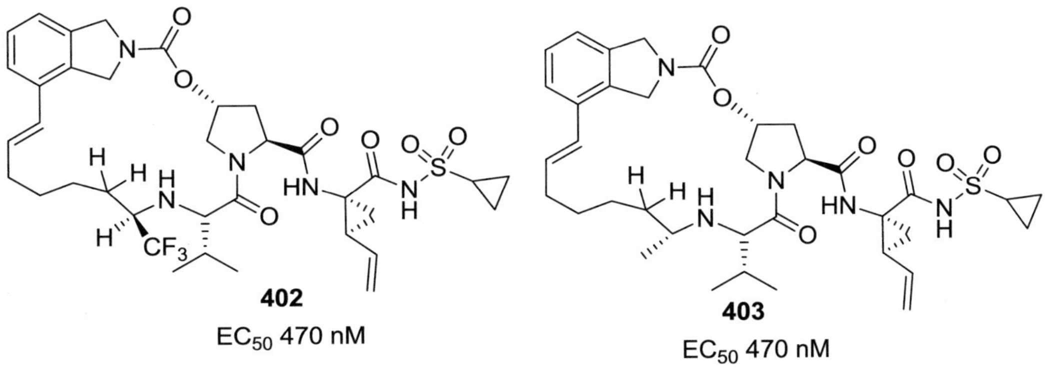

Fig. 42 contd.....

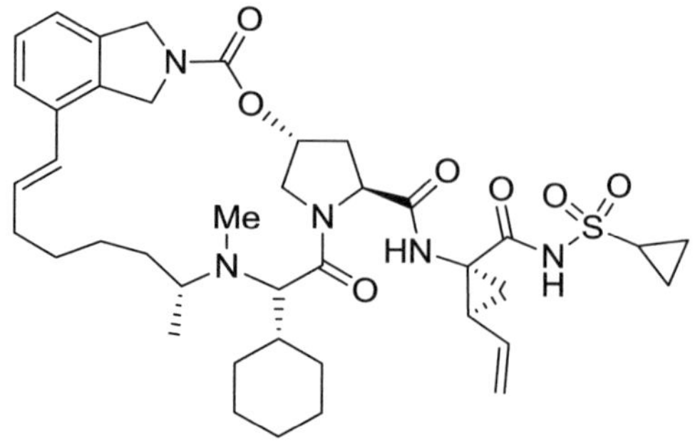

404

EC_{50} 3 nM

Fig. (42). P2-P4 amine and trifluoroethyl amine amide and isostere inhibitors.

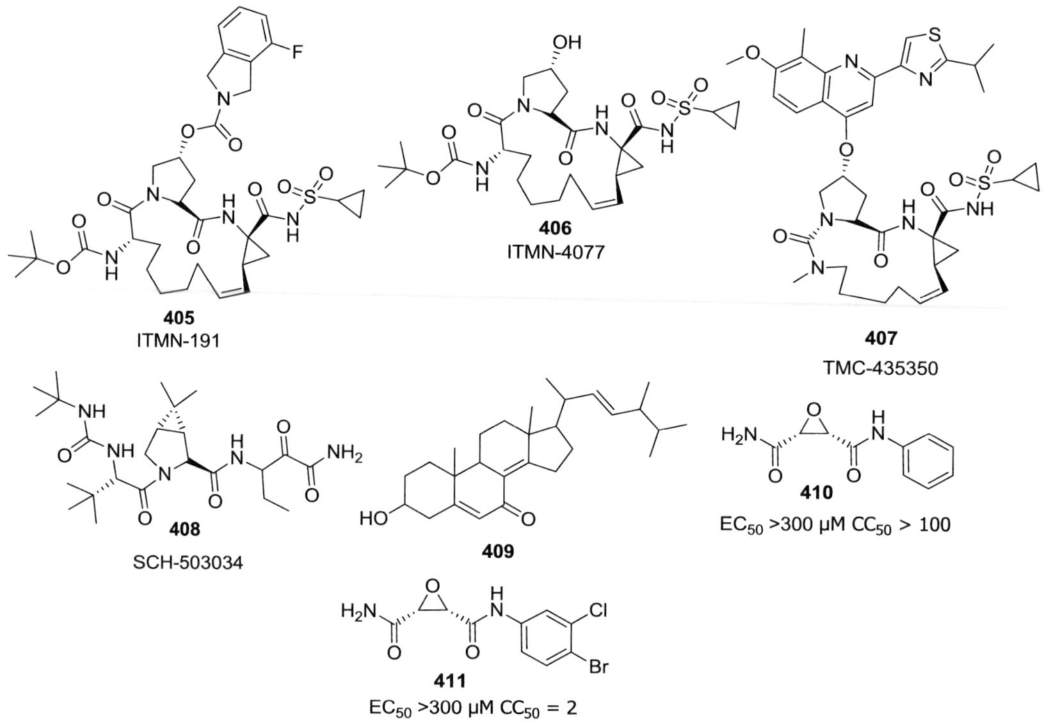

Fig. (43). Anti-HCV NS3 protease inhibitors..

Ergosta-5, 8 (14), 22-trien-7-one, 3-hydroxy-(3*β*, 22E) **405** isolated from the fermentation of *Fusarium oxysporum* has NS3 protease inhibitory activity [166].

4.7. Synthetic Products

Different epoxide-containing molecules are capable of blocking NS2–NS3 proteolysis, have demonstrated a potential selectivity towards the NS2 auto-protease [167]. ITMN-191, a macrocyclic inhibitor of the NS3 protease active site during replication, promoted rapid multilog viral load reductions in chronic HCV patients (Fig. **44**) [168]. Inhibitors of P4 pocket and optimization of P1′-capping led to the discovery of new ketoamide inhibitors of the HCV NS3 serine protease with improved *in vitro* potency [169].

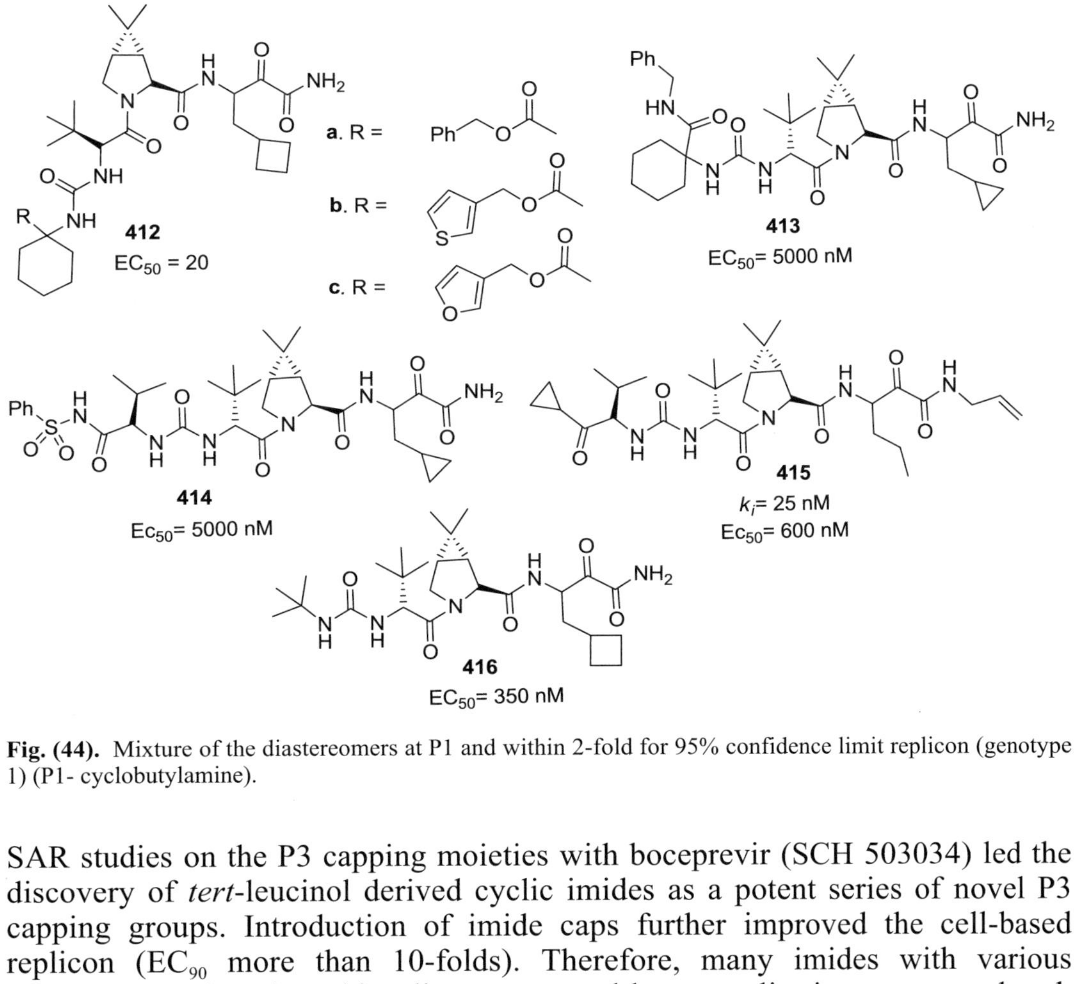

Fig. (44). Mixture of the diastereomers at P1 and within 2-fold for 95% confidence limit replicon (genotype 1) (P1- cyclobutylamine).

SAR studies on the P3 capping moieties with boceprevir (SCH 503034) led the discovery of *tert*-leucinol derived cyclic imides as a potent series of novel P3 capping groups. Introduction of imide caps further improved the cell-based replicon (EC_{90} more than 10-folds). Therefore, many imides with various substitutions, ring sizes, bicyclic systems and heterocyclic rings were explored. The x-ray structure-enzyme study of inhibitor **427** revealed that there is an additional hydrogen bonding interaction between one of the imide carbonyls and Cys159 [170]. The vinyl-ACCA is the first reported carboxylic acid containing P1 residue that produced NS3 protease inhibitors are significantly more active than the inhibitors containing a cysteine at the same position (Fig. **45**) [171].

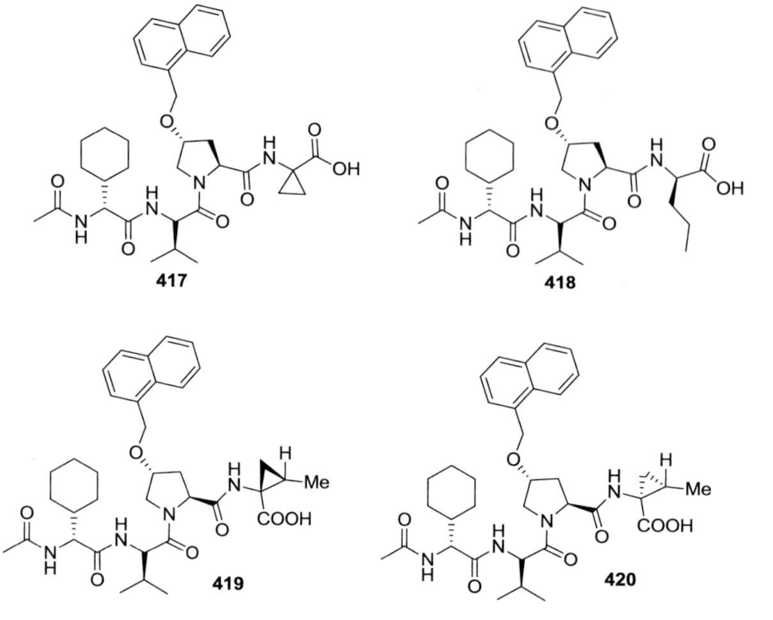

Fig. (45). ACCA optimization.

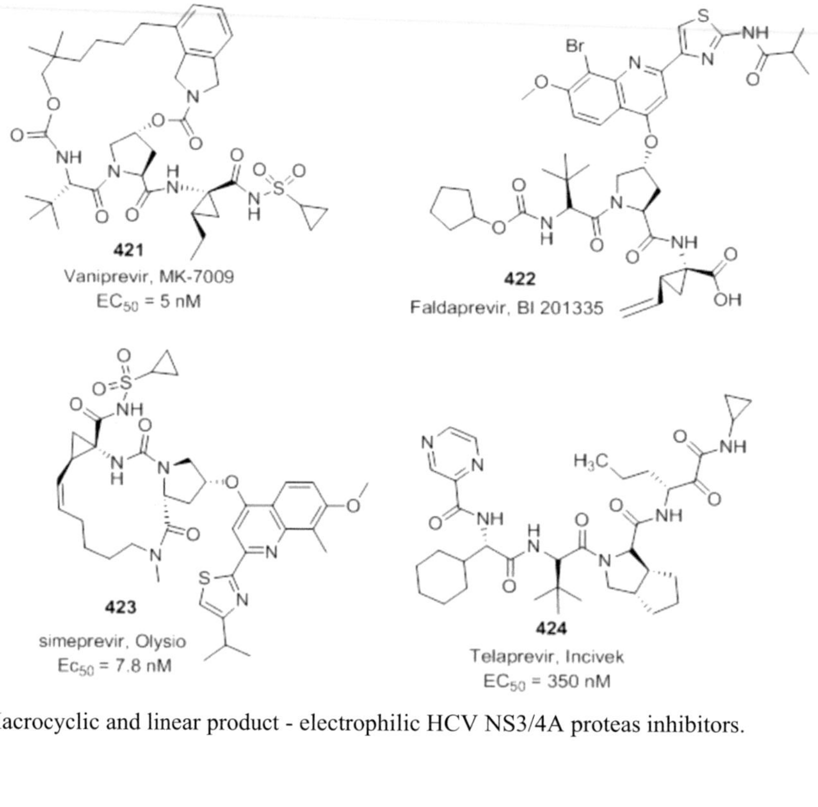

Fig. (46). Macrocyclic and linear product - electrophilic HCV NS3/4A proteas inhibitors.

A linear and macrocyclic P2 pyrimidinyloxyphenylglycine based inhibitors are reported based on vinyl substituents in P3, P2 and P10 positions of original probes (Fig. **46**). Drug resistant variants (*e.g.*, R155 K) indicated that P3–P10 macrocyclization, leaving the P2 substituent in a flexible mode as a promising approach. Also, the study demonstrated that phenylglycine based inhibitors benefit from p-phenylpyrimidinyloxy and m-vinyl groups as well as the combination with an aromatic P1 motif with alkenylic P10 elongations were found promising inhibitory potencies and drug like properties (Fig. **47**) [172].

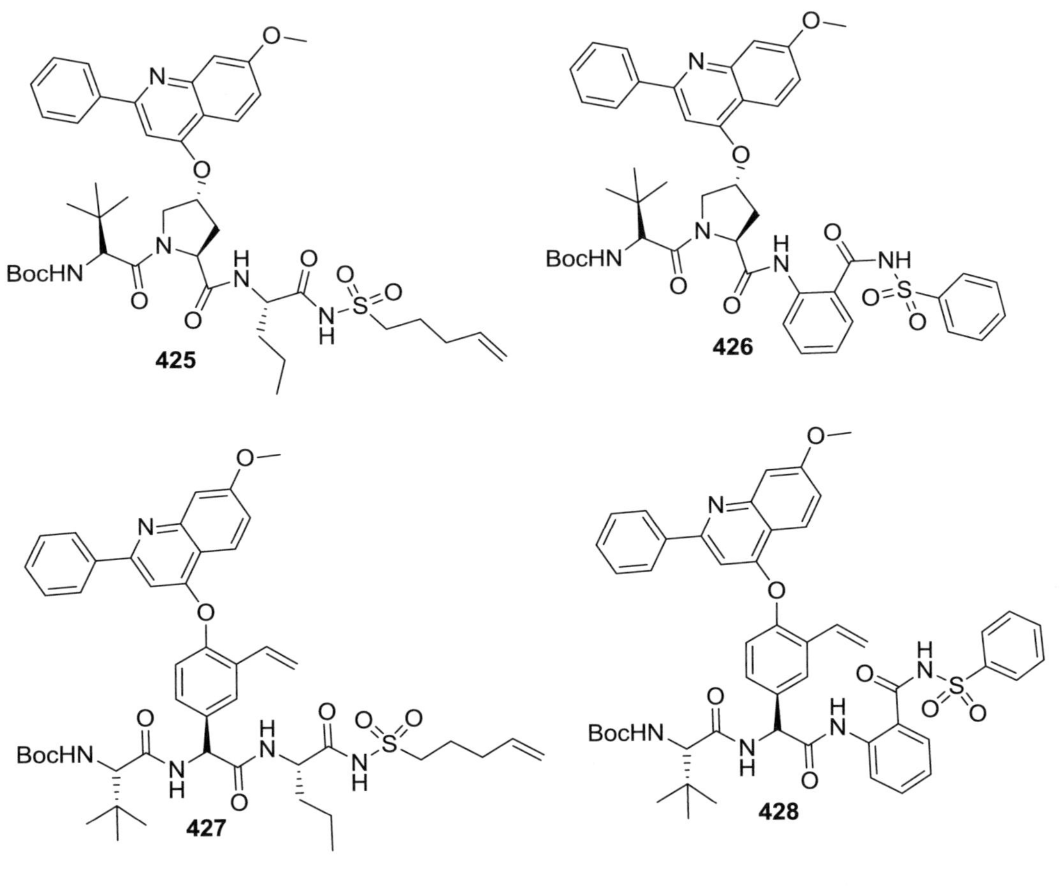

Fig. (47). Example of fragments better suited with phenylglycine than proline. (1) alkenylic P1' elongations (425 *vs* 426) (2) aromatic P1 moiety (427 *vs* 428).

2-Phenyl-4-methoxy-pyrimidinyloxy substituent is an interesting candidate for a P2 substituent. Pyrimidine based P2 substituent synthesis opened up for diversification of the P2 substituent such as vinyl functionalities for macrocyclization to the P2 substituent from P3 which is an interesting option with a better understanding of the binding mode of phenylglycine-based inhibitors a diverse series of linear and macrocyclic HCV NS3/ 4A protease inhibitors (Fig. **48**) [173].

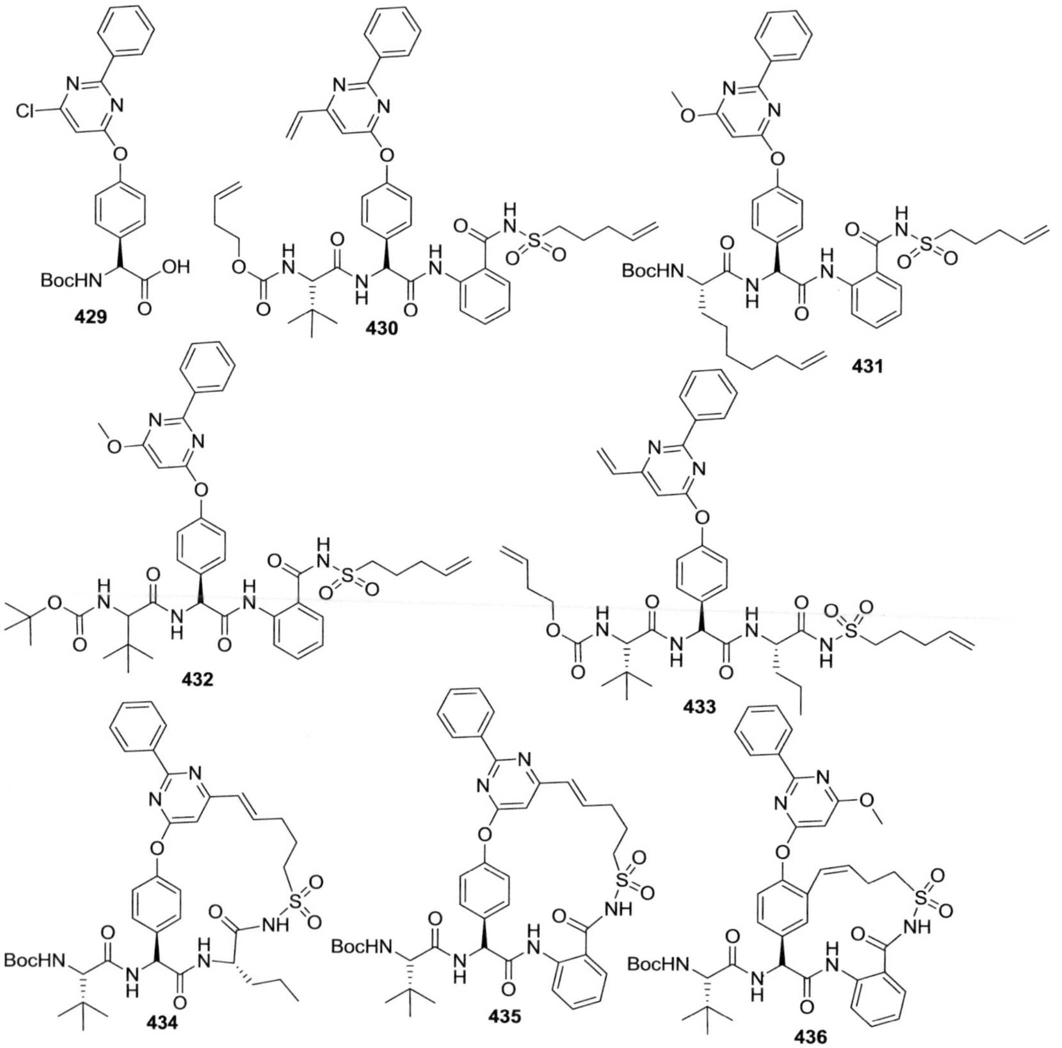

429 **430** **431** **432** **433** **434** **435** **436**

Fig. 48 contd.....

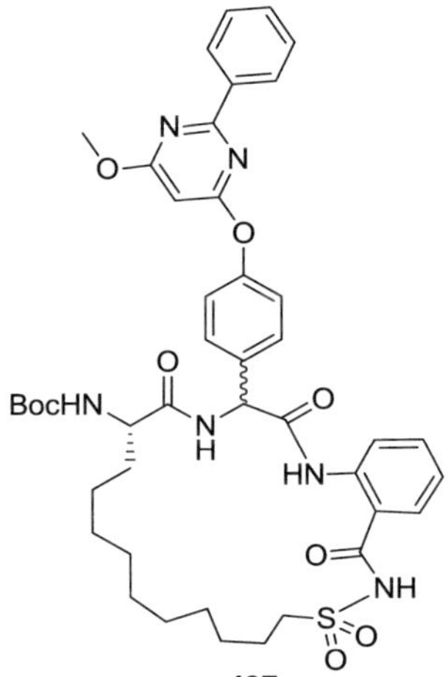

437

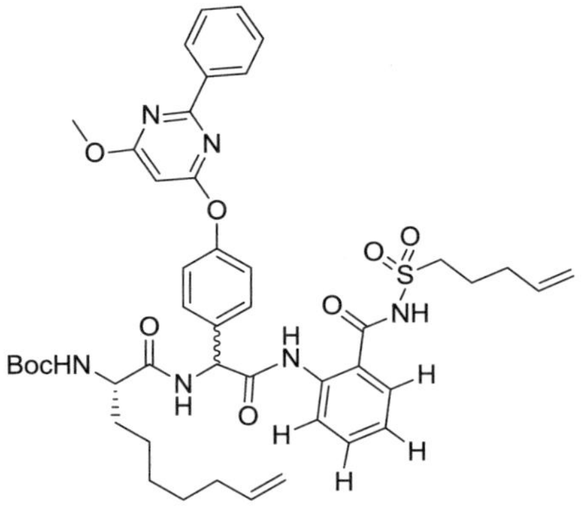

438

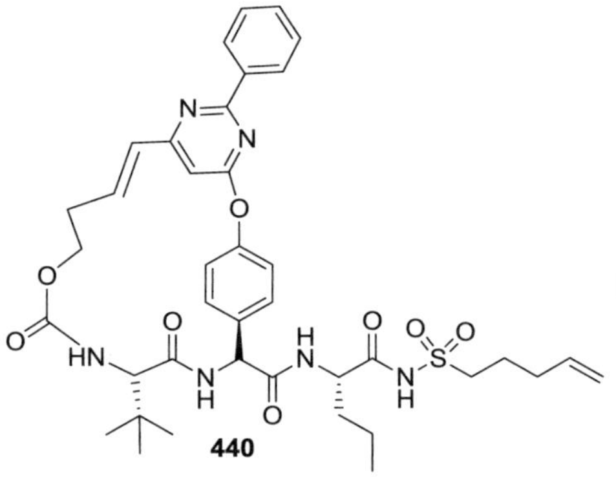

440

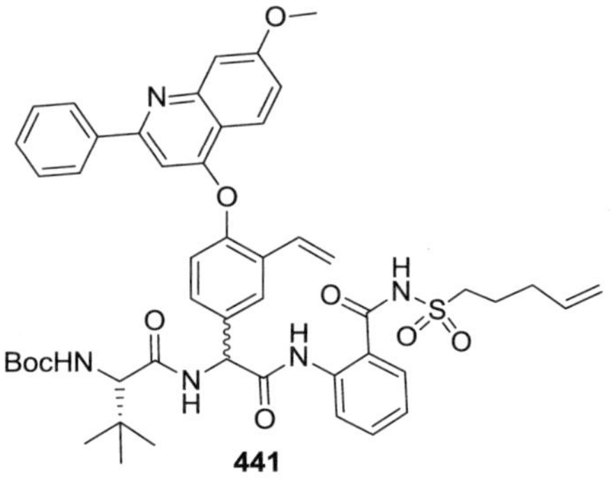

441

Fig. (48). Pyrimidine based derivatives for P2 substituent protease inhibitors.

The NS3 protease x-ray crystal structure showed to be monomeric with two domains: a trypsin-like fold and a structural zinc-binding site. Substrate specificity is different from the cellular serine proteases with a cysteine residue in the P1 position of peptide substrates (Fig. **49**) [174].

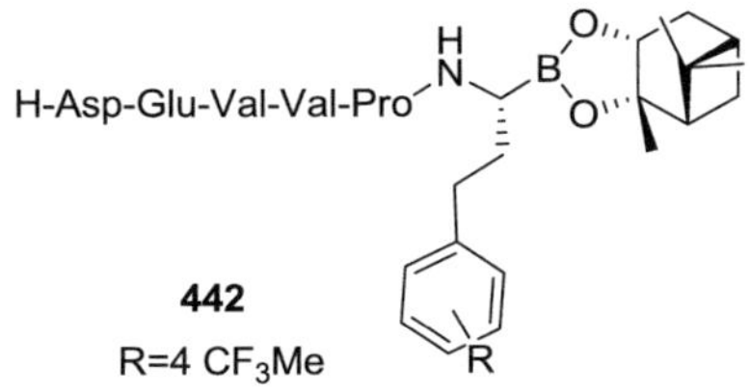

442

R=4 CF_3Me

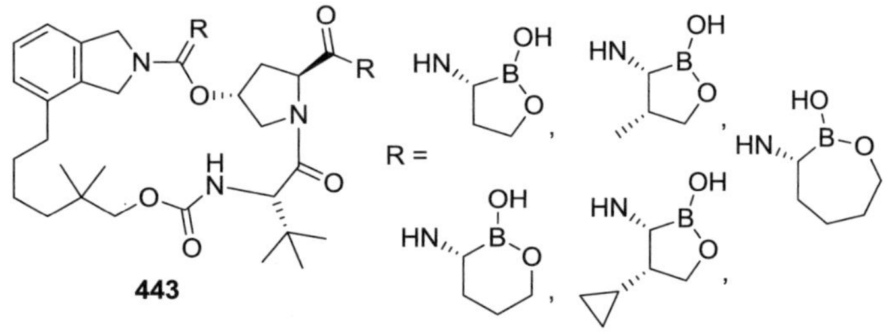

443

Fig. 49 contd.....

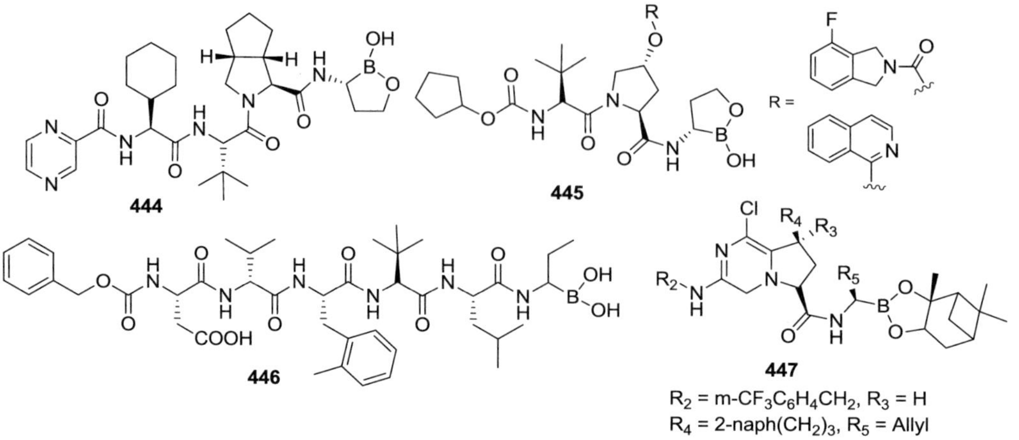

Fig. (49). Peptidyl and nonpeptide boronic acids HCV NS3 protease inhibitors.

R-Ketoamide-type electrophiles were synthesized to bind serine hydroxyl of protease. However, these inhibitors imitated the structures of the peptides (Fig. **50**). For depeptidize the inhibitors, strategies like hydrazine urea replacement of amide bonds and P2 to P4 and P1 to P3 macrocyclizations were examined for the enhanced potency (Fig. **51**) [175].

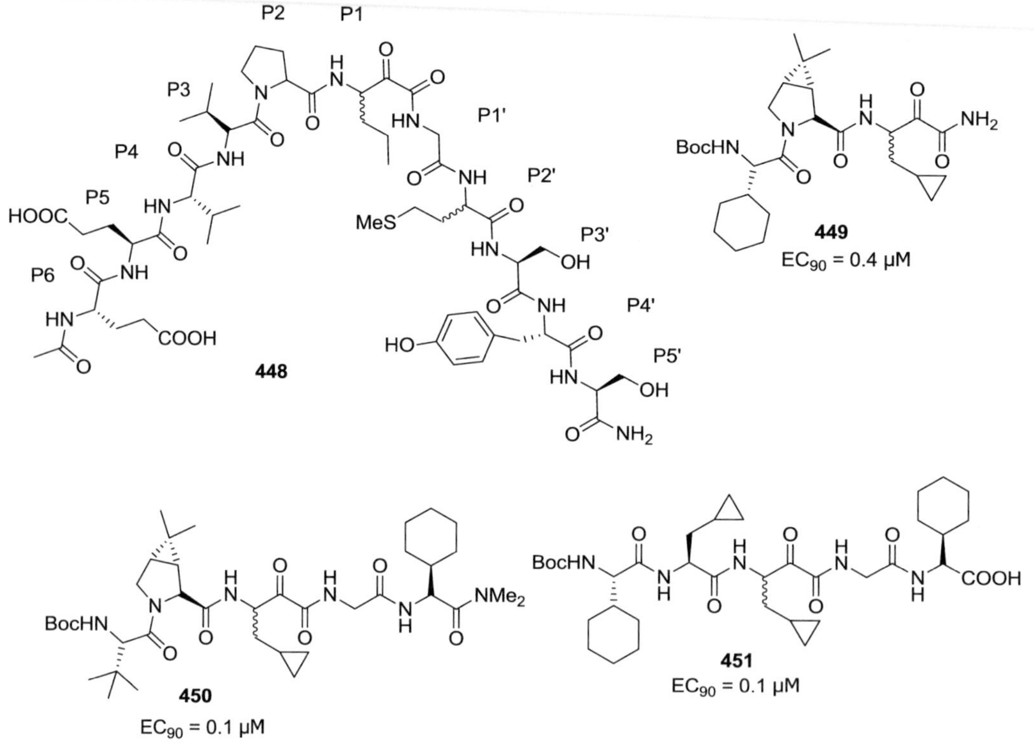

Fig. 50 contd.....

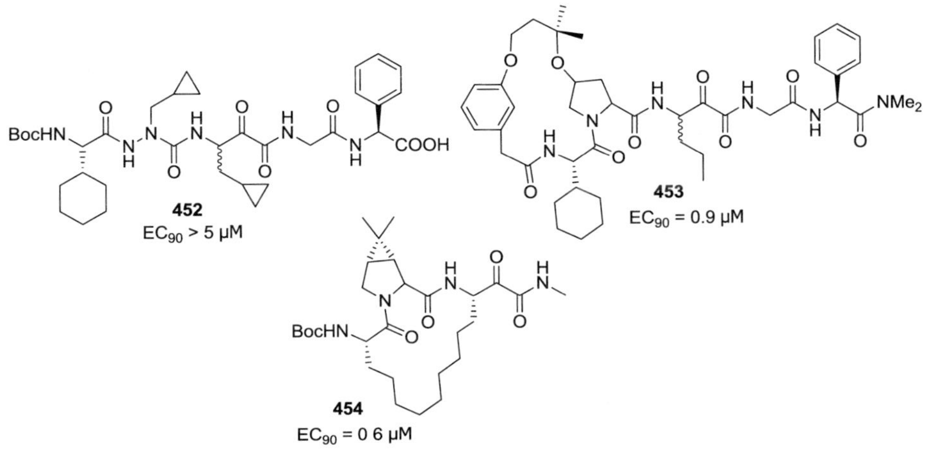

Fig. (50). Undecapeptide to pentapeptide HCV NS3 protease inhibitors.

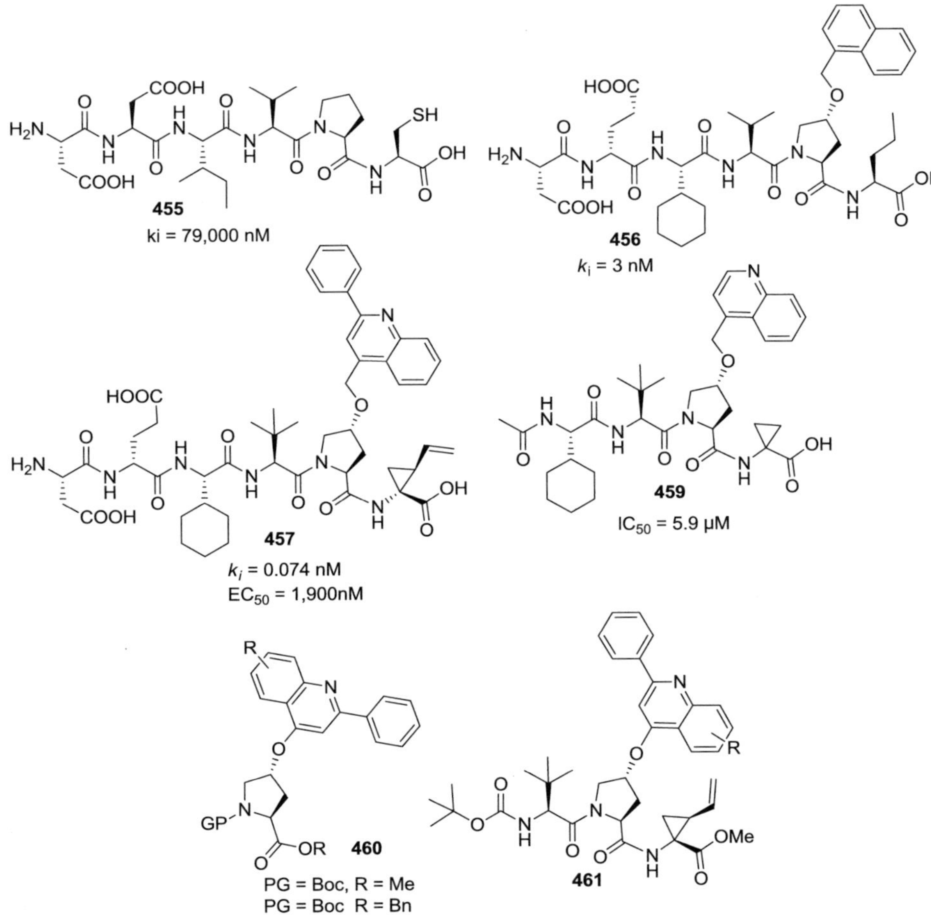

Fig. (51). Hexapeptide inhibitors of the NS3 protease.

The replacement of a hydrogen atom by a fluorine atom is a common and promising strategy in medicinal chemistry to alter the pharmacological properties of bioactive compounds such as solubility, lipophilicity, metabolic stability and binding properties. Thus, the fluorinated analogue of the cyclopropyl core: methyl α-amino-β-fluoro-β-vinyl cyclopropane carboxylate building block (±)-cis-6 is reported. Because of the total synthesis of a fluorinated analogue **483** developed by Janssen Pharmaceutica which was recently approved by the FDA is reported as a HCV NS3/4A protease inhibitor (Fig. **52**) [176]. The Bristol-Myers Squibb's NS3 protease inhibitors asunaprevir (Sunvepra), the NS5A replication complex inhibitor daclatasvir (Daklinza) and the allosteric NS5B polymerase inhibitor beclabuvir are used in chronic HCV infection, may also be cured by treatment with DAAs alone in the absence of interferon [177].

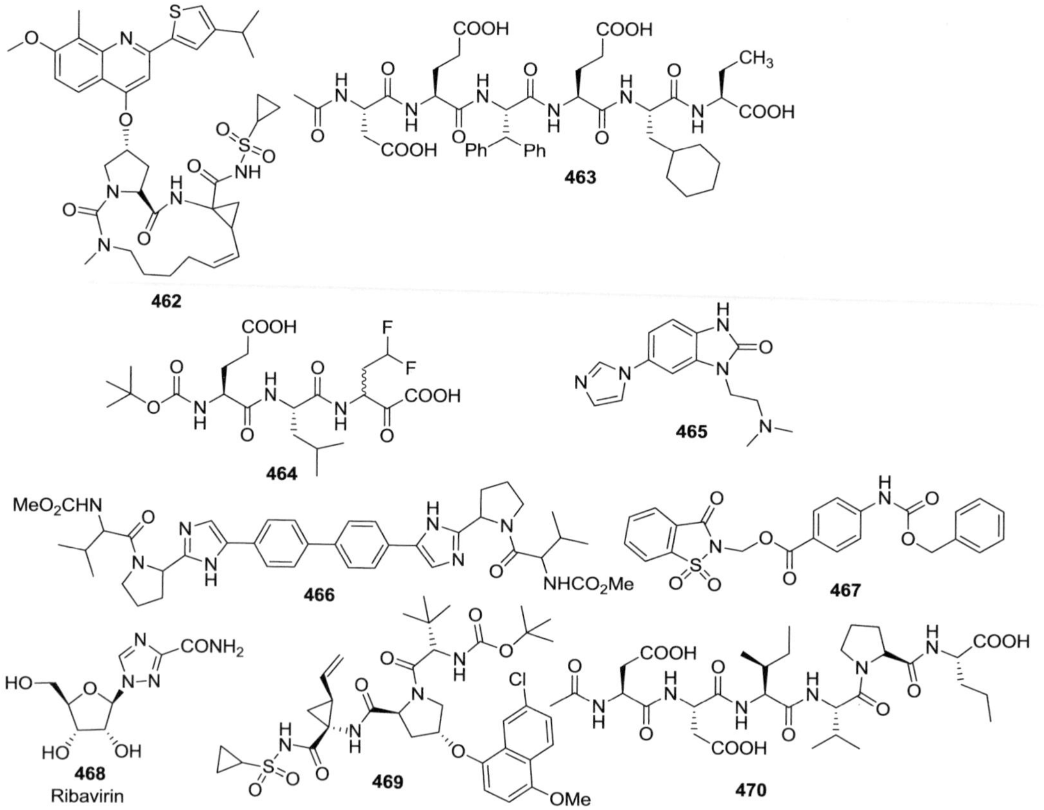

Fig. 52 contd.....

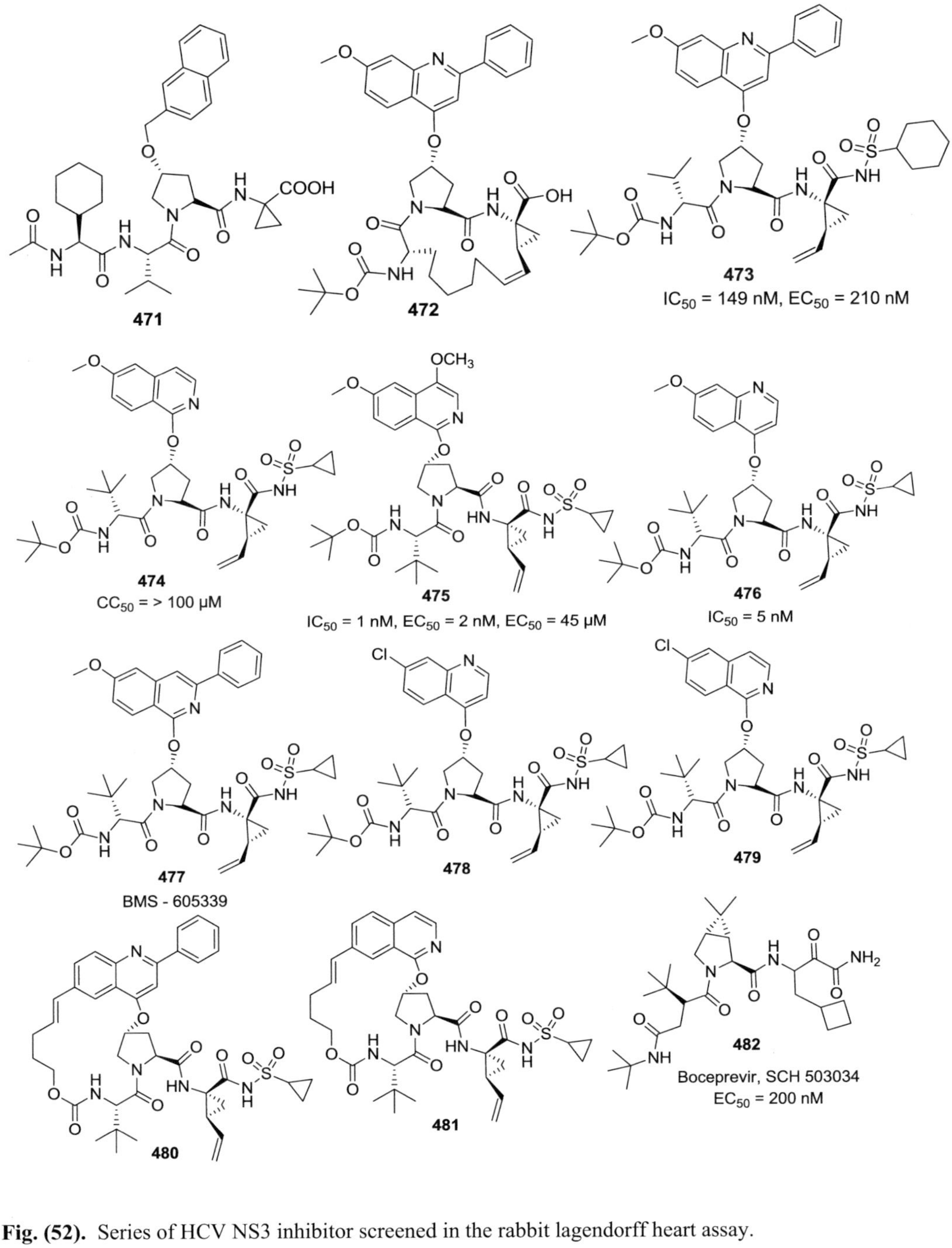

Fig. (52). Series of HCV NS3 inhibitor screened in the rabbit lagendorff heart assay.

Microwave-assisted an efficient one-pot and two-step protocol is reported to afford N-1 and C-6 functionalized 3,5-dichloro-2(1H)-pyrazinones for NS3 protease inhibition property (Fig. **53**) [178].

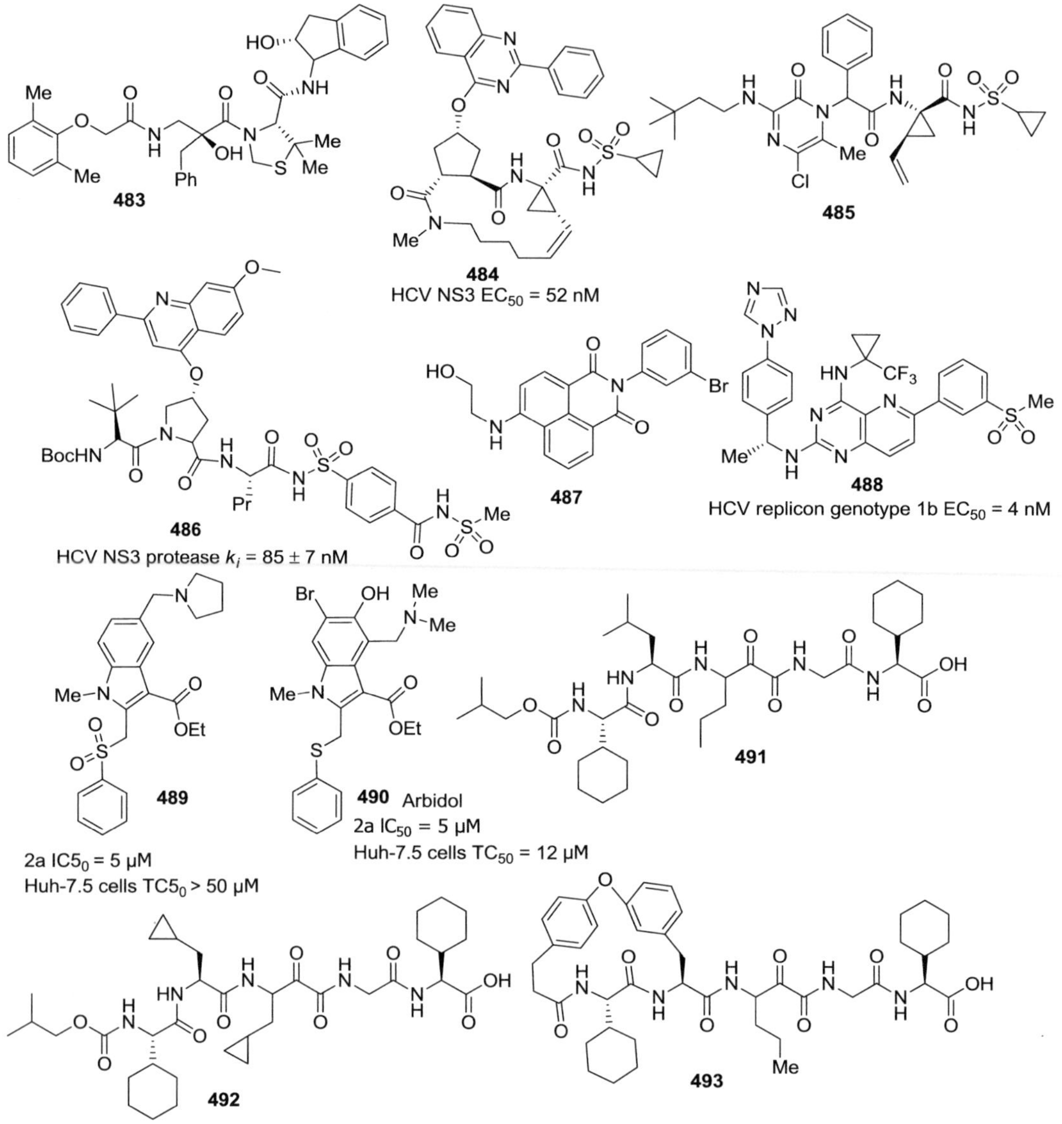

Fig. (53). Structures of NS3 protease inhibitors.

A 7-methoxy-2-phenyl-4-quinolinoxy substituted moiety afforded substantial increase in anti-HCV potency. Similarly, SAR studies led to the identification of carbamate-containing tripeptides that are able to inhibit replication of sub-genomic RNA in the cell culture [179].

4.8. Resistance to NS3/4A Inhibitors

RNA-dependent RNA polymerase and numerous variants (quasi-species) are produced during HCV replication because of elevated replication rate and the poor fidelity. These variants carrying mutations, altered the conformation of the binding sites for DAA compounds. The pre-existing drug-resistant variants have a fitness advantage and can be selected to become the dominant viral quasi-species in the treatment with specific anti-virals. The quasi-species resistant to NS3/4A protease or non-nucleoside polymerase inhibitors can be detected at low levels (about 1%) even patients have never been treated with these specific anti-virals [180].

4.9. Inhibitors of NS4A Binding

NS4A analogues alone or linked to an NS5A/NS5B peptide strategy has been developed to connect both domains simultaneously [181].

4.9.1. Peptidomimetic Protease Inhibitors

A biochemical studies showed that the N-terminal products obtained after cleavage are competitive inhibitors of the natural enzyme, a hexapeptide with residues P6-P1 generally displayed low *K*i-value. Therefore, the natural substrates may be the starting points for rational design and lead optimization of peptidomimetic inhibitors [182]. For example, VX-950 (Vertex/Mitsubishi) is used as peptidomimetic inhibitor for NS3/4A protease that is stabilized into the enzyme's active site with the inclusion of an R-ketoamide [183]. Many others are at various stages of development. Since the cross-resistance to diverse protease inhibitors can be achieved with the mutation of a single amino acid, the combination of multiple protease inhibitors could turn out to have limited value in the clinical practice.

4.9.2. Non-covalent Peptidomimetic Inhibitors

A hexapeptide inhibitor optimal binding required an acidic anchor at the N-terminus and the carboxylic at the C-terminus as per SAR studies. Thus, a free carboxylic acid present on the P1 residue contributes to potency and imparts selectivity with respect to other serine protease. The researchers focused on alternating P1 residue as the first step in lead optimization, starting from hexapeptide inhibitors derived from the N-terminal NS3 cleavage product [184]. Several non-covalent product-based inhibitors obtained with C-terminal moieties like carboxylic acid, acyl sulphonamide and phenethyl amide as (1*R*,2*S*)-1-ami-o-2-vinylcyclopropane carboxylic acid, led to the discovery of bioavailable tripeptide inhibitor, BILN-2061. It binding to the active site of the NS3/4A protease, resulted in the distortion of catalytic triad and disruption of H-bonds which gave potent and competitive inhibition of protease genotypes 1a and 1b (*K*i 0.3 and 0.66 nM) respectively [185].

4.9.3. Non-peptidic Protease Inhibitors

Poor bioavailability of peptidomimetic derivatives resulted in failure of protease inhibitors. Thus, non-peptidic, small molecules have been adopted such as thiazolidine phenanthrenequinone, aryl-alkylidene rhodanines and benzimidazole derivatives and isolated RNA aptamers to demonstrate *in vitro* NS3 inhibitory. They are competitive inhibitors of the HCV protease and their mechanisms of action remain unclear.

4.9.4. Covalent Substrate-based Inhibitors

Generally, NS3 protease–substrate interactions have H-bonds on substrate backbone and electrostatic contacts along the binding site. The peptidic inhibitors that interact with the catalytic serine residues as reversibly or irreversibly. They are derived from known substrates after replacing the scissile amide bond with an electrophilic moiety such as α-ketoamides, boronic acids, aldehydes, α-ketoacids, azapeptides or pyrrolidine-5,5-*trans* lactams. Among them, the α-ketoamides have been extensively explored for VX-950 drug [186].

4.9.5. Nucleic-acid-based Antiviral Agents

During the past few years, synthetic nucleic acids drugs has received increasing attention for therapeutic agents as anti-sense oligonucleotides, ribozymes and siRNAs. But failed due to their adverse effects and limited efficacy [187].

4.10. Natural Products

Tripeptide dienes with (1*R*,2*S*)-vinyl amino cyclopropylcarboxylate residue were cyclized under ring-closing metathesis (RCM) to afford α-strand scaffolds [188]. The peptidic scaffolds were revealed similar to BILN 2061 have clinically validated inhibitors of the HCV [189].

4.10.1. RNA Interference Approach to HCV Antivirals

In the nucleic acid based approaches to explore HCV therapy, RNA interference (RNAi) is the latest addition [190]. The siRNA and vector-encoded short hairpin RNA (shRNA) used against the viral genome effectively which blocks the replication of HCV replicons in tissue culture. But not all siRNAs showed the same efficiency. It was found that all regions including conserved sequences of the HCV genome were susceptible to RNAi [191]. A pH-triggered (at pH 5.5) PEGylated siRNA nanoparticles stable with respect to aggregation in 80% serum can still release siRNA payload within 30 min. This is used in delivery to cultured murine hepatocyte cells *in vitro* even with high degree of PEGylation (5 mol%). A pH triggered PEGylated siRNA nanoparticles entered cells by clathrin-coated pit endocytosis but functional delivery requires membrane fusion events (fusogenicity) and more that 70% of administered nanoparticles are present in the liver hepatocytes and post intravenous administration (Fig. **54**). Similarly, proof-of-concept experiment also supported the possibility of RNAi therapy for HCV infections for pH-triggered PEGylated siRNA nanoparticles [192].

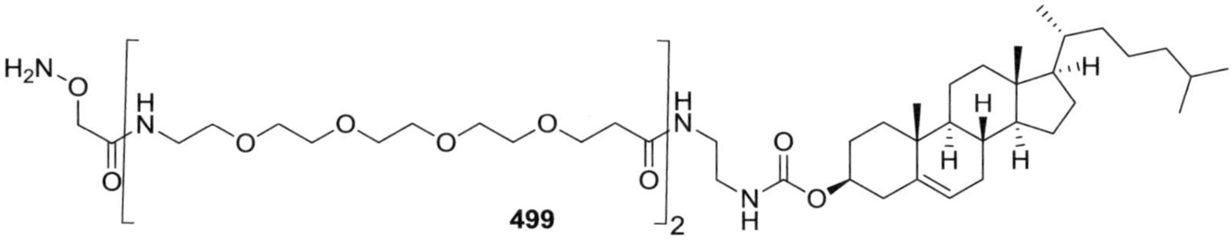
499
CPA 6

Fig. (54). Lipid structures as anti-HCV.

The conserved 5'-untranslated region (UTR) of HCV RNA is targeted with siRNA using a liver-targeted dendritic nano-vector functionalized with a galactopyranoside ligand (DG). The complexation of DG with siRNA is revealed by the physico-chemical characterization and molecular dynamic simulations which demonstrated sugar moieties projecting "out" in the complex. A highly specific ligand–receptor interaction between dendritic galactose and asialoglycoprotein receptor supported in releasing of siRNA to the liver to form the siRNA-DG complex as perinuclear localization in liver cells and co-localization with viral proteins [193].

4.10.2. Nucleoside Inhibitors

During inhibition of virus replication, nucleoside inhibitors act as either chain terminators or non-chain terminators. After entry, they are converted to nucleotide triphosphates (NTP). The synthetic nucleoside inhibitors served as competitive substrates for the polymerase and integrated into the nascent chain by the viral polymerase, led to a premature termination of the elongation process and cause base-mis-match in subsequent rounds of replication, resulting in accumulated mutations in the viral genome so-called "error catastrophe". Several sugar- and base-modified nucleosides have been reported to inhibit the RdRp enzymatic activity and HCV replication in the replicon systems. Among these, the most promising derivatives are of 2α- and 3α-substituted ribonucleoside analogs. Merck Research Laboratory described 2'-*C*-methyladenosine **500** and 2'-*O*-methyl-cytidine **501** inhibitory activity in NS5B polymerase *in vitro* assay. 2α-*C*-methylguanosine **502** and other nucleosides also act in similar mode to 2α-*C*-methyladenosine and 2α-*O*-methylcytidine [194]. Nucleoside analogs with *C*-2--methyl group reported to have good anti-HCV activity. For example, 2α-Deox--2α-fluoro-2α-*C*-methylcytidine **503** has been evaluated in several systems (Fig. **55**) [195]. Furthermore, a series of 3α-deoxyribonucleosides and 3α-deoxy-cytidine **504** exhibited chain terminators activity in a biochemical assay. NM283 **506** developed by idenix is a promising orally bioavailable pro-drug of 2α-*C*-methylcytidine, NM107 **505** where NM283 targets the RNA polymerase in two ways.

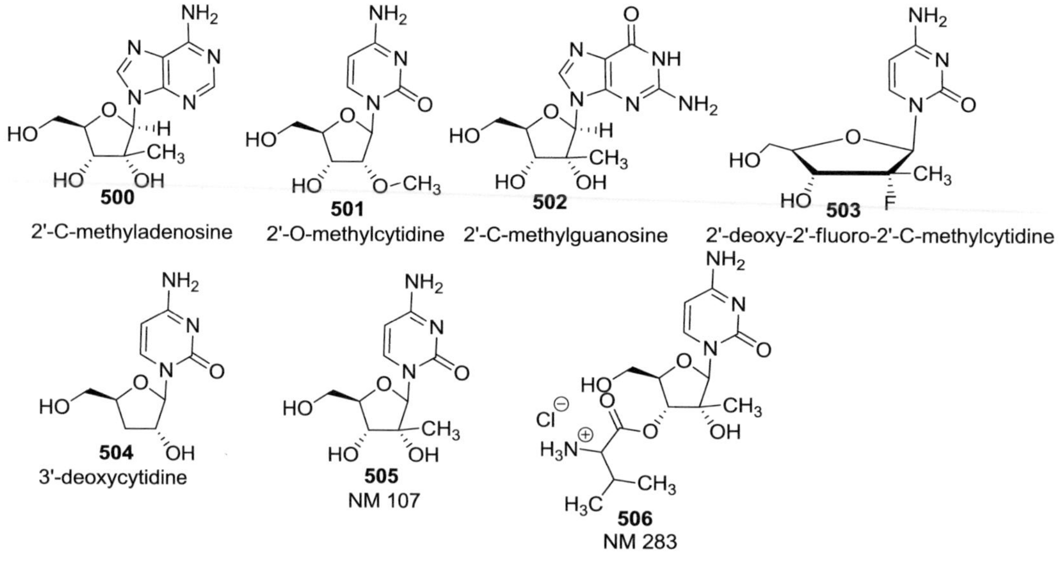

Fig. (55). Sugar-modified and base-modified nucleoside analogs.

4.10.3. Non-nucleoside Inhibitors

Besides active site, the x-ray derived co-crystal structures revealed distinct allosteric regulatory sites, located distant of compounds bound to NS5B might be the targets for developing anti-viral agents [196]. Thus, many α,α-diketoacids have been synthesized as HCV polymerase inhibitors. SAR studies also indicated that the diketoacid moiety are essential for activity and the substitution of aryl to thienyl group at the α-position is necessary for selectivity and potency (Fig. **56**).

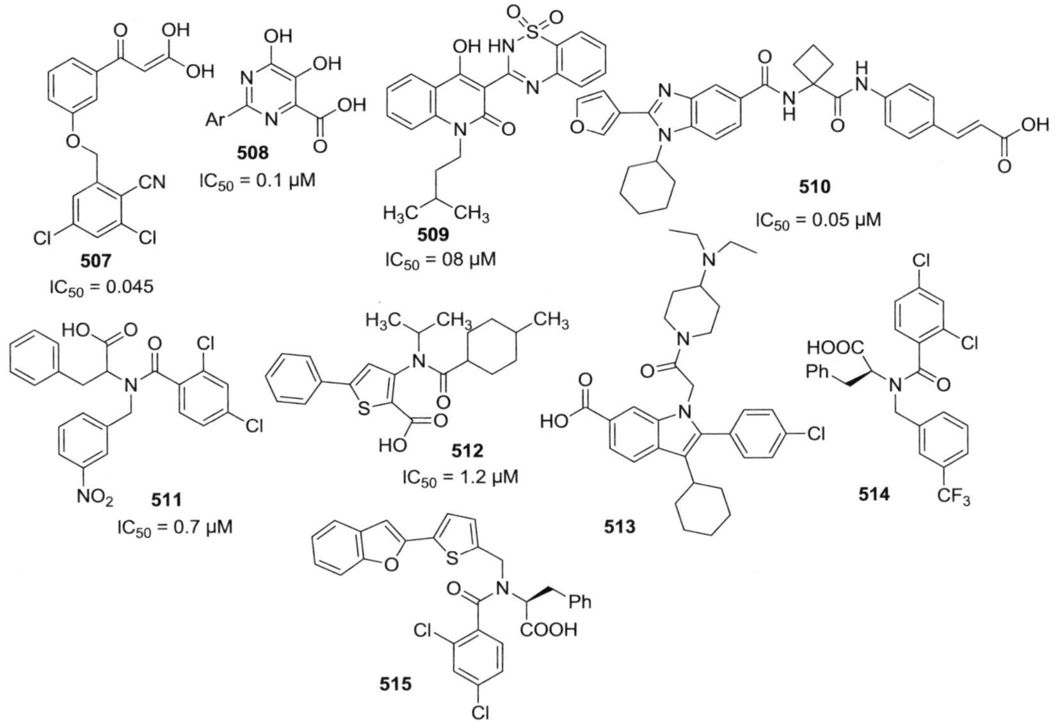

Fig. (56). Structure of non-nucleoside NS5B polymerase inhibitor.

Benzothiadiazine derivatives are highly selective for HCV RdRp but failed to inhibit other viral and mammalian polymerases. Similarly, benzimidazole derivatives, the first non-nucleoside inhibitors disclosed to be active against the HCV polymerase by Japan Tobacco. Cross-resistance studies and synergistic inhibition of HCV polymerase in combinations of benzimidazole and benzothiadiazine which further showed the two structurally distinct classes of inhibitors had non-overlapping binding sites and different mode of action. Compound HCV-796, a novel non-nucleoside HCV polymerase inhibitor is evaluated in clinical trials in combination with PEG-IFN by ViroPharma and Wyeth showed that it was well tolerated with no serious adverse events. The structural work with **507** bound to the enzyme has indicated that the molecule acts as allosteric inhibitor by contacts between two domains on the enzyme [197]. Non-nucleoside inhibitors, (2*S*)-2-[(2,4-dichlorobenzoyl)-(3-trifluoromethyl benzyl) amino]-3-phenylpropionic acid **508** and (2*S*)-2-[(5-benzofuran-2-yl thiophen-2-ylmethyl)-(2,4-dichlorobenzoyl)amino]-3-phenyl propionic acid **509** bound to HCV polymerase indicated that the binding site of the NNIs is located at the base of the thumb sub-domain [198] with two hydrophobic pockets and a pair of adjacent main chain amide groups. The predominate binding interaction is hydrophobic and exists between the primary binding pocket and the 2,4-dichlorophenyl group of both inhibitors. SAR study of benzimidazole derivatives indicated that a 1,2-disubstituted benzimidazole 5-carboxylic acid scaffold **510** is the minimum core required for biological activity (Fig. **57**) [199].

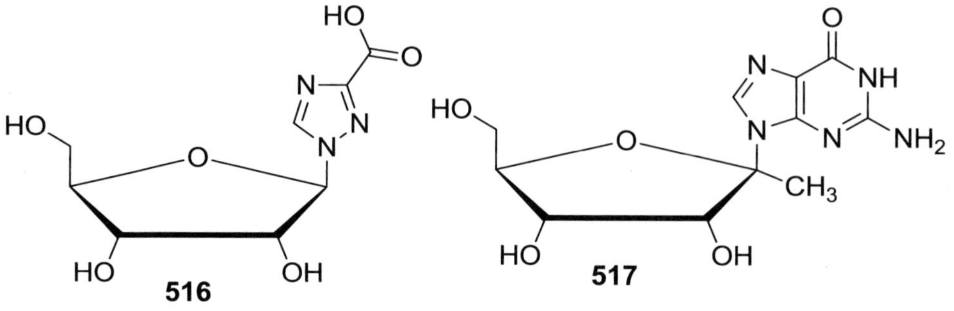

Fig. (57). Structure of two nucleoside analogue inhibitors of HCV polymerase: ribavirin **516** and α-D-2'-methylribofuranosylguanosine **517**.

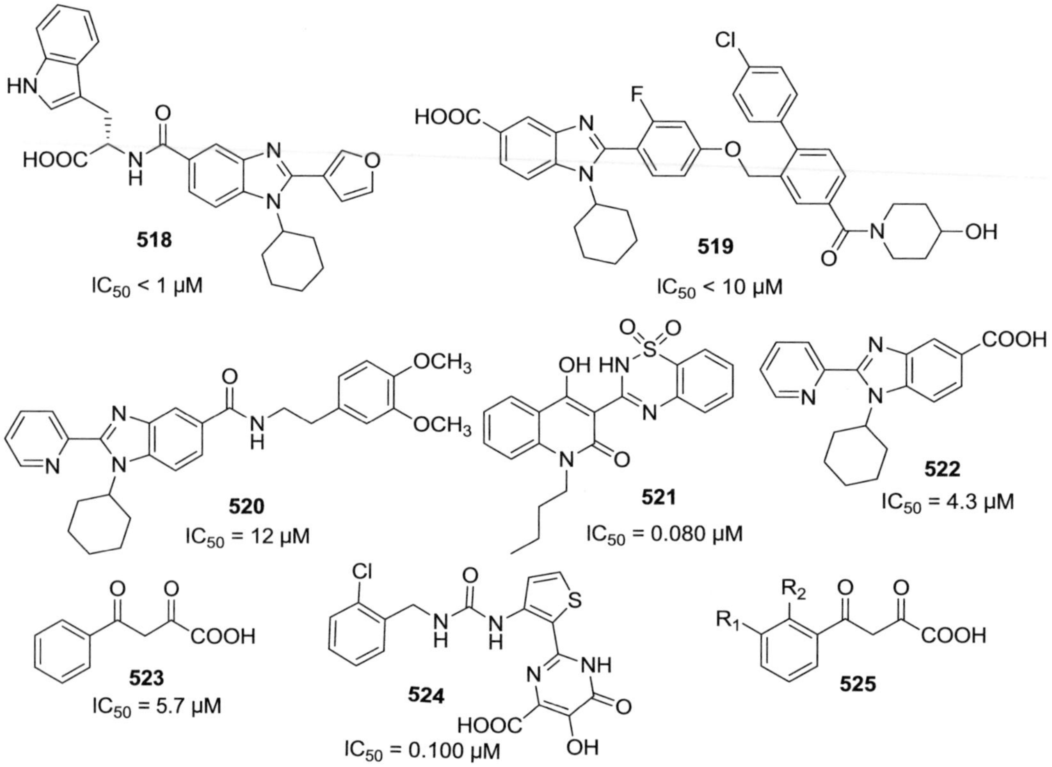

Fig. (58). Structures of benzimidazole and diketo acid inhibitors of HCV polymerase.

4.10.4. RNA Aptamers

Aptamers are single-stranded nucleic acids which directly inhibit protein's function by folding into a specific 3D-structure that dictates high affinity binding to the targeted protein [200]. They are similar to monoclonal antibodies or small molecule drugs which inhibits the activity of existing proteins directly and greatly increased the number of clinical indications that are potentially treatable by nucleic acid based compounds (Fig. **58**) [201].

4.10.5. Pyrophosphate Mimics

Like nucleoside inhibitors of HCV polymerase, pyrophosphate mimics are structurally and chemically homogeneous class with compounds that possessing a diketo acid moiety. Novel class of substituted dihydroxypyrimidine carboxylates are also believed to act as pyrophosphate mimics [202].

4.11. NS5A Inhibitors

HCV NS5A protein has important role in HCV replication, assembly and release in the early formation of the replication complex interaction with intracellular lipid membranes and initiates viral assembly at the surface of lipid droplets with the HCV core. It also serves as a channel to protect and direct viral RNA within the membranes of the replication complex and interact with NS5B, results in an enhanced activity of RNA polymerase. Besides HCV replication impact, NS5A also modulates host cell signaling pathways with interferon resistance [203]. NS5A inhibitors daclatasvir, ledipasvir and ombitasvir are used for the hepatitis C treatment even at low doses of daclatasvir and ledipasvir demonstrate high anti-viral efficacy in all HCV genotypes exception HCV genotype 3 with higher EC_{50} concentrations. NS5A inhibitors are only be used in combination with other DAAs like PEG-IFN α and ribavirin due to mutations. Elbasvir, a NS5A inhibitor is used as broad genotype coverage with grazoprevir, a NS3/4A inhibitor as a fixed combination. Other NS5A inhibitors are velpatasvir, ABT-450, MK-8408, BMS-824393 and PPI-461 [204].

4.11.1. Natural Products

Daclatasvir (DCV; known as BMS-790052 and Daklinza), an NS5A replication inhibitor is the most potent direct-acting anti-HCV agents. The co-operative interaction of a pair of compounds suggests that one inhibitor binds to resistant NS5A causing conformational changes and transmitted to adjacent NS5As which resensitize resistant NS5A, so that the second inhibitor can act to restore inhibition. This synergistic anti-HCV activity enhanced the resistance barrier for

DCV which provides options for combination therapy and new insight into the role of NS5A in the replication cycle (Fig. **59**) [205].

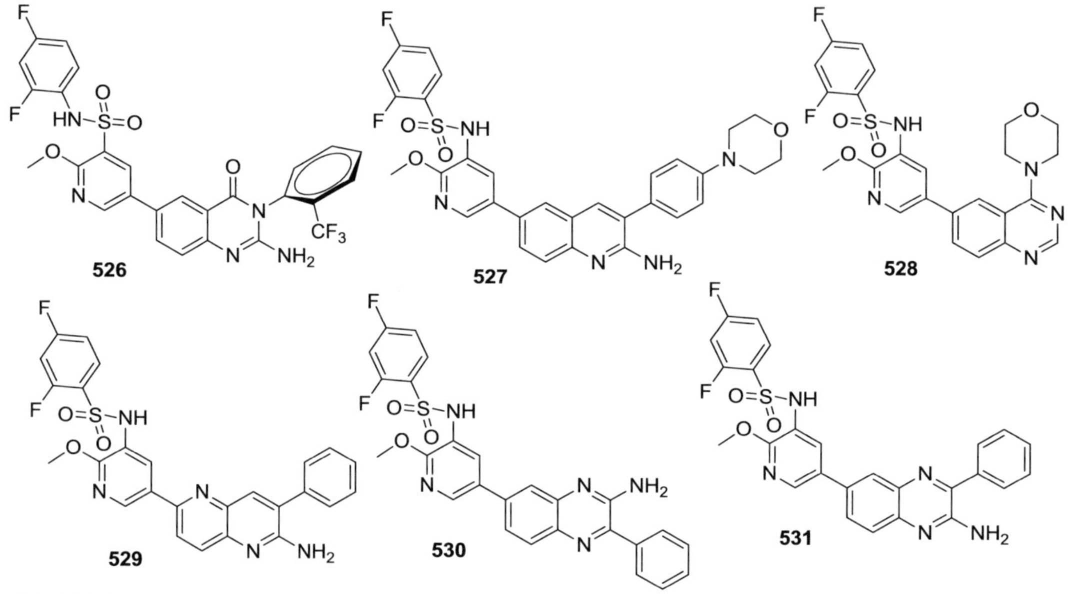

Fig. (59). Structures of HCV NS5A inhibitors.

4.11.2. Synthetic Products

Lipid kinase, PI4KIIIα contacts with RNA interference and results in breakdown of the replication complex and termination of HCV replication observed in Huh-7 cells. However, PI4KIIIα and HCV NS5A interaction, enriched the HCV replication complex with product phosphoinositol 4-phosphate (PI4P) which led to elevation of PI4P at the endoplasmic reticulum that linked to HCV infection in the liver. Compound quinazolinone **526** displayed high selectivity for PI4KIIIα and so potent inhibitor of HCV replication *in vitro* [206].

2-Pyrrolidin-2-yl-5-{4-[4-(2-pyrrolidin-2-yl-1H-imidazol-5-yl)buta-1,3-diynyl] phenyl}-1H-imidazole derivatives were designed as NS5A inhibitors based on SAR studies. Compound **532** (AV4025) with (S,S,S,S)-stereochemistry (EC_{50} 3.4 pM, HCV replicon genotype 1b) was found more active than the compounds with two (S)- and two (R)-chiral centers (Fig. **60**) [207].

Based on phenotypic screening, benzothiazole scaffolds were synthesized. They have better oral bioavailability due to low molecular weight and hydrophobicity. The benzothiazole-disulfoamide derivatives were found potent anti-HCV selectivity in targeting NS5A (Fig. **61**) [208].

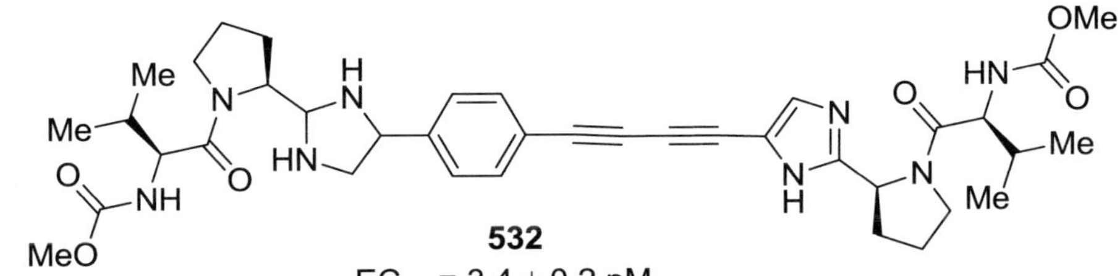

532

EC_{50} = 3.4 ± 0.2 pM

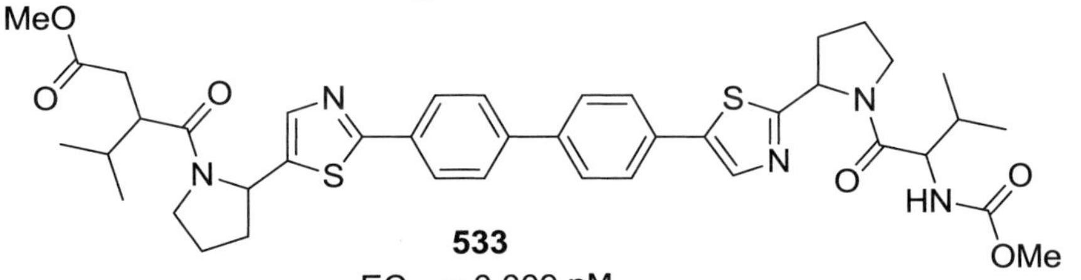

533

EC_{50} = 0.009 nM

Fig. (60). Inhibitors of HCV genotype 1b replicon.

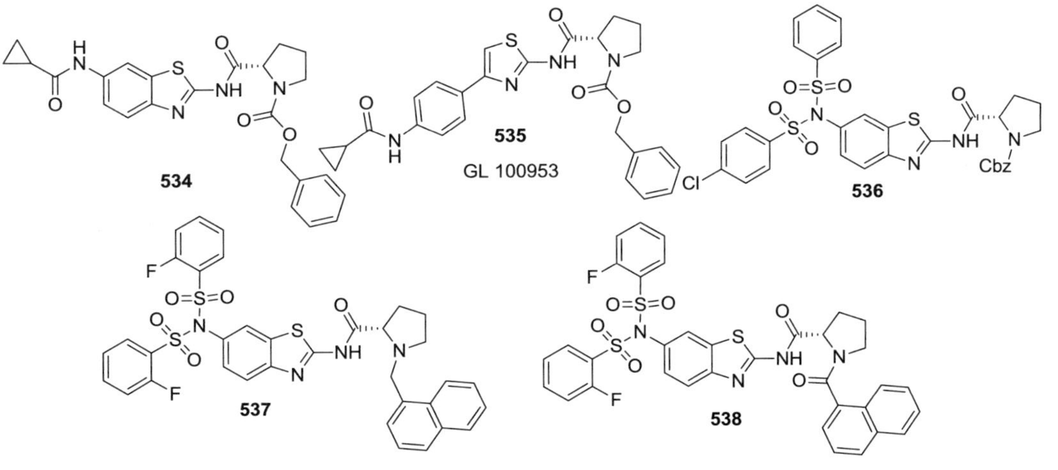

534, **535** (GL 100953), **536**, **537**, **538**

Fig. (61). Structures of Inhibitors of HCV NS5A.

RG7128, an inhibitor of the NS5B polymerase; BMS-790052, an inhibitor of NS5A and alisporivir, an inhibitor of human cyclophilins are directly acting and host targeting anti-virals against chronic HCV patients. In combination with inhibitors of HCV NS3/4A protease produce additively or synergistically an improved rate of virologic response, more than the pegylated interferon plus ribavirin therapy [209]. They interfere with host factors that support viral replication distinct from agents that modulate the host innate immune response (*e.g.* alternative interferons, nitazoxanide).

4.11.3. Inhibition of NTPase Activity by Allosteric Mechanisms

The competitive NTPase inhibitors may be partially circumvented by utilizing chemically unrelated compounds to NTP which reduce the accessibility to the NTP-binding site through a non-competitive manner [210]. For example, the calmodulin antagonist trifluoroperazine is interacted with domain 1 of HCV helicase, resulted from conformational changes or from blockage of the ATP-binding site (Fig. **62**) [211].

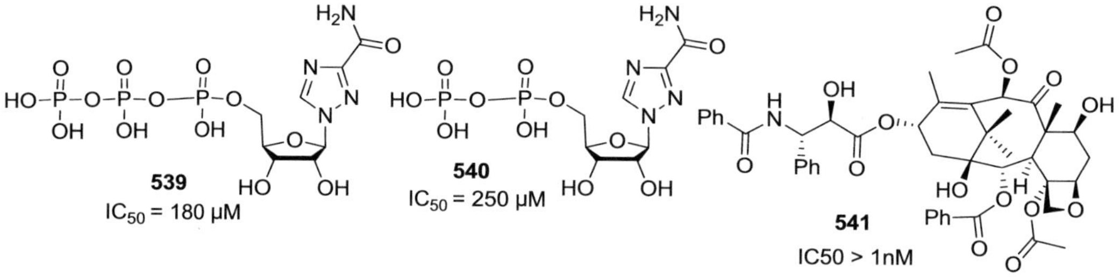

Fig. (62). Structure of three competitive HCV helicase inhibitors ribavirin 5'-triphosphate **539**, ribavirin 5'-diphosphate **540**, and paclitaxel **541**.

Bromo-and morpholinomethyl-tropolone analogues were synthesized which showed anti-HCV activity against helicase and NTPase in the fluorometric helicase assay. These derivatives have higher inhibitory activities than those of the non-modified analogues and 3,7-dibromo-5-morpholinomethyl tropolone are exceptionally high. Further modification needed to develop potent inhibitors of HCV helicase and viral replication (Fig. **63**) [212].

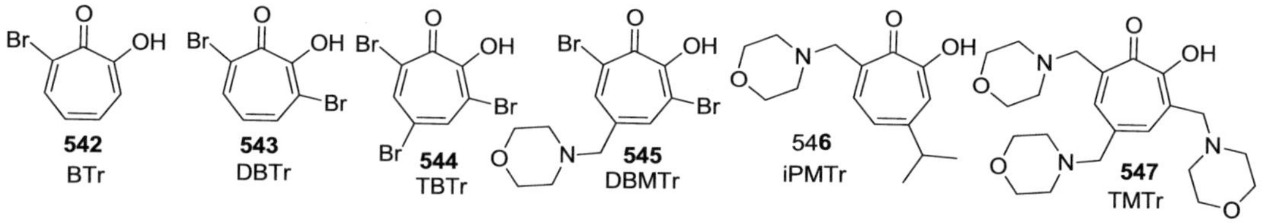

Fig. (63). Tropolone analogues as anti-HCV helicase and NTPase activities.

4.11.4. Competitive Inhibition of RNA Binding

The initial studies in HCV helicase activity gave numerous polynucleotides as inhibitors (Fig. **64** & Fig. **65**). Their inhibition resulted from the competition of the polynucleotides with DNA or RNA substrates that may be mimic by synthetic macromolecules. SAR study also indicated that benzimidazole ring or benzene group at the C2 position of benzimidazole moiety and the nature of linker are essential for inhibitory activity (Fig. **66**) [213].

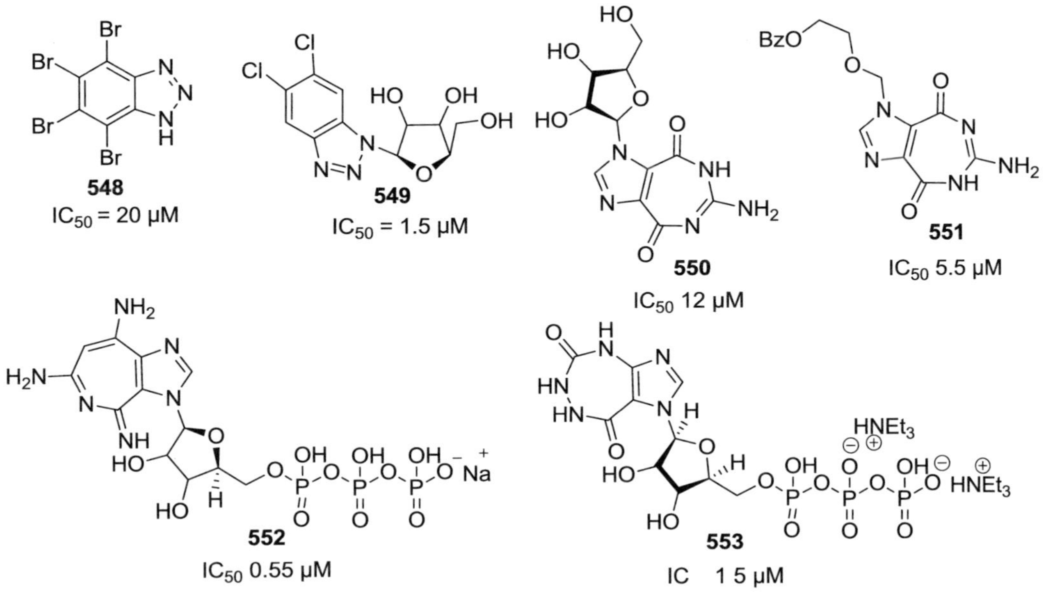

Fig. (64). Structure of the halogenated benzotriazoles DRBT **549** and TBBT **548** and the ring-expanded nucleosides **550** and **551** in addition to the ring-expanded 5'-triphosphate nucleosides **552** and **553**.

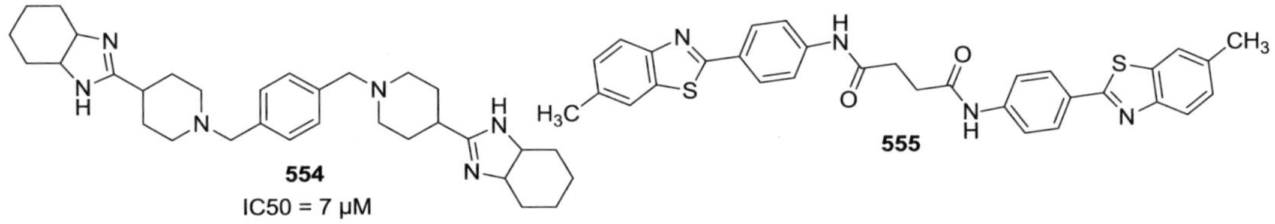

Fig. (65). Structures of aminophenylbenzimidazole **554** and aminophenylbenothiazole **555** HCV helicase competitive inhibitors.

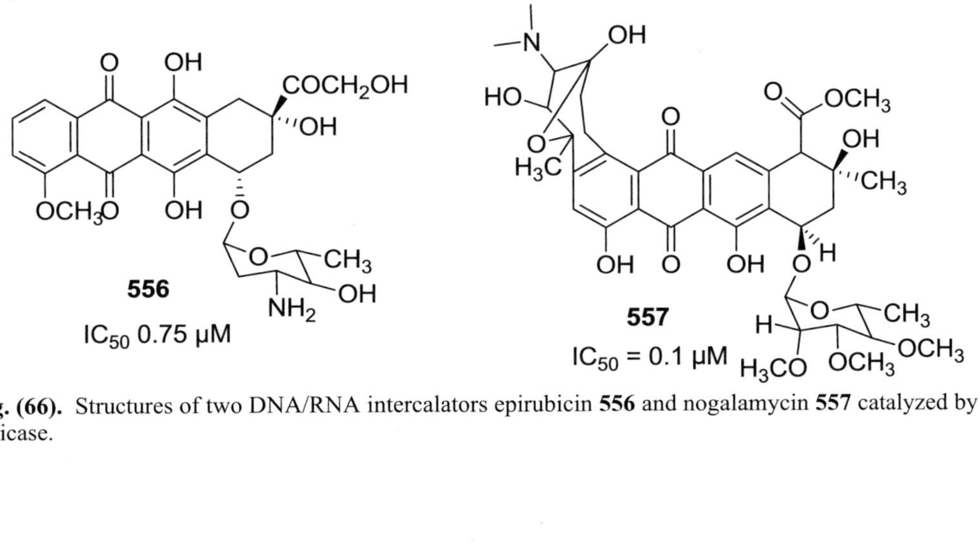

Fig. (66). Structures of two DNA/RNA intercalators epirubicin **556** and nogalamycin **557** catalyzed by HCV helicase.

4.11.5. Inhibition of the Unwinding through Intercalation of Polynucleotide Chain

Duplexes of DNA or RNA with an intercalated agent are more stable than the unbound counterparts which increases the energy required for duplex unwinding. For example, epirubicin and nogalamycin are members of anthracycline family (anticancer/antibiotics) are effective inhibitors of the unwinding reaction catalyzed by the helicase enzyme (Fig. **67**) [214].

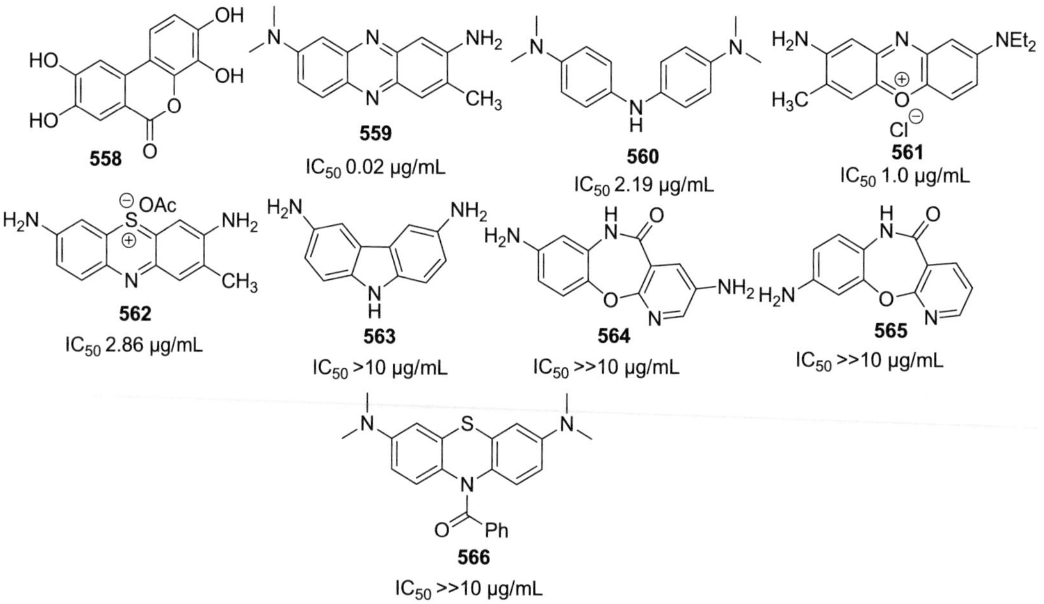

Fig. (67). Compounds with anti HCV IRES activity.

4.12. Other Targets

Other structural and non-structural proteins (NS2 and NS2/3 proteases) are responsible for a cleavage in the viral polyprotein between non-structural proteins NS2 and NS3 [215]. For example, the minimal protein region needed to catalyze NS2 and NS3 that includes most of NS2 and N-terminal of one-third NS3. The NS2-NS3 protease sequence homology does not share with any known protease, leading to conflicting opinions as it is a metalloprotease or a zinc-dependent cysteine protease. Thus, it has little attention as an anti-viral target because the protease acts co-translationally. Inhibition of NS2/3 by NS4A peptides can be rationalized from the organizing effect of NS4A on the N-terminus of NS3 (the NS2/3 cleavage point), suggested by the known 3D structure of the NS3 protease domain [216]. Recently, the HCV envelope protein E2 binds specifically to CD81 (CD81 located on the surfaces of hepatocytes) indicating that CD81 acts as putative receptor for viral attachment [217].

4.13. Novel Immunomodulatory Agents

Generally, the synthetic molecules are agonists for toll-like receptors (TLRs) 7 and 9 which showed potency in controlling HCV infection. They also sense the presence of invading micro-organisms on the basis of molecular patterns of pathogens (bacteria, viruses and parasites). They are also articulated by immune cells such as macrophages, monocytes, dendritic cells and B cells [218]. So far, ten TLRs have been identified in humans that recognize molecular patterns associated with a specific class of microbial agents. TLRs 3, 7, 8 and 9 are intracellular receptors specialized in the recognition of viral nucleic acids and detect respectively double-stranded RNA (TLR-3), single-stranded RNA (TLR-7 and -8) and unmethylated deoxycytosine-deoxyguanosine (CpG) DNA sequences (TLR-9) in late endosomes and lysosomes [219]. TLR-9 and TLR-7 in humans are expressed in B cells and plasmacytoid dendritic cell (PDCs). Short synthetic oligonucleotides with one or more unmethylated CpG motifs flanked by specific sequences are potent agonists of TLR-9. TLR-7 which recognizes several synthetic compounds that are structurally related to nucleic acids such as imidazoquinolines, loxoribine (7-allyl-7,8-dihydro-8-oxoguanosine) and bropirimine (2-amin-5-bromo-6-phenyl-4(3)-pyrimidinone). The anti-viral properties of synthetic TLR-7 ligands is known for long time which induce a potent, broad-spectrum anti-viral response owing to their ability to induce the release of inflammatory cytokines like IFN-α ANA245 (7-thia-8-oxoguanosine or Isatoribine; Anadys Pharmaceuticals), is a guanine nucleoside analogue whose immunostimulatory activity depends upon its agonistic activity on TLR-7 [220].

4.14. NS4B Inhibitors

NS4B is less characterized HCV NS protein due to its integral membrane association. It plays a structural role in HCV RNA replication due to the ability to reorganize the intracellular membranes into new membranous structures for the HCV replication complex (Fig. **68**). The high-throughput-screening (HTS) identified most of NS4B ligands due to HCV replicon. In particular, the identification of mutations in the NS4B sequence, conferring drug viral resistance which confirmed NS4B protein as target for anti-HCV compounds.

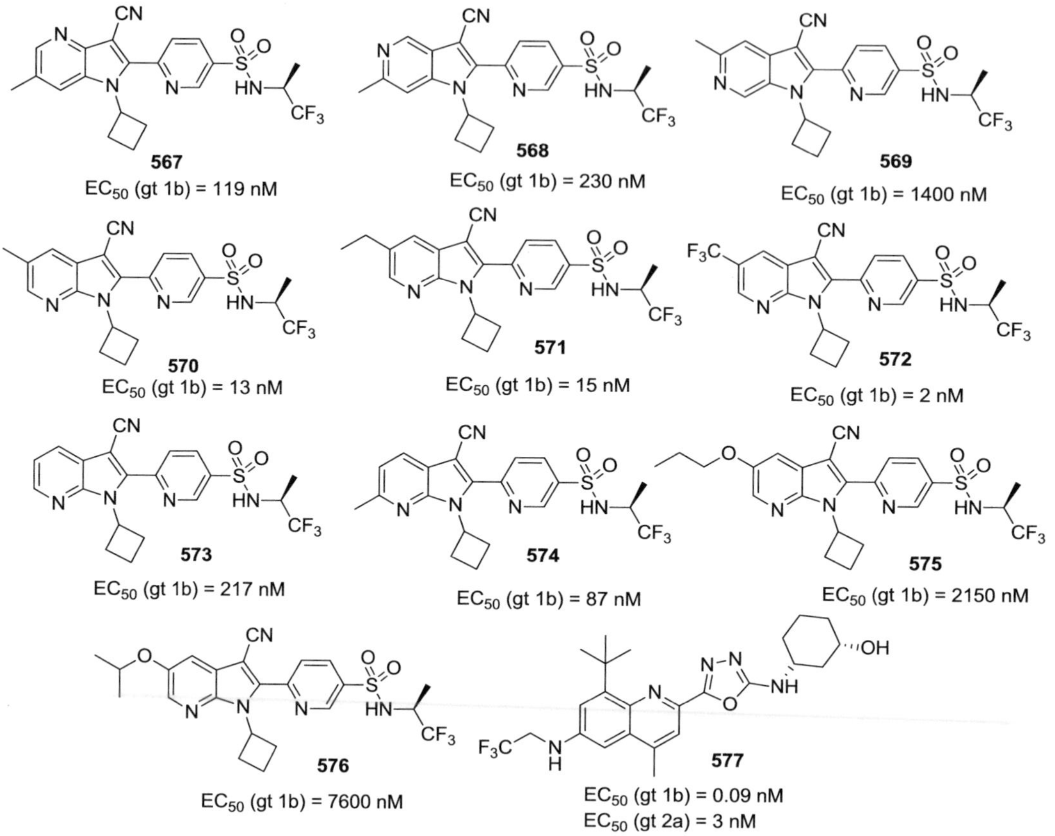

Fig. (68). Structures and activities of 6-(6-azaindol-2-yl)pyridine-3-sulfonamides **567-655** and pan-gt HCV inhibitor **577**.

4.14.1. Synthetic Products

Spirocyclic piperidine analogs were synthesized based on pyrazolo[1,5-a]pyridine core and evaluated for anti-HCV activity. Different piperidine ketals afforded dispiro compounds which showed excellent *in vitro* anti- genotype 1a and 1b replicons activities (EC_{50} 1.5 nM and 1.2 nM) respectively (Fig. **69**). Also, piperidine oxazolidinones afforded anti-genotype 1a and 1b replicons activities (EC_{50} 10.9 nM and 6.1 nM) respectively. These compounds bound directly to NS4B protein *in vitro* (IC_{50} 10.2 and 30.4 nM) respectively and exhibited reduced potency in replicons containing resistance mutations encoding changes in the NS4B protein (Fig. **70**) [221].

Many NS4B inhibitors were synthesized on hit identification, hit-to-lead optimization, ADME profile evaluation and the structure-activity relationship data (Fig. **71**) [222].

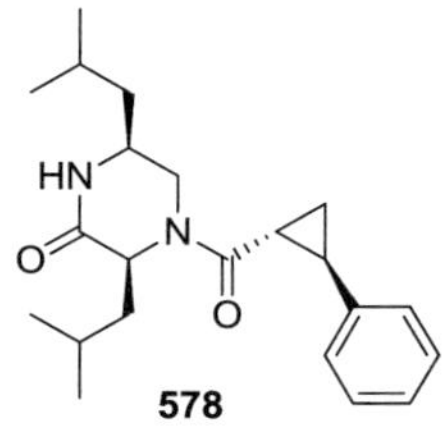

578

EC_{90} (gt 1a) = 1.0 μM
EC_{90} (gt 1b) = 0.8 μM
CC_{50} range = 40-76 μM

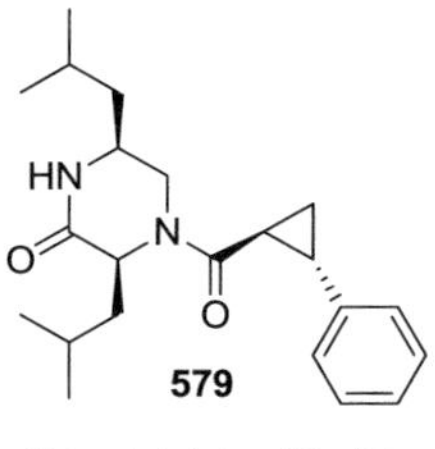

579

EC_{90} (gt 1a) > 10 μM
EC_{90} (gt 1b) > 10 μM

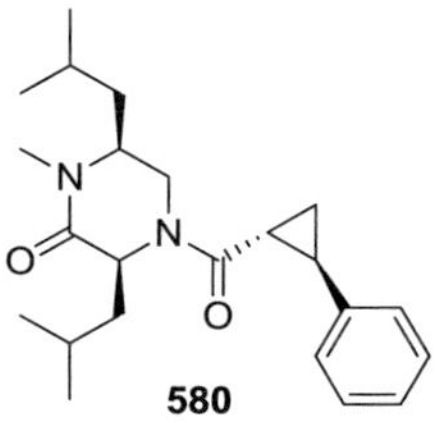

580

EC_{90} (gt 1b) = 8.8 μM

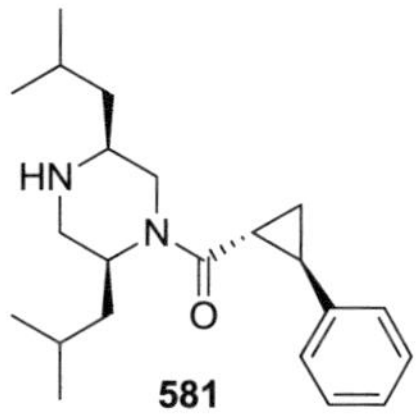

581

EC_{90} (gt 1b) > 10 μM

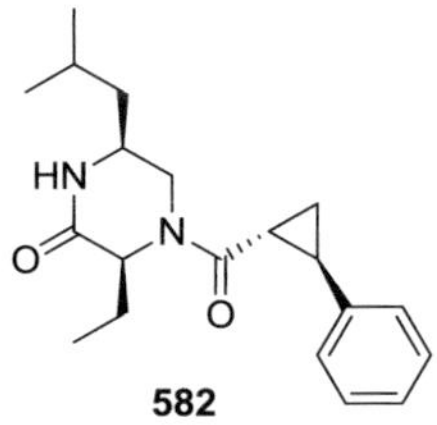

582

EC_{90} (gt 1b) > 10 μM

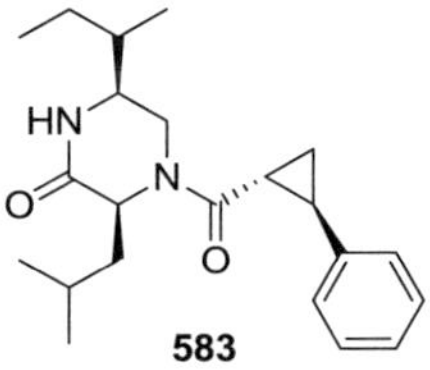

583

EC_{90} (gt 1b) > 10 μM

Fig. (69). Structures of piperazinone its isomers activities in cell lines (Huh7, HepG2, BxPC3 and CEM)..

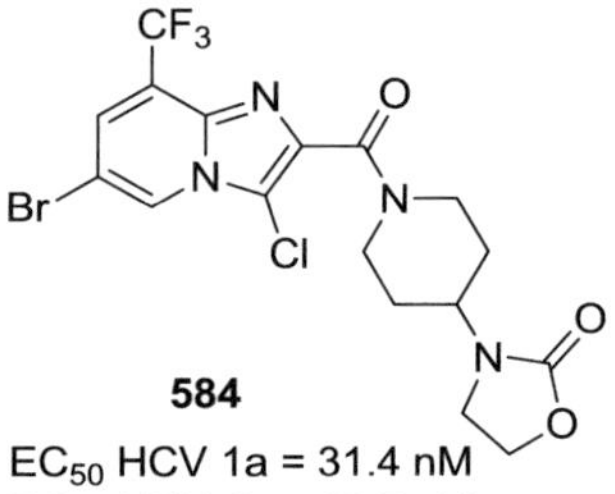

584

EC_{50} HCV 1a = 31.4 nM
EC_{50} HCV 1b = 45.5 nM

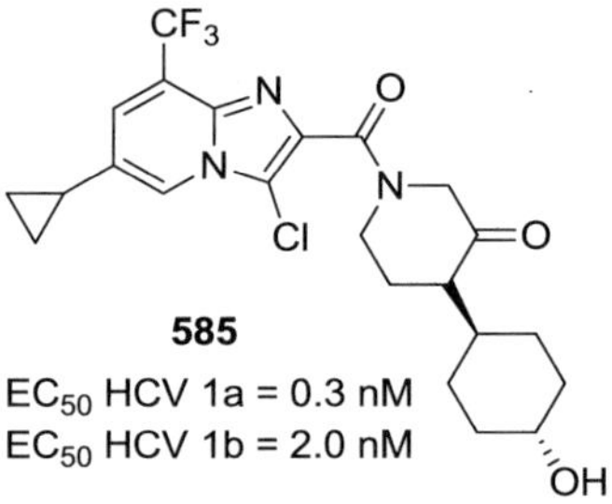

585

EC_{50} HCV 1a = 0.3 nM
EC_{50} HCV 1b = 2.0 nM

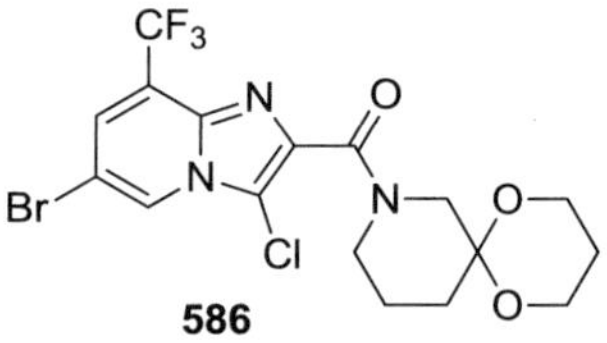

586

EC_{50} (gt 1a and1b) > 5000 nM

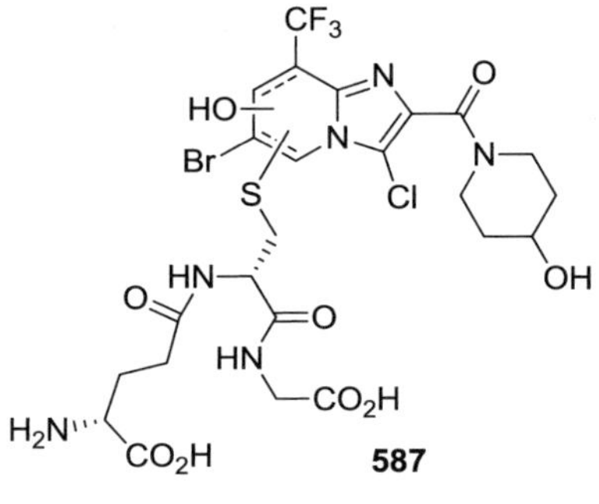

587

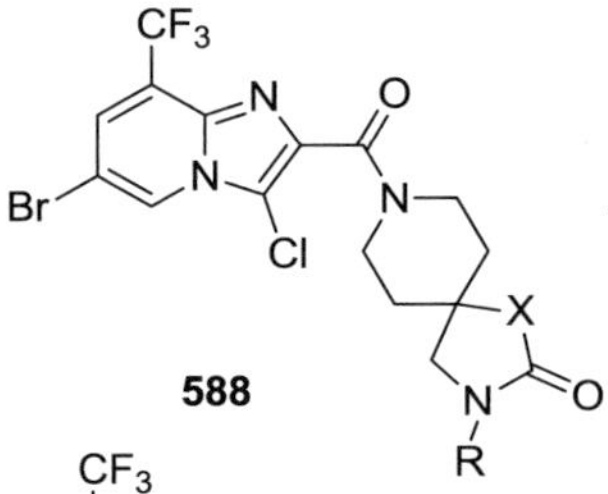

588

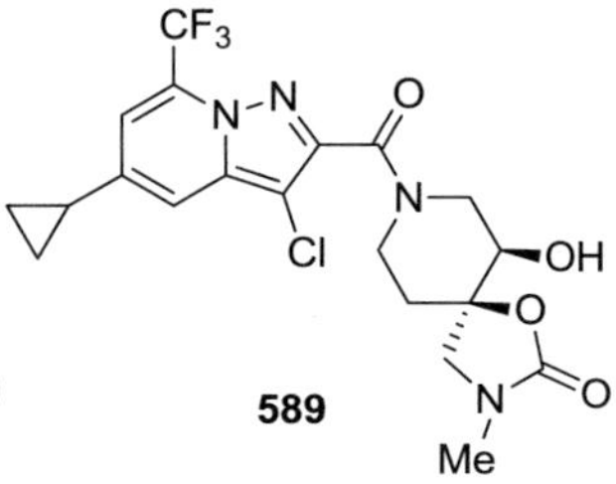

589

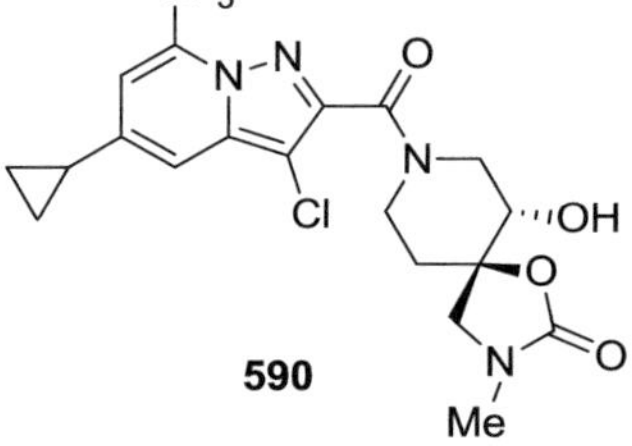

590

Fig. (70). Anti-HCV 1a and HCV 1b replicon of spiro analogs.

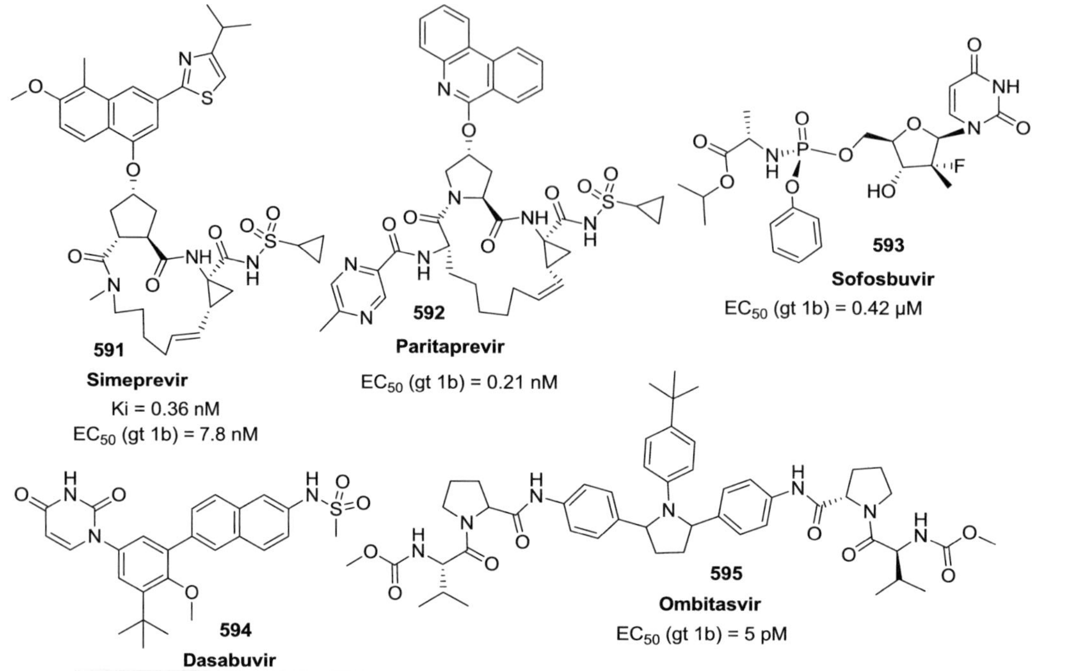

591 **Simeprevir** Ki = 0.36 nM EC_{50} (gt 1b) = 7.8 nM

592 **Paritaprevir** EC_{50} (gt 1b) = 0.21 nM

593 **Sofosbuvir** EC_{50} (gt 1b) = 0.42 μM

594 **Dasabuvir** IC50 = 10.7 nm EC_{50} (gt 1b) = 1.8 nM

595 **Ombitasvir** EC_{50} (gt 1b) = 5 pM

Fig. (71). Latest approved drugs for NS4B inhibitors.

These developments open the possibility for future combination therapies with other DAAs [223] even the less characterized NS4B protein is emerging as potentially attractive target for anti-viral drug discovery. Although, no anti-NS4B molecule found to be efficacious in clinical trials yet but there is increasing evidence from *in vitro* studies that small molecules could suppress HCV replication by altering one of the recently described functions of NS4B (Fig. **72**).

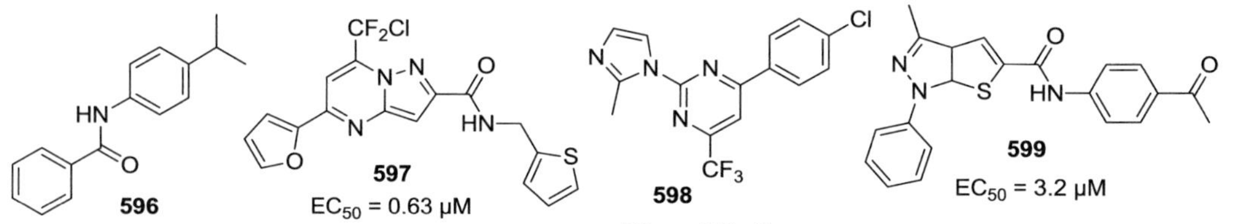

596 EC_{50} = 2.8 μM

597 EC_{50} = 0.63 μM

598 EC_{50} = 2.2 μM

599 EC_{50} = 3.2 μM

Fig. 72 contd.....

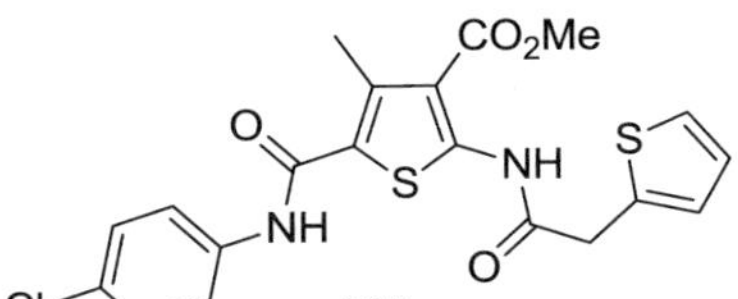

600

EC_{50} = 0.7 µM

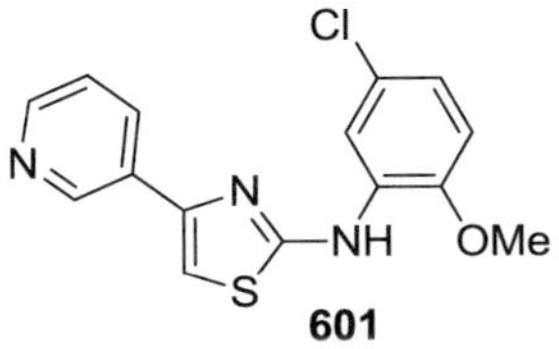

601

EC_{50} = 1.5 µM

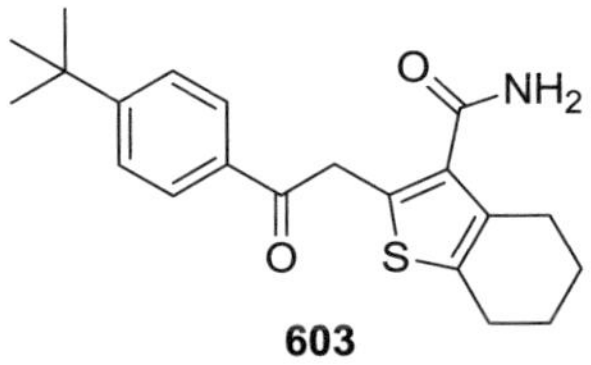

603

EC_{50} = 0.87 µM

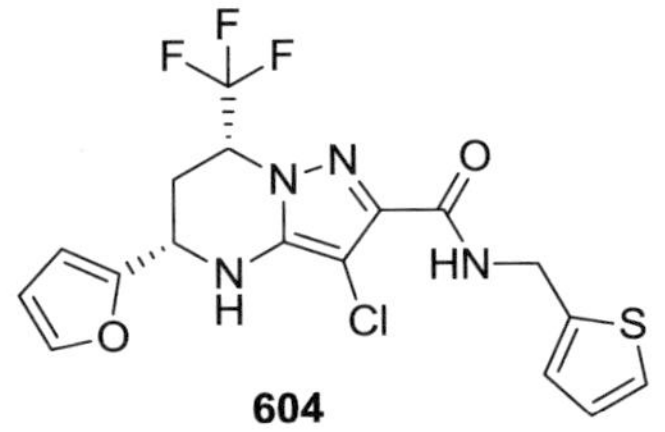

604

EC_{50} = 0.45 µM

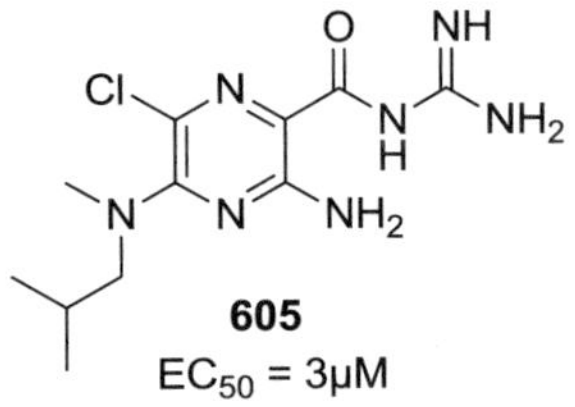

605

EC_{50} = 3µM

Fig. (72). Compounds identified as NS4B binding molecules.

4.15. Biological Functions of NS4B in HCV Replication

Electron microscopy helped in revealing that the cytoplasm alterations in hepatic tissues from HCV infected, caused by the presence of an intracellular membranous web during HCV replication [224].

4.15.1. The Pyrazolopyrimidines and other ViroPharma Inc. Compounds

Both pyrazolopyrimidine and pyrazolopyrimidines were discovered by Apath LLC as anti-HCV NS4B inhibitors. The company claimed analogs of the tetrahydropyrazolo[1,5-a]pyrimidine scaffold resulting from a partial saturation of ViroPharma's pyrazolopyrimidine core. Compound (AP 80978) is the most potent with 1b replicon (EC_{50} 0.45µM and EC_{50} <2µM against the genotype 1a) replicon. Resistance selection experiments identified a change at position 98 (F98L/V) and **238** (S238Y) that were associated with a loss in the sensitivity of compound (Fig. **73**).

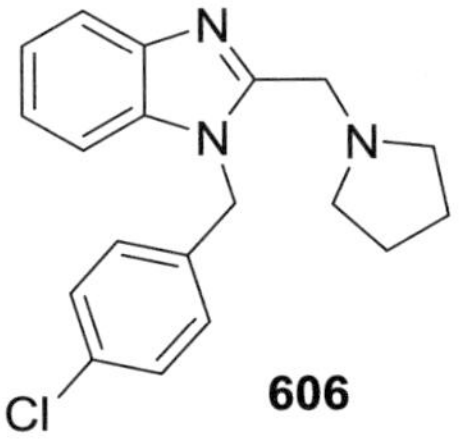

606

EC_{50} > 20 µM

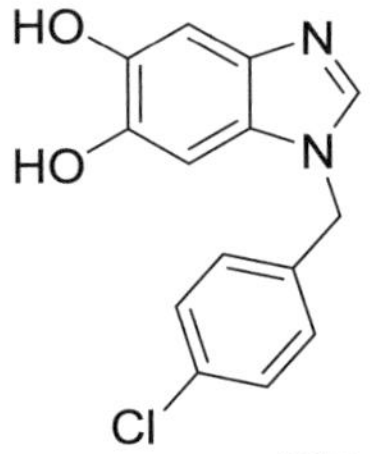

607

EC_{50} < 5 µM

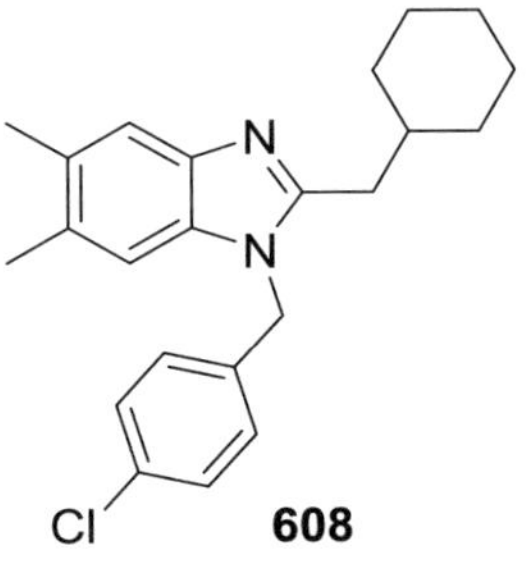

608

EC_{50} = 8 µM

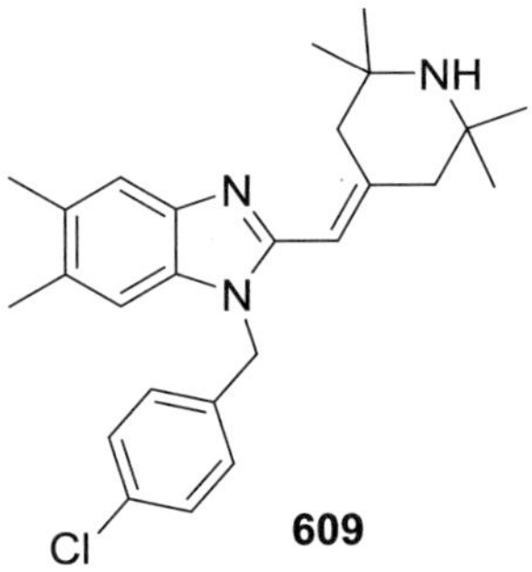

609

EC_{50} = 2.7 µM

Fig. 73 contd.....

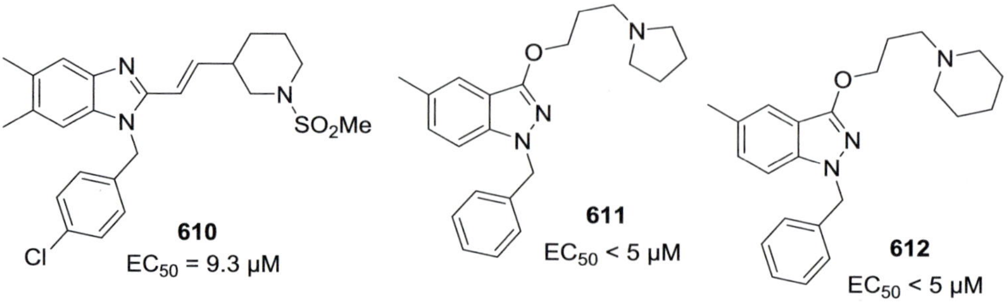

610
EC_{50} = 9.3 μM

611
EC_{50} < 5 μM

612
EC_{50} < 5 μM

Fig. (73). Compounds identified as NS4B RNA binding inhibitors.

4.15.2. The Discovery of Clemizole Hydrochloride

RNA binding with clemizole hydrochloride afforded anti-activity (IC_{50} 24 nM) that translated to an EC_{50} 8μM against the infectious virus of genotype 2a (JFH1). Also, clemizole-related molecules with improved *in vitro* potency have recently emerged. Based on indazole core substitution, the benzimidazole of the clemizole family afforded compounds of novel, potent and orally bioavailable inhibitor of hepatitis C RNA replication targeting NS4B. Compound **615** (PTC725) has also been identified through chemical optimization of the 6-(indol-2-yl)pyridi-e-3-sulfonamide to improve DMPK and safety properties. Compound **615** has excellent potency against the HCV 1b replicon (EC_{50} 2 nM) with respect to cellular GAPDH (Fig. **74**) [225].

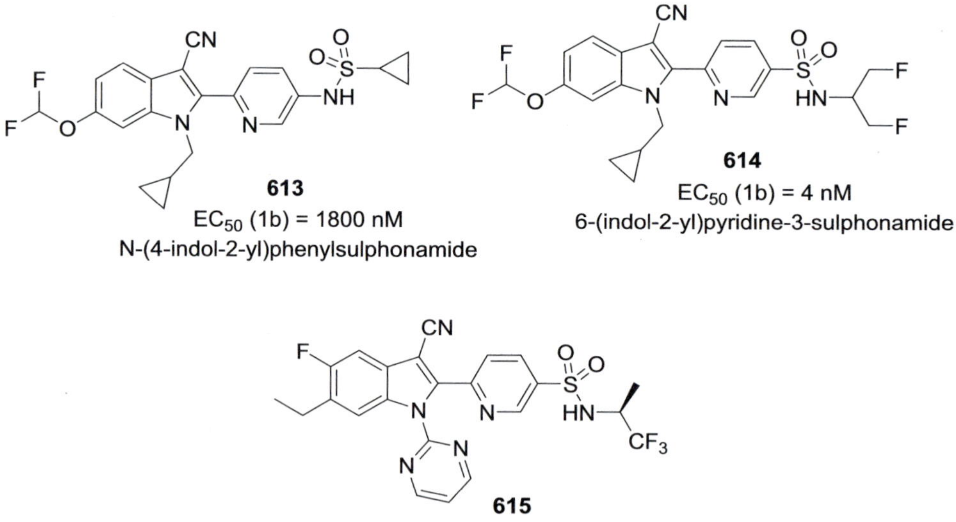

613
EC_{50} (1b) = 1800 nM
N-(4-indol-2-yl)phenylsulphonamide

614
EC_{50} (1b) = 4 nM
6-(indol-2-yl)pyridine-3-sulphonamide

615
(PTC725)
EC_{50} (1b) = 2 nM
6-(indol-2-yl)pyridine-3-sulphonamide

Fig. (74). HCV inhibitors and their activity against the HVC 1b replicon.

4.16. NS5B Inhibitors

Unlike the NS3-4A protease, the N5B RNA-dependent RNA polymerase (RdRp) is an excellent target in drug discovery. Therefore, several compounds have been reported as the NS5B polymerase inhibitors [226]. They are classified into the following categories on the basis of core structure: (i) Nucleosides/Nucleotides [227]. (ii) sulfonamides [228] (iii) fatty acids [229] (iv) aromatic acids [230]. (v) phenols [231]. (vi) quinolinones [232]. (vii) others [233]. The synthesis and the future direction of the NS5B polymerase inhibitors are given below (Fig. **75**):

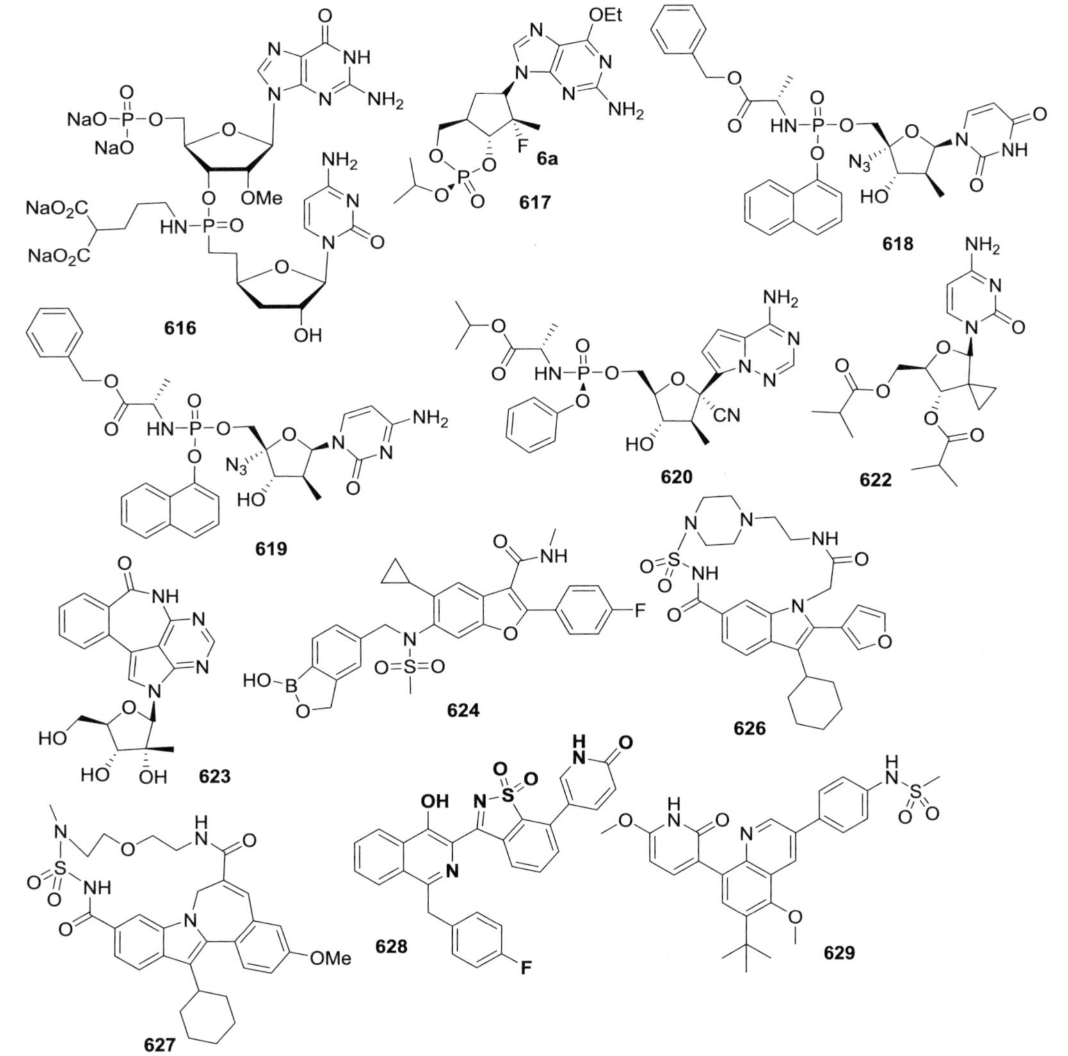

Fig. 75 contd.....

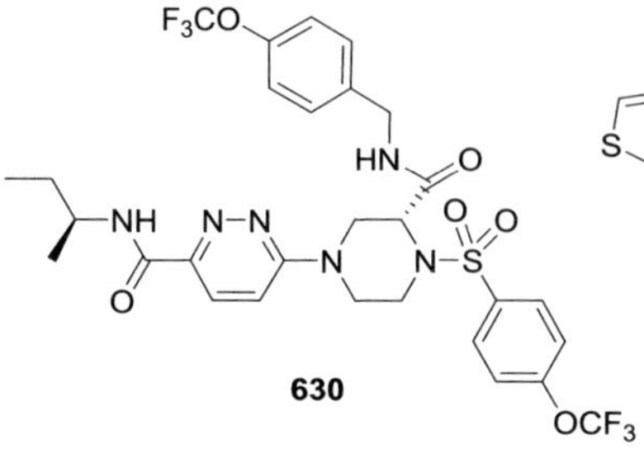

630

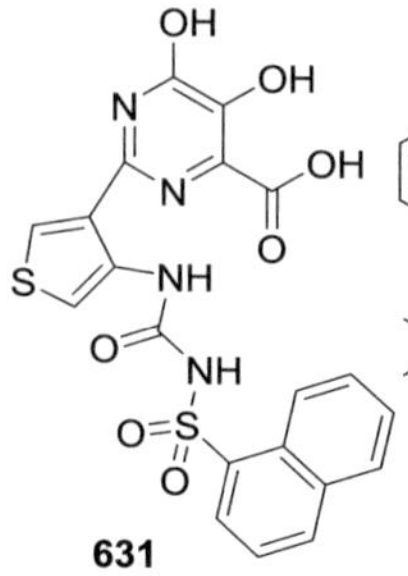

631

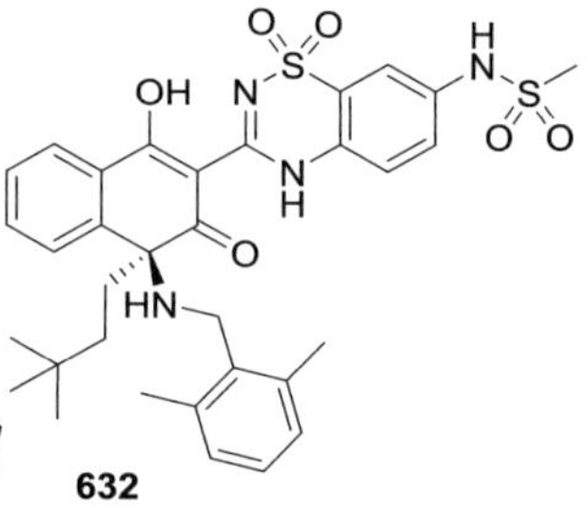

632

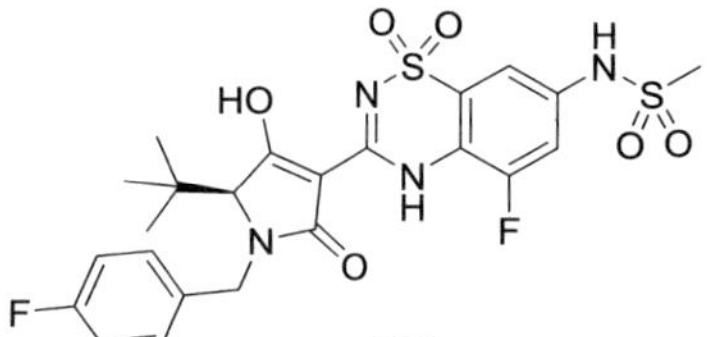

633

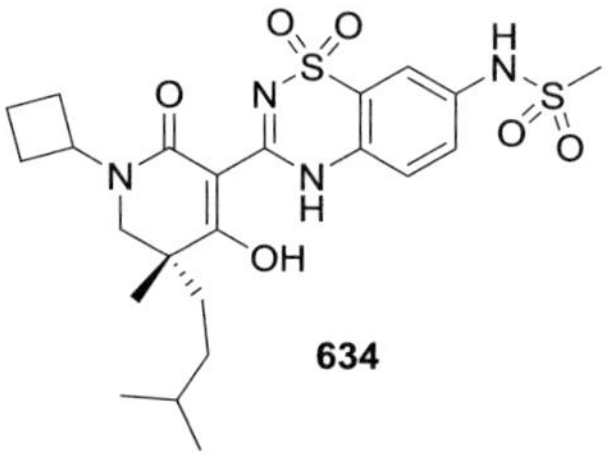

634

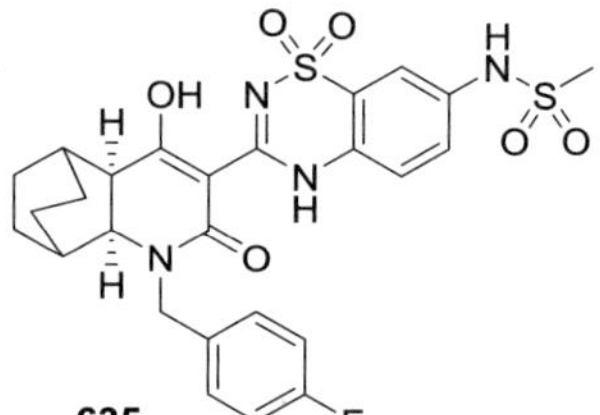

635

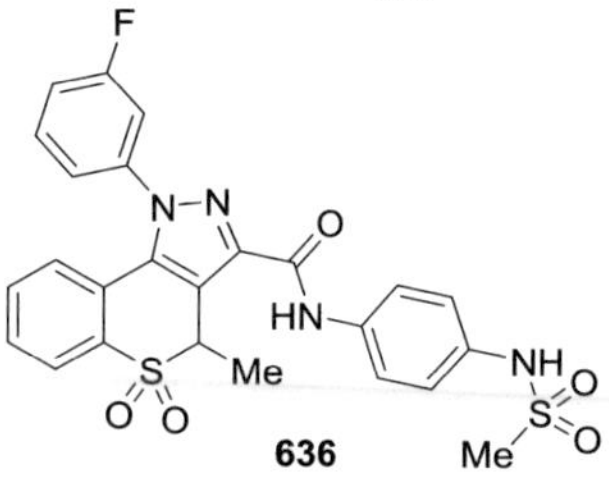

636

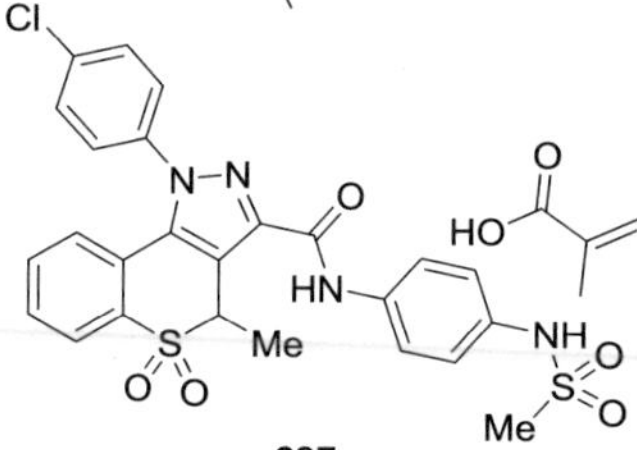

637

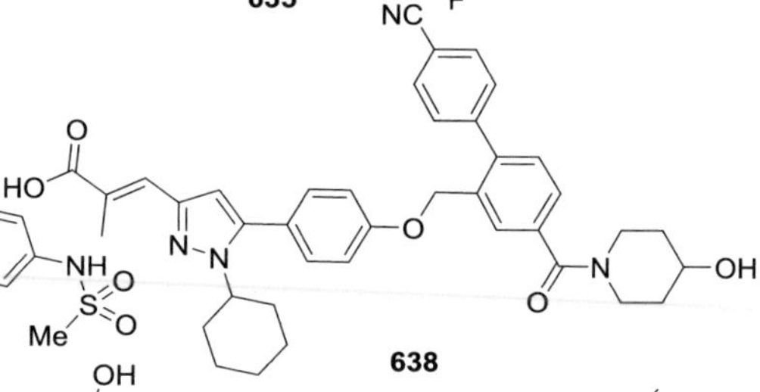

638

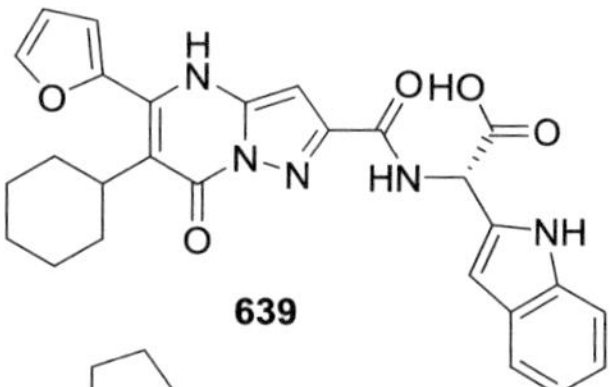

639

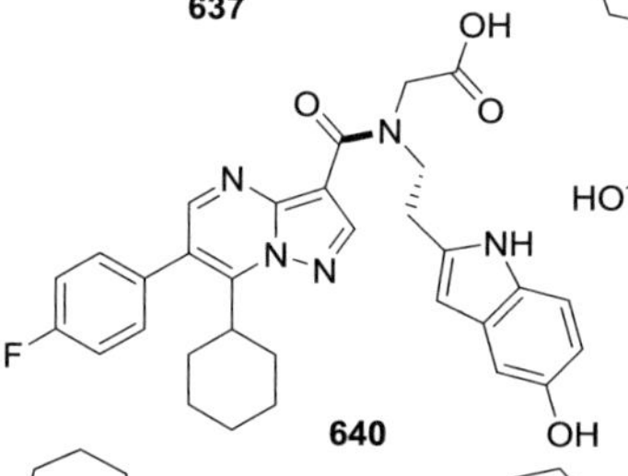

640

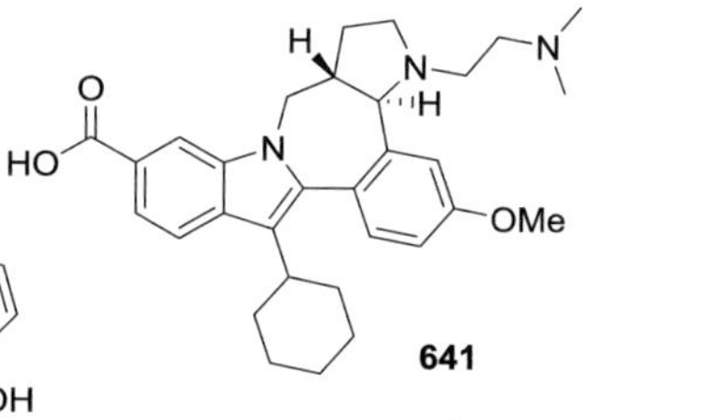

641

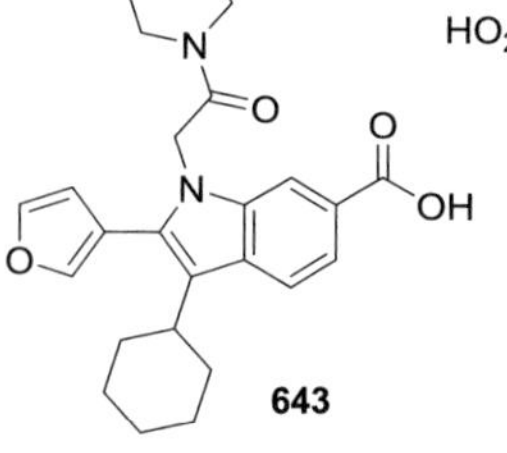

643

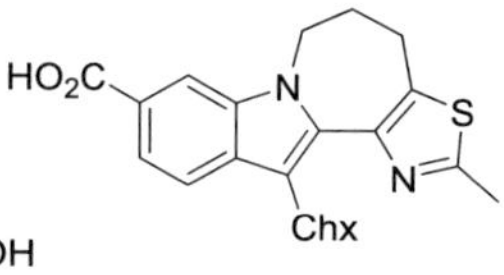

644

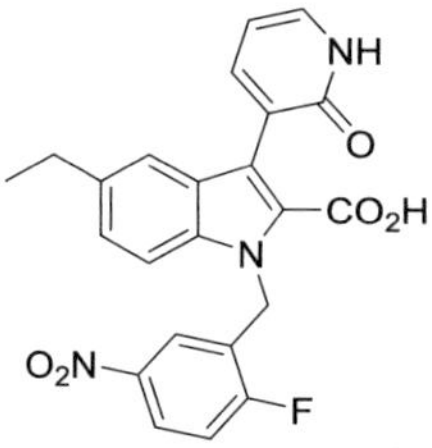

645

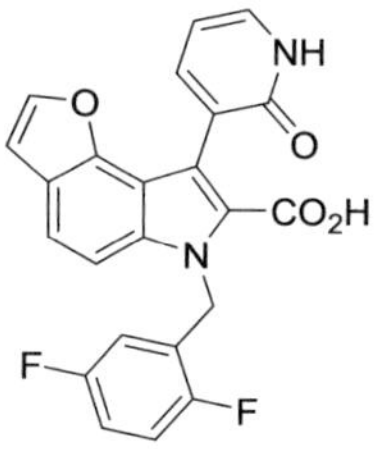

646

Fig. 75 contd.....

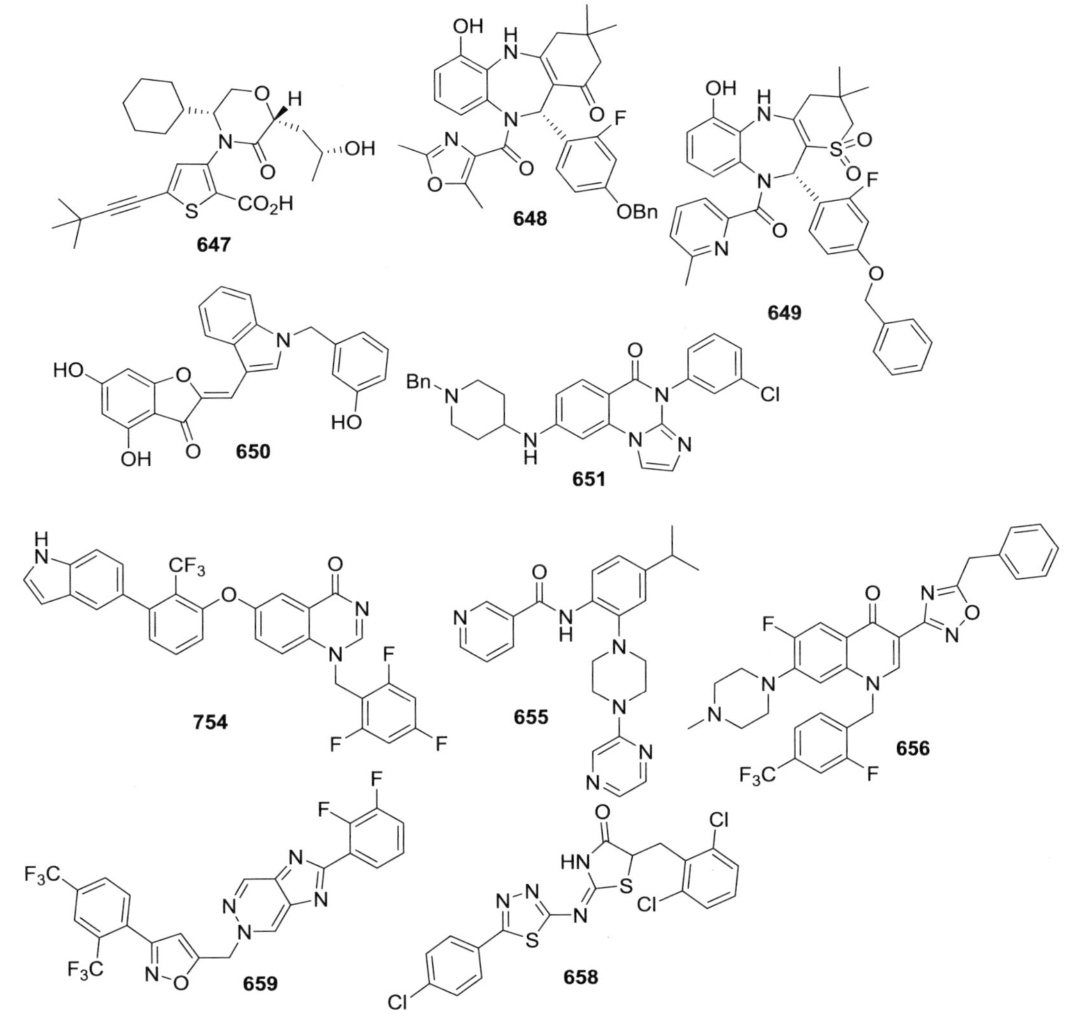

Fig. (75). Some anti- NS5B inhibitors.

Two major groups of NS5B inhibitors are: the nucleoside and nucleotide inhibitors (NIs) that bind to the polymerase active site and the non-nucleoside inhibitors (NNI) that bind in one of four allosteric binding sites (NNI sites 1–4) on the polymerase. The substrate analogues that led to the identification of several nucleoside and non-nucleoside inhibitors (NNIs) are high throughput screening. Nucleoside analogues need to be converted to the corresponding nucleotides by the host-cell machinery which in turn inhibit synthesis of viral RNA as chain terminators (*i.e.*, substrate analogues that are incorporated by the viral polymerase in the nascent RNA molecule and induce premature termination of the RNA synthesis). Conversely, NNIs are almost invariably allosteric inhibitors to block the enzyme preventing a conformational transition which is needed for initiation of RNA synthesis [234]. Interestingly, different binding sites for NNIs exist on the HCV polymerase. Further, several classes of nucleoside analogues and NNIs elicit diverse patterns of resistance. Although, these agents target the same viral enzyme which offer to be developed for combination therapy.

Replication of HCV genome is catalyzed by NS5B, an RNA-RdRp which forms an active replicase after complexed with other viral and cellular proteins. NS5B is highly conserved across HCV genotypes and adopts a right-handed 3D-structure with fingers, palm and thumb domains analogous to those of the RdRps of other RNA viruses (Fig. **76**) [235]. Due to high degree of conservation in the NS5B active site, NIs of NS5B exhibit broad spectrum activity against the HCV genotypes with high barriers to resistance due to the fitness costs associated with the mutations that confer resistance [236].

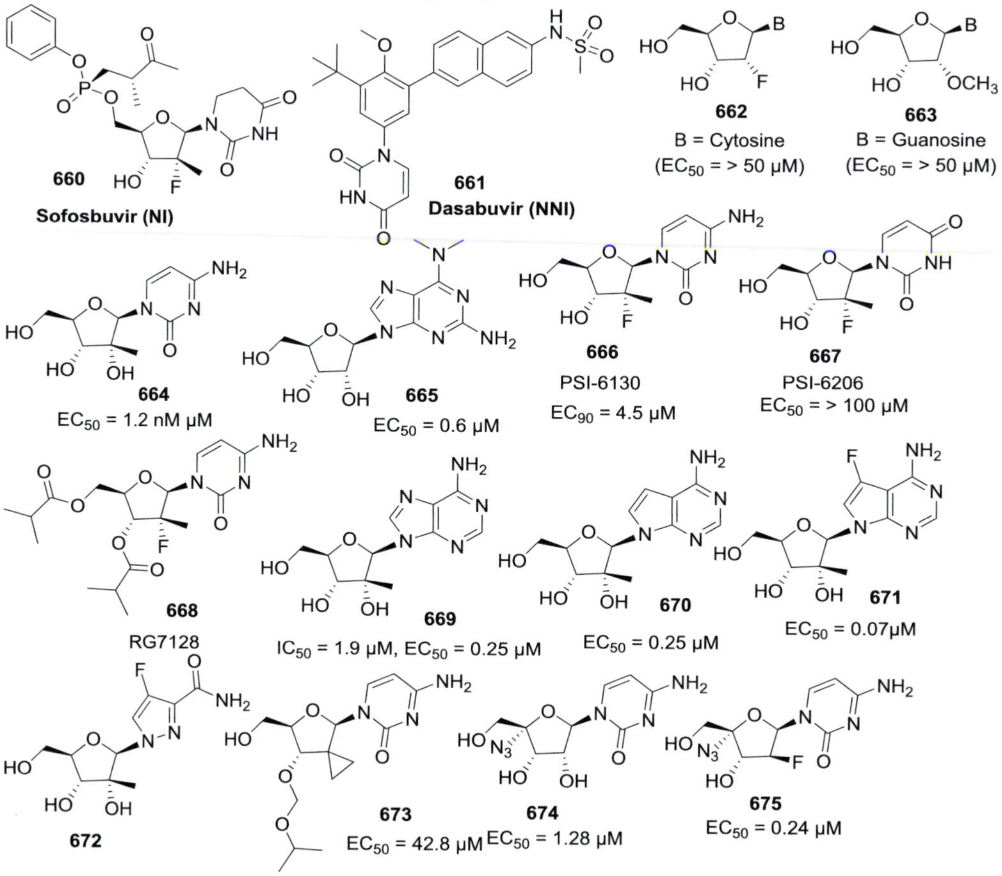

Fig. 76 contd.....

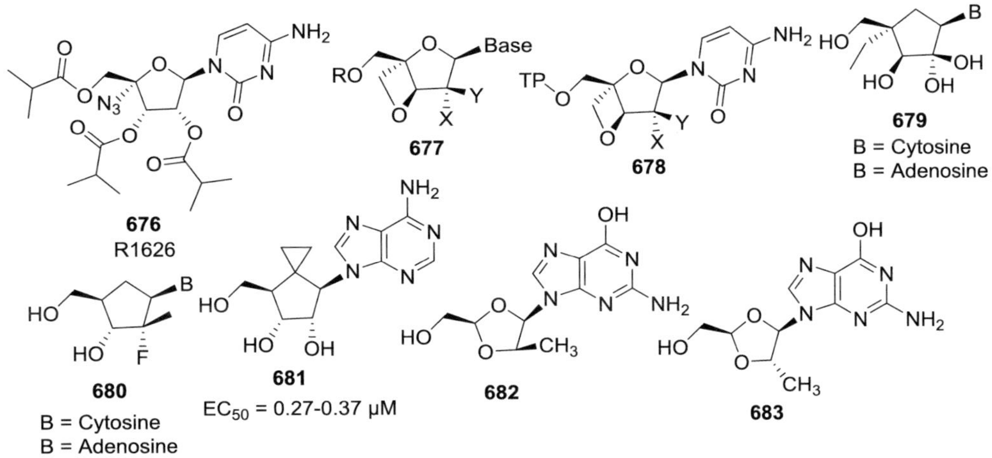

676 R1626; **677**; **678**; **679** B = Cytosine, B = Adenosine; **680** B = Cytosine, B = Adenosine; **681** EC_{50} = 0.27-0.37 μM; **682**; **683**

Fig. (76). Different class of selected compounds NS5B polymerase inhibitors [237].

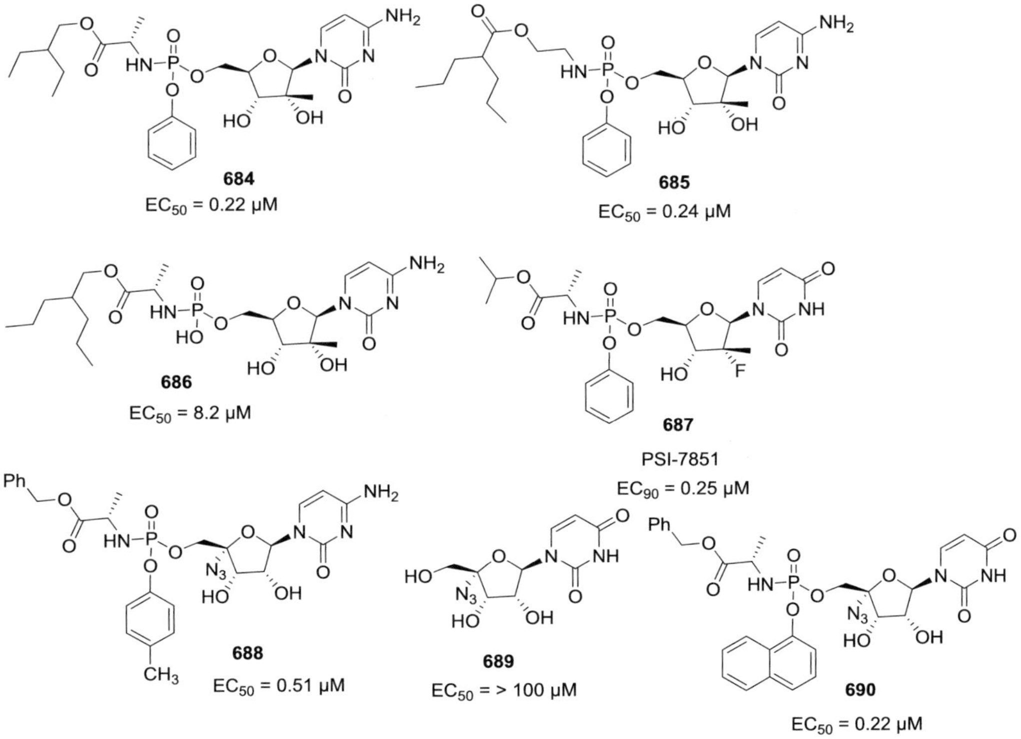

684 EC_{50} = 0.22 μM

685 EC_{50} = 0.24 μM

686 EC_{50} = 8.2 μM

687 PSI-7851 EC_{90} = 0.25 μM

688 EC_{50} = 0.51 μM

689 EC_{50} = > 100 μM

690 EC_{50} = 0.22 μM

Fig. 77 contd.....

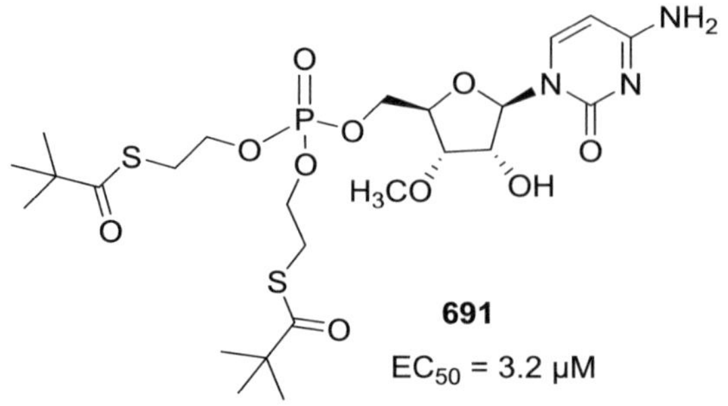

691

EC_{50} = 3.2 μM

Fig. (77). Nucleosides based prodrugs as inhibitors of NS5B.

4.17. Nucleotide Prodrug Inhibitors

Nucleosides have to convert intracellularly to their 5′-triphosphate derivatives to be active inhibitors of viral polymerases but many nucleosides failed in whole cell assays because of poor substrates for one or more of the kinases in the phosphorylation cascade (Fig. **77**).

Thus, it was hypothesized that a 5′-monophosphate pro-drug could increased potency by accomplishing kinase bypass, improve cell penetration and block deamination. The phosphoramidate pro-drug **693** of 2′-C-methyladenosine showed no improved activity (EC_{50} 0.25 μM) than the parent nucleoside. Similarly, 2′-α-F-2′-β-C-methyl-7-ethynyl-7-deazaadenosine **694** (Fig. **16**) reported for low replicon activity (EC_{50} 24 μM) and many other phosphoramidate pro-drugs **695** were prepared but gave no anti-viral activity (Fig. **78**).

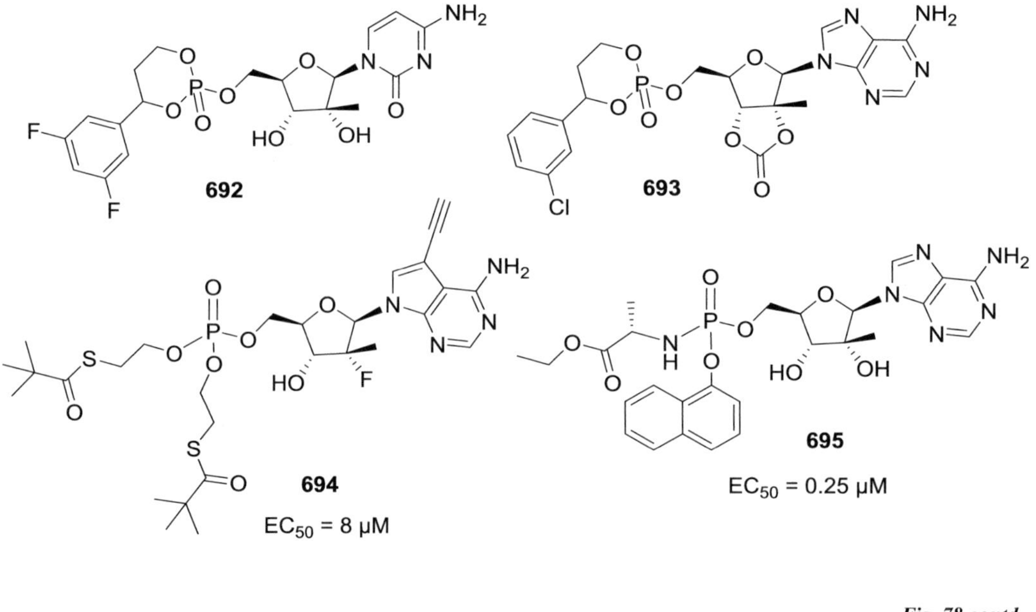

692 **693**

694 EC_{50} = 8 μM

695 EC_{50} = 0.25 μM

Fig. 78 contd.....

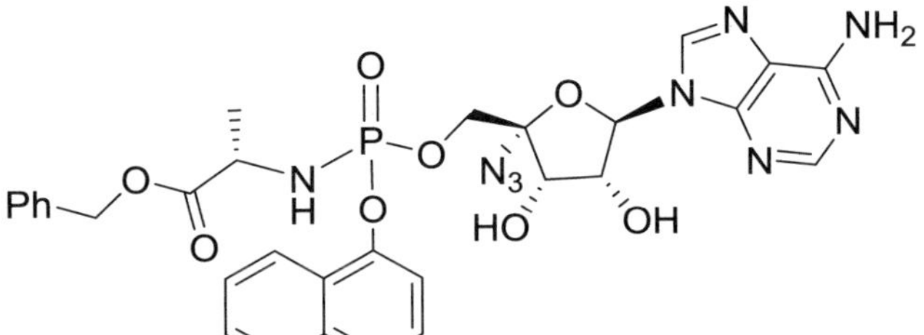

696

EC_{50} = 0.22 μM

Fig. (78). Phosphoramidate prodrug as inhibitors of NS5B.

The bis-SATE pro-drug strategy is used to deliver 2′-α-F-2′-β-C-m-thyl-7-ethynyl-7-deazaadenosine and 3′,5′-cyclic-SATE ester pro-drug of 2′---methyladenosine entailed the application to a 4′-substituted carbocyclic nucleoside **703** which employed a phosphonate that ultimately produce a stable form of the nucleoside 5′-monophosphate (Fig. **18**). The resulting 2′---methyladenosine 3′,5′-cyclic phosphonate SATE pro-drug **704** was only moderately active (EC_{50} 27.6 μM) in the HCV replicon assay, a <3-fold more potent than the phosphonate product intended to deliver and >14-fold less active than 2′-C-methyadenosine (Fig. **79**).

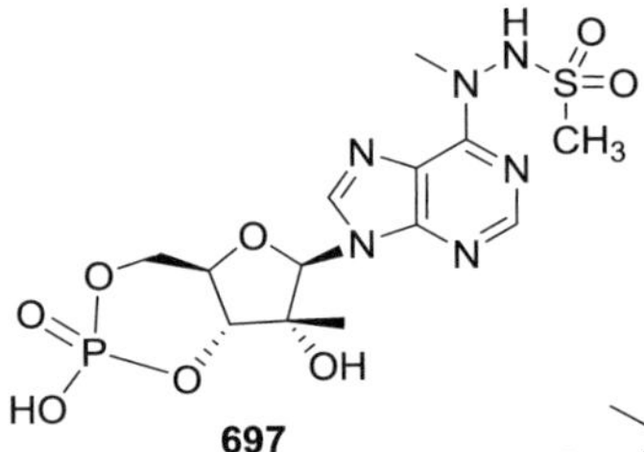

697

EC_{50} = 68.5 μM

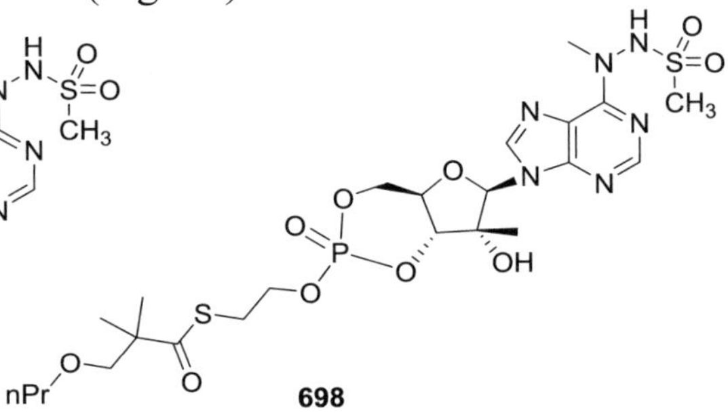

698

EC_{50} = 0.039 μM

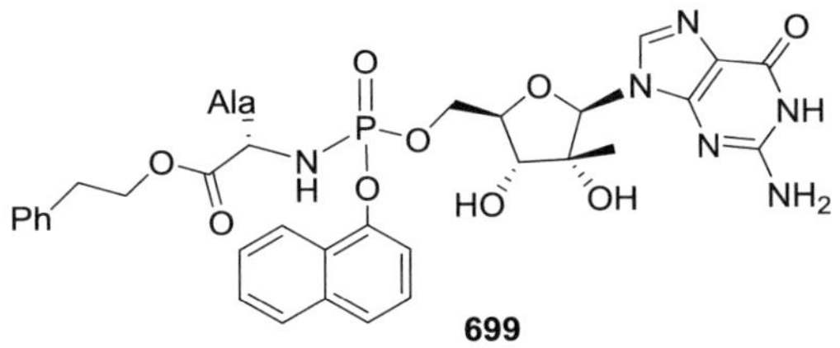

699

EC_{50}= 0.08 μM

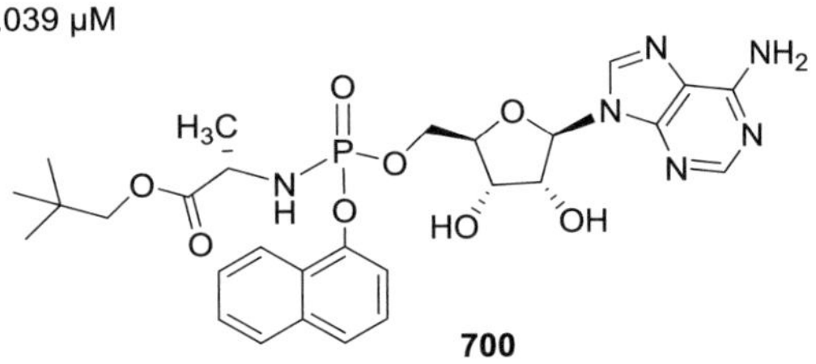

700

INX-08189

EC_{50} = 0.010 μM

Fig. 79 contd.....

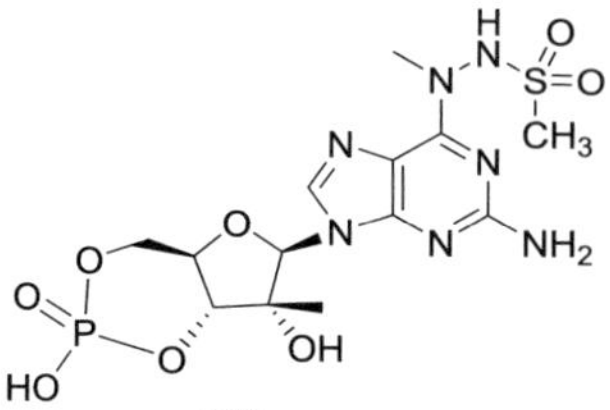

702
EC_{50} = 1.7 μM

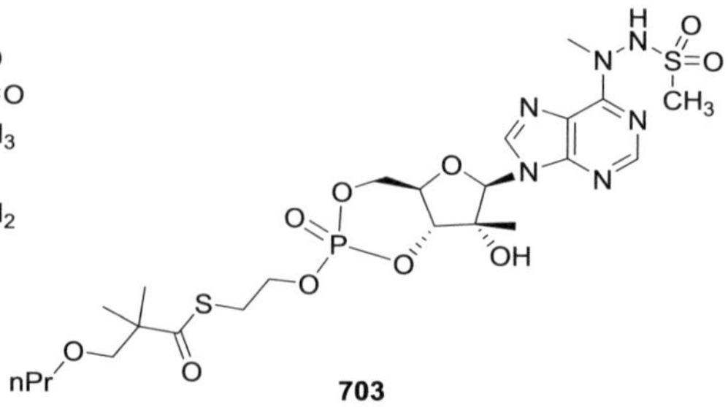

703
EC_{50} = 0.008 μM

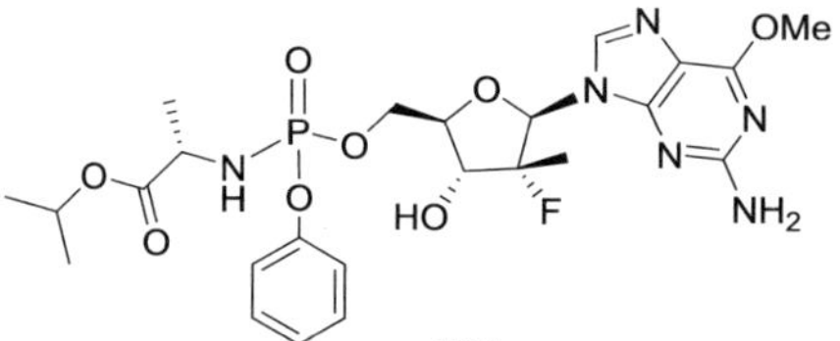

704
EC_{50} = 0.020 μM

Fig. (79). Phosphate prodrug as anti-NS5B inhibitors.

Nucleosides and nucleotides are also known to inhibit HCV during the elongation phase of viral RNA synthesis *via* a non-obligate chain termination mechanism. It was found that dinucleotides have the potential to inhibit RNA replication at the initiation phase as primer molecules are used as inhibitors of HCV replication (Fig. **80**).

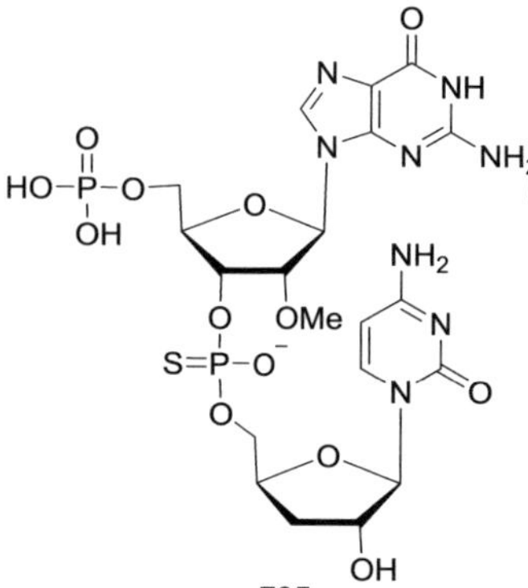

705
IC_{50} = 20 μM

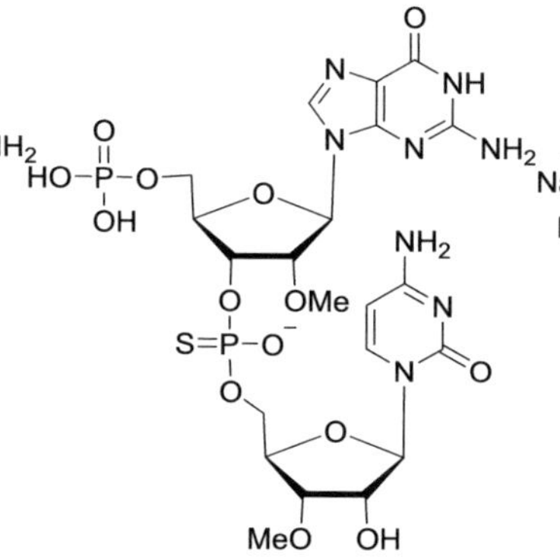

706
IC_{50} = 65 μM

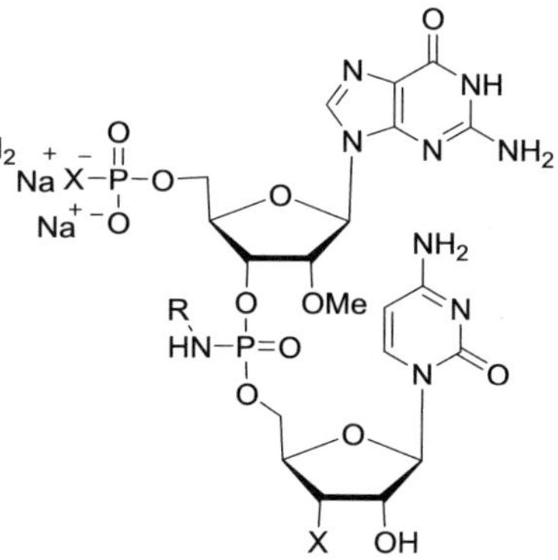

707
X = S, R = $-(CH_2)_5CO_2^-Na^+$, Y = OH,
Sp isomer EC_{50} = 9 μM

Fig. (80). Dinucleotide inhibitors of NS5B enzyme.

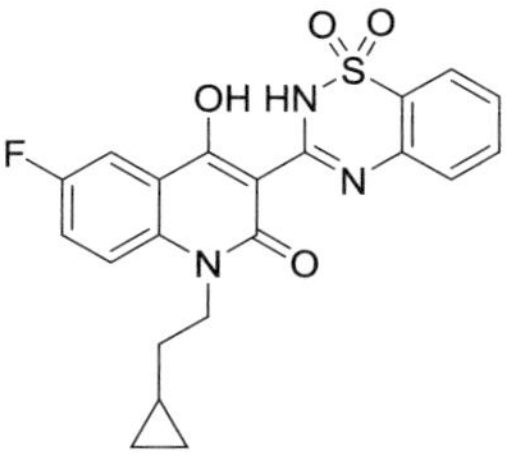

708
SB711845
IC_{50} = 0.010 μM, EC_{50} = 0.38 μM

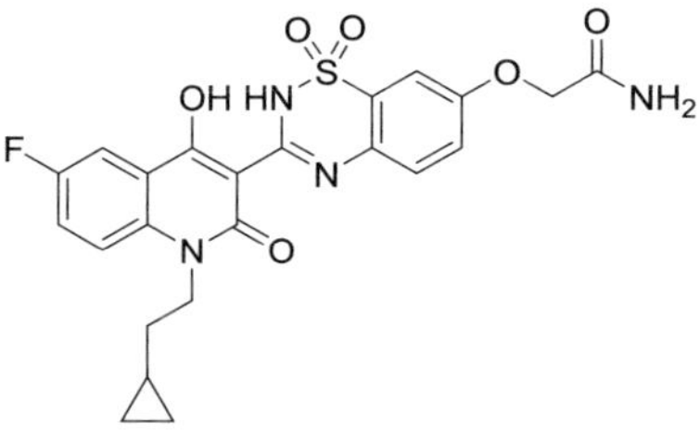

709
SB-750330
IC_{50} < 0.005 μM, C_{50} = 0.002 μM

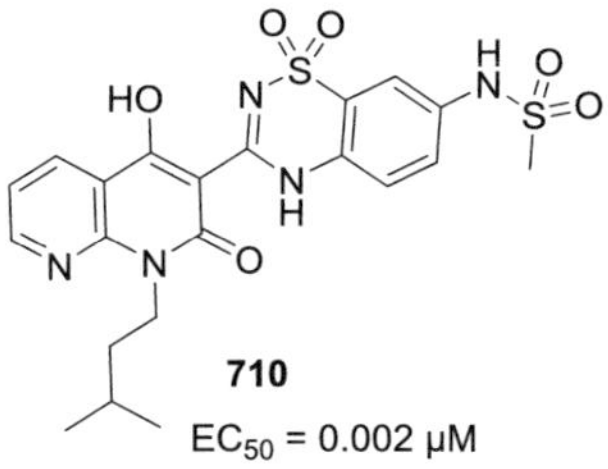

710
EC_{50} = 0.002 μM

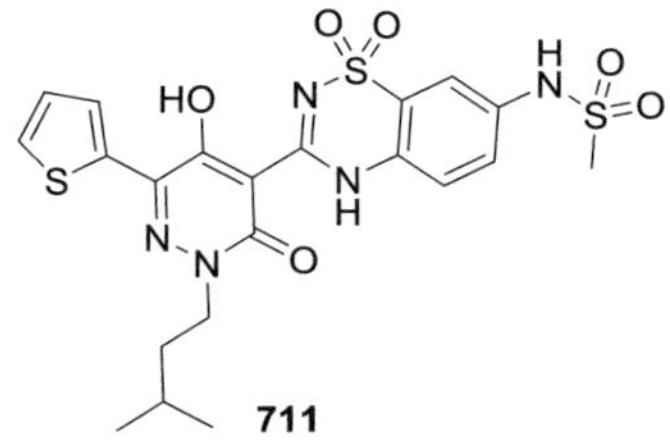

711
IC_{50} < 0.010 μM, C_{50} = 0.005 μM

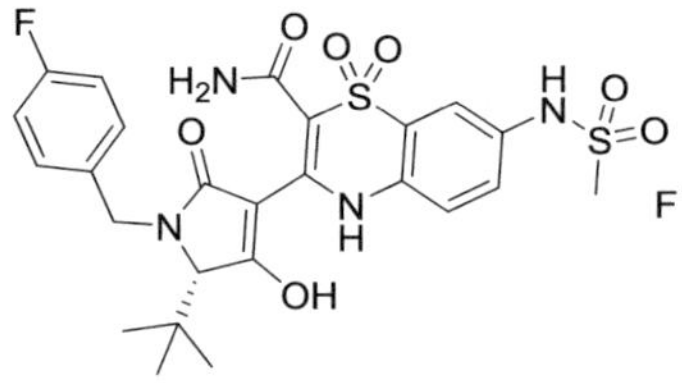

712
EC_{50} = 0.016μM

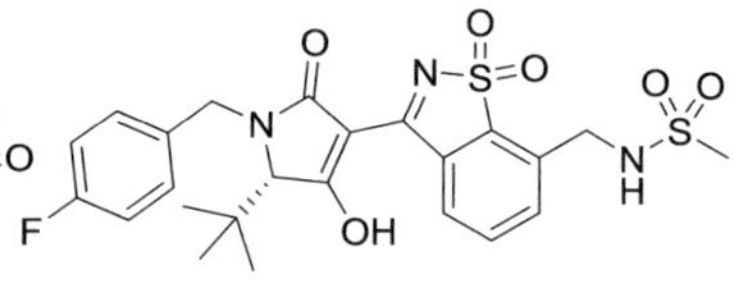

713
EC_{50} = 0.076μM

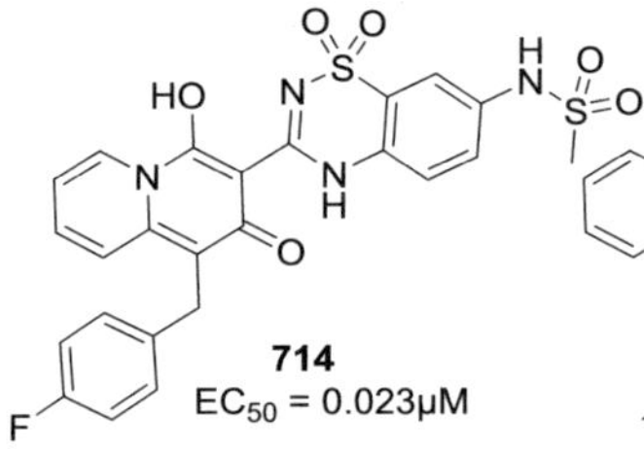

714
EC_{50} = 0.023μM

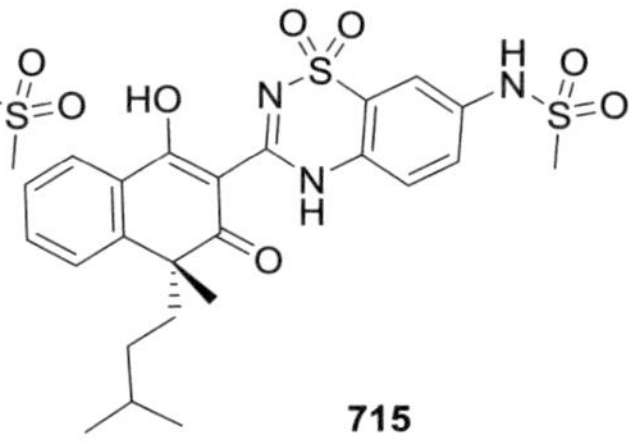

715
IC_{50} = 0.0009 μM, EC_{50} = 0.003μM

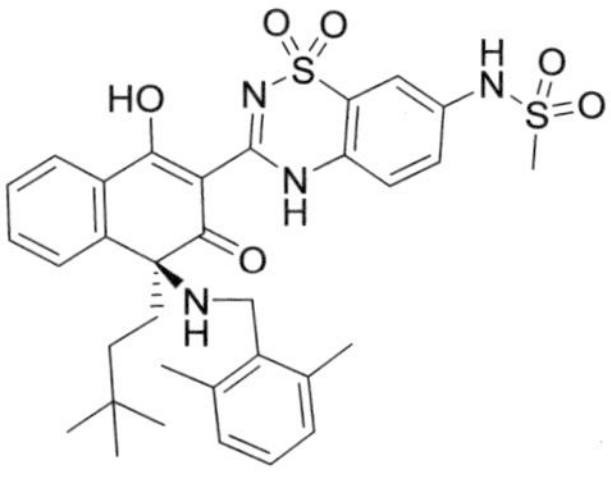

716
IC_{50} = 0.019 μM, EC_{50} = 0.006μM

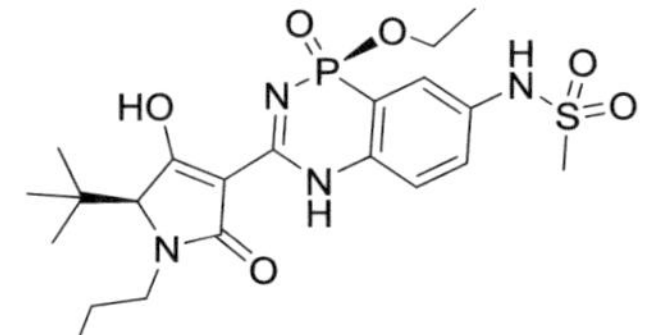

717
IC_{50} = 0.0005 μM, EC_{50} = 0.0018μM

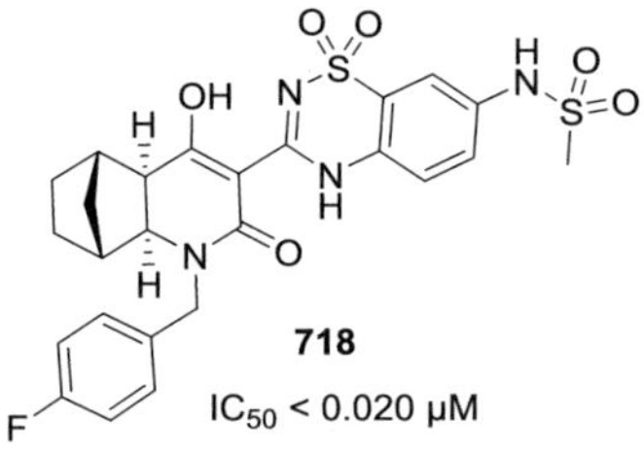

718
IC_{50} < 0.020 μM

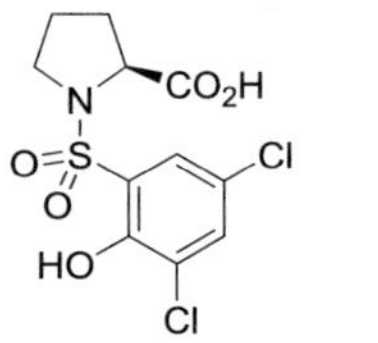

719
IC_{50} = 0.08 μM

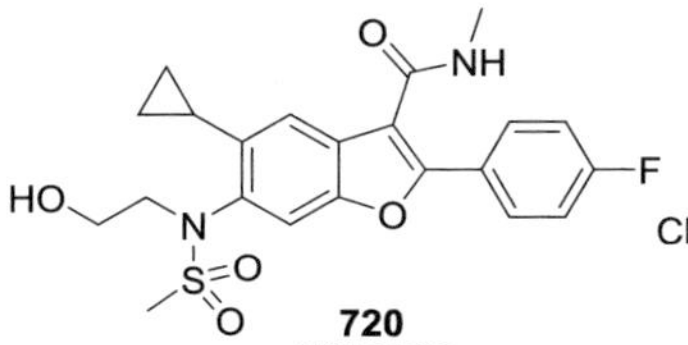

720
HCV-796
EC_{50} = 0.013 μM

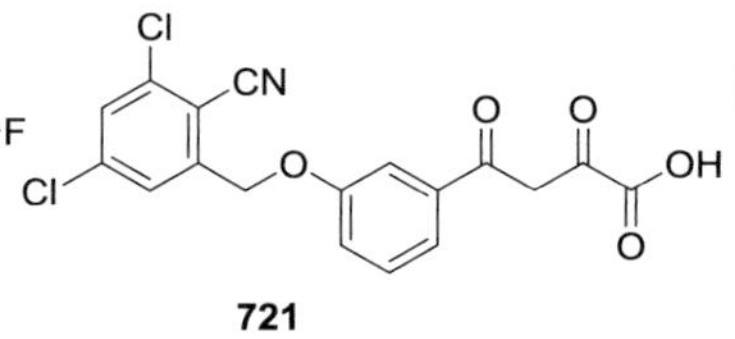

721
IC_{50} = 0.045 μM

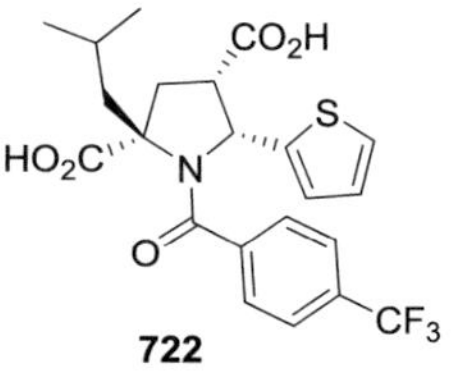

722
IC_{50} = 0.3 μM

Fig. 81 contd.....

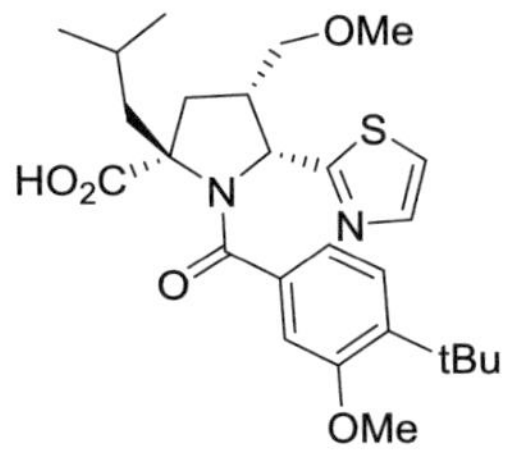

723

IC_{50} = 0.44 μM, EC_{50} = 0.39 μM

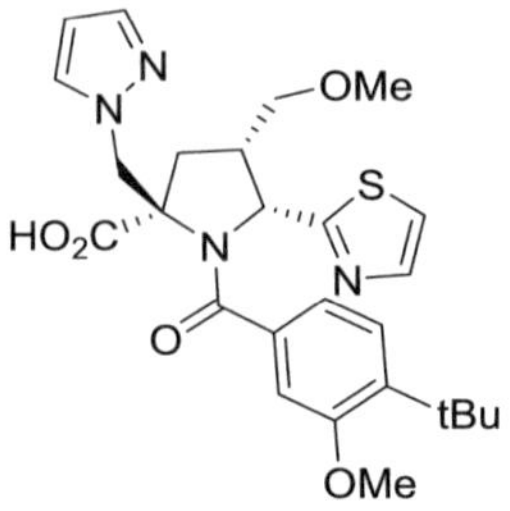

724

GSK625433

IC_{50} = 0.028 μM, EC_{50} = 0.003 μM

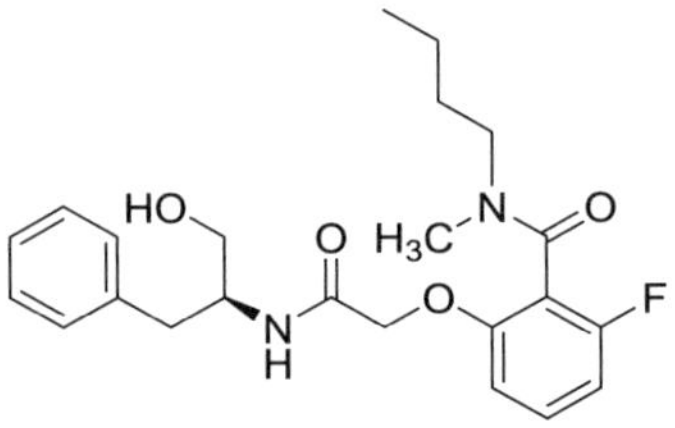

725

IC_{50} = 0.8 μM

Fig. (81). Molecules of NS5B palm site inhibitors.

4.18. Non-Nucleoside Inhibitors (Palm Domain Inhibitors)

The palm site allosteric binding pocket is located at the interface of the thumb and palm domains near the polymerase active site. The hairpin loop that links the palm region to thumb residues 363-369 is sometimes referred as the primer grip site because of its intrusion into the catalytic region of the palm and its similarity to interactions, observed in RNA-dependent DNA polymerases (Fig. **81**).

4.19. Thumb Domain Site I Inhibitors

The example of important thumb domain site I inhibitors are given in Fig. (**82**).

4.20. Thumb Domain Site II Inhibitors

Sofosbuvir is used as NS5B inhibitor, strongly effective against all HCV genotypes and has high genetic fitness barrier to develop resistance. Thus far, S282T is the only known variant in NS5B, associated with a reduced susceptibility to sofosbuvir. However, S282T has been identified in less than 1% of patients. ACH-3422, a novel uridine nucleotide analogue as NS5B inhibitor is used in HCV genotype 3 compared to sofosbuvir. IDX21437, another uridine nucleotide analogue as NS5B inhibitor is potent anti-viral activity against all HCV genotypes. It was safe and well tolerated which decreases HCV viral maximum load (HCV gentoypes 1, 2 and 3) in monotherapy. Further, development of ACH-3422 and IDX21437 may increased substantially future therapeutic repertoire in hepatitis C. PF-00868554 is a potent non-nucleoside inhibitor (NNI) that binds to the Thumb II allosteric pocket of NS5B polymerase but several PF-00868554 resistant mutants have been identified where M423 variants are the most common NS5B mutations, occurred after PF-00868554 monotherapy (Fig. **83**) [238]. Some other NNI NS5B inhibitors of the thumb site I include deleobuvir, BMS-791325, TMC-647055 (site 1) and GS-9669 (site 2) and the palm site binders GSK-5852 and RG-7109 [237].

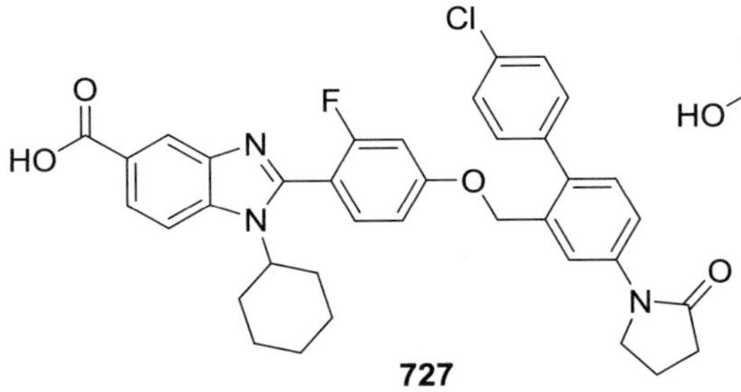

727
JTK-109
IC_{50} = 0.017 μM, EC_{50} = 0.32 μM

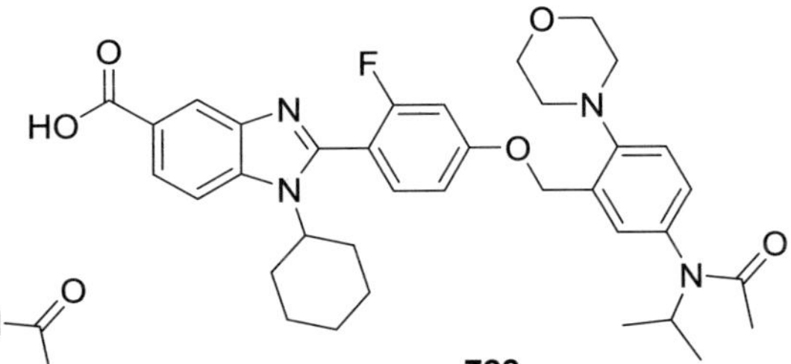

728
IC_{50} = 0.042 μM, EC_{50} = 0.27 μM

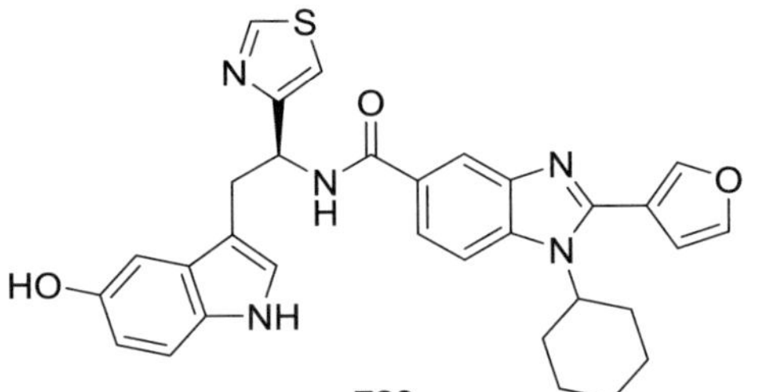

729

IC_{50} = 0.3 μM, EC_{50} = 1.7 μM

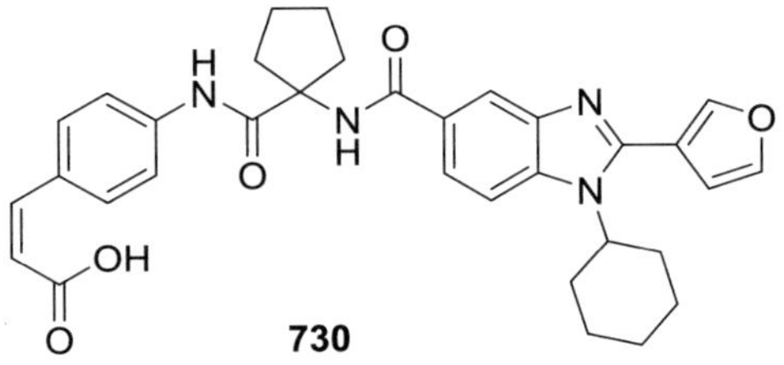

730
EC_{50} = 0.55 μM

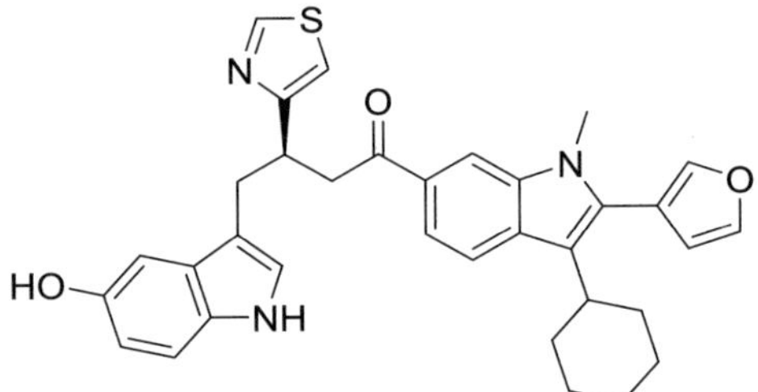

731
EC_{50} = 0,05 μM

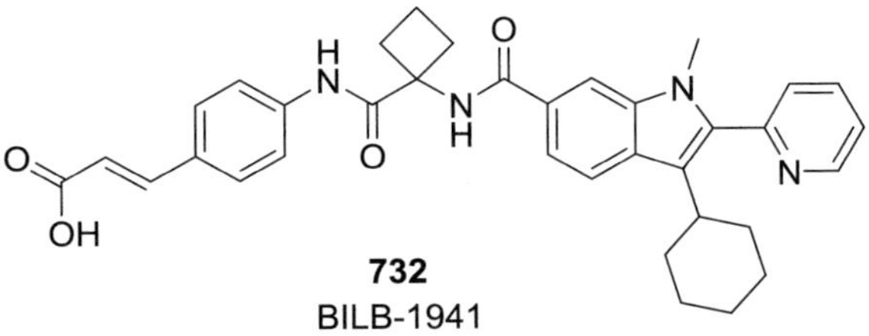

732
BILB-1941
(EC_{50} = 0.0845 μM)

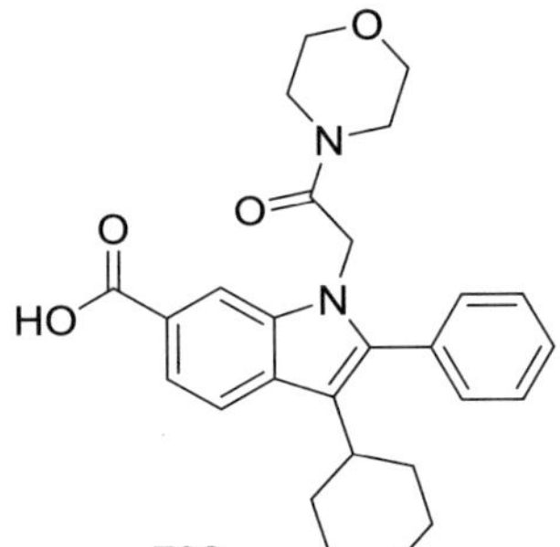

733
(EC_{50} = 0.08 μM)

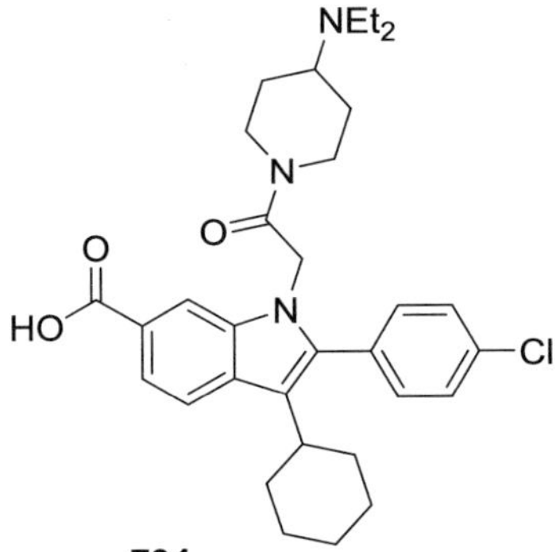

734
EC_{50} = 0.127 μM

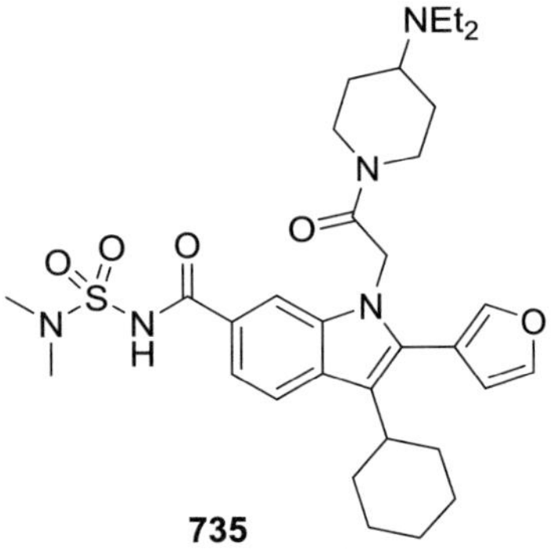

735
EC_{50} = 0.12 μM

Fig. 82 contd.....

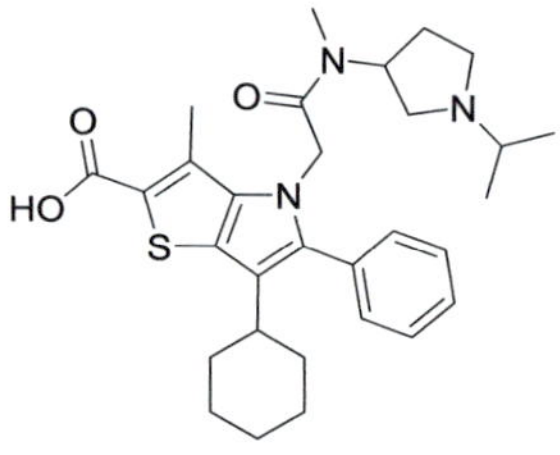

736

IC_{50} = 0.010 μM, EC_{50} = 0.13μM

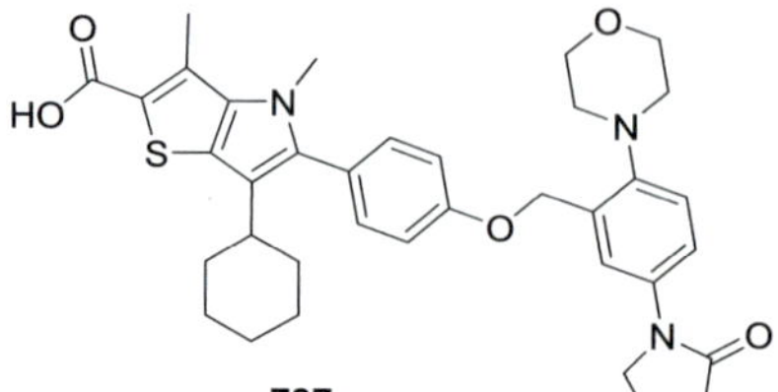

737

IC_{50} = 0.010 μM, EC_{50} = 0.52 μM

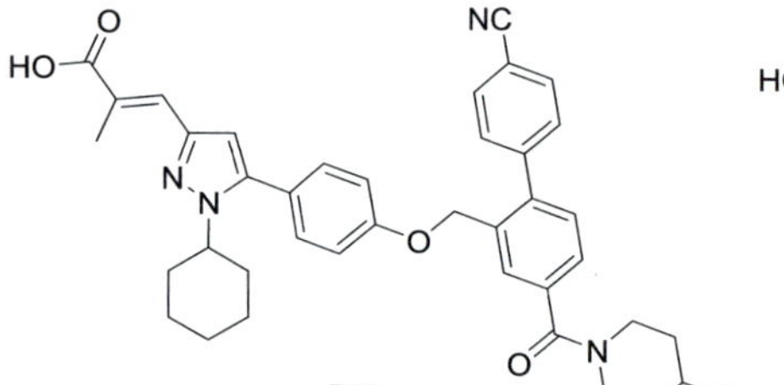

738

IC_{50} = 0.034 μM, EC_{50} = 0.4 μM

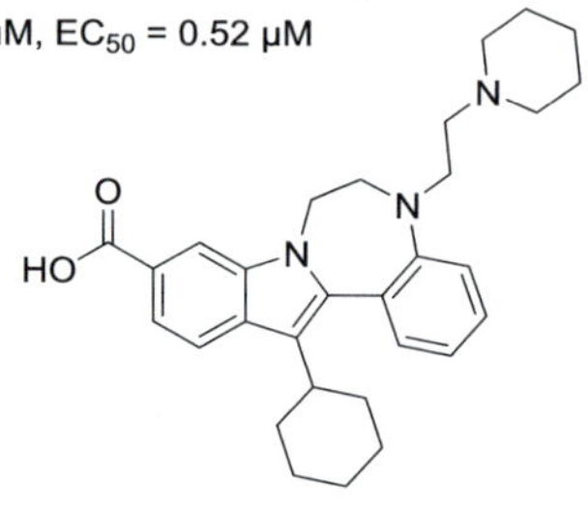

739

IC_{50} = 0.009 μM, EC_{50} = 0.35 μM

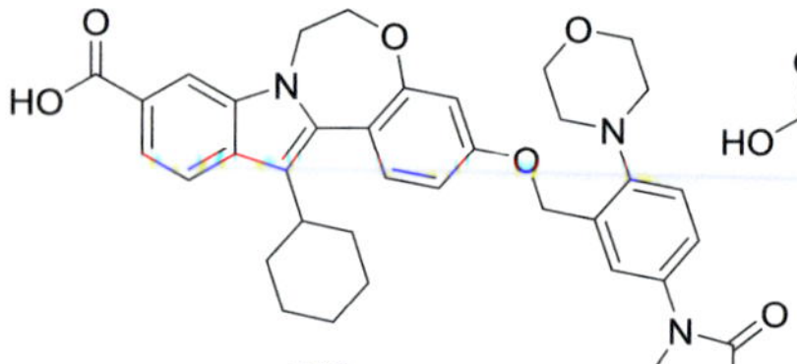

740

IC_{50} = 0.0072 μM, EC_{50} = 0.0076 μM

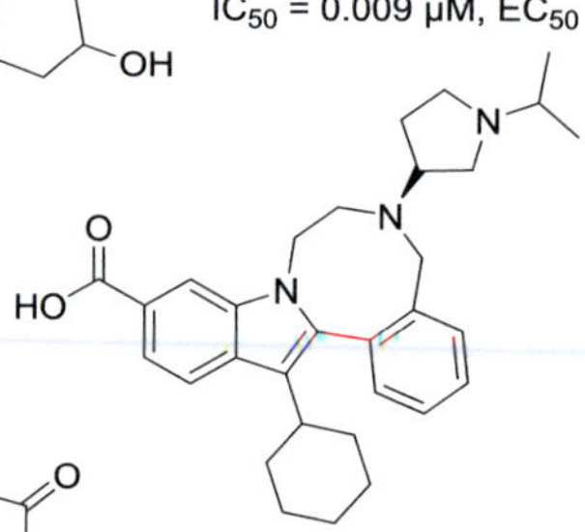

741

IC_{50} = 0.019 μM, EC_{50} = 0.15 μM

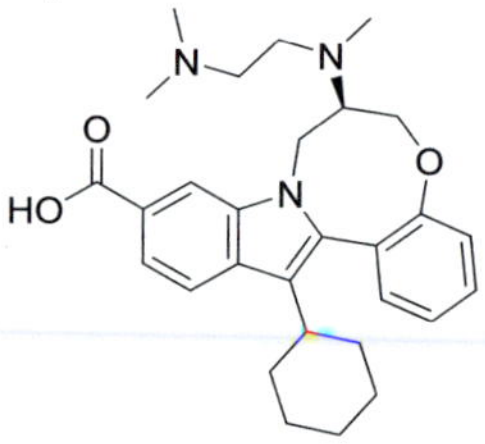

742

MK-3281

IC_{50} = 0.006 μM, EC_{50} = 0.039 μM

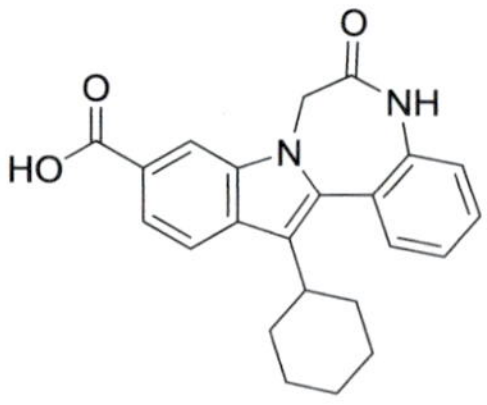

743

IC_{50} = 0.07 μM, EC_{50} = 0.24 μM

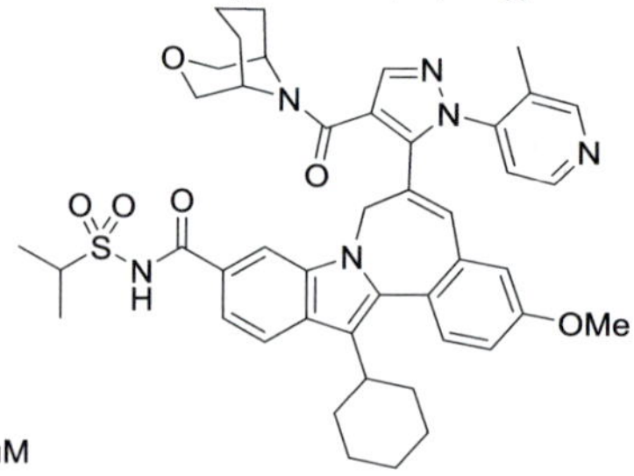

744

IC_{50} = 0.0043 μM, EC_{50} = 0.004 μM

Fig. (82). Molecules of NS5B thumb site I inhibitors.

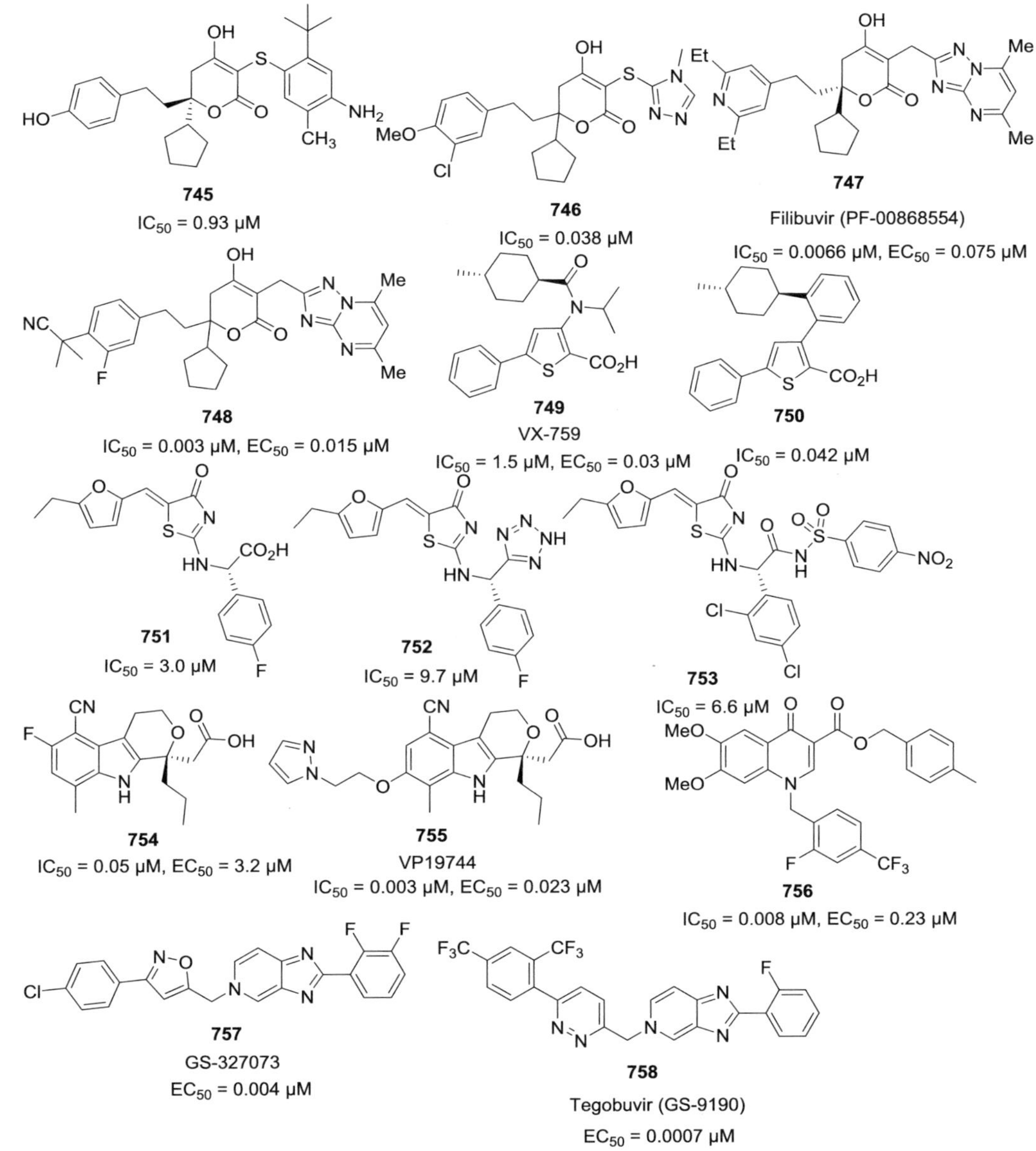

Fig. (83). Molecules of NS5B thumb site II inhibitors.

4.20.1. Discovery of Benzimidazole 5-carboxylic Acid Scaffold

Several indole core modified were reported to afford antiviral agents: (i) Modifications at C-2 and C-5 position of benzimodazole core for NS5B thumb site I inhibitors [239]. The gem-dimethyl analogue and cyclopentyldiamide compounds exhibited remarkable increased potency compared to the naked glycine analogues which highlighted the importance of conformational selection and flexibility in the inhibitors (Fig. **84**) [240].

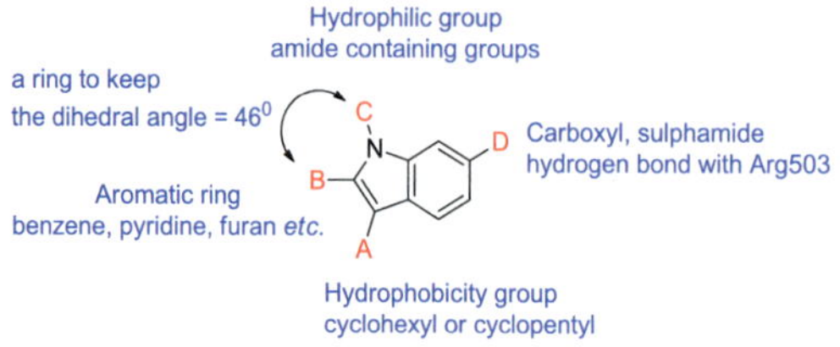

Fig. (84). General SARs model of indole thumb site Iinhibitors.

(ii) Modifications at the N-1 position of indole core for NS5B thumb site I inhibitors (Fig. **85**) [241]:

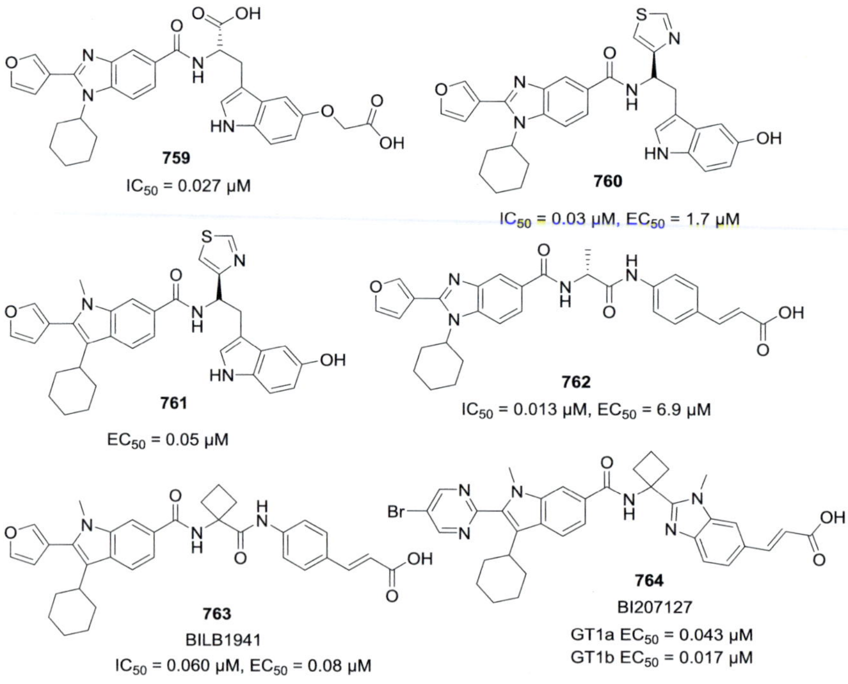

Fig. (85). Modifications at the N-1 position of NS5B thumb site I inhibitors and benzimidazole to indole scaffold.

(iii) Conformationally restricted multi-cyclic indole scaffolds [242]:
(iv) Variations of indole scaffolds [243]:
(v) General SARs of indole thumb site I inhibitors: (Fig. **86** and **87**)

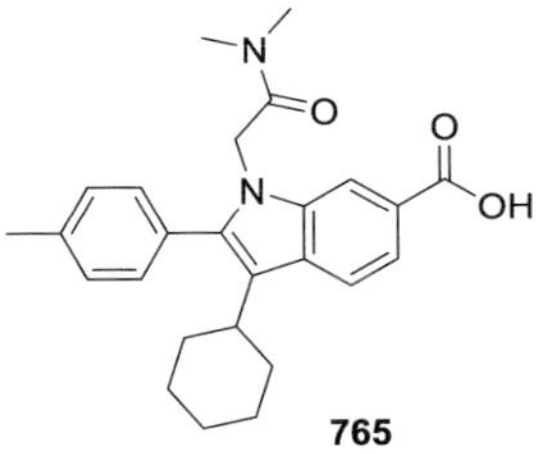

765
IC_{50} = 0.017 μM, EC_{50} = 0.5 μM

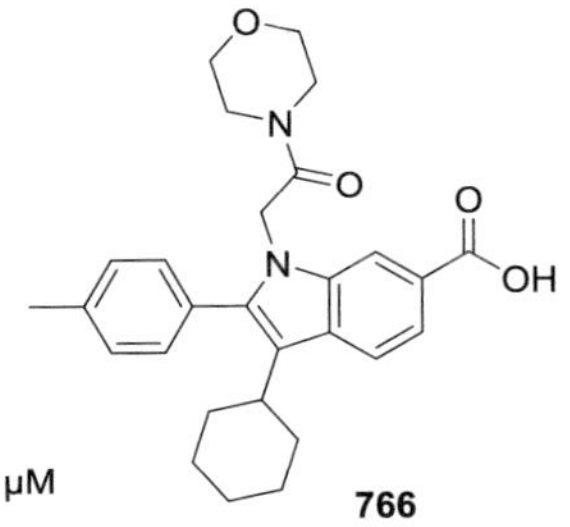

766
IC_{50} = 0.011 μM, EC_{50} = 0.3 μM

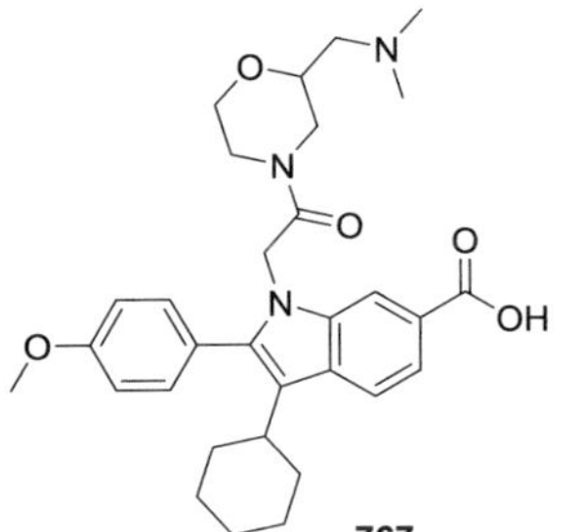

767
IC_{50} < 0.006 μM, EC_{50} = 0.15 μM

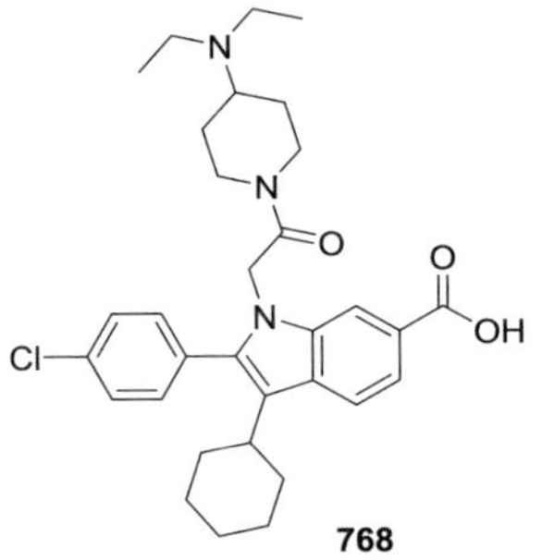

768
IC_{50} = 0.004 μM, EC_{50} = 0.12 μM

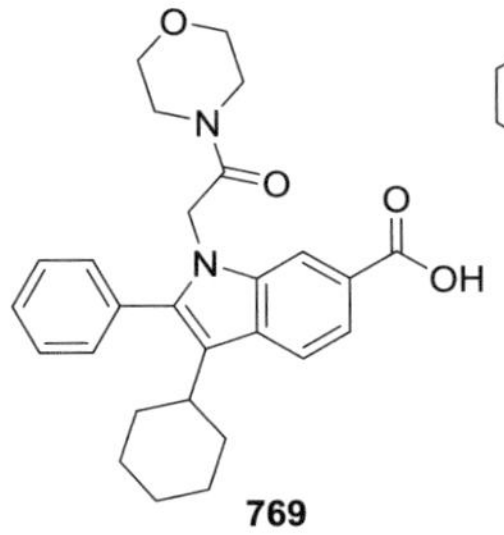

769
EC_{50} = 0.8 μM

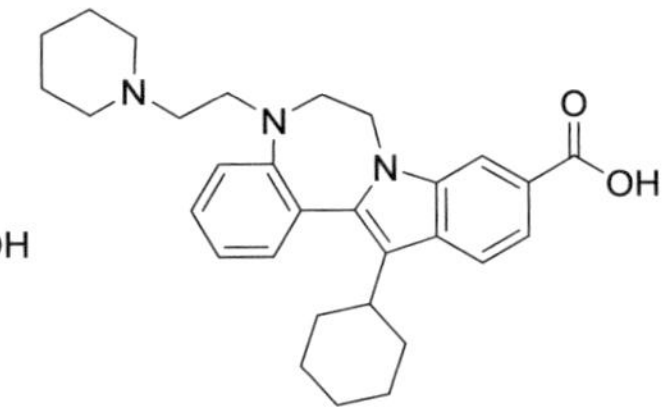

917
IC_{50} = 0.009 μM, EC_{50} = 0.35 μM

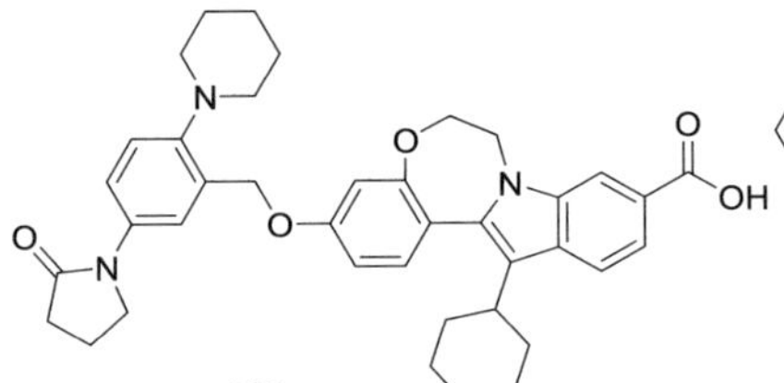

918
IC_{50} = 0.0072 μM, EC_{50} = 0.0076 μM

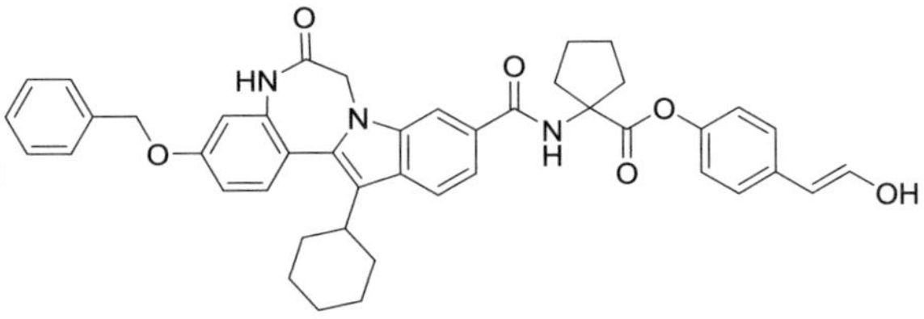

919
IC_{50} = 0.02 μM, EC_{50} = 0.01 μM

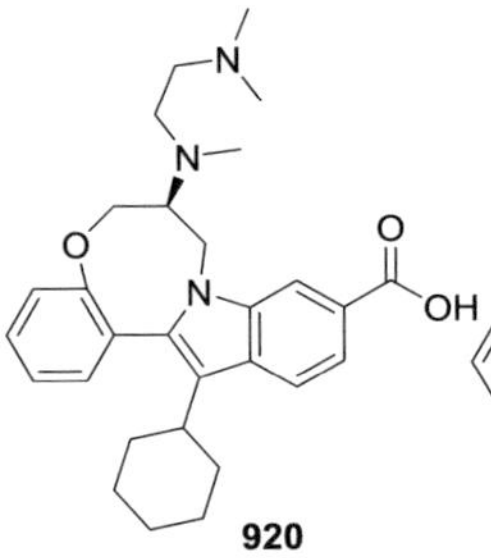

920
MK-3281
IC_{50} = 0.006 μM, EC_{50} = 0.038 μM

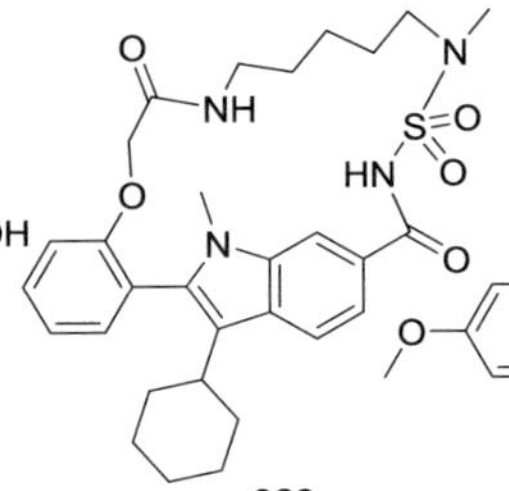

923
EC_{50} = 0.18 μM

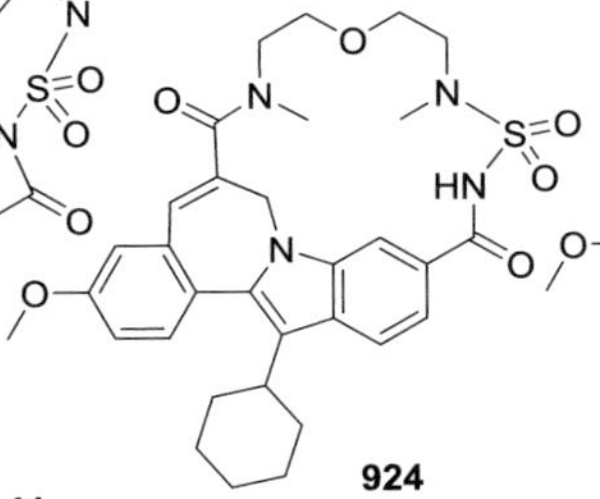

924
TMC-647075
EC_{50} = 0.077 μM

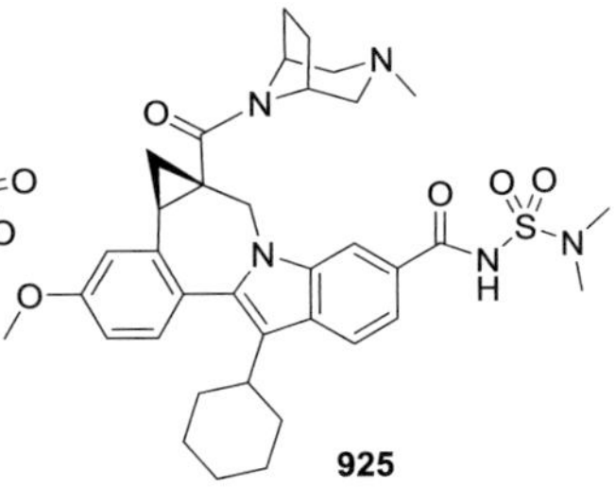

925
BMS-791325
GT 1a EC_{50} = 0.003 μM
GT 1b EC_{50} = 0.006 μM

Fig. (86). N-1 position modified indole core and conformationally restricted multicyclic indole analouges targating NS5B thumb site I inhibitors

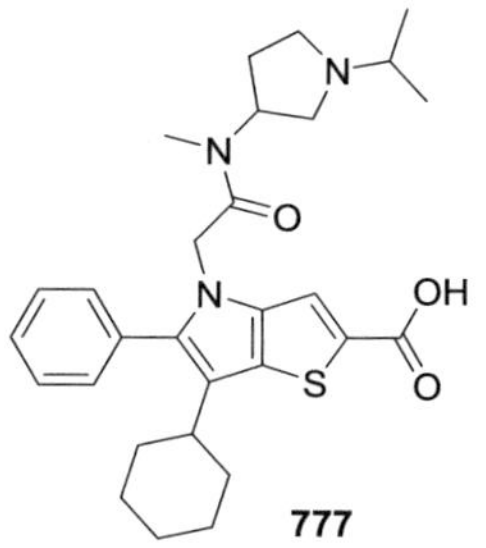

777

IC_{50} = 0.010 μM, EC_{50} = 0.13 μM

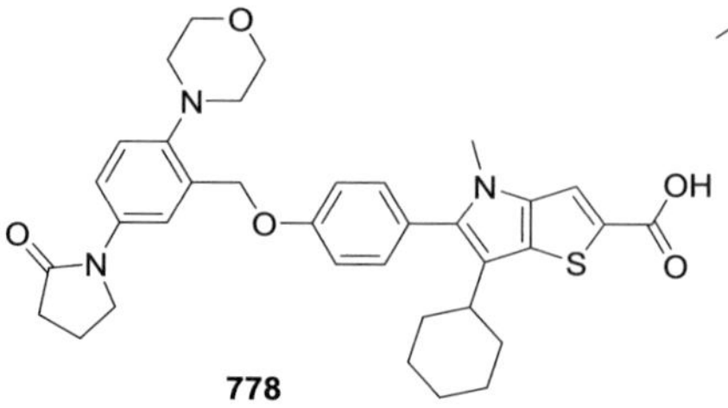

778

IC_{50} = 0.010 μM, EC_{50} = 0.052 μM

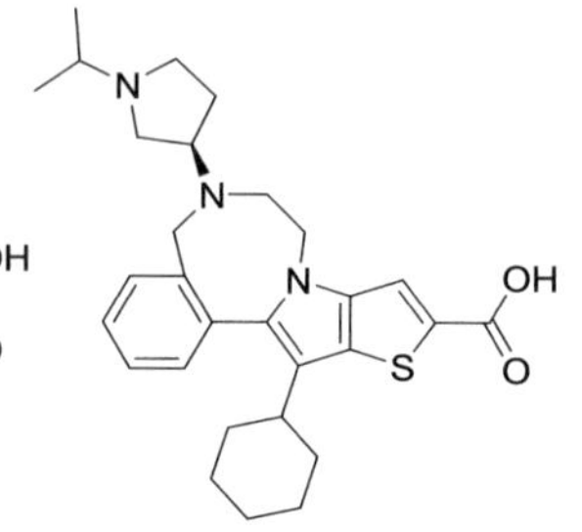

779

IC_{50} = 0.019 μM, EC_{50} = 0.150 μM

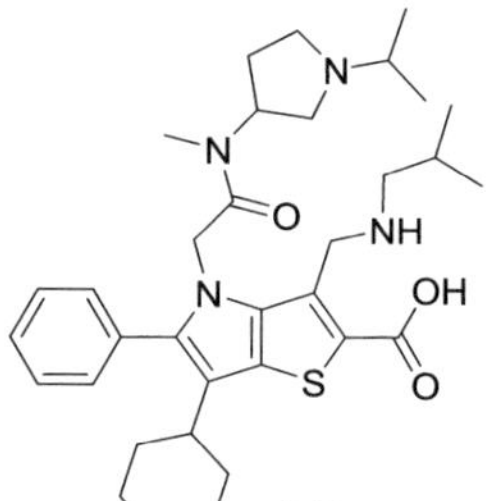

780

IC_{50} = 0.011 μM, EC_{50} = 0.51 μM

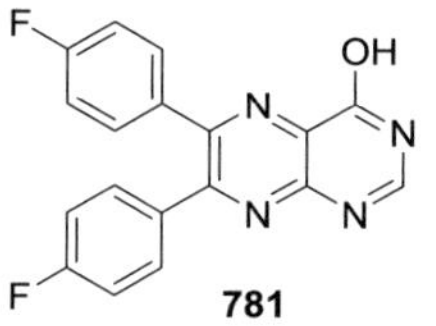

781

IC_{50} = 0.5 μM

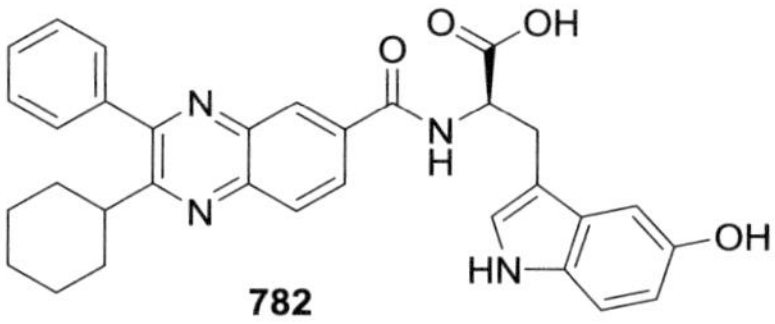

782

IC_{50} = 0.6 μM

Fig. (87). Representative NS5B thumb site I inhibitors.

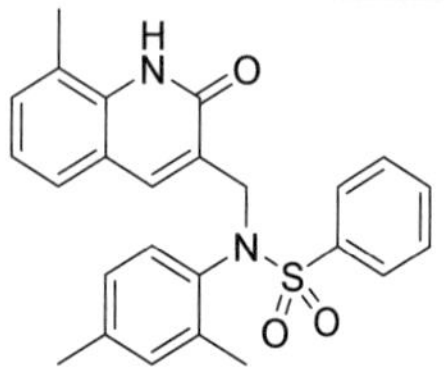

784

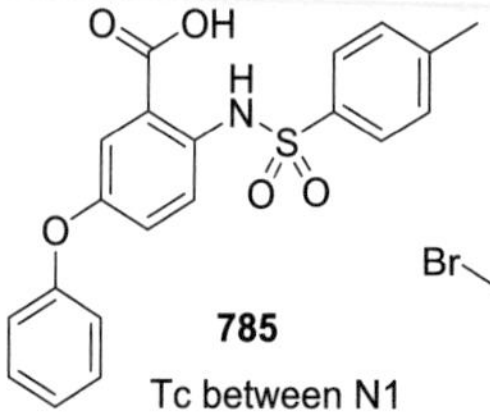

785

Tc between N1 and K1: 0.24

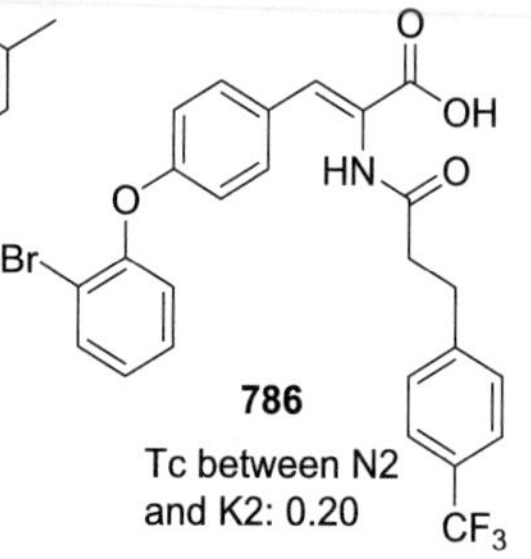

786

Tc between N2 and K2: 0.20

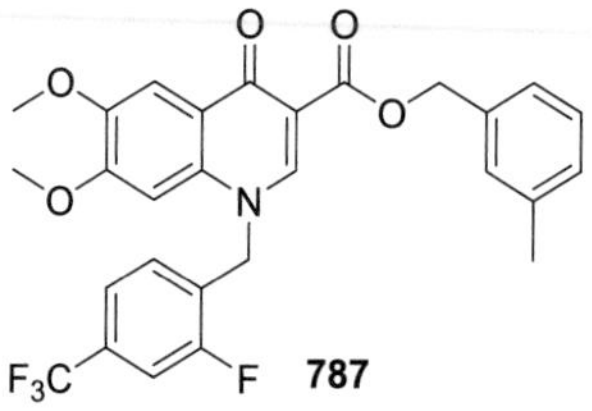

787

Tc between N3 and K3: 0.20

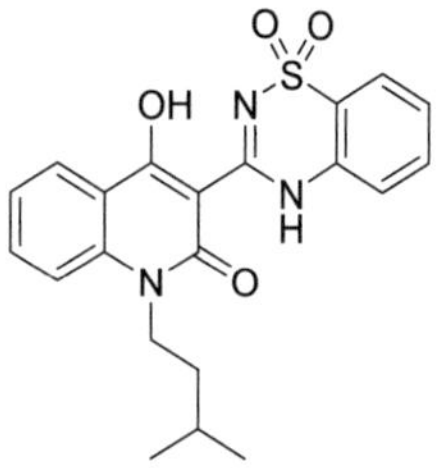

788

Tc between N5 and K5: 0.29

Fig. (88). The structure of known NS5B inhibitors (KI-K5) these inhibitors have highest N1-N5 respectively.

A chemical library of 441,574 compounds were screened for virtual screening approach which gave 5 compounds as hits for further anti-HCV and cellular cytotoxicity assay. These showed inhibitory potency against NS5B polymerase inhibitory activities (IC_{50} 2.01–23.84 μM) without cellular cytotoxicity. Further, optimization and development needed for potent and highly active NS5B polymerase inhibitors (Fig. **88**) [244].

Indole-*N*-acetamides **789** are potent allosteric inhibitors of HCV NS5B polymerase enzyme, established by crystal structure as a proof in the design of a 2D-compound array for zwitterionic inhibitors. They showed strong intracellular potency and pregnane X receptor (PXR) activation, linked to a structural feature of the inhibitor. However, optimized analogues devoid of PXR activation (*e.g.*, **793**, EC_{50} 127 nM) and retain strong cell-based efficacy under high serum conditions (Fig. **89**) [245].

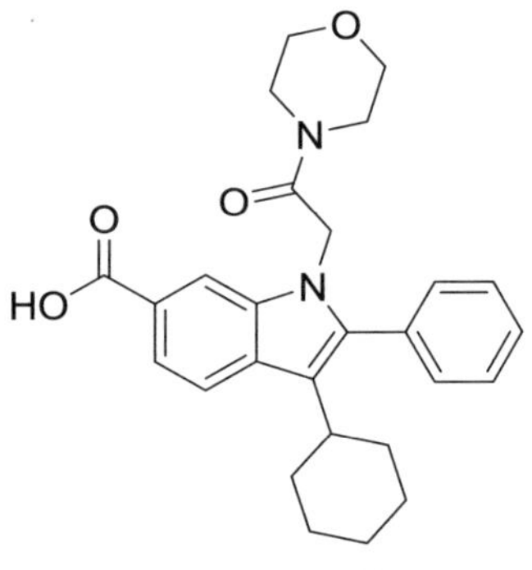

789
IC_{50} = 26 nm, EC_{50} = 0.8 μM

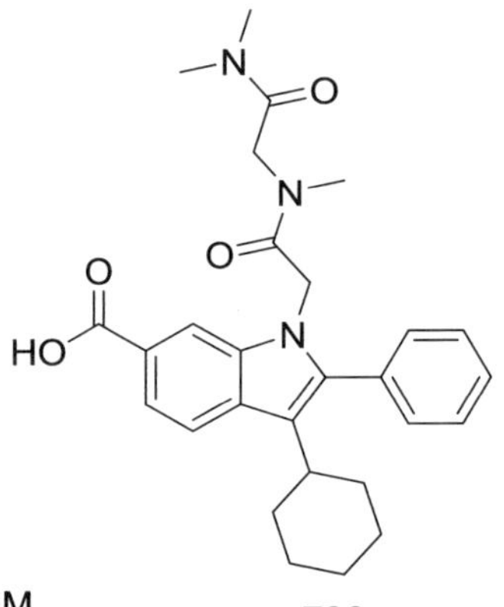

790
IC_{50} = 26 nm, EC_{50} = 1.9 μM

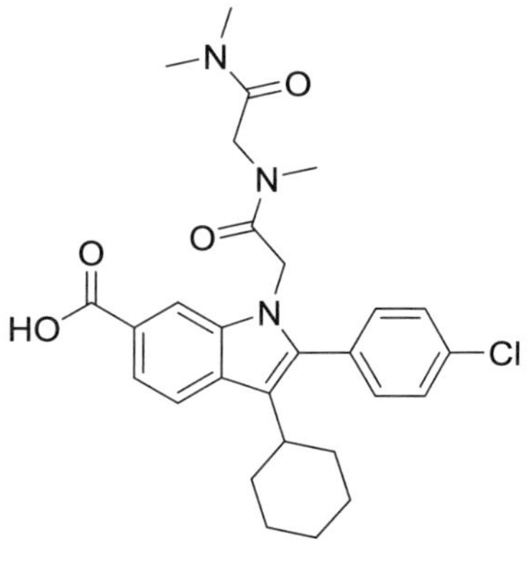

791
IC_{50} = 17 nm, EC_{50} = 1.1 μM

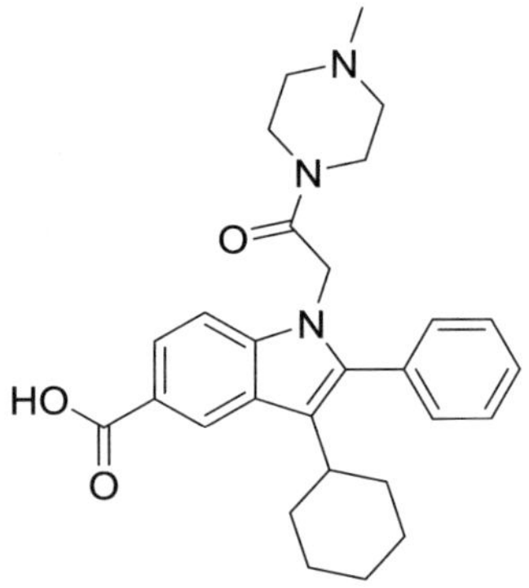

792
IC_{50} = 448 nm, EC_{50} = 3.5 μM

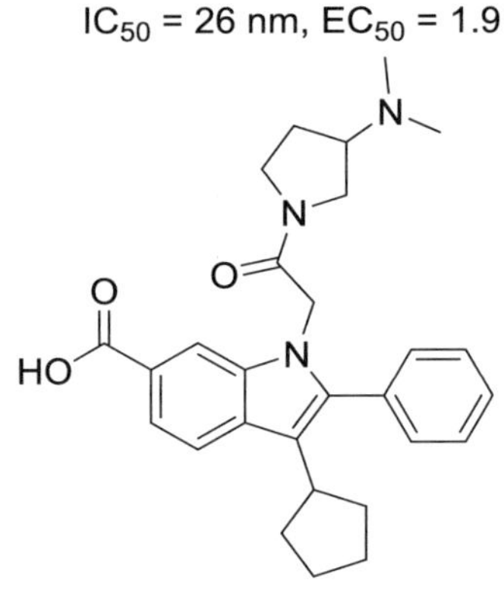

793
IC_{50} = 78 nm, EC_{50} = 1.5 μM

Fig. (89). Potent allosteric inhibitors of HCV NS5B polymerase enzyme.

In viral replication, NS5B RNA-dependent RNA polymerase is important thus a potent target for drug discovery. The leaves methanol extract of *T. officinale* is rich in flavonoids and ecaluated in human hepatoma (Huh-7) and CHO cell lines for anti-HCV activity which helped in blocking the viral replication and NS5B gene expression without any toxic effect on normal fibroblast cells (Fig. **90**) [246].

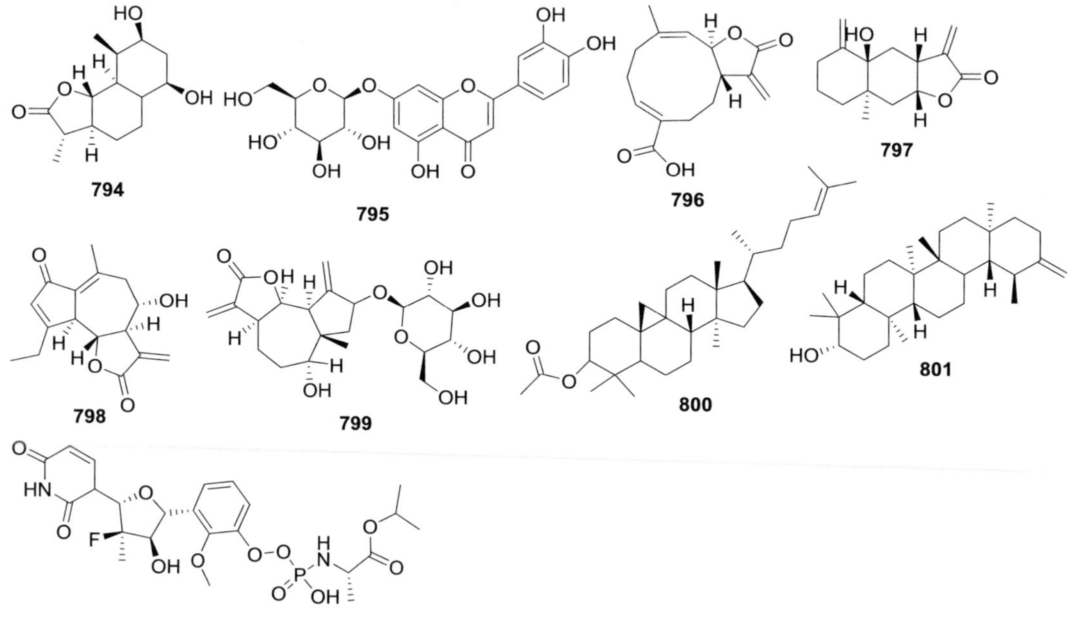

794 **795** **796** **797** **798** **799** **800** **801** **802**

Fig. (90). Chemical structures of *Taraxacum officinale* phytochemicals.

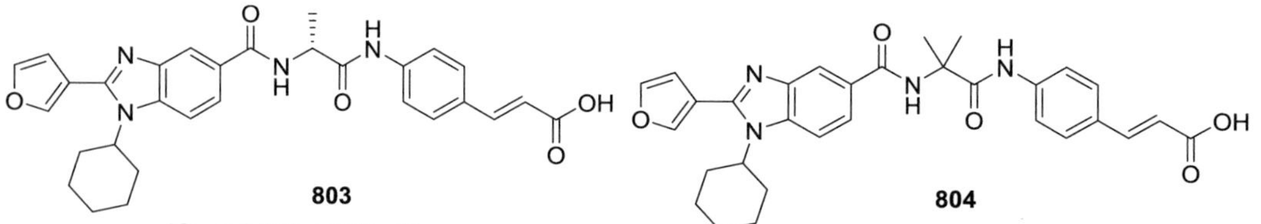

803

IC_{50} = 0.013 ± 0.02 μM
EC_{50} = 6.9 ± 0.8 μM (1b replicon)

804

IC_{50} = 0.04 ± 0.01 μM
EC_{50} = 1.85 ± 0.4 μM (1b replicon)
Calcd LogP = 4.4

Fig. (91). Thumb Pocket I benzimidazole inhibitors of HCV NS5B polymerase.

In the allosteric Thumb Pocket 1 HCV NS5B finger loop inhibitors, the benzimidazole core was replaced by more lipophilic indole core which gave up to 30-fold improvements in potency against cell-based sub-genomic replicon assays. Modifications at C-2 position in the indole core, led to many analogs with EC_{50} <100 nM (Fig. **91**) [247].

Novel benzothiazine-substituted quinolinediones were synthesized and evaluated as HCV NS5B polymerase inhibitors. SAR studies also revealed that the methyl sulfonamide group has high affinity like compound **2** showed promising low micro-molar potency, slightly improved solubility and significantly enhanced pharmacokinetic properties (Fig. **1**). A methyl group at meta-position in the p-fluorobenzyl series also provided additional boost potency in PS replicon assay. Several alkyl groups were also synthesized and evaluated like compound **806** a key lead structure (Fig. **92**) [248].

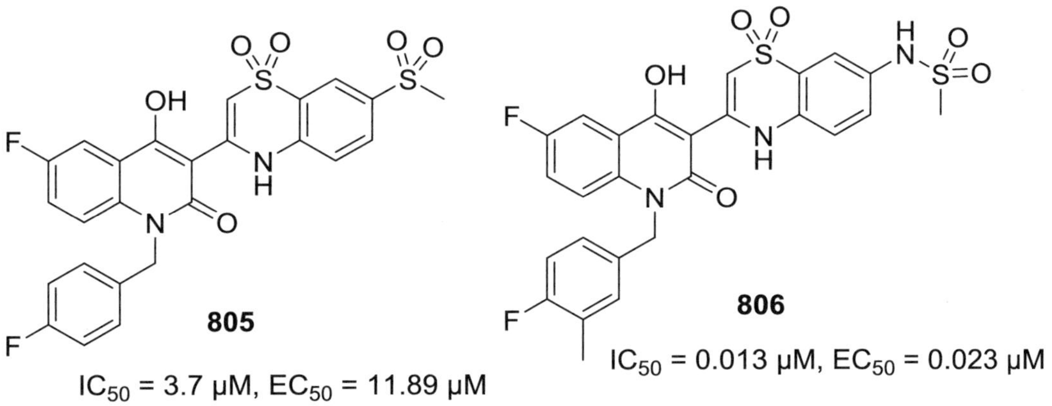

Fig. (92). Benzothiazine-substituted quinolinediones.

The non-nucleoside inhibitors of allosteric thumb pocket 1 inhibited replication of HCV NS5B polymerase during replicon. The optimization of indole-based inhibitors afforded better metabolic liability than the many previously reported inhibitors. In the parallel synthesis techniques, matrix of same inhibitors was used to collect the inhibitors for satisfactory potency criteria which improved *in vitro* ADME profiles. "Cassette" screening for oral absorption in rat also provided a short list of potential candidates and their evaluation led to the discovery of the first thumb pocket 1 NS5B inhibitor, BILB 1941 which demonstrated anti-viral activity in patients chronically infected with genotype 1 HCV (Fig. **93**) [249].

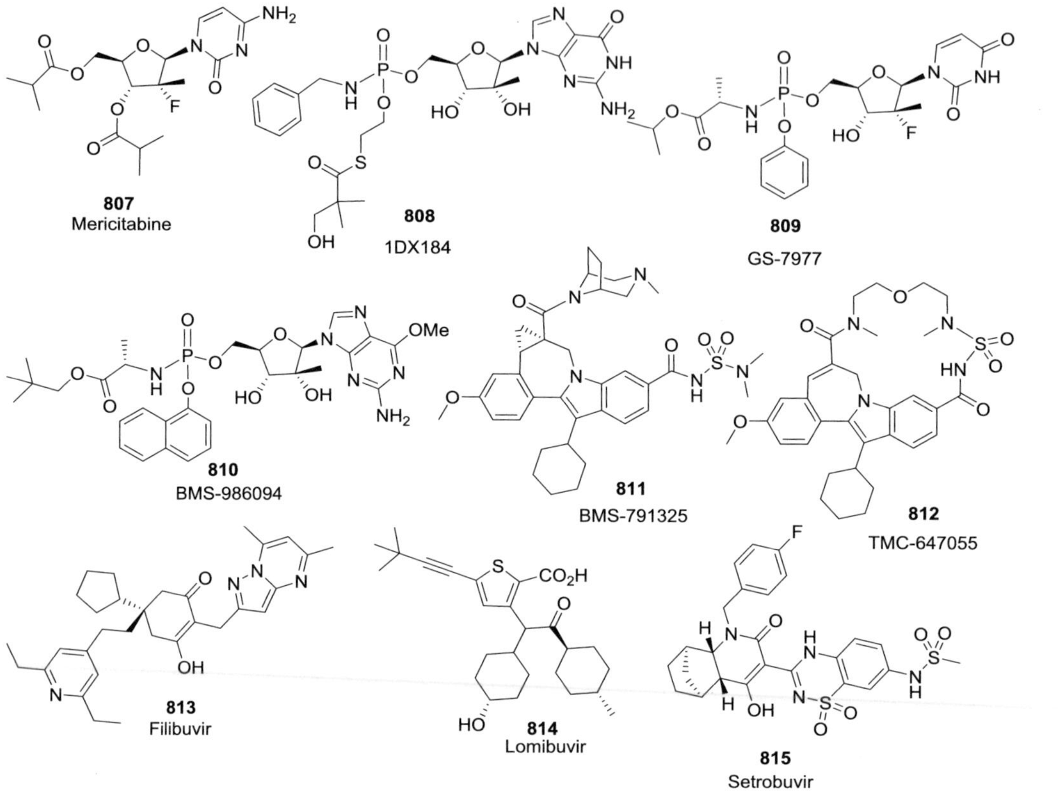

Fig. (93). Active site nucleoside and nucleotide **807-810**, Thumb pocket I **811-812**, Thumb pocket II **813-814** and Palm site I **815** NS5B inhibitors currently in clinical development.

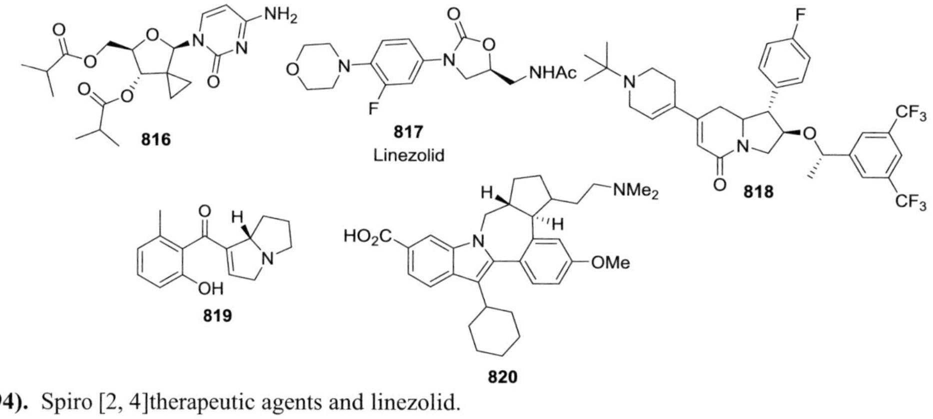

Fig. (94). Spiro [2, 4]therapeutic agents and linezolid.

2'-Deoxy-2'-spirocyclopropylcytidine derivatives were used as inhibitor for HCV NS5B polymerase (Figs. **24** & **94**). For example, imidazo[1,2-a]pyridines derivatives created the core moieties of anti-HCV agents (EC_{50} < 20 nM) in HCV genotypes 1a and 1b replicon [250].

1′-Cyano-2′-C-methyl 4-aza-7,9-dideaza adenosine showed a potent and selective inhibitor of NS5B target. Thus, a series of monophosphate pro-drug compounds synthesized for HCV replicon assays. Further, pharmacokinetic optimization for better oral absorption and liver triphosphate loading, led to identification of a clinical development candidate GS-6620 (Fig. **95**) [251].

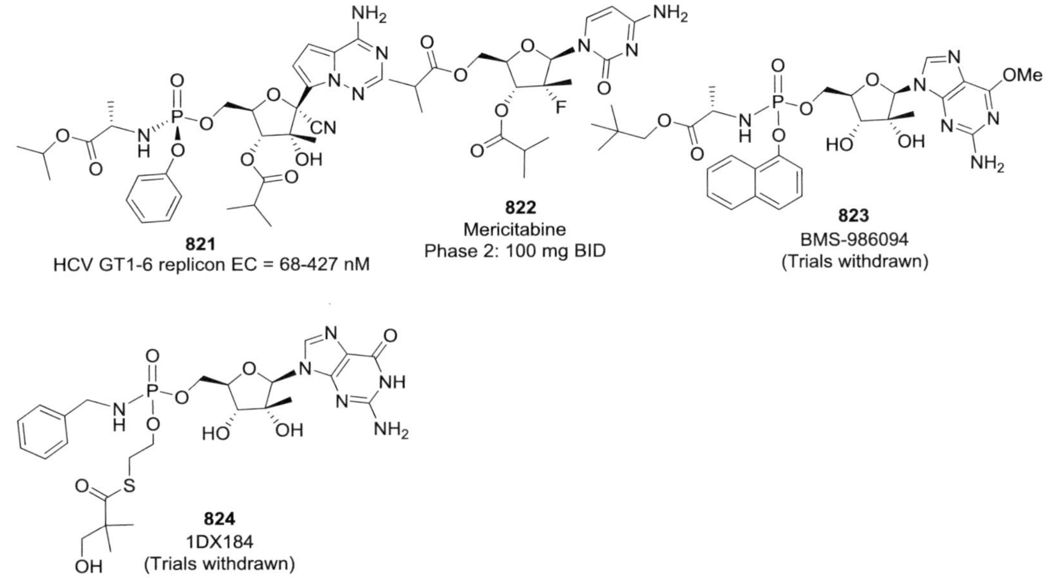

Fig. (95). Nucleoside polymerase inhibitors in clinical development.

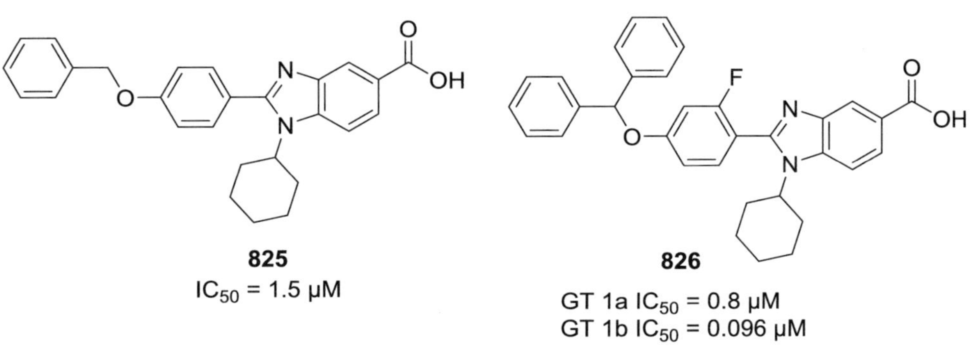

Fig. (96). Benzimidazole 5-carboxylic acid scaffold targating NS5B thumb site I.

Nucleoside and non-nucleoside inhibitors have demonstrated efficacy in targeting different allosteric sites compared to thumb site I, better than many other allosteric target inhibitors. For example, indole analogues are most important series of NS5B thumb site I inhibitors (Fig. **96**) [252].

The 6-amino-7-[4-(2-pyridinyl)-1-piperazinyl]quinolone derivative **827** is the best compound against NS5B polymerase (IC_{50} 0.069 μM) and selective (EC_{50} 3.03 μM) anti-viral effect without cytostatic effect (CC_{50} > 163 μM) in Huh 9–13 cells against HCV genotype 1b in MTS assay (Fig. **97**) [253].

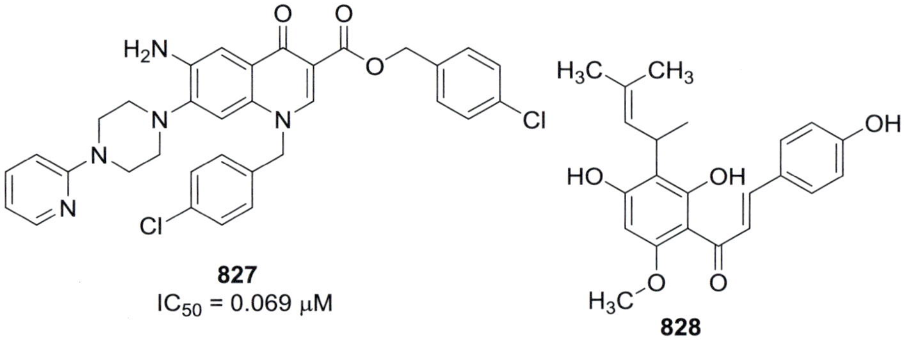

827
IC_{50} = 0.069 μM

828

Fig. (97). Anti-NS5B quinolone and xanthohumol derivative.

Xanthohumol (XN) **991**, a natural compound showed cytopathic effects (CPE) by inhibiting BVDV E2 expression and viral RNA levels in a dose-dependent manner [254]. The inhibitory activity of XN on CPE, BVDV E2 expression and viral RNA levels was stronger than that of RBV but weaker than IFN-α. Conformationally restricted 2′-spironucleosides and their pro-drugs were synthesized as potential anti-HCV agents and triphosphate of a 2′-oxetane cytidine analogue and demonstrated potent intrinsic biochemical activity against the NS5B polymerase (IC_{50} 8.48 μM) with reduced S282T mutation. Phosphoramidate pro-drugs of 2′-oxetane 2-amino-6-O-methylpurine nucleoside demonstrated potent anti-HCV activity *in vitro* and the corresponding triphosphate retained similar potent activity against both wild-type and S282T HCV NS5B polymerase (Fig. **98**) [255].

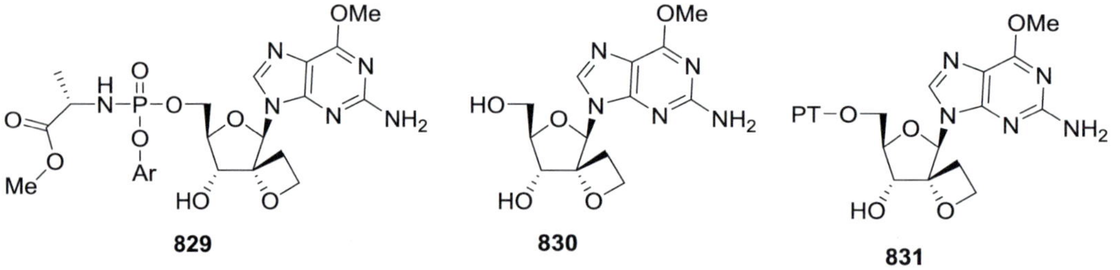

829 **830** **831**

Fig. (98). Anti-NS5B 2′-spironucleosides.

Several quinoline derivatives were synthesized substituting benzothiadiazine moiety as potential bioisosteric for anti-HCV NS5B polymerase inhibitors which exhibited potent activity in enzymatic and replicon assays (Fig. **99**). SAR studies also showed that the modification of N-alkyl-4-hydroxy-3,4-dihydroquino-ine-2-one moiety of 1,1 such as the gem-dialkyl derivative 2,2 have profound effects on both the anti-viral activity and pharmacological properties [256].

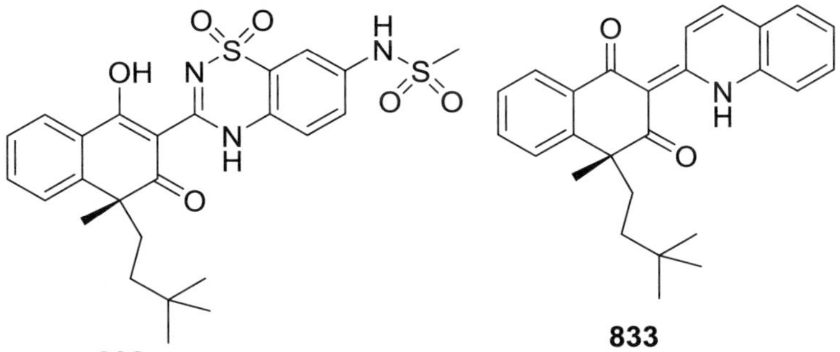

832
IC_{50} = 3 nm

833
IC_{50} = 5550 nm

Fig. (99). Benzothiadiazine and quinoline derivatives..

Many diarylmethyl containing benzimidazole derivatives afforded anti-HCV NS5B RNA-dependent RNA polymerase (HCV NS5B RdRp). SAR study also showed analogues bearing a substituted biphenyl group are better in activity. Compound optimization by modification of the A, B and C rings afforded potent inhibitors with low nanomolar potency against genotype 1b. Compounds with a substituent carbonyl function at 4-position of the B-ring efficiently blocked sub-genomic viral RNA replication in the replicon cell assay at low sub-micromolar concentrations. Among them, compound **836** (JTK-109) exhibited high selectivity for NS5B in the treatment of hepatitis C (Fig. **100**) [257].

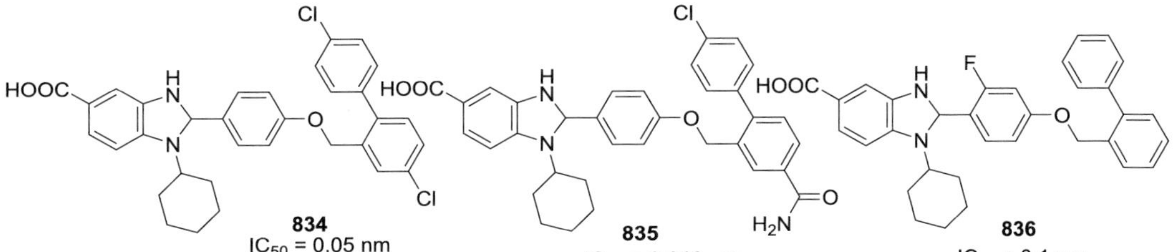

834
IC_{50} = 0.05 nm

835
IC_{50} = 0.013 μm

836
IC_{50} = 0.1 μm

Fig. (100). Anti-NS5B inhibitor.

SAR studies were carried out at different atoms in the indole core which afforded the indole-based C-3 pyridone inhibitor **2** as anti-HCV polymerase. The C-5 positions were found more compact and nonpolar than the C-6 attachments without affecting potency. An N-1 benzyl-type substituent studies indicated that the best substituents are fluoro or methyl groups at 2′ or 5′ positions of the benzyl group and acylsulfonamides as acid isosteres at the C-2 position. Further, optimization of the combination at N-1, C-2, C-5 and C-6 resulted in the identification of compound **839** which has an excellent potency in both NS5B enzyme (IC_{50} 0.008 μM) and cell-based replicon (EC_{50} 0.02 μM) assays (Fig. **101**) [258].

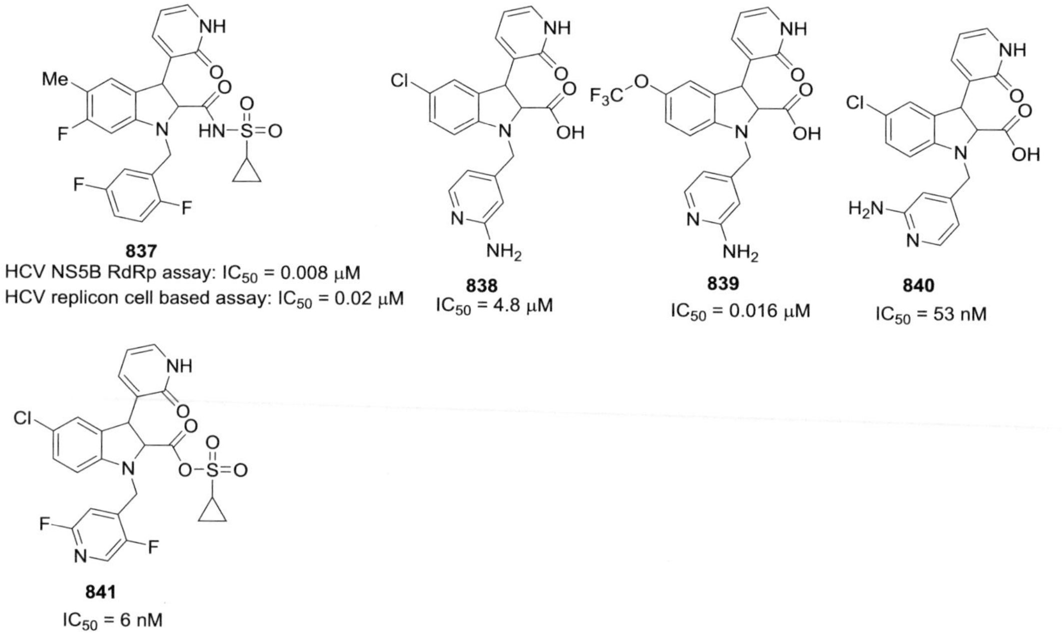

Fig. (101). Indole-based C-3 pyridone lead HCV polymerase inhibitor.

Also, SAR study of indole N-1 benzyl moiety was performed which gave indole-based C-3 pyridone as HCV NS5B polymerase inhibitor. This led to the discovery of irreversible inhibitors having p-fluoro-sulfone- or p-fluoro-nitro-substituted N-1 benzyl groups for excellent replicon assay potency (EC_{50} 1 nM). The C-5 ethyl C-2 carboxylic acid derivative **840** has an excellent oral area-under the curve (AUC) of 18 μM·h (10 mg/kg) [259]. The RNA-dependent RNA NS5B polymerase is one of the attractive and validated targets for development of new drugs to block HCV infection which gave benzothiadiazines as HCV NS5B polymerase inhibitors (Fig. **102**) [260].

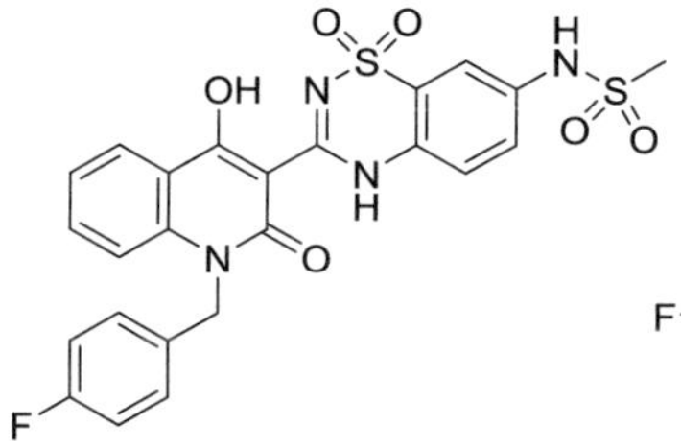

842
IC_{50} = 0.005 μM

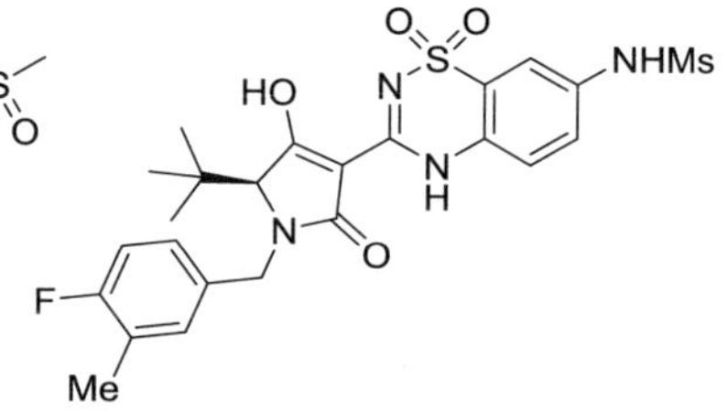

843
IC_{50} = 0.003 μM

Fig. (102). Thiazine and Quinoline analogs.

The enzymatic and cellular characterization of pyrazolobenzothiazines as anti-HCV inhibitors is reported which was mapped to NS5B palm site I employing a mutant counter screen assay. Derivative **844** proved to be the best anti-HCV derivative (IC_{50} 7.9 I1/4M) against NS5B polymerase in HCV replicon assay [261]. Similarly, enzymatic and cellular characterization of 6-aminoquinolone derivatives as potent inhibitors of NS5B polymerase is reported. The 6-amino-7-[4-(2-pyridinyl)-1-piperazinyl] quinolone derivative **846** proved to be the best compound (IC_{50} 0.069 I1/4M) against NS5B polymerase in HCV genotype 1b in MTS assay (Fig. **103**) [255].

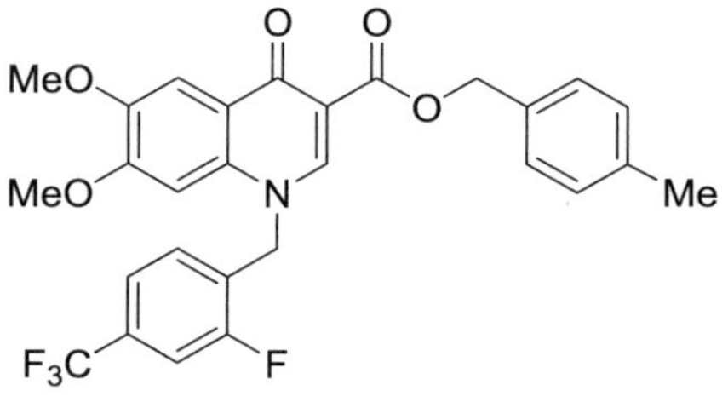

844

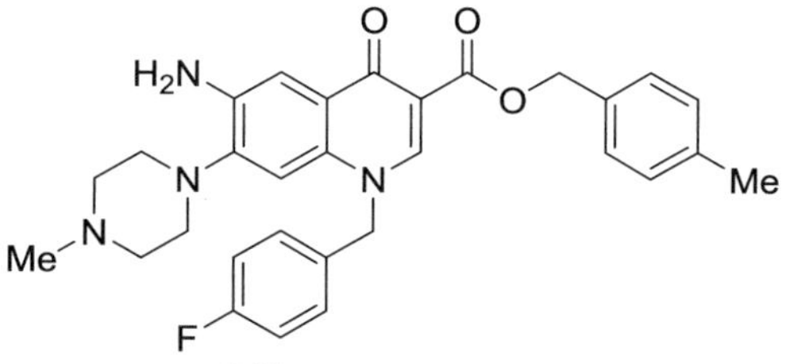

845
IC_{50} = 0.04 ± 0.004 μM

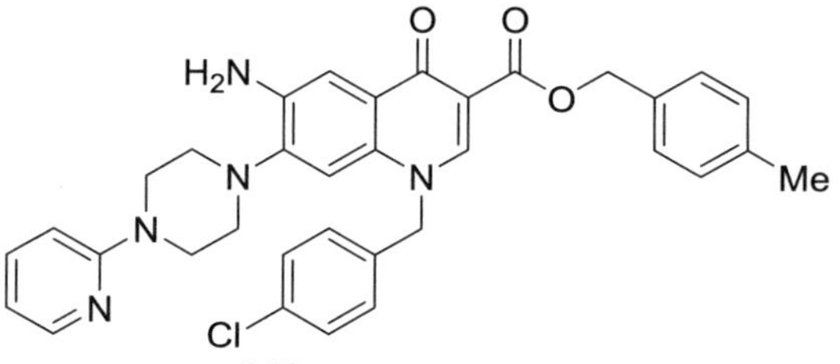

846
IC_{50} = 0.069 ± 0.002 μM

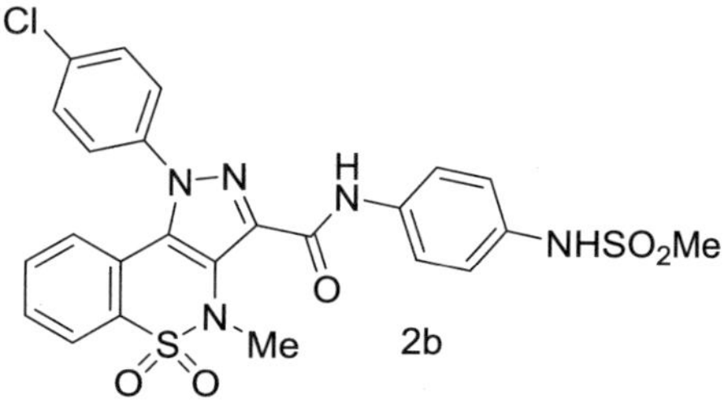

847

Fig. (103). Anti-NS5B polymerase in HCV genotype 1b.

Tri-substituted acylhydrazine as isostere of a tertiary amide was explored in a series of HCV NS5B thumb site II inhibitors which is located 35 Å away from the active site (Fig. **104**) [262]. The importance of this aspect of the inhibitor conformation was further exemplified by the optimized tertiary amide series which incorporated branched N-substituents to enhance and maintain the perpendicularity of the (4-Me) cyclohexyl moiety with respect to the thiophene scaffold in the conformation of 3 bound to the NS5B protein (Fig. **2**). It is postulated that other structural motifs might perform a more effective scaffolding function and initiated a program to identify novel NS5B inhibitors of the thiophenecarboxylic acids [263].

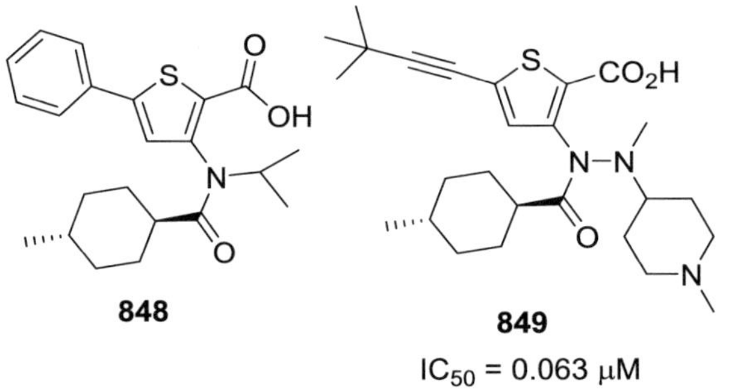

Fig. (104). Thiophenecarboxylic acid NS5B thumb site II inhibitors.

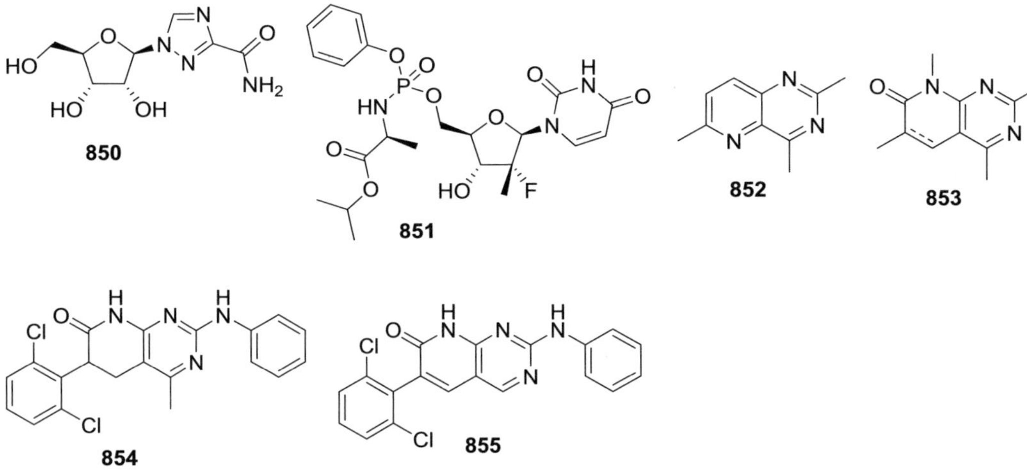

Fig. (105). Anti-HCV NS3 protease inhibitors.

Pyrido[2,3-d]pyrimidin-7(8H)-ones (more than 121 compounds) have been synthesized and evaluated for inhibitory activity against HCV genotype 1b replicon which afforded compounds **854** and **855** with very high activities (EC_{50} 0.027 mM and EC_{50} 0.034 mM) respectively, similar to the EC_{50} reported for sofosbuvir (0.048 mM). In silico studies, compounds **854** and **855** inhibited NS5B polymerase by allosteric site binding (Fig. **105**) [264].

Pyrazolobenzothiazine scaffold is reported as a suitable template for novel anti-HCV agents targeting the NS5B polymerase. The meta-fluoro-N-1-phenyl pyrazolobenzothiazine derivative **857** (EC_{50} 3.6 µM, EC_{90} 25.6 µM) was best compound showed in the Huh 9–13 replicon assay (Fig. **106**) [265].

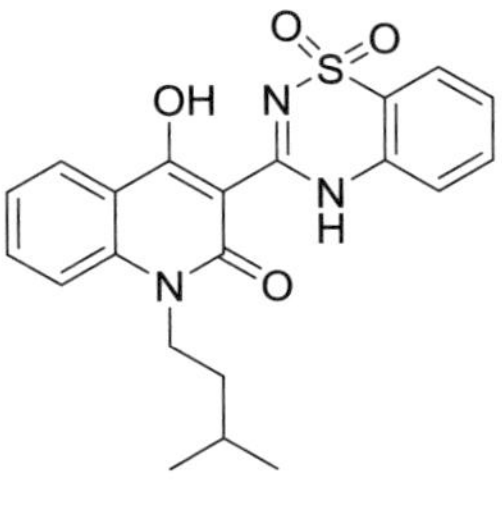

856

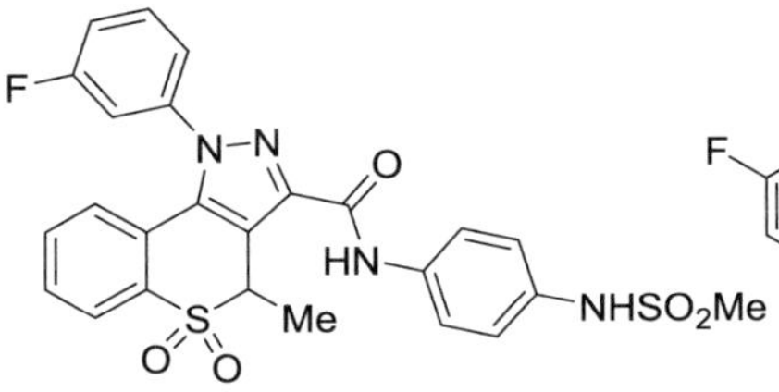

857

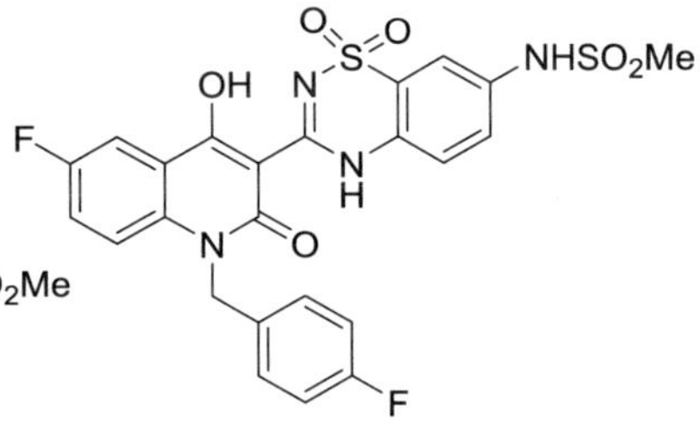

858

Fig. (106). NNIs analogues.

2'-C-Methylcytidine (NM107) a pro-drug is nucleoside based phosphoramidate inhibitor for HCV NS5B polymerase. NM107 and its valyl ester (NM283) pro-drug was effective in reducing the viral load in HCV infected patients. Based on this, many phosphoramidates were synthesized which showed 10-200-fold superior potency with respect to the parent nucleoside in the cell-based replicon assay (Fig. **107**) [266].

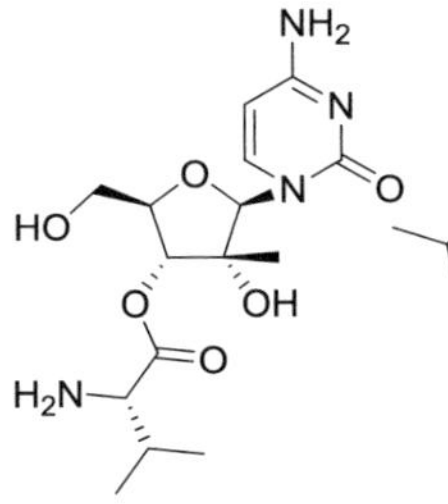

859

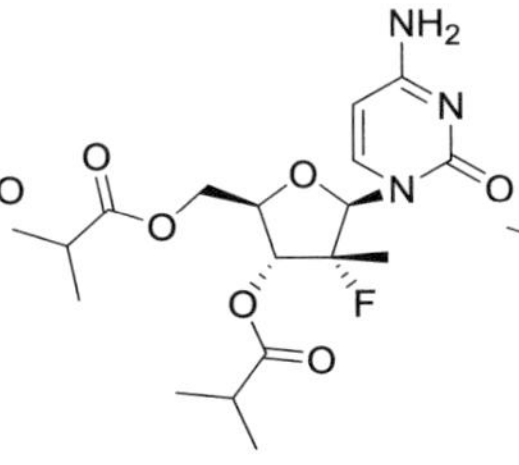

860

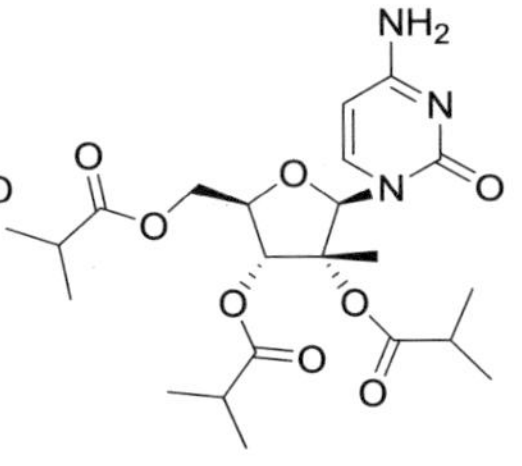

861

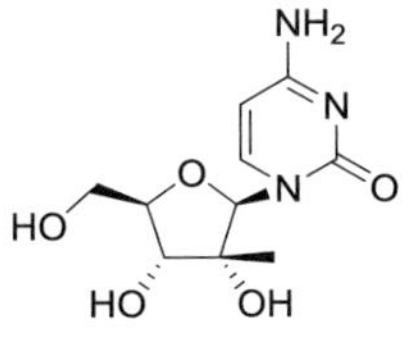

862

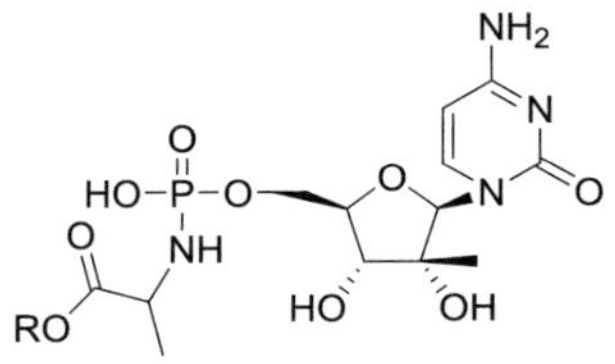

863

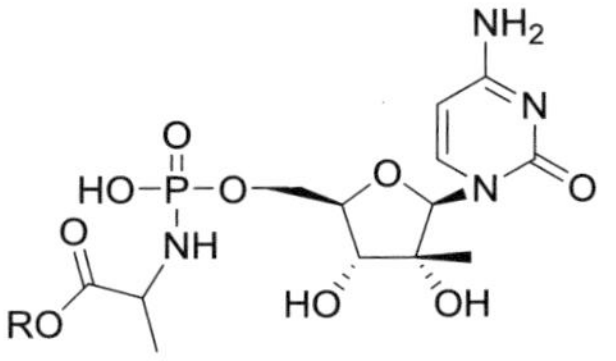

864

Fig. (107). HCV NS5B polymerase inhibitors.

Non-nucleoside NS5B polymerase allosteric inhibitors in combination with DAAs have a complementary mechanism of action. Compound (BI 207524, **27**) gave the first thumb pocket 1 NS5B inhibitor to demonstrate antiviral activity in genotype 1 HCV infected patients, BILB 1941 (1) (Fig. **108**). Thus, ADME-PK optimization lead to **27**, a predicted low clearance compound in man [267].

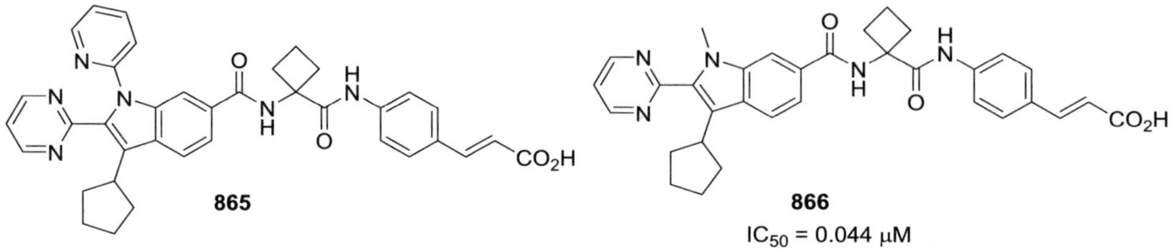

Fig. (108). Cinnamic acid derivatives.

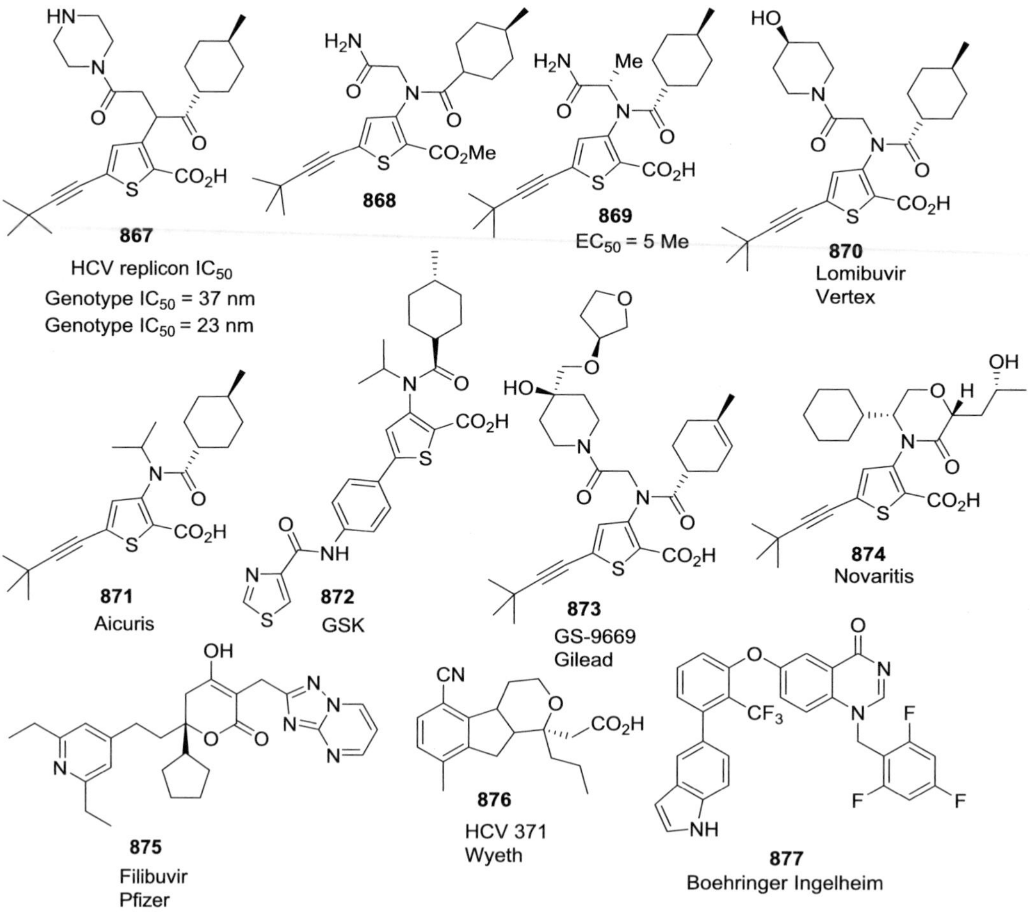

Fig. (109). Thiophene carboxylate allosteric inhibitors.

Many thiophene carboxylate allosteric inhibitors bound at the thumb pocket 2 site of NS5B polymerase. For example, Lomibuvir (VCH-222 and VX-222) is an allosteric has demonstrated excellent anti-HCV NS5B inhibitor activity and potential clinical utility in combination with DAA agents (Fig. **109**) [268]. Lomibuvir is a non nucleoside that binds to the so-called thumb pocket 2, a distance of 35 A... from the active site. Other inhibitors act at the same allosteric site include related thiophene carboxylic acids [269, 270] as well as the structurally unrelated compounds Filibuvir (HCV-371). The trans--methylcyclohexyl group is known to be deeply buried in a hydrophobic pocket, while the isopropyl or the trans-4-hydroxycyclohexyl substituent appears to extend into more open space.

Gilead's Sofosbuvir have investigated as unique 2′-sugar modification (2′-Me, 2′-F) of nucleoside analogues to exploit the biological activity. In this regard, a combined tricyclic "expanded" purine base motif with the 2′-Me, 2′-F sugar have been modified for interesting biological activity [271]. Further the potential of this scaffold with the 2′-modified sugar was found in Sofosbuvir to give corresponding tricyclic Sofosbuvir analogues **878-883** (Fig. **110**) [272].

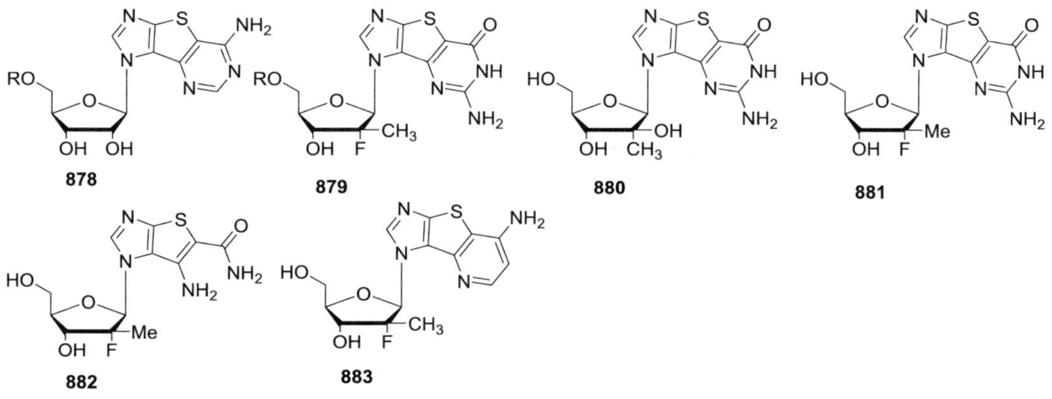

Fig. (110). Tricyclic and bicyclic targets.

The structural modifications of indole-based anti-HCV NS5B polymerase inhibitors were reported with multiple substituents on indole to further improve potency and pharmacokinetic (PK) properties. Bicyclic quinazolinone substituent at indole nitrogen and 4,5-furanylindole were identified as the best core. Compound **886** demonstrated excellent potency and C-2 N,N-dimethylaminoethyl ester pro-drug **885** (SCH 900188) demonstrated significant improvement in PK values (Fig. **111**) [273].

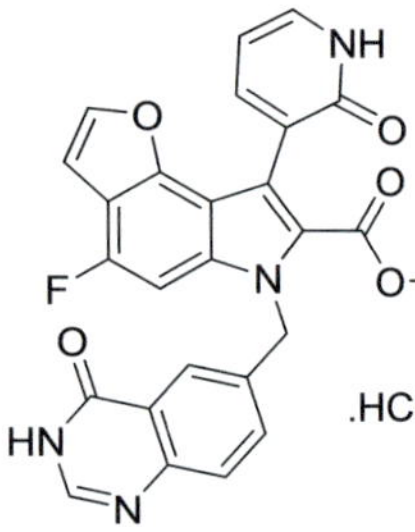

885
(900188, Prodrug)

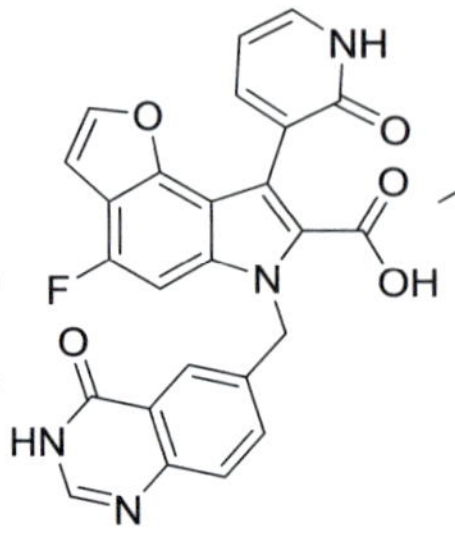

886
IC_{50} = 5 nm, EC_{50} = 6 nm

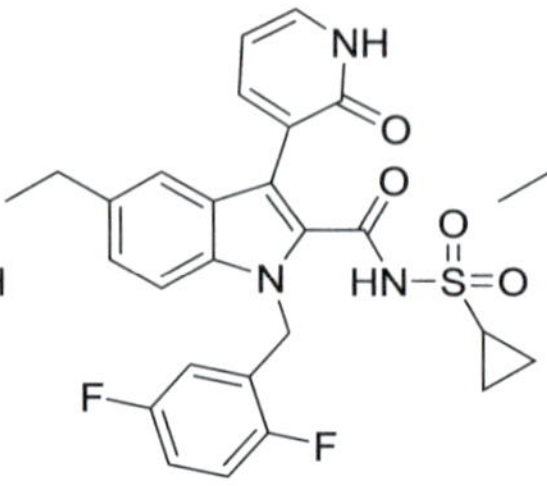

887
IC_{50} = 3 nm
EC_{50}= 40 nm

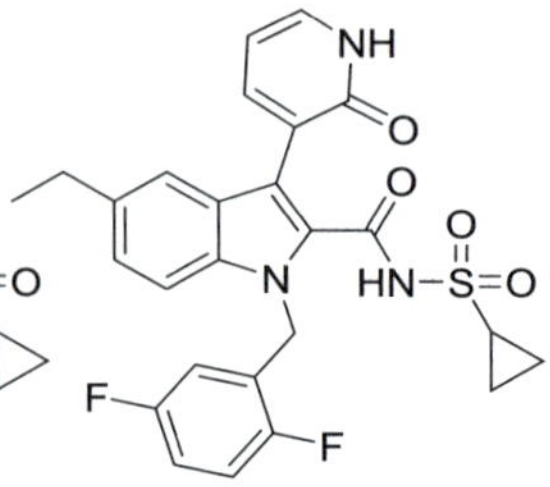

888
IC_{50} = 3 nm
EC_{50}= 40 nm

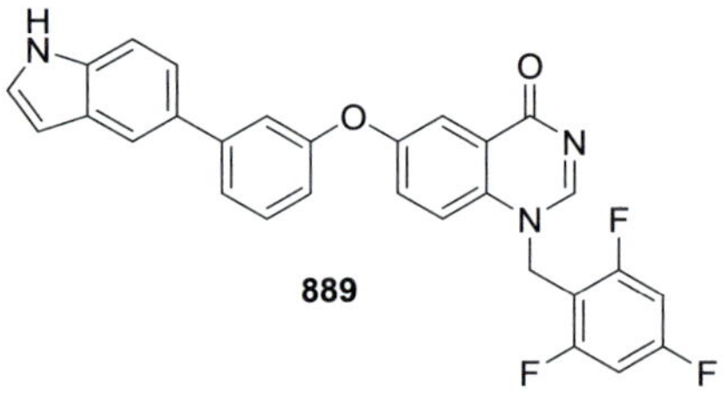

889

Fig. (111). Anti-NS5B polymerase inhibitor.

Many 1H-quinazolin-4-ones **889** allosteric HCV NS5B thumb pocket 2 (TP-2) inhibitors are reported. On the MD protocol guideline, the design of inhibitors were utilized in the novel H-bond interactions with the two backbone carbonyl groups which led to the first thumb pocket 2 NS5B inhibitor in genotype (gt) 1a and 1b replicons (EC_{50} 120 and 110 pM) respectively [274]. SAR study at the C-2 position of benzimidazole-based Thumb Pocket I inhibitors of HCV NS5B polymerase revealed parallel activity for 5-hydroxytryptophan amides, neutral thiazole isosteres and cinnamic acid diamides (Fig. **112**). New inhibitors with sub-micromolar cell-based replicon potency and improved 'drug-like' features are disclosed along with preliminary characterization of their ADME-PK profile [275].

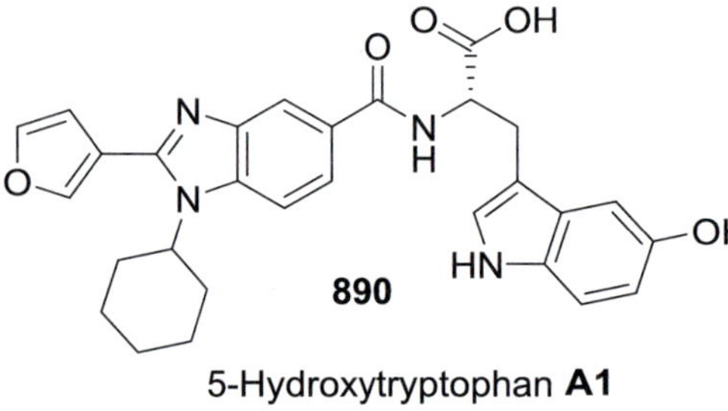

890
5-Hydroxytryptophan **A1**
IC_{50} = 0.03 μM

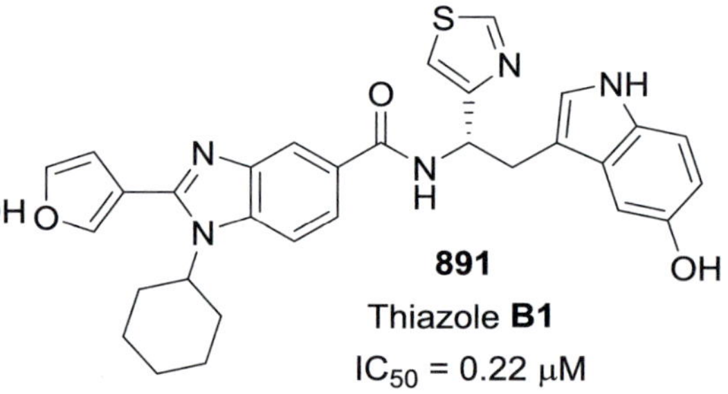

891
Thiazole **B1**
IC_{50} = 0.22 μM

Fig. 112 contd.....

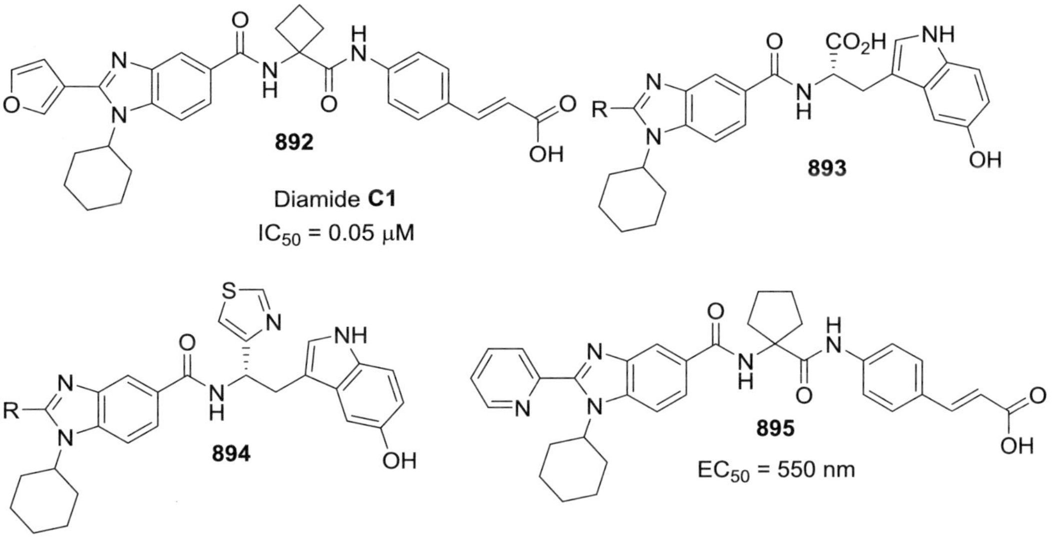

Fig. (112). Cyclopentyl diamide derivatives.

Tetracyclic indole-based compounds showed the inhibition property against allosteric sites on the thumb domain and their SAR studies around an indolo-benzoxazocine scaffold led to the compound **898** (MK-3281) as good HCV inhibitor in sub-genomic replication assay (Fig. **113**) [276].

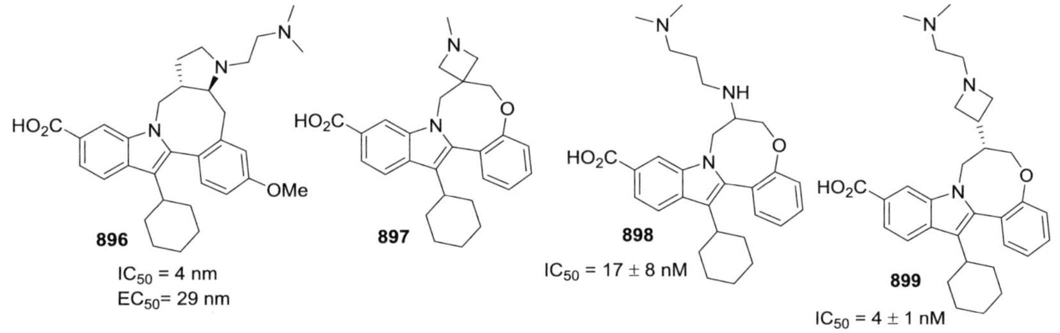

Fig. (113). Tti- and tetracyclic indole inhibitors.

A natural alkaloids compounds, APS **900-909** (EC_{50} 2.3 lM) is isolated from *Maytrenus ilicifolia* and lignans 3⁄43 (EC_{50} 4.0 lM), 3⁄20 (EC_{50} 8.2 lM) and 5⁄362 (EC_{50} 38.9 lM) isolated from *Peperomia blanda*. These have shown anti-HCV inhibition property in replication by reductions in luciferase activity and HCV protein expression in both the sub-genomic and infectious systems (Fig. **114**) [277].

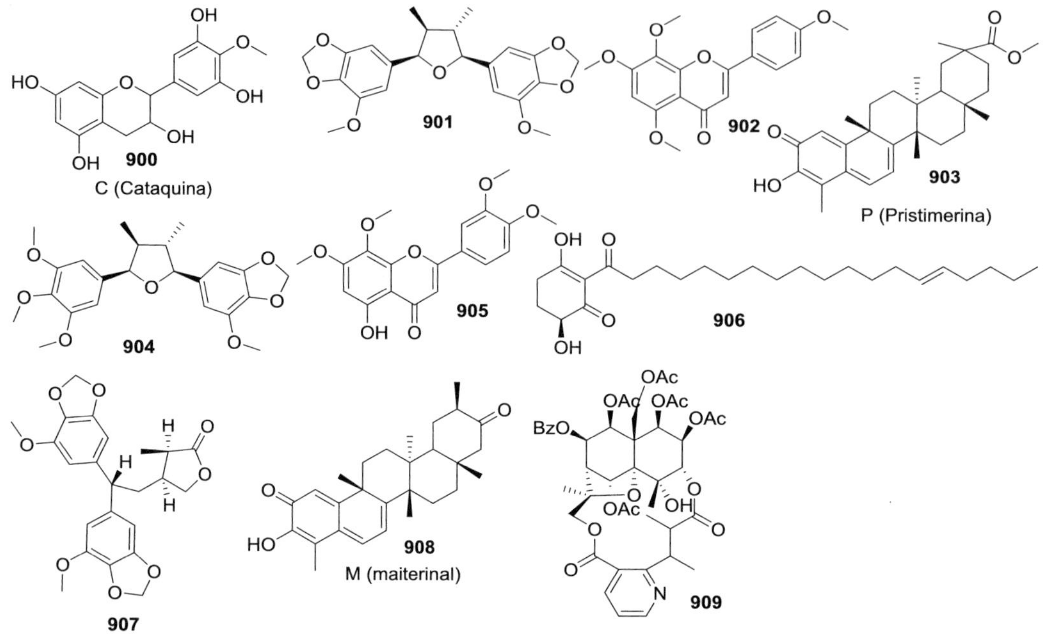

Fig. (114). Alkaloid isolated from *Maytrenus ilicifolia* and *Peperomia blanda*.

The synthesis of galloyl (3,4,5-trihydroxybenzoyl), its isomer 2,3,4-trihydroxybenzoyl and other mono- or dihydroxybenzoyl compounds with two, three or five units of moieties have been reported. The activity of tripodal compounds with 2,3,4-trihydroxybenzoyl moieties were found better than the linear compounds. However, the linear compounds **910** and **911** containing a 12 polymethylene chain and two 2,3-di- or 2,3,4-tri-hydroxybenzoyl groups at the ends of the molecule, showed good anti-HCV efficiency (Fig. **115**) [278].

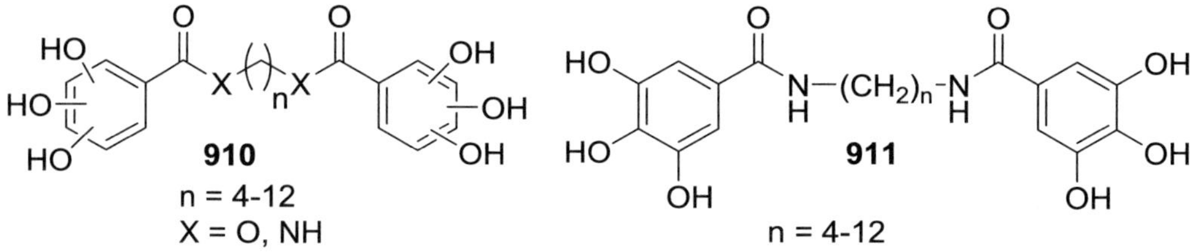

Fig. 115 contd.....

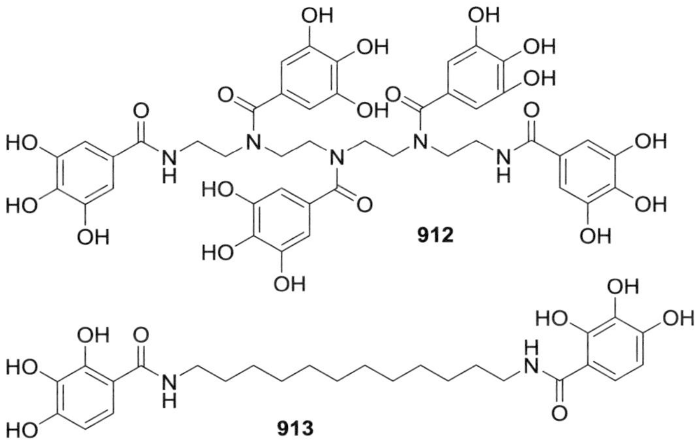

Fig. (115). Linear and branched polyphenols.

Several 1,2,4-triazole and imidazole based L-ascorbic acid and imino-ascorbic acid derivatives **914-917** were prepared and evaluated for their inhibitory activity against HCV replication (Fig. **116**) [279].

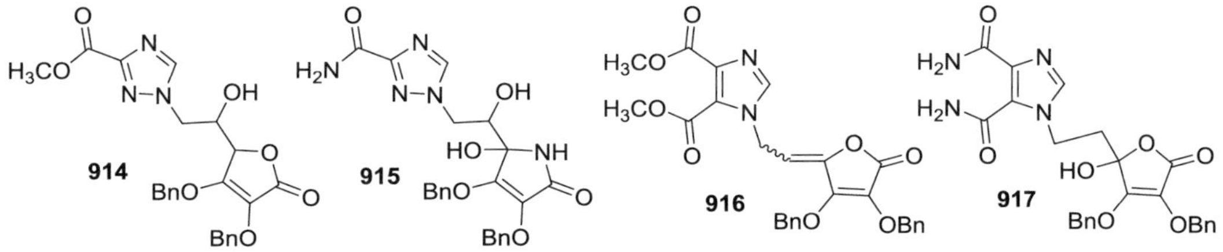

Fig. (116). 1,2,4-triazole, imidazole L-ascorbic acid and imino-ascorbic acid derivatives.

The most important secondary structure in nucleic acids is G-quadruplex (G4). Their stabilization is a promising new strategy for anti–hepatitis C drug development in the genome of hepatitis C [280]. The multi-functional DNAzyme (Dz) delivery system is developed on nano-sized graphene oxide (nGO) for simultaneous detection and knockdown of the target gene. The Dz/nGO complex allowed convenient monitoring of HCV mRNA in living cells and silencing of the HCV gene expression by Dz-mediated catalytic cleavage [281]. Similarly, copper-catalysed nucleoside analogues (NAs) diastereoselectively is synthesized as P-chiral phosphoramidate pro-drugs (ProTides) [282]. A novel lipocyclo-depsipeptide, MA026 was isolated from fermentation broth of *Pseudomonas sp.* and RtIB026, a cyclodepsipeptide with a peptide chain and an N-terminal (R)---hydroxydecanoic acid have shown anti-HCV activity in cell culture assay and revealed that MA026 **918** suppresses HCV infection into host hepatocytes by inhibiting the entry process in a dose-dependent manner (Fig. **117**) [283].

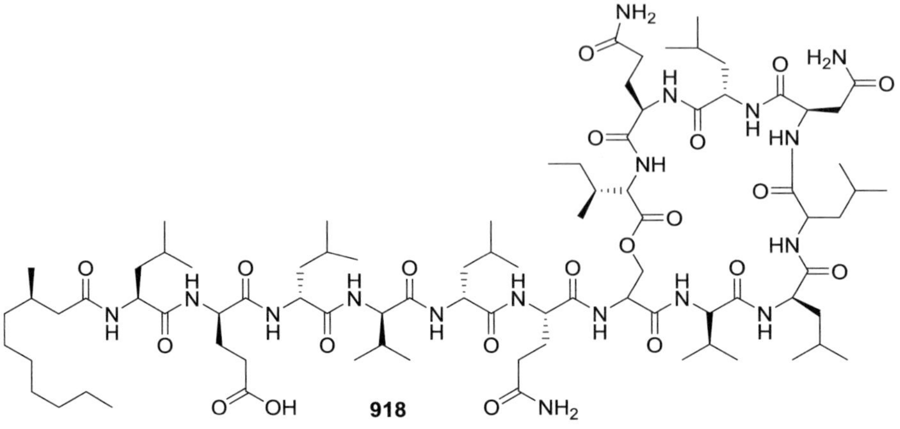
918

Fig. (117). MA026 hepatitis C virus entry inhibitor.

Many water-soluble triazole-bridged acyclodextrin-pentacyclic triterpene conjugates were synthesized and their anti-HCV entry activities were determined based on HCVpp/VSVGpp entry assays. Compounds **921** and **922** gave the best anti-HCV entry activities (IC_{50} 1.18 mM and 0.25 mM), respectively. The anti-HCV entry activity of pentacyclic triterpenes is widely found in plants as potent HCV inhibitors (Fig. **118**) [284].

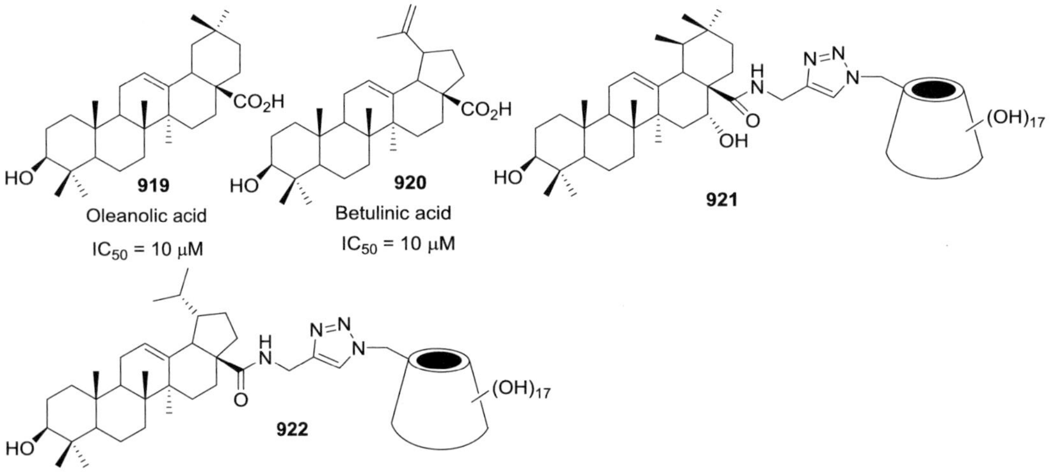
919 Oleanolic acid IC_{50} = 10 μM

920 Betulinic acid IC_{50} = 10 μM

921

922

Fig. (118). Pentacyclic triterpines derivatives as HCV entry inhibitor..

Camel milk is found as alternative medicine to control the HCV infection. It contains proteins (including lactoperoxidase, LPO) with a broad spectrum of activity against pathogenic micro-organisms and viruses. Camel and bovine LPOs showed activity against HCV genotype 4 assayed [285]. Over 500 compounds are randomly selected and rationally designed small molecules where 1-boraadamantane L-phenylalanine methyl ester complex **5**, 1-boraadamantane ethanolamine complex and (*S*)-2-[(adamantane-1-carbonyl)amino]-3-phenyl-propionic acid **923-928** showed a dose-dependent selective anti-proliferative activity in the concentration of 0.1-10 μM (Fig. **119**). The values are consistent with the binding and activation of CD81 and gave a 2-fold improvement compared to the clinically prescribed anti-HCV drug, amantidine in the same concentration range (Fig. **120**) [286].

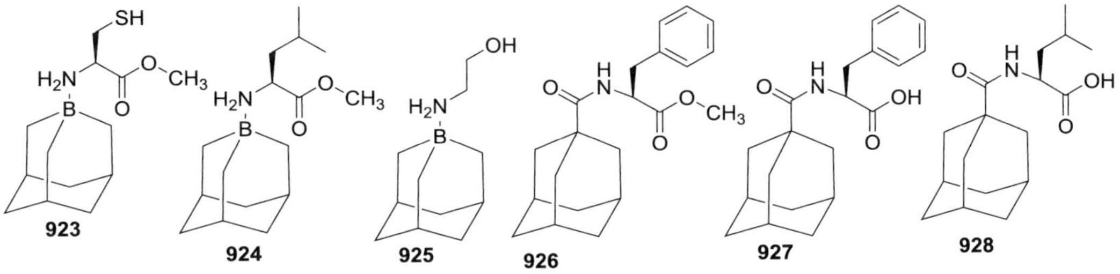

Fig. (119). 1-boraadamantane L-phenylalanine methyl ester derivatives.

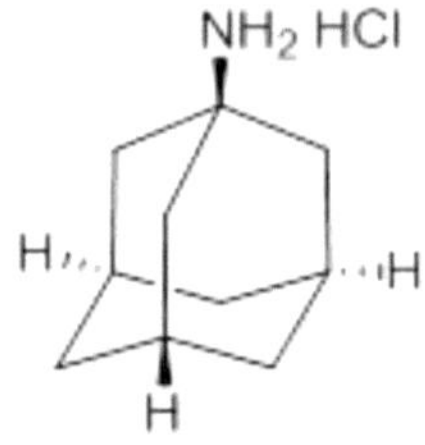

Fig. (120). Anti-HCV drug, amantidine.

PSI-352938 is a novel 2'-deoxy-2'-α-fluoro-2'-β-C-methyl 3',5'-cyclic phosphate nucleotides pro-drug **929-939** currently under investigation for the treatment of hepatitis C virus infection (Fig. **121**) [287].

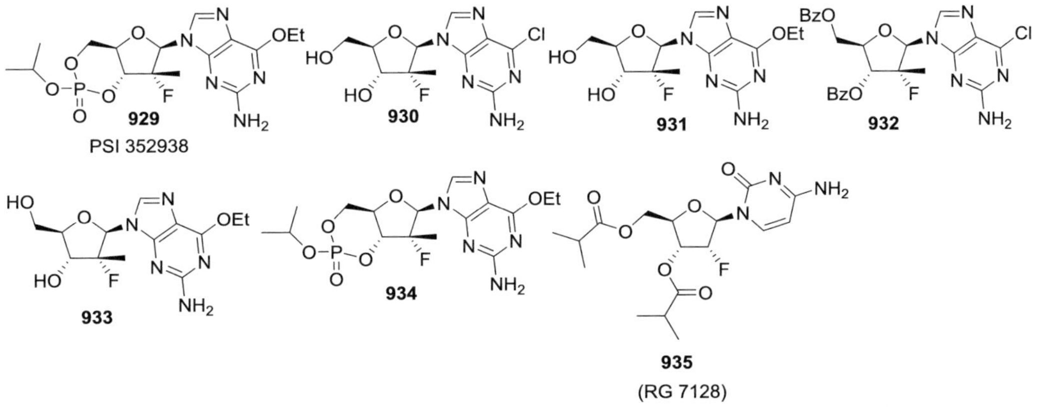

Fig. 121 contd.....

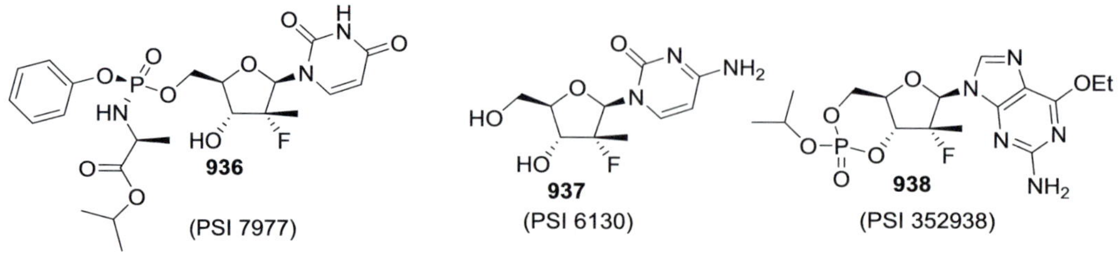

Fig. (121). 2'-deoxy-2'-α-fluoro-2'-β-C-methyl 3',5'-cyclic phosphate nucleoside /tide inhibitor of HCV.

RO8191, a newly discovered small molecule of IFN-like agent displayed potent anti-HCV activity. Thus, several compounds bearing imidazo[1,2-α] [1, 8]naphthyridine core and amide group linked side chain were designed and synthesized. Compounds **939-940** were evaluated against HCV cell culture (HCVcc-hRluc-JFH1) where some of them exhibited remarkable anti-HCV activity (EC_{50} 0.017–0.159 μM) and low toxicity (CC_{50} > 25 μM) (Fig. **122**) [288].

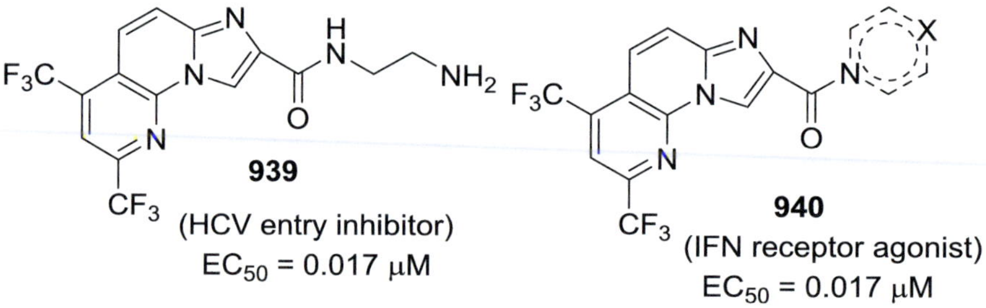

Fig. (122). Imidazo[1,2-α] [1, 8]naphthyridine derivatives.

Non-structural protein 2 (NS2) in HCV encodes an autoprotease activity which is necessary for replication are an attractive anti-viral target. Epoxide-containing compounds **941** known for potent inhibitors of the clotting factor, FXIII, also inhibit NS2-mediated proteolysis *in vitro* and have anti-viral activity in cell culture models [289]. Similarly, spirooxindoles **942** have been identified as privileged chemotypes for antiviral drug development. Among them, spiropyrazolopyridone oxindoles have been reported as potent inhibitors of dengue virus, NS4B, *etc.* leading to the discovery of an orally bioavailable candidate (Fig. **123**). The development of biologically active spirooxindoles for their antiviral potential, primarily focusing on the SARs and modes of action as well as future directions to achieve more potent analogues toward a viable antiviral therapy [290].

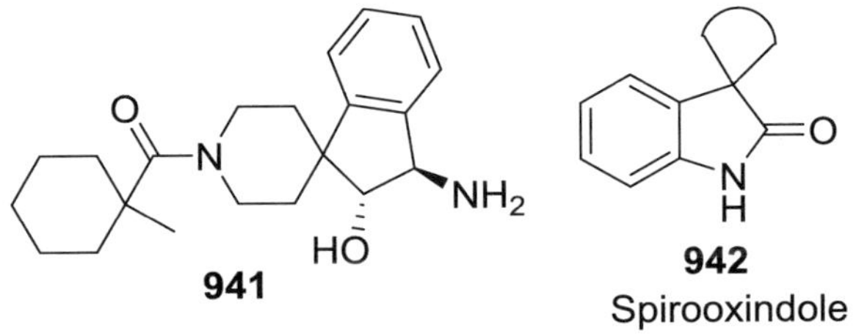

Fig. (123). Anti-NS2 **941** and anti-NS4B **942** compounds.

2'-C-Me-branched ribo-C-nucleoside adenosine analogues, a nucleoside inhibitors (NIs) contains a pyrrolo[2,1-f] [1, 2, 4]triazin-4-amine heterocyclic base and an imidazo[2,1-f] [1, 2, 4]triazin-4-amine heterocyclic base as two compounds with promising anti-HCV *in vitro* activity. Synthesis and evaluation of these compounds substituted at the 2-, 7- and 8-positions of the heterocyclic bases gave many compounds. However, 7-fluoro analogue displayed good potency and triple combination therapy is poorly tolerated with serious adverse side-effects [291]. Also, amidino urea compounds were designed as isosteric analogues of the anti-viral drug moroxydine. Derivatives **943** and **944** showed excellent HCV inhibition activity and proved to inhibit a step(s) of the RNA replication (Fig. **124**) [292].

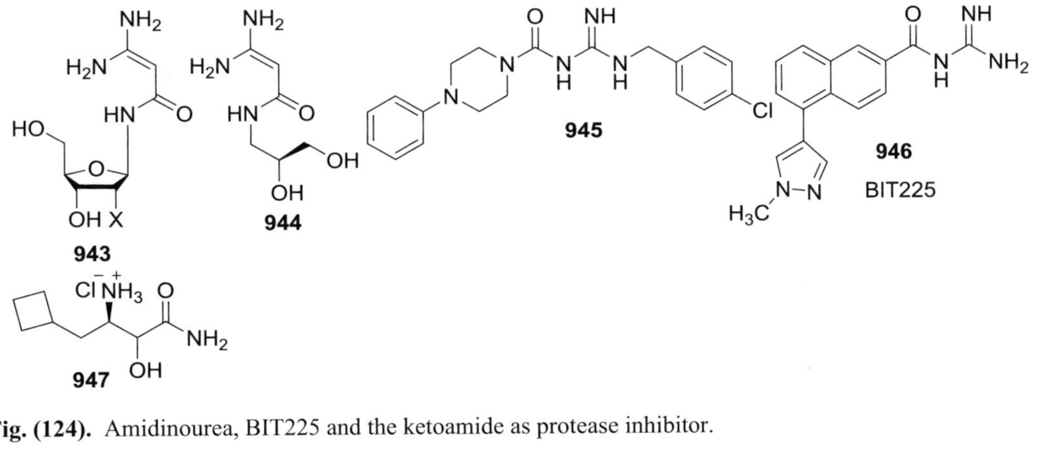

Fig. (124). Amidinourea, BIT225 and the ketoamide as protease inhibitor.

(N-[5-(1-Methyl-1H-pyrazol-4-yl)-napthalene-2-carbonyl]-guanidine: CAS No. 917909-71-8), BIT225 **946** was identified as HCV inhibitor of p7 ion channel activity. It has also potent anti-viral activity against the HCV model pesti-virus, bovine viral, diarrhea virus (BVDV). Combinations of BIT225 with recombinant interferon alpha-2b (rIFNα-2b) showed synergistic anti-viral action against BVDV. Synergic effect was also observed between BIT225 and two nucleoside analogues which inhibit the HCV RNA-dependent RNA polymerase [293].

Similarly, stereoselective addition of 2-phenyloxazol-4-yl trifluoromethane sulfonate to N-sulfinylimines is obtained for the synthesis of ketoamide **947** fragment of the protease inhibitor boceprevir [294]. These protease inhibitors contain a β-amino-α- ketoamide **948-949** that binds to the NS3 protease at S1 pocket and forms covalent and reversible complex with Ser139.3. In the case of boceprevir, the amino stereocenter of the β-amino-α-ketoamide undergoes rapid equilibration under cellular conditions (Fig. **125**) [295].

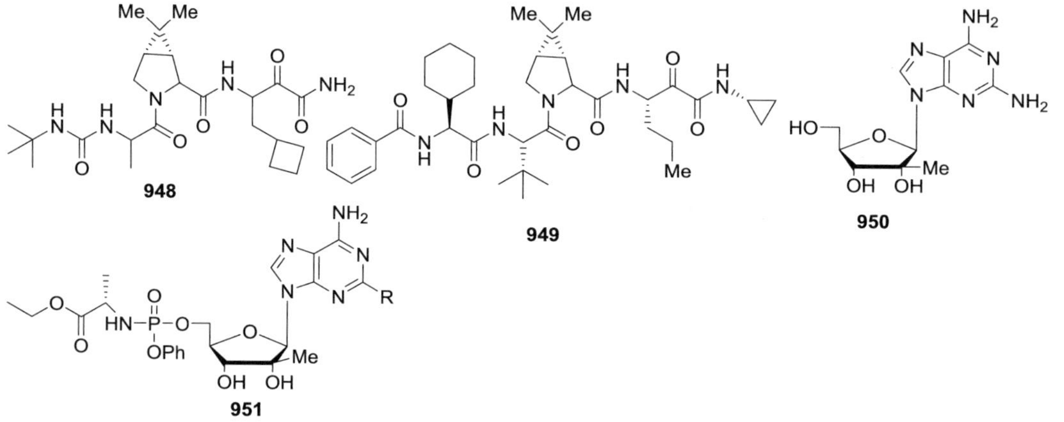

Fig. (125). Protease inhibitors.

Several 2,6-modified purine 2′-C-methylribonucleosides and their phosphoramidate pro-drugs **950-951** were synthesized and screened for inhibition of HCV RNA replication in Huh-7 cells [296]. Piperazine drugs **952-956** based chlorcyclizine (CCZ, Rac-2) has anti-HCV activity (Fig. **126**) [297].

Imidazo[1,2-α] [1, 8]naphthyridine derivatives like RO8191 analogues **957-959** were synthesized (Fig. **127**). Some of them displayed promising anti-HCV activities in the HCV cell culture [298].

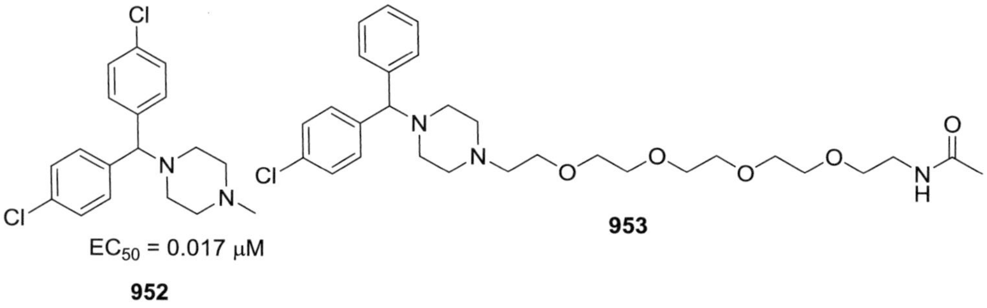

Fig. 126 contd.....

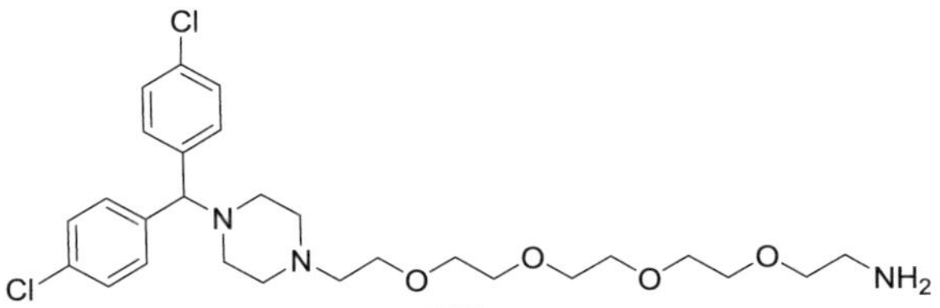

954

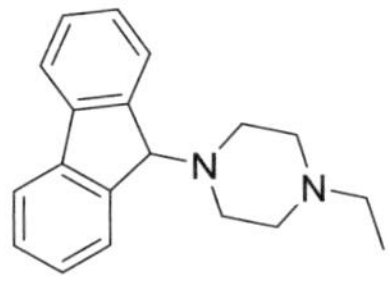

955

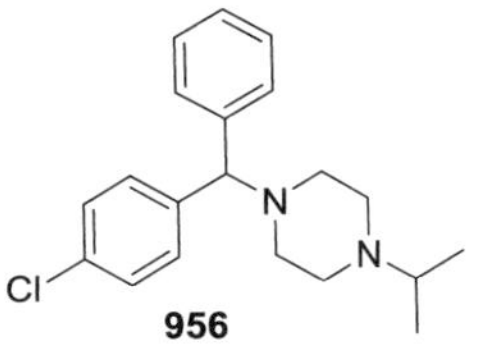

956

Fig. (126). Chlorcyclizine (CCZ, Rac-2) and analogue.

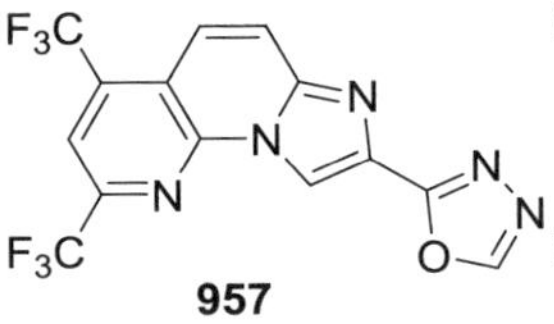

957
RO8191

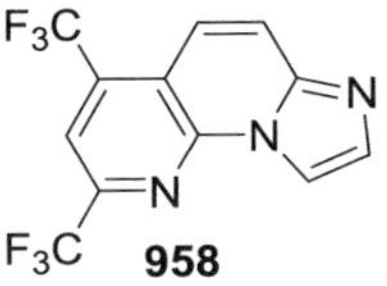

958

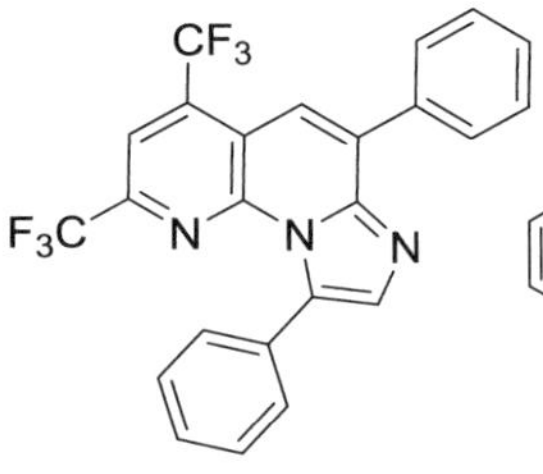

959

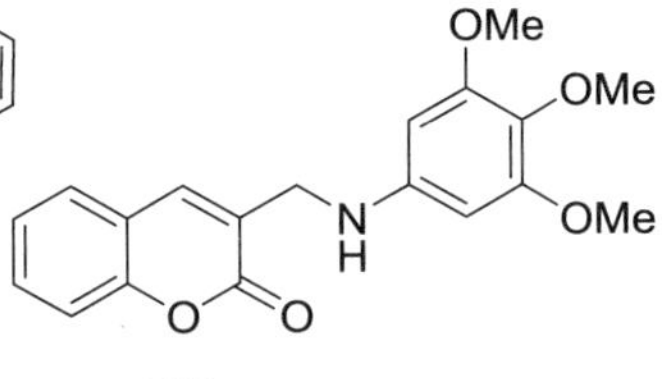

960

Fig. (127). RO8191 and analogue and 3-(3’,4’,5’-trimethoxyanilin-1’-yl)-methylaminocoumarin.

Novel anilinocoumarins were synthesized and their efficacy against HCV replication was evaluated. 3-(3’,4’,5’-Trimethoxyanilin-1’-yl)-methylamino coumarin **960** was exhibited strong anti-HCV activity against HCV RNA levels (EC_{50} 12.0 μM). A combination treatment of compound **960** and interferon-α with telaprevir also induced a significant decrease in HCV RNA levels [299]. Aspartic acid (Asp) and iminodiacetic acid (IDA) esters of amidate counterparts as 2’-- -methyl containing nucleosides, 2’-C-Me-cytidine, 2’-C-Me-uridine and 2’-C--e-2’-fluoro-uridine were reported for anti-HCV properties where Asp-based phosphoramidates are found 550-fold more potent than the parent nucleosides. The inhibitory activity of Asp-ProTides was higher than the Ala-ProTides recommended that Asp would be a potential amino acid candidate for developing novel anti-viral pro-drugs [300].

Quinoxalin-2(1H)-one derivative, N-(7-(cyclohexyl-(methyl) amino)-3-oxo--,4-dihydro quinoxalin-6-yl carbamothioyl) benzamide **962** gave potent anti-HCV activity *in vitro*. Further, SAR study of N-(7-(cyclohexyl (methyl)amino)-3-o-o-3,4-dihydroquinoxalin-6-yl carbamothioyl)-furan-2-carboxamide (EC_{50} 1.8 μM), 6-(cyclohexyl-(methyl) amino)-7-(4-phenylthiazol-2-ylamino)quino-alin-2(1H)-one (EC_{50} 1.67 μM), 2-(cyclo hexyl(methyl)amino)-3-(4-phenyl-thiazol-2-ylamino)-7,8,9,10-tetrahydro-5H-pyrido[1,2-a] quinoxalin-6(6aH)-one (EC_{50} 1.19 μM), 8-(cyclohexyl (methyl) amino)-7-(4-phenylthiazol-2-ylamino) pyrrolo [1,2-a]quinoxalin-4(5H)-one (EC_{50} 1.82 μM) and 6-(diethylamino)-7-(4-phenylthiazol-2-ylamino) quinoxalin-2(1H)-one (EC_{50} 1.27 μM) showed anti-HCV activities (Fig. **128**) [301].

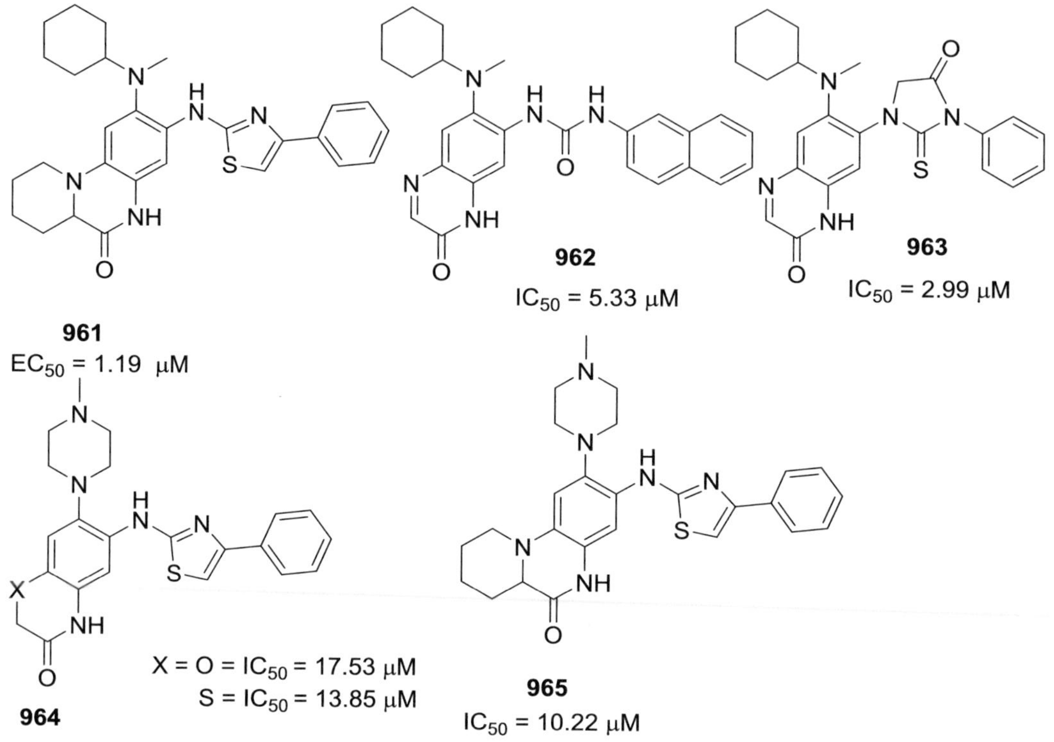

Fig. (128). Quinoxalin-2(1H)-one derivatives for HCV infections..

In the synthesis of benzoxaborole, a byproduct as macrocyclic urea **2** was found to be a novel and potent HCV protease inhibitor. Compounds **966** was established to be more potent in HCV replicon assays than leading second generation inhibitors danoprevir and TMC-435350 [302].

Sixty-seven phosphorodiamidates are reported as both symmetrical and asymmetric phosphorodiamidates of two 6-*O*-alkyl 2′-*C*-methyl guanosines with significant variation in the diamidate structure. They have various esterified amino acids in both D- and L-forms along with simple amines. They were evaluated against hepatitis C virus in replicon assay. Many compounds were non-cytotoxic at 100 μM, leading to high anti-viral selectivities [303]. Parthenolide **967** was found an active compound for fever and migraine and also a lead compound against HCV replication in a sub-genomic RNA replicon assay (Fig. **129**) (EC_{50} 2.21 μM). It has ability to potentiate the interferon-α and SAR study elucidated that the spatial arrangement of the terpenoid skeleton fused with α-methylene-γ-lactone moiety, produces maximal anti-HCV activity. In addition, a strong anti-HCV potency may be due to a possibility of secondary amino adducts converting back to parthenolide or being replaced by the nucleophilic residues of proteins inside the cells [304].

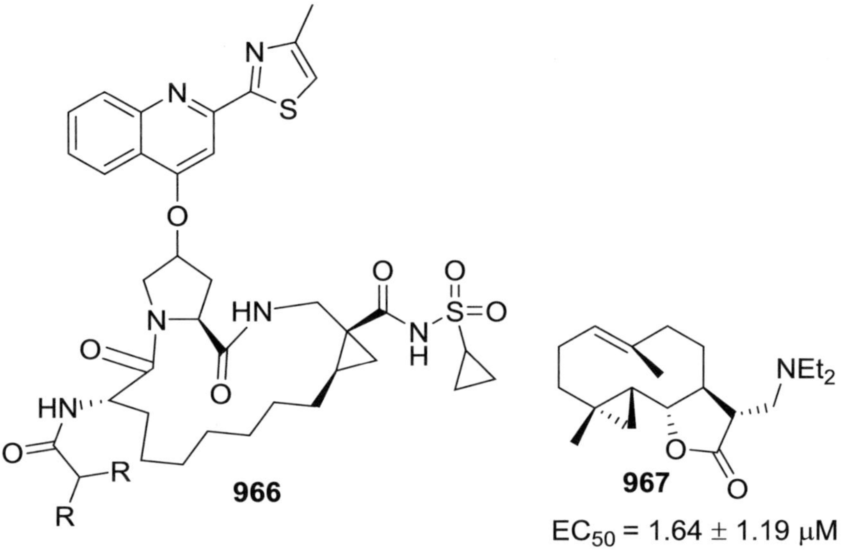

Fig. (129). Potent HCV replicon inhibitors.

In the replicon assays, thiazolides [2-hydroxyaroyl-*N*-(thiazol-2-yl)amides **968-970** were shown as anti-HCV genotypes 1a and 1b (Fig. **130**). However, the SARs study gave better anti- HBV properties than the HCV for these thiazolides although an electron-with-drawing group at C(5′) afforded similar potency. Among the salicyloylanilides, the *m*-fluorophenyl analogue was found most promising; niclosamide and close analogues showed very low solubility and bioavailability [305].

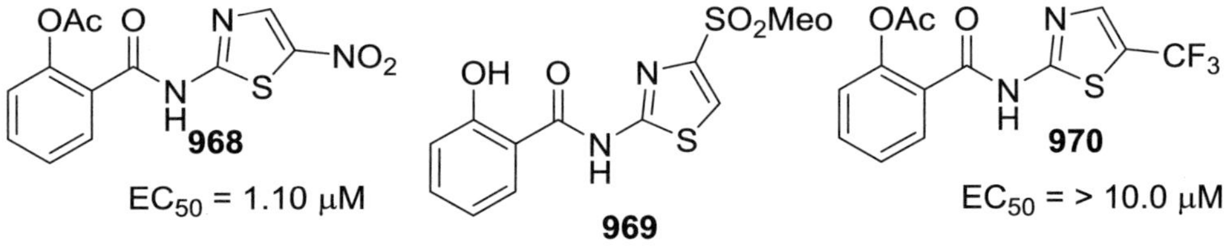

Fig. (130). Thiazolides [2-hydroxyaroyl-*N*-(thiazol-2-yl)amides] anti-HCV genotypes 1a and 1b.

New induced-fit docking program (GENIUS) was used to the discovery of a new class of NS3-4A protease inhibitors **971-976** (IC_{50} 1–10 lM) (Fig. **131**). Further, the docking models and preliminary structure–activity relationships revealed as new inhibitors [306].

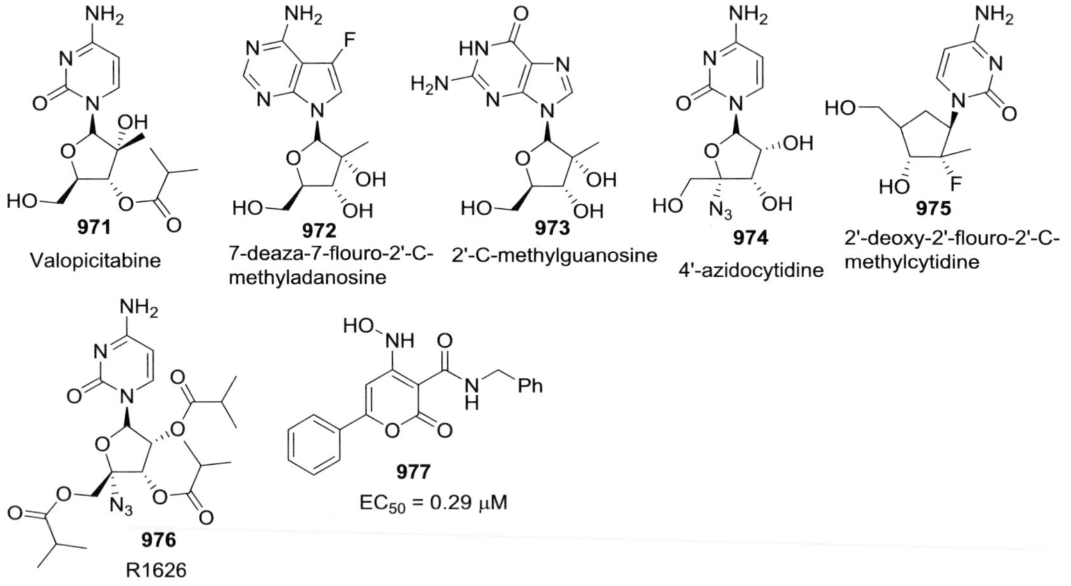

Fig. (131). Various NRRIs possessing anti-HCV activity..

The three dimensional-quantitative structure activity relationship (3D-QSAR) study was performed on a series of 4-hydroxyamino α-pyranone carboxamide analogues using comparative molecular similarity indices analysis (COMSIA) to develop a satisfactory model, providing a reliable prediction based on 4-hydroxyamino α-pyranone carboxamide analogues **977** as anti-HCV inhibitors [307, 308]. Different small-molecule compound collection (300,000 compounds) were screened using high-throughput method in cell-based HCV luciferase reporter assay, where benzofuran compounds **978-980** identified as HCV potent inhibitors (EC_{50} <100 nM) of HCV, low cytotoxicity and excellent selectivity (selective index CC_{50}/EC_{50} >371-fold) (Fig. **132**). Further, the design and synthesis of 45-compounds library were explored as anti-HCV activity through SAR studies [309]. In the drug discovery process, computer-aided drug design techniques and in particular, de novo methodologies found useful to identify putative ligands for a specific target, relying only on the structural information of the target [310].

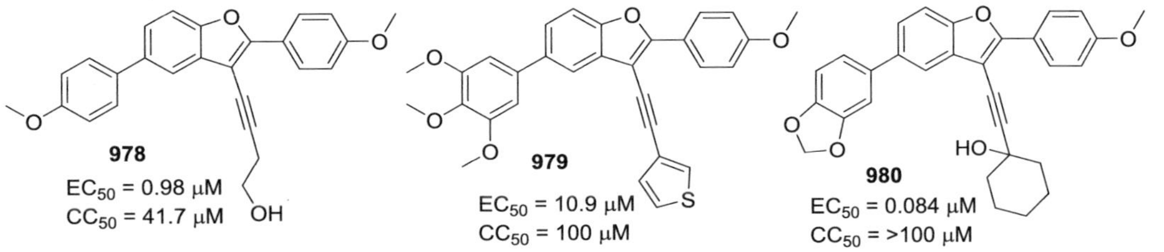

Fig. (132). Benzofuran based qHTS compounds.

4.21. Adherence Therapy

Adherence therapy is the most important factors associated with the success of anti-viral treatment. It was used in the PEG-IFN era as the "80/80 rule", *i.e.*, patients who receive > 80% of the medication are treated for > 80% of the planned duration of treatment known as adherent. One study showed that a cumulative ribavirin dose of > 60% is important to achieve SVR. For the IFN based triple therapy, adherence to the DAA becomes even more important. For some patient populations, they are treated under DOT (directly observed therapy) condition to guarantee adherence. Another important issue is drug-drug interactions that can diminish the effectiveness of the DAAs or induce toxicity of medications which may lead to discontinuation of all drugs and helps in the optimal management of patients receiving DAA treatment [311].

5. FUTURE PERSPECTIVES

The development of direct targeting anti-viral agents on viral life cycle, have shown effective treatment. Unlike non-specific anti-virals (IFN-R and ribavirin) and immune based therapies (anti-HCV immunoglobulins, interleukin-2, interleukin-10 and several T-cell vaccines), target-specific anti-virals directly blocked the viral replication and so prevent infection in the hepatocytes. Therefore, efforts have been done to yield a diverse set of anti-hepatitis agents which inhibit HCV replication *via* both viral and host targets. Theoretically, it was found that for IFN-free cure, anti-HCV drugs should have distinct mechanistic path and work additively and/or synergistically with orthogonal resistance profiles against HCV in combination.

The researches are mainly focused on the inhibition of key viral enzymes like two proteolytic enzymes NS2/3 and NS3/NS4A. In addition, NS3 possesses an RNA helicase domain and the NS5B RNA-dependent RNA polymerase (RdRp) are another attractive therapeutic target. It is a virus specific enzyme with no functional homologues in the host and so may be less toxic to the host. The 5'-non-translated region of the RNA genome constitutes an internal ribosomal entry site (IRES) that binds to the ribosomes or ribosome-like structures of the infected cell and allowed translation of the pro-viral DNA genome. It is highly conserved but an outstanding target too for the drug development. HCV NS3 serine protease based inhibitors of *N*-terminal cleavage products of peptide substrates have prospective to become efficacious anti-viral agents. HCV replicons with dual resistance to the PI and NNI is selected *in vitro,* suggested that a cure will require more than two agents. Inhibitors of NS5B polymerase are an excellent foundation in the new inhibitor discovery. Similarly, silico methods have been applied to discover and develop new NS5B polymerase inhibitors including quantitative structure-activity relationships (QSAR), pharmacophore modeling, molecular dynamics (MD) simulation and molecular docking. Novel small molecule NS5B polymerase inhibitors lead a virtual screening workflow such as random forest (RB-VS), e-pharmacophore (PB-VS) and molecular docking (DB-VS) methods. In the virtual screening, the NS5B polymerase is one of the most attractive targets for developing new drugs to block HCV infection. Molecular modelling methodologies are also considered an essential component of drug discovery and lead optimization. Among different methodologies, de novo drug design can often provide researcher with new ideas for targeting less exploited biological targets or to generate new IP around well-established therapies.

The natural products obtained from plants are potential anti-viral agents. However, some other natural compounds, do not target the virus directly, might also be used to improve HCV therapy. Several novel synthetic drugs have entered or will enter soon in clinical evaluation for their clinical usefulness. Aside from the safety and efficacy requirements of all new drugs, the success of targeted agents will be heavily influenced by their ability to inhibit all viral variants and prevent the emergence of escape mutants. Although the agents targeting host rather than viral factors are less likely to fail owing to this problem, but no drug can be considered totally exempt from the risk of resistance development. The first wave of experimental targeted drugs, yielding promising results in the clinical trials however wider novel anti-viral agents needed. For this, drug discoverers must consider and pursue all other known viral targets for which there are not yet clinically useful inhibitors such as p7 ion channel, the NS2/3 cysteine protease and the NS3 helicase. The advancement in the field of therapeutic RNAi made it conceivable to target, a variety of host factors that are essential for viral replication or persistence for which development of small molecule inhibitors may turn out to be prohibitively difficult.

6. HEPATITIS D

Worldwide an estimated 350 millions people are chronically HBV infected and 15-20 millions of them are also found hepatitis delta virus (HDV) positive annually. Hepatitis D virus is a defective RNA virus which requires HBV surface antigen (HBsAg) for complete replication and transmission. Hepatitis D infection occurs only in the case of HBsAg-positive individuals as acute co-infection or super-infection. Chronic HDV infection leads to more severe liver disease than chronic HBV mono-infection with fibrosis progression and a slightly increased risk of hepatocellular carcinoma and cirrhosis. Thus far, only interferon-α treatment has been revealed to exert some anti-viral activity against HDV. While pegylated interferon lead to prolonged virological off-treatment responses in 25% patients but long-term HDV RNA relapses may occur [312].

Hepatitis D virus is a single-stranded RNA virus of 36 nm in size, having HDV RNA and delta antigens. It is high base-paired (about 1700 nucleotides), circular and smallest known genome of all animal virus, coated with an envelope protein derived from the pre-S and S antigens of the HBV [313]. It contains six open reading frames (ORFs) of which three on the genomic and three on the anti-genomic strand. A single nucleotide change (A-G) in the small HDAg sequence led to the synthesis of large HDAg. The small HDAg accelerates genome synthesis while the large HDAg inhibits HDV RNA synthesis which is necessary for virion morphogenesis. Mostly, hepatitis cases were induced by genotype 3 delta virus. Acute HBV/HDV co-infection in adults led to the recovery in more than 90% of cases but frequently causes severe acute hepatitis with a high risk for developing a fulminant course. In contrast, HDV is cleared spontaneously in minority of patients with HDV super-infection of chronic HBsAg carriers.

In the treatment of HBV infections, several nucleoside and nucleotide analogs have been used effectively but they are ineffective against HDV. Famciclovir was used in 1990 to treat HBV infection which had no significant anti-viral activity against HDV. Lamivudine is ineffective in trials of hepatitis delta [314]. Ribavirin alone or in combination with interferon also failed to increase rate of HDV RNA clearance. Similarly, short-term entecavir treatment failed to show significant activity against HDV and very long treatment with HBV polymerase inhibitors may lead to beneficial effects in hepatitis delta possibly due to the reduction of HBsAg levels. It is also interesting to note that HDV RNA decline was not associated with HBsAg decline [315]. Both PEG-IFN groups showed a significant higher reduction in HDV RNA levels than the adefovir monotherapy however it is better than PEG-IFN α-2a and adefovir monotherapy. Lonafarnib and Myrcludex-B is also being developed for hepatitis delta where Myrcludex-B is a lipopeptide, derived from preS1 domain of the HBV envelope, has delayed HDV infection in mice transplanted with human hepatocytes [316].

7. HEPATITIS E

Globally an estimated 56,000 deaths are reported each year due to Hepatitis E virus (HEV) infection. It causes an inflammatory liver disease to be endemic in many tropical countries due to poor sanitary conditions [317]. Hepatitis E virus is a non-enveloped single-stranded RNA virus of the Hepeviridae genus and *Hepevirus* family. The size of genome is 7.2 kb with three ORFs and 3′ and 5′ cis elements which play a major role in HEV transcription and replication [318]. There are four HEV human pathogenic genotypes cause endemic and epidemic infections in different part of the world. These genotypes are usually transmitted fecal-orally by contaminated drinking water under poor sanitary conditions. In contrast, genotype 3 can be found in humans and animals in Europe, US and Asia. For this genotype, zoonotic transmission, foodborne transmission or *via* contact with infected animals has been depicted [319]. The natural host for HEV is humans while animals are possible reservoir in the amplification of the virus. The mode of transmission could be through transfusion. No specific treatment for HEV infection is recommended, but ribavirin therapy has been effective in some persons although it is contraindicated with pregnant women. In chronically infected patients, a combination of ribavirin and interferon-α has also been used. Sofosbuvir was used as a modest inhibitor of HEV and a recombinant HEV vaccine was approved for the use in China since 2012.

CONCLUSION

In the development of anti-viral agents, enormous work has been done in relatively short span of time. Further avenues are possible to arise as more and more information has been revealed about virus life-cycle. For the best possible future therapy of chronic hepatitis at least four criteria should be fulfilled. Firstly, it should be IFN-free to reduce side effects; Secondly, it should adopt a high barrier of drug-resistance; Thirdly, it should require a short duration of treatment and Forthly, SVR should be more than 90%.

A combination therapy is well-tolerated by patients where novel all-oral combinations may be superior for the treatment of patients with decompensated cirrhosis which further permit ultra-short duration of treatment and reduce the costs of anti-viral therapy. Finding of new receptors has also revealed useful anti-viral targets, enabled the foundation of much needed cell-culture system for the infection and stimulated enthusiasm for the development of new and curative drugs. Similarly, agents such as siRNA, HBsAg and capsid inhibitors have accomplished clinical trials with diverse mechanism of action as compared to the current therapies. The new delivery technologies such as lipid nanoparticles have breathed new life in the siRNA approach. Innovative technologies, screening and profiling have made possible the development of many agents such as entry inhibitors, use of novel chimeric epitopes, selective killing of infected hepatocytes and novel vaccines. There is much anticipation that these agents have novel mechanisms for inhibition, replication which used alone or in combination with the existing therapies, would helpful in better management of chronic hepatitis. The great challenge is to reduce intrahepatic viral DNA levels and to eradicate cccDNA. In addition to the DAAs, it is thought that agents that can boost the immune response against the virus, can play an important role in sustained off drug virological responses. Thus, new HTAs are in development for therapeutic vaccines, ligand pathway inhibitors, novel chimeric antigens and enhancement of antigen might be beneficial.

The essential component in drug discovery and lead optimization are SAR study, molecular modeling and virtual screening methodologies. An advancement in computer software can effectively speed up the design and optimization of novel and active molecules. The de novo drug design can often provide researchers with new thoughts for targeting less exploited biological targets or to generate new IP for well-established therapies. Without de novo drug design consideration, the computer-based methods have been used successfully in the viral infections. The constant validation and identification of novel targets and rapidly increasing number of 3D-structures from different viruses which are present in the Protein Data Bank, offering new exciting opportunities in the anti-viral drug discovery [320]. In this context, it is easy to see that de novo approaches with the most advanced algorithms and software could play an increasingly important role in the design of the future anti-viral agents. Furthermore, the proof-of-concept investigational drugs are entering into clinical studies with promising potency and good pharmacokinetic profiles.

CONFLICT OF INTEREST

The author (editor) declares no conflict of interest, financial or otherwise.

ACKNOWLEDGEMENTS

Thanks to my PhD students Mr. Mohammad Waheed and Mr. Danish Khan for immense support. The reviewer's valuable comments are highly appreciated.

ABBRAVIATIONS

AVP	Antiviral protein
HAV	Hepatitis A virus
HBV	Hepatitis B virus
HCV	Hepatitis C virus
HDV	Hepatitis D virus
HEV	Hepatitis E virus
HBsAg	Surface HBV antigen

R-IFN	R-Interferon
cccDNA	Covalently closed circular DNA
rcDNA	Relaxed circle DNA
TLR7/8/9	Toll-like receptors
STING	Stimulator of interferon genes
PAMPs	Pathogen-associated molecular patterns
Nod	Nucleotide-binding oligomerization domain
CLRs	C-type lectin receptors
c-di-AMP	Cyclic di-adenosine monophosphate
c-di-GMP	Cyclic di-guanosine monophosphate
cGAS	Cyclic guanosine monophosphate-adenosine monophosphate synthase
RT	Reverse transcriptase
NK	Natural killer
TDF	Tenofovir disoproxil fumarate
pgRNA	Pre-genomic mRNA
HBcAg	Hepatitis B core antigen
HBeAg	Hepatitis B e. antigen
HBxAg	Hepatitis B x. antigen
TP	Terminal protein
HTA-i	HTA immunomodulators
HTA-hf	HTA host functions
NTCP	Sodium taurocholate cotransporting polypeptide
CsA	Cyclosporine A
DAAs	Direct-acting antivirals
FOXO1	Forkhead transcription factor
SAR	Structure-activity relationship
D-FMAU	2'-fluoro-5-methyl-β-D-arabinofuranosyluracil
RNAi	RNA interference
GAG	Glycosaminoglycans
VLDL	Very low density lipoproteins
NS	Non-structural
RdRp	RNA-dependent RNA polymerase
PI	Protease inhibitor
EGCG	(–)-Epigallocatechin-3-gallate
HTS	High-throughput-screening

NS5B	Non-structural protein 5B
Nis	Nucleotide inhibitors
NNIs	Non-nucleoside inhibitors
PRR	Pattern recognition receptors
HepG2 2.2.15	Human hepatoblastoma cell line

REFERENCES

[1] Furman PA, Lam AM, Murakami E. Nucleoside analog inhibitors of hepatitis C viral replication: recent advances, challenges and trends. Future Med Chem 2009; 1: 1429-52.

[2] Mauss BM, Wedemeyer SR. Hepatology. A clinical textbook. 7th ed., 2016.

[3] Faillon S, Martinot A, Hau I, *et al.* Impact of travel on the seroprevalence of hepatitis A in children. J Clin Virol 2013; 56(1): 46-51.

[4] Collier MG, Khudyakov YE, Selvage D, *et al.* Outbreak of hepatitis A in the USA associated with frozen pomegranate arils imported from Turkey: an epidemiological case study. Lancet Infect Dis 2014; 10: 976-81.

[5] Choi HK, Song YG, Han SH, *et al.* Clinical features and outcomes of acute kidney injury among patients with acute hepatitis A. J Clin Virol 2011; 52: 192-7.

[6] Drexler JF, Corman VM, Lukashev AN, *et al.* Evolutionary origins of hepatitis A virus in small mammals. Proc Natl Acad Sci USA 2015; 112: 15190-5.

[7] Feng Z, Li Y, McKnight KL. Hensley. L.; Lanford, R. E.; Walker, C. M.; Lemon, S. M. Human pDCs preferentially sense enveloped hepatitis A virions. J Clin Invest 2015; 125: 169-76.

[8] Schulte I, Hitziger T, Giugliano S, *et al.* Characterization of CD8+ T-cell response in acute and resolved hepatitis A virus infection. J Hepatol 2011; 54: 201-8.

[9] Tseng YT, Chang SY, Liu WC, *et al.* Comparative effectiveness of two doses *versus* three doses of hepatitis a vaccine in HIV-infected and HIVuninfected men who have sex with men. Hepatology 2013; 57(5): 1734-41.

[10] Esser-Nobis K, Harak C, Schult P, *et al.* Novel perspectives for hepatitis A virus therapy revealed by comparative analysis of hepatitis C virus and hepatitis A virus RNA replication. Hepatology 2015; 62(2): 397-408.

[11] Montuclard C, Hamza S, Rollot F, *et al.* Causes of death in people with chronic HBV infection: A population-based cohort study. J Hepatol 2015; 62: 1265-71.

[12] Asselah T, Lada O, Moucari R, Martinot M, Boyer N, Marcellin P. Title???. Clin Liver Dis 2007; 11: 839-49.

[13] Liu J, Zhang E, Ma Z, *et al.* Enhancing virus-specific immunity *in vivo* by combining therapeutic vaccination and PD-L1 blockade in chronic hepadnaviral infection. PLoS Pathog 2014; 10(1): e1003856.

[14] Ning X, Nguyen D, Mentzer L, *et al.* Secretion of genome-free hepatitis B virus-single strand blocking model for virion morphogenesis of para-retrovirus. PLoS Pathog 2011; 7: e1002255.

[15] Pierson EE, Keifer DZ, Selzer L, *et al.* Detection of late intermediates in virus capsid assembly by charge detection mass spectrometry. J Am Chem Soc 2014; 136: 3536-41.

[16] Burg JS, Ingram JR, Venkatakrishnan AJ, *et al.* Structural biology. Structural basis for chemokine recognition and activation of a viral G protein-coupled receptor. Science 2015; 347: 1113-7.

[17] Chang J, Guo J-T. Treatment of chronic hepatitis B with pattern recognition receptor agonists: Current

status and potential for a cure. Antiviral Res 2015; 121: 152-9.

[18] Takeuchi O, Akira S. Pattern recognition receptors and inflammation. Cell 2010; 140(6): 805-20.

[19] Ishikawa H, Barber GN. STING is an endoplasmic reticulum adaptor that facilitates innate immune signalling. Nature 2008; 455(7213): 674-8.

[20] Guo F, Han Y, Zhao X, *et al.* STING agonists induce an innate antiviral immune response against hepatitis B virus. Antimicrob Agents Chemother 2015; 59(2): 1273-81.

[21] Iwasaki A, Medzhitov R. Control of adaptive immunity by the innate immune system. Nat Immunol 2015; 16(4): 343-53.

[22] Shlomai A, Schwartz RE, Ramanan V, *et al.* Modeling host interactions with hepatitis B virus using primary and induced pluripotent stem cell-derived hepatocellular systems. Proc Natl Acad Sci USA 2015; 111(33): 12193-8.

[23] Sato S, Li K, Kameyama T, *et al.* The RNA sensor RIG-I dually functions as an innate sensor and direct antiviral factor for hepatitis B virus. Immunity 2015; 42(1): 123-32.

[24] Gao LH, Trinh N. Li; J.; Nguyen, M. H. Tenofovir Is superior to Entecavir for achieving complete viral suppression in HBeAg-positive chronic hepatitis B patients with high HBV DNA. Aliment Pharmacol Ther 2014; 39(6): 629-37.

[25] Dando T, Plosker G. Adefovir dipivoxil: a review of its use in chronic hepatitis B. Drugs 2003; 63: 2215-34.

[26] Menne S, Tumas DB, Liu KH, *et al.* Sustained efficacy and seroconversion with the Toll-like receptor 7 agonist GS-9620 in the Woodchuck model of chronic hepatitis B. J Hepatol 2015; 62(6): 1237-45.

[27] Jo J, Tan AT, Ussher JE, *et al.* Toll-like receptor 8 agonist and bacteria trigger potent activation of innate immune cells in human liver. PLoS Pathog 2014; 10(6): e1004210.

[28] Lee JM, Park JY. Long-term adefovir dipivoxil monotherapy for up to 5 years in lamivudine-resistant chronic hepatitis B. Antivir Ther 2010; 15: 235-41.

[29] Tian Y, Chen WL, Ou JH. Effects of interferon-alpha/beta on HBV replication determined by viral load. PLoS Pathog 2011; 7: e1002159.

[30] Papatheodoridis G, Buti M, Cornberg M, Janssen H, Mutimer D. Easl clinical practice guidelines: Management of chronic hepatitis B virus infection. J Hepatol 2012; 57: 167-85.

[31] Liaw YF, Gane E, Leung N, *et al.* 2-year globe trial results: Telbivudine is superior to lamivudine in patients with chronic hepatitis B. Gastroenterology 2009; 136: 486-95.

[32] Erik De Clercq. Antivirals past, present and future. Biochem Pharmacol 2013; 85: 727-44.

[33] Milich DR, Jones JE, Hughes JL, Price J, Raney AK, McLachlan A. Is a function of the secreted hepatitis B e antigen to induce immunologic tolerance in utero? Proc Natl Acad Sci USA 1990; 87: 6599-603.

[34] Jansen K, Thamm M, Bock CT, *et al.* High prevalence and high incidence of coinfection with hepatitis B, hepatitis C, and syphilis and low rate of effective vaccination against hepatitis B in HIV-positive men who have sex with men with known date of HIV seroconversion in Germany. PLoS One 2015; 10: e0142515.

[35] Zhang L, Gui XE, Teter C, *et al.* Effects of hepatitis B immunization on prevention of mother-to-infant transmission of hepatitis B virus and on the immune response of infants towards hepatitis B vaccine. Vaccine 2014; 32: 6091-7.

[36] Papatheodoridis GV, Chrysanthos N, Hadziyannis E, Cholongitas E, Manesis EK. Longitudinal changes in serum HBV DNA levels and predictors of progression during the natural course of HBeAg-negative chronic hepatitis B virus infection. J Viral Hepat 2008; 15: 434-41.

[37] Polizzotto MN, Wood EM, Ingham H, Keller AJ. Reducing the risk of transfusion-transmissible viral

infection through blood donor selection: the Australian experience 2000 through 2006. Transfusion 2008; 48: 55-63.

[38] Borzooy Z, Jazayeri SM, Mirshafiey A, *et al.* Identification of occult hepatitis B virus (HBV) infection and viral antigens in healthcare workers who presented low to moderate levels of anti-HBs after HBV vaccination. Germs 2015; 5: 134-40.

[39] Niu Y, Chen X, Feng L, *et al.* Anti-HBc-positive/HBsAg-negative liver donors pose a higher risk of occult HBV infection but do not cause severe histological damage in liver grafts. Clin Res Hepatol Gastroenterol 2014; 38: 475-80.

[40] Ganem D, Prince AM. Hepatitis B virus infection-natural history and clinical consequences. N Engl J Med 2004; 350: 1118-29.

[41] Kang L, Pan J, Wu J, Hu J, Sun Q, Tang J. Anti-HBV drugs: Progress, unmet needs, and new hope. Viruses 2015; 7: 4960-77.

[42] Block TM, Rawat S, Brosgart CL. Chronic hepatitis B: A wave of new therapies on the horizon. Antiviral Res 2015; 121: 69-81.

[43] Yeh SF, Hong CY, Huang YL, *et al.* Effect of an extract from Phyllanthus amarus on hepatitis B surface antigen gene expression in human hepatoma cells. Antiviral Res 1993; 20: 185-92.

[44] Zlotnick A, Venkatakrishnan B, Tan Z, *et al.* Core protein: A pleiotropic keystone in the HBV lifecycle. Antiviral Res 2015; 121: 82-93.

[45] Blanchet M, Sureau C. Infectivity determinants of the hepatitis b virus pre-s domain are confined to the N-terminal 75 amino acid residues. J Virol 2007; 81: 5841-9.

[46] Bock CT, Schwinn S, Locarnini S, *et al.* Structural organization of the hepatitis B virus Minichromosome J. Med Biol 2001; 307: 183-96.

[47] Harms ZD, Haywood DG, Kneller AR, *et al.* Single-particle electrophoresis in nanochannels. Anal Chem 2015; 87: 699-705.

[48] Zhang Y, Mao R, Yan R, *et al.* Transcription of hepatitis B virus covalently closed circular DNA is regulated by CpG methylation during chronic infection. PLoS One 2014; 9: e110442.

[49] Qian G, Jin F, Chang L, Yang Y, Peng H, Duan C. NIRF, a novel ubiquitin ligase, interacts with hepatitis B virus core protein and promotes its degradation. Biotechnol Lett 2012; 34: 29-36.

[50] Yan H, Peng B, Liu Y, *et al.* Viral entry of hepatitis b and d viruses and bile salts transportation share common molecular determinants on sodium taurocholate cotransporting polypeptide. J Virol 2014; 88: 3273-84.

[51] Slijepcevic D, Kaufman C, Wichers CG, *et al.* Impaired uptake of conjugated bile acids and hepatitis b virus pres1-binding in na(+) -taurocholate cotransporting polypeptide knockout mice. Hepatology 2015; 62: 207-19.

[52] Tsukuda S, Watashi K, Iwamoto M, *et al.* Dysregulation of retinoic acid receptor diminishes hepatocyte permissiveness to hepatitis b virus infection through modulation of sodium taurocholate cotransporting polypeptide (NTCP) expression. J Biol Chem 2015; 290: 5673-84.

[53] Bouezzedine F, Fardel O, Gripon P. Interleukin 6 inhibits HBV entry through NTCP down regulation. Virology 2015; 481: 34-42.

[54] Isogawa M, Robek MD, Furuichi Y, Chisari FV. Toll-like receptor signaling inhibits hepatitis b virus replication *in vivo.* J Virol 2005; 79: 7269-72.

[55] Yan H, Peng B, Liu Y, *et al.* Viral Entry of Hepatitis B and D Viruses and Bile Salts Transportation Share Common Molecular Determinants on Sodium Taurocholate Cotransporting Polypeptide. Journal of Virology 2014; 88(6): 3273-84.

[56] Gane EJ, Lim YS, Gordon SC, *et al.* The oral toll-like receptor-7 agonist gs-9620 in patients with chronic hepatitis b virus infection. J Hepatol 2015; 63: 320-8.

[57] Zhang E, Lu M. Toll-like receptor (tlr)-mediated innate immune responses in the control of hepatitis b virus (HBV) infection. Med Microbiol Immunol (Berl) 2015; 204: 11-20.

[58] Kapoor R, Kottilil S. Strategies to eliminate hbv infection. Future Virol 2014; 9: 565-85.

[59] Slijepcevic D, Kaufman C, Wichers CG, *et al.* Impaired uptake of conjugated bile acids and Hepatitis B Virus preS1-binding inNa+-taurocholate cotransporting polypeptide knockout mice. Hepatology 2015; 65: 207-19.

[60] Peng L, Zhao Q, Li Q, *et al.* The p.Ser267Phe variant in SLC10A1 is associated with resistance to chronic hepatitis B. Hepatology 2014; 61: 1251-60.

[61] Zeisel MB, Lucifora J, Mason WS, *et al.* Towards an HBV cure: state-of-the-art and unresolved questions-report of the ANRS workshop on HBV cure. Gut 2015; 64: 1314-26.

[62] Lin Z, Liao W, Ren J. Physicochemical Characterization of a Polysaccharide Fraction from Platycladus orientalis (L.) Franco and Its Macrophage Immunomodulatory and Anti-Hepatitis B Virus Activities. J Agric Food Chem 2016; 64: 5813-23.

[63] Volz T, Allweiss L, Ben MM, *et al.* The entry inhibitorMyrcludex-B efficiently blocks intrahepatic virus spreading in humanizedmice previously infected with hepatitis B virus. J Hepatol 2013; 58: 861-7.

[64] Jiang W. Blockade of b7-h1 enhances dendritic cell-mediated T cell response and antiviral immunity in HBV transgenic mice. Vaccine 2012; 30: 758-66.

[65] Tian Y, Chen WL, Ou JH. Effects of interferon-alpha/beta on HBV replication determined by viral load. PLoS Pathog 2011; 7: e1002159.

[66] Liaw YF, Kao JH, Piratvisuth T, Chien RN. Asian-pacific consensus statement on the management of chronic hepatitis B: A 2012 update. Hepatol Int 2012; 6: 531-61.

[67] Xiang XG, Xie Q. IL-35: A potential therapeutic target for controlling hepatitis B virus infection. J Dig Dis 2015; 16: 1-6.

[68] Tang J, Zhang ZH, Liu GL. A systematic analysis of the predicted human la protein targets identified a hepatitis b virus infection signature. J Viral Hepat 2013; 20: 12-23.

[69] Zhang F, Wang G. A review of non-nucleoside anti-hepatitis B virus agents. Eur J Med Chem 2014; 75: 267-81.

[70] Bouezzedine F, Fardel O, Gripon P. Interleukin 6 inhibits HBV entry through NTCP down regulation. Virology 2015; 481: 34-42.

[71] Kaneko M, Watashi K, Kamisuki S, *et al.* A Novel Tricyclic Polyketide, Vanitaracin A, Specifically Inhibits the Entry of Hepatitis B and D Viruses by Targeting Sodium Taurocholate Cotransporting Polypeptide. J Virol 2015; 89: 11945-53.

[72] Huang RL, Huang YL, Ou JC, Chen CC, Hsu FL, Chang C. Screening of 25 compounds isolated from Phyllanthus species for anti-human hepatitis B virus *in vitro.* Phytother Res 2003; 17: 449-53.

[73] Shin MS, Kang EH, Lee YI. A flavonoid from medicinal plants blocks hepatitis B virus-e antigen secretion in HBV-infected hepatocytes. Antiviral Res 2005; 67: 163-8.

[74] Li J, Huang H, Zhou W, Feng M, Zhou P. Anti-hepatitis B virus activities of Geranium carolinianum L. extracts and identification of the active components. Biol Pharm Bull 2008; 31: 743-7.

[75] Zembower DE, Zhang H. Total Synthesis of Robustaflavone, a Potential Anti-Hepatitis B Agent. J Org Chem 1998; 63: 9300-5.

[76] Rechtman MM, Har-Noy O, Bar-Yishay I, *et al.* Curcumin inhibits hepatitis B virus *via* down-regulation of the metabolic coactivator PGC-1alpha. FEBS Lett 2010; 584: 2485-90.

[77] Lu LG, Zeng MD, Mao YM, *et al.* Inhibitory effect of oxymatrine on serum hepatitis B virus DNA in HBV transgenic mice. World J Gastroenterol 2004; 10: 1176-9.

[78] Wang YP, Zhao W, Xue R, *et al.* Oxymatrine inhibits hepatitis b infection with an advantage of overcoming drug-resistance. Antiviral Res 2011; 89: 227-31.

[79] Xu WS, Zhao KK, Miao XH, *et al.* Effect of oxymatrine on the replication cycle of hepatitis B virus *in vitro.* World J Gastroenterol 2010; 16: 2028-37.

[80] Chinese Society of Hepatology and Chinese Society of Infectious Diseases, Chinese Medical Association. The guidelines of prevention and treatment for chronic hepatitis B. Zhonghua Gan Zang Bing Za Zhi 2005; 13: 881-91. [In Chinese].

[81] Li J, Huang H, Zhou W, Feng M, Zhou P. Anti-hepatitis B Virus Activities of Geranium carolinianum L. Extracts and Identification of the Active Components Biol. Pharm Bull 2008; 31: 743-7.

[82] Yeo H, Li Y, Fu L, *et al.* Synthesis and Antiviral Activity of Helioxanthin Analogues J Med Chem 2005; 48: 534-46.

[83] Janmanchi D, Lin CH, Hsieh JY, *et al.* Synthesis and biological evaluation of helioxanthin analogues. Bioorg Med Chem 2013; 21: 2163-76.

[84] Zhang Q, Jiang ZY, Luo J, *et al.* Anti-HBV agents. Part 1: Synthesis of alisol A derivatives: A new class of hepatitis B virus inhibitors. Bioorg Med Chem Lett 2008; 18: 4647-50.

[85] Wang S, Li J, Huang H, *et al.* Anti-hepatitis B virus activities of astragaloside IV isolated from radix astragali Biol Pharm Bull 2009; 32: 132-5.

[86] Gao LM, Han YX, Wang YP, *et al.* Design and synthesis of oxymatrine analogues overcoming drug resistance in hepatitis B virus through targeting host heat stress cognate 70. J Med Chem 2011; 54: 869-76.

[87] Du NN, Li X, Wang YP, *et al.* Synthesis, structureactivity relationship and biological evaluation of novel N-substituted matrinic acid derivatives as host heat-stress cognate 70 (Hsc70) down-regulators. Bioorg Med Chem Lett 2011; 21: 4732-5.

[88] Cheng P, Ma YB, Yao SY, *et al.* Two new alkaloids and active anti-hepatitis B virus constituents from Hypserpa nitida. Bioorg Med Chem Lett 2007; 17: 5316-20.

[89] Wu YR, Ma YB, Zhao YX, *et al.* Two Two new quaternary alkaloids and anti-hepatitis B virus active constituents from *Corydalis saxicola.* Planta Med 2007; 73: 787-91.

[90] Peng YR, Li YB, Liu XD, Zhang JF, Duan J. A Antitumor activity of C-21 steroidal glycosides from Cynanchum auriculatum Royle ex Wight. Phytomedicine 2008; 15: 1016-20.

[91] Wang LJ, Geng CA, Ma YB, *et al.* Synthesis, structure-activity relationships and biological evaluation of caudatin derivatives as novel anti-hepatitis B virus agents. Bioorg Med Chem 2012; 20: 2877-88.

[92] Guo RH, Geng CA, Huang XY, *et al.* Synthesis of hemslecin A derivatives: A new class of hepatitis B virus inhibitors. Bioorg Med Chem Lett 2013; 23: 1201-5.

[93] Lv Z, He W, Tian X, *et al.* Design, synthesis, and biological evaluation of new N4-Substituted 20-deoxy-20-fluoro-40-azido cytidine derivatives as potent anti-HBV Agents. Eur J Med Chem 2015; 101: 103-10.

[94] Permi RB, Conway SC, Ladner SK, *et al.* Phenylpropenamide derivatives as inhibitors of hepatitis B virus replication. Bioorg Med Chem Lett 2000; 10(23): 2687-90.

[95] King RW, Ladner SK, Miller TJ, *et al.* Antimicrob. Agents. Chemother 1998; 42: 3179-86.

[96] Dong WL, Liu ZX, Liu XH, Li ZM, Zhao WG. Synthesis and antiviral activity of new acrylamide derivatives containing 1,2,3-thiadiazole as inhibitors of hepatitis B virus replication. Eur J Med Chem 2010; 45: 1919-26.

[97] Mehta A, CarrouA(c)e S, Conyers B, *et al.* Inhibition of hepatitis B virus DNA replication by imino sugars without the inhibition of the DNA polymerase: Therapeutic implications. Hepatology 2001; 33: 1488-95.

[98] Ei-Barbary AA, Abou-Ei-Ezz AZ, Abdel-Kader AA, Ei-Daly M, Nielsen C. Synthesis Of Some New 4-Amino-1,2,4-Triazole Derivatives As Potential Anti-Hiv And Anti-Hbv. Phosphorus Sulfur Silicon Relat Elem 2004; 179: 1497-508.

[99] Zhao WG, Wang JG, Li ZM, Yang Z. Synthesis and antiviral activity against tobacco mosaic virus and 3D-QSAR of a-substituted-1,2,3-thiadiazoleacetamides. Bioorg Med Chem Lett 2006; 16: 6107-11.

[100] Asif-Ulah M, Choi KJ, Choi KI, Jeong YJ, Yu YG. Identification of compounds that inhibit the interaction between core and surface protein of hepatitis B virus. Antiviral Res 2006; 70: 85-90.

[101] Li YF, Wang GF, He PL, Huang WG. Synthesis and anti-hepatitis B virus activity of novel benzimidazole derivatives. J Med Chem 2006; 49: 4790-4.

[102] Luo Y, Yao JP, Yang L, *et al.* Design and synthesis of novel benzimidazole derivatives as inhibitors of hepatitis B virus. Bioorg Med Chem 2010; 18: 5048-55.

[103] Zhao YF, Liu YJ, Chen D, Wei ZQ, Liu WZ, Gong P. Synthesis and biological evaluation of 1H-benzimidazol-5-ols as potent HBV inhibitors. Bioorg Med Chem Lett 2010; 20: 7230-3.

[104] Zhong Q, Yang Z, Liu Y, *et al.* Antiviral activity of Arbidol against Coxsackie virus B5 *in vitro* and *in vivo*. Arch Virol 2009; 154: 601-7.

[105] Boriskin YS, Leneva IA, Pecheur EI, Polyak SJ. Arbidol: A broad-spectrum antiviral compound that blocks viral fusion. Curr Med Chem 2008; 15: 997-1005.

[106] Guo RH, Zhang Q, Ma YB, *et al.* Structureeactivity relationships study of 6-chloro-4-(2-chlorophenyl)- 3-(2-hydroxyethyl) quinolin-2(1H)-one derivatives as novel non-nucleoside anti-hepatitis B virus agents. Eur J Med Chem 2011; 46: 307-19.

[107] Liu Y, Zhao Y, Zhai X, *et al.* Synthesis and anti-HBV activities evaluation of new ethyl 8-imidazolylmethyl-7-hydroxyquinoline-3-carboxylate derivatives *in vitro*. Arch Pharm (Weinheim) 2008; 341: 446-52.

[108] Liu Y, Zhao Y, Zhai X, Feng X, Wang J, Gong P. Synthesis and anti-hepatitis B virus evaluation of novel ethyl 6-hydroxyquinoline-3-carboxylates *in vitro*. Bioorg Med Chem 2008; 16: 6522-7.

[109] Guo RH, Zhang Q, Ma YB, *et al.* Synthesis and biological assay of 4-aryl-6-chloro-quinoline derivatives as novel non-nucleoside anti-HBV agents. Bioorg Med Chem 2011; 19: 1400-8.

[110] Jia W, Liu YJ, Li W, *et al.* Synthesis and *in vitro* anti-hepatitis B virus activity of 6*H*-[1]benzothiopyrano[4,3-*b*]quinolin-9-ols. Bioorg Med Chem 2009; 17: 4569-74.

[111] Bourne CR, Lee S, Venkataiah B, *et al.* Small-molecule effectors of hepatitis B virus capsid assembly give insight into virus life cycle. J Virol 2008; 82: 10262-70.

[112] Stray SJ, Bourne CR, Punna S, *et al.* A heteroaryldihydropyrimidine activates and can misdirect hepatitis B virus capsid assembly. Proc Natl Acad Sci USA 2005; 102(23): 8138-43.

[113] Crosby IT, Bourke DG, Jones ED, *et al.* Antiviral agents 3. Discovery of a novel small molecule non-nucleoside inhibitor of hepatitis B virus (HBV). Bioorg Med Chem Lett 2011; 21: 1644-8.

[114] Stachulski AV, Pidathala C, Row EC, *et al.* Thiazolides as novel antiviral agents. 1. inhibition of hepatitis B virus replication. J Med Chem 2011; 54: 4119-32.

[115] Wang X-j, Hu W, Zhang T-y, *et al.* Irbesartan, an FDA approved drug for hypertension and diabetic nephropathy, is a potent inhibitor for hepatitis B virus entry by disturbing Na+-dependent taurocholate cotransporting polypeptide activity. Antiviral Res 2015; 120: 140-6.

[116] Forsman JJ, Leino R. L-Pentoses in biological and medicinal applications. Chem Rev 2011; 111: 3334-57.

[117] Kumar R, Semaine W, Johar M, Tyrrell DL, Agrawal B. Effect of various pyrimidines possessing the 1-[(2-hydroxy-1-(hydroxymethyl) ethoxy)methyl] moiety, able to mimic natural 2-deoxyribose, on wild-type and mutant hepatitis B virus replication. J Med Chem 2006; 49: 3693-700.

[118] Ye B, Liu X, Li X, Kong H, Tian L, Chen Y. T-cell exhaustion in chronic hepatitis B infection: current knowledge and clinical significance. Cell Death Dis 2015; 6: e1694.

[119] Gish RG, Yuen M-F, Chan HL, *et al.* Synthetic RNAi triggers and their use in chronic hepatitis B therapies with curative intent. Antiviral Res 2015; 121: 97-108.

[120] Weiser BM, Tellinghuisen TL. Structural biology of the hepatitis C virus proteins. Drug Discov Today Technol 2012; 9(3): e195-204.

[121] Belouzard S, Cocquerel L, Dubuisson J. Hepatitis C virus entry into the hepatocyte. Cent Eur J Biol 2011; 6: 1-13.

[122] Meredith LW, Wilson GK, Fletcher NF, McKeating JA. Hepatitis C virus entry: Beyond receptors. Rev Med Virol 2012; 22: 182-93.

[123] Huanga M, Jianga J-D, Peng Z. Recent advances in the anti-HCV mechanisms of interferon. Acta Pharm Sin B 2014; 4(4): 241-7.

[124] Farci P, Shimoda A, Coiana A, *et al.* The outcome of acute hepatitis C predicted by the evolution of the viral quasispecies. Science 2000; 288: 339-44.

[125] C.L. Murray, C.M. Rice. An unsuspected drug target for HCV. Nature 2010; 465: 42-4.

[126] Tellinghuisen TL, Evans MJ, von Hahn T, You S, Rice CM. Studying hepatitis C virus: Making the best of a bad virus. J Virol 2007; 81: 8853-67.

[127] Meanwell NA. Improving drug design: An update on recent applications of efficiency metrics, strategies for replacing problematic elements, and compounds in nontraditional drug space. Chem Rev Toxicol 2016; 29: 564-616.

[128] De Francesco R, Carfí A. Advances in the development of new therapeutic agents targeting the NS3-4A serine protease or the NS5B RNA-dependent RNA ploymerase of the hepatitis C virus. Adv Drug Deliv Rev 2007; 59: 1242-62.

[129] Zhang X. Direct anti-HCV agents. Acta Pharm Sin B 2016; 6(1): 26-31.

[130] Sainz B, Barretto N, Martin DN, *et al.* Identification of the Niemann-Pick C1-like 1 cholesterol absorption receptor as a new hepatitis C virus entry factor. Nat Med 2012; 18: 281-5.

[131] Poordad F, Dieterich D. Treating hepatitis C: Current standard of care and emerging direct-acting antiviral agents. J Viral Hepat 2012; 19: 449-64.

[132] Pembrey L, Newell ML, Tovo PA. The management of HCV infected pregnant women and their children European paediatric HCV network. J Hepatol 2005; 43: 515-25.

[133] Roth D, Zucker K, Cirocco R, *et al.* The impact of hepatitis C virus infection on renal allograft recipients. Kidney Int 1994; 45: 238-44.

[134] Boesecke C, Grint D, Soriano V, *et al.* Hepatitis C seroconversions in HIV infection across Europe: which regions and patient groups are affected? Liver Int 2015; 35(11): 384-91.

[135] Romero-Gutierrez M, del Campo TS, Moreno ZA, *et al.* Does low-dose prolonged steroid therapy affect the natural history of chronic hepatitis C? J Med Virol 2014; 86(5): 758-64.

[136] Sarrazin C, Berg T, Ross RS, *et al.* Prophylaxis, diagnosis and therapy of hepatitis C virus (HCV) infection: the German guidelines on the management of HCV infection. Z Gastroenterol 2010; 48: 289-351.

[137] Chu CM, Yeh CT, Liaw YF. Fulminant hepatic failure in acute hepatitis C: increased risk in chronic carriers of hepatitis B. virus Gut 1999; 45: 613-7.

[138] He XS, Rehermann B, López-Labrador FX, *et al.* Quantitative analysis of hepatitis C virus-specific CD8+ T cells in peripheral blood and liver using peptide-MHC tetramers. Proc Natl Acad Sci USA 1999; 96: 5692-7.

[139] Beaulieu PL, Tsantrizos YS. Inhibitors of the HCV NS5B polymerase: new hope for the treatment of hepatitis C infections. Curr Opin Investig Drugs 2004; 5: 838-50.

[140] Pisarev AV, Shirokikh NE, Hellen CU. Translation initiation by factor-independent binding of eukaryotic ribosomes to internal ribosomal entry sites. C R Biol 2005; 328: 589-605.

[141] Tellinghuisen TL, Rice CM. Interaction between hepatitis C virus proteins and host cell factors. Curr Opin Microbiol 2002; 5: 419-27.

[142] Urbani A, Bianchi E, Narjes F, *et al.* Substrate specificity of the hepatitis C virus serine protease NS3. J Biol Chem 1997; 272: 9204-9.

[143] Yan Y, Li Y, Munshi s, *et al.* Complex of NS3 protease and NS4A peptide of BK strain hepatitis C virus: a 2.2 A resolution structure in a hexagonal crystal form. Protein Sci 1998; 7: 837-47.

[144] Gentile I, Buonomo AR, Zappulo E, *et al.* Asunaprevir, a protease inhibitor for the treatment of hepatitis C infection. Ther Clin Risk Manag 2014; 10: 493-504.

[145] Lamarre D, Anderson PC, Bailey M, *et al.* An NS3 protease inhibitor with antiviral effects in humans infected with hepatitis C virus. Nature 2003; 426: 186-9.

[146] (a) Goudreau N, Cameron DR, Bonneau P, *et al.* NMR structural characterization of peptide inhibitors bound to the Hepatitis C virus NS3 protease: design of a new P2 substituent. J Med Chem 2004; 47: 123-32.; (b) Tsantrizos YS, Bolger G, Bonneau P, *et al.* Macrocyclic inhibitors of the NS3 protease as potential therapeutic agents of hepatitis C virus infection. Angew Chem Int Ed Engl 2003; 42: 1356-60.

[147] Ingallinella P, Altamura S, Bianchi E, *et al.* Potent Peptide Inhibitors of Human Hepatitis C Virus NS3 Protease Are Obtained by Optimizing the Cleavage Products. Biochemistry 1998; 37: 8906-14.

[148] Johansson A, Hubatsch I, Akerblom E, *et al.* Inhibition of hepatitis C virus NS3 protease activity by product-based peptides is dependent on helicase domain. Bioorg Med Chem Lett 2001; 11: 203-6.

[149] Sudo K, Matsumoto Y, Matsushima M, *et al.* Novel hepatitis C virus protease inhibitors: 2,4,6-trihydroxy, 3-nitro-benzamide derivatives. Antivir Chem Chemother 1997; 8: 541-4.

[150] Polyak SJ, Morishima C, Lohmann V, *et al.* Identification of hepatoprotective flavonolignans from silymarin. Proc Natl Acad Sci USA 2010; 107: 5995-9.

[151] Rutter K, Scherzer TM, Beinhardt S, *et al.* Intravenous silibinin as "rescue treatment" for on-treatment non-responders to pegylated interferon/ribavirin combination therapy. Antivir Ther (Lond) 2011; 16: 1327-33.

[152] Chow HH, Cai Y, Hakim IA, *et al.* Pharmacokinetics and safety of green tea polyphenols after multiple-dose administration of epigallocatechin gallate and polyphenon E in healthy individuals. Clin Cancer Res 2003; 9: 3312-9.

[153] Bhat R, Adam AT, Lee JJ, *et al.* Rotella Structure–activity studies of (-)-epigallocatechin gallate derivatives as HCV entry inhibitors. Bioorg Med Chem Lett 2014; 24: 4162-5.

[154] Haid S, Novodomská A, Gentzsch J, *et al.* A plant-derived flavonoid inhibits entry of all HCV genotypes into human hepatocytes. Gastroenterology 2012; 143: 213-22.

[155] Nahmias Y, Goldwasser J, Casali M, *et al.* Apolipoprotein B-dependent hepatitis C virus secretion is inhibited by the grapefruit flavonoid naringenin. Hepatology 2008; 47: 1437-45.

[156] Gonzalez O, Fontanes V, Raychaudhuri S, *et al.* The heat shock protein inhibitor Quercetin attenuates hepatitis C virus production. Hepatology 2009; 50: 1756-64.

[157] Liu M-M, Zhou L, He P-L, *et al.* Discovery of flavonoid derivatives as anti-HCV agents *via* pharmacophore search combining molecular docking strategy. Eur J Med Chem 2012; 52: 33-43.

[158] Lan K-H, Wang Y-W, Lee W-P, *et al.* Multiple effects of Honokiol on the life cycle of hepatitis C virus. Liver Int 2012; 32: 989-97.

[159] Wu SF, Lin CK, Chuang YS, *et al.* Anti-hepatitis C virus activity of 3-hydroxy caruilignan C from *Swietenia macrophylla* stems. J Viral Hepat 2012; 19: 364-70.

[160] Suzuki M, Sasaki K, Yoshizaki F, Oguchi K, Fujisawa M, Cyong J-C. Anti-hepatitis C virus effect of citrus unshiu peel and its active ingredient nobiletin. Am J Chin Med 2005; 33: 87-94.

[161] Zuo G-Y, Li Z-Q, Chen L-R, Xu X-J. *In vitro* anti-HCV activities of *Saxifraga melanocentra* and its related polyphenolic compounds. Antivir Chem Chemother 2005; 16: 393-8.

[162] Duan D, Li Z, Luo H, Zhang W, Chen L, Xu X. Antiviral compounds from traditional Chinese medicines *Galla Chinese* as inhibitors of HCV NS3 protease. Bioorg Med Chem Lett 2004; 14: 6041-4.

[163] Craxía A, Pernob CF, Viganó M, *et al.* From current status to optimization of HCV treatment: Recommendations from an expert panel. Dig Liver Dis 2016; 48: 995-1005.

[164] Harper S, Ferrara M, Crescenzi B, *et al.* Inhibitors of the Hepatitis C Virus NS3 Protease with Basic Amine Functionality at the P3-Amino Acid N-Terminus: Discovery and Optimization of a New Series of P2-P4 Macrocycles. J Med Chem 2009; 52: 4820-37.

[165] Li-Yuan Y, Jun L, Bin Z, Yan-Gang L, Bao-Quan Z. Inhibitors of the Hepatitis C Virus NS3 Protease with Basic Amine Functionality at the P3-Amino Acid N-Terminus: Discovery and Optimization of a New Series of P2-P4 Macrocycles. J Med Chem 2016; 52: 4820-37.

[166] Shaw J, Fishwick CW, Harris M. Epoxide based inhibitors of the hepatitis C virus non-structural 2 Autoprotease. Antiviral Res 2015; 117: 20-6.

[167] Rajagopalan R, Misialek S, Stevens SK, *et al.* Inhibition and Binding Kinetics of the Hepatitis C Virus NS3 Protease Inhibitor ITMN-191 Reveals Tight Binding and Slow Dissociative Behavior. Biochemistry 2009; 48: 2559-68.

[168] Bogen SL, Pan W, Ruan S, *et al.* Toward the Back-Up of Boceprevir (SCH 503034): Discovery of New Extended P4-Capped Ketoamide Inhibitors of Hepatitis C Virus NS3 Serine Protease with Improved Potency and Pharmacokinetic Profiles. J Med Chem 2009; 52: 3679-88.

[169] Chen KX, Nair L, Vibulbhan B, *et al.* Second-Generation Highly Potent and Selective Inhibitors of the Hepatitis C Virus NS3 Serine Protease. J Med Chem 2009; 52: 1370-9.

[170] Rancourt J, Cameron DR, Gorys V, *et al.* Peptide-Based Inhibitors of the Hepatitis C Virus NS3 Protease: Structure-Activity Relationship at the *C*-. Terminal Position J Med Chem 2004; 47: 2511-22.

[171] Lampa A, Alogheli H, Ehrenberg AE, *et al.* Vinylated linear P2 pyrimidinyloxyphenylglycine based inhibitors of the HCV NS3/4A protease and corresponding macrocycles. Bioorg Med Chem 2014; 22: 6595-615.

[172] Liverton NJ, Holloway MK, McCauley JA, *et al.* Molecular modeling based approach to potent P2–P4 macrocyclic inhibitors of hepatitis C NS3/4A protease. J Am Chem Soc 2008; 130: 4607.

[173] Smoum R, Rubinstein A, Dembitsky VM, Srebnik M. Boron containing compounds as protease inhibitors. Chem Rev 2012; 112: 4156-220.

[174] Njoroge FG, Chen KX, Shih N-Y, Piwinski JJ. Challenges in modern drug discovery: A case study of boceprevir, an HCV protease inhibitor for the treatment of hepatitis C virus infection. Acc Chem Res 2008; 41: 50-9.

[175] Milanole G, Andriessen F, Lemonnier G, *et al.* Toward the synthesis of fluorinated analogues of HCV NS3/4A serine protease inhibitors using methyl α-amino-β-fluoro-β-vinylcyclopropanecarboxylate as key intermediate. Org Lett 2015; 17: 2968-71.

[176] Meanwell NA, Philip S. Portoghese Medicinal Chemistry Lectureship.. Curing hepatitis C virus infection with direct-acting antiviral agents: The arc of a medicinal chemistry triumph. J Med Chem 2016; 59: 7311-51.

[177] Gising J, Odell LR, Larhed M. Microwave-assisted synthesis of small molecules targeting the

infectious diseases tuberculosis, HIV/AIDS, malaria and hepatitis C. Org Biomol Chem 2012; 10: 2713-29.

[178] Llina`s-Brunet M, Bailey MD, Ghiro E, *et al.* A systematic approach to the optimization of substrate-based inhibitors of the hepatitis C virus NS3 protease: Discovery of potent and specific tripeptide inhibitors. J Med Chem 2004; 47: 6584-94.

[179] Jacobson I, Dore GJ, Foster G, *et al.* Simeprevir (TMC435) with peginterferon/ribavirin for treatment of chronic HCV genotype 1 infection in treatment-naive patients: efficacy in difficult-to-treat patient sub-populations in the QUEST-1 and 2 Phase III trials. Hepatology 2013; 58: 756.

[180] Butkiewicz NJ, Wendel M, Zhang R, *et al.* Enhancement of hepatitis C virus NS3 proteinase activity by association with NS4A-specific synthetic peptides: identification of sequence and critical residues of NS4A for the cofactor activity. Virology 1996; 225: 328-38.

[181] Chen SH, Tan SL. Discovery of small molecule inhibitors of HCV NS3-4A protease as potential therapeutic agents against HCV infection. Curr Med Chem 2005; 12: 2317-42.

[182] Chen S-H, Lamar J, Yip Y, *et al.* P1 and P1'-optimization of [3,4]-bicycloproline P2 incorporated tetrapeptidyl α-ketoamide based HCV protease inhibitors. Lett Drug Des Discov 2005; 2: 118-23.

[183] Campbell JA, Good AC, Scola PM, Sin N, Venables B. Hepatitis C virus inhibitors. International Patent 2004.WO 04032827 Bristol-Myers Squibb Co.

[184] Lamarre D, Anderson PC, Bailey M, *et al.* An NS3 protease inhibitor with antiviral effects in humans infected with hepatitis C virus. Nature 2003; 426: 186-99.

[185] Perni RB, Almquist SJ, Byrn RA, *et al.* Preclinical profile of VX-950, a potent, selective, and orally bioavailable inhibitor of hepatitis C virus NS3-4A serine protease. Antimicrob Agents Chemother 2006; 50: 899-909.

[186] Foster GR. Past, present, and future hepatitis C treatments. Semin Liver Dis 2004; 24 (Suppl. 2): 97-104.

[187] Poirier M, Aubry N, Boucher C, *et al.* RCM of Tripeptide Dienes Containing a Chiral Vinylcyclopropane Moiety: Impact of Different Ru-Based Catalysts on the Stereochemical Integrity of the Macrocyclic Products. J Org Chem 2005; 70: 10765-73.

[188] Goudreau N, Brochu C, Cameron DR, *et al.* Potent inhibitors of the hepatitis C virus NS3 protease: Design and synthesis of macrocyclic substrate-based β-strand mimics. J Org Chem 2004; 69: 6185.

[189] Kronke J, Kittler R, Buchholz F, *et al.* Alternative approaches for efficient inhibition of hepatitis C virus RNA replication by small interfering RNAs. J Virol 2004; 78: 3436-46.

[190] Randall G, Grakoui A, Rice CM. Clearance of replicating hepatitis C virus replicon RNAs in cell culture by small interfering RNAs. Proc Natl Acad Sci USA 2003; 100: 235-40.

[191] Kolli S, Wong S-P, Harbottle R, *et al.* pH-Triggered Nanoparticle Mediated Delivery of siRNA to Liver Cells *in vitro* and *in vivo*. Bioconjugate Chem 2013; 24: 314-32.

[192] Lakshminarayanan A, Reddy BU, Raghav N, *et al.* A galactose-functionalized dendritic siRNA-nanovector to potentiate hepatitis C inhibition in liver cells. Nanoscale 2015; 7: 16921-31.

[193] Migliaccio G, Tomassini JE, Carroll SS, *et al.* Characterization of resistance to non-obligate chain-terminating ribonucleoside analogs that inhibit hepatitis C virus replication *in vitro.* J Biol Chem 2003; 278: 49164-70.

[194] Clark JL, Hollecker L, Mason JC, *et al.* Design, synthesis, and antiviral activity of 2α-deoxy--α-fluoro-2α-*C*-methylcytidine, a potent inhibitor of hepatitis C virus replication. J Med Chem 2005; 48: 5504-8.

[195] Love RA, Parge HE, Yu X, *et al.* Crystallographic identification of a noncompetitive inhibitor binding site on the hepatitis C virus NS5B RNA polymerase enzyme. J Virol 2003; 77: 7575-81.

[196] Di Marco S, Volpari C, Tomei L, *et al.* Interdomain communication in hepatitis C virus polymerase

abolished by small molecule inhibitors bound to a novel allosteric site. J Biol Chem 2005; 280: 29765-70.

[197] Hashimoto H, Mizutani K, Yoshida A. Interdomain communication in hepatitis C virus polymerase abolished by small molecule inhibitors bound to a novel allosteric site. J Biol Chem 2001; 280: 29765-70.

[198] Beaulieu PL, Bos M, Bousquet Y, *et al.* Nonnucleoside inhibitors of the hepatitis C virus NS5B polymerase: discovery and preliminary SAR of benzimidazole derivatives. Bioorg Med Chem Lett 2004; 14: 119-24.

[199] Urvil PT, Kakiuchi N, Zhou D-M, Shimotohno K, Kumar PK, Nishikawa S. Selection of RNA aptamers that bind specifically to the NS3 protease of hepatitis C virus. Eur J Biochem 1997; 248: 130-8.

[200] Fukuda K, Vishinuvardhan D, Sekiya S, *et al.* Specific RNA aptamers to NS3 protease domain of hepatitis C virus. Nucleic Acids Symp Ser 1997; 37: 237-8.

[201] Summa V, Petrocchi A, Pace P, *et al.* Discovery of R,ç-Diketo Acids as Potent Selective and Reversible Inhibitors of Hepatitis C Virus NS5b RNA-Dependent RNA Polymerase. J Med Chem 2004; 47(1): 14-7.

[202] Wohnsland A, Hofmann WP, Sarrazin C. Viral determinants of resistance to treatment in patients with hepatitis C. Clin Microbiol Rev 2007; 20: 23-38.

[203] Lange CM, Jacobson IM, Rice CM, *et al.* Emerging therapies for the treatment of hepatitis C. EMBO Mol Med 2014; 6: 4-15.

[204] Sun J-H, O'Boyle DR II, Fridell RA, *et al.* Resensitizing daclatasvir-resistant hepatitis C variants by allosteric modulation of NS5A. Nature 2015; 527: 245-60.

[205] Leivers AL, Tallant M, Shotwell JB, *et al.* Discovery of Selective Small Molecule Type III Phosphatidylinositol 4-Kinase Alpha (PI4KIIIα) Inhibitors as Anti Hepatitis C (HCV) Agents. J Med Chem 2014; 57: 2091-106.

[206] Ivachtchenko AV, Mitkin OD, Yamanushkin PM, *et al.* Discovery of Novel Highly Potent Hepatitis C Virus NS5A Inhibitor (AV4025). J Med Chem 2014; 57: 7716-30.

[207] Liu N, Zhu S, Zhang X, *et al.* The discovery and characterization of a novel scaffold as a potent hepatitis C virus inhibitor. Chem Commun (Camb) 2016; 52: 3340-3.

[208] Yang PL, Gao M, Lin K, Liu Q, Villareal VA. Anti-HCV drugs in the pipeline. Curr Opin Virol 2011; 1: 607-16.

[209] Kuang W-F, Lin Y-C, Jean F, *et al.* Hepatitis C virus NS3 RNA helicase activity is modulated by the two domains of NS3 and NS4A. Biochem Biophys Res Commun 2004; 317: 211-7.

[210] Borowski P, Mueller O, Niebuhr A, *et al.* ATP-binding domain of NTPase/helicase as a target for hepatitis C antiviral therapy. Acta Biochim Pol 2000; 47: 173-80.

[211] Boguszewska-Chachulska AM, Krawczyk M, Najda Z, *et al.* Searching for a new anti-HCV therapy: Synthesis and properties of tropolone derivatives. Biochem Biophys Res Commun 2006; 341: 641-7.

[212] Phoon CW, Ng PY, Ting AE, Yeo SL, Sim MM. Biological evaluation of hepatitis C virus helicase inhibitors. Bioorg Med Chem Lett 2001; 11: 1647-50.

[213] Borowski P, Schalinski S, Schmitz H. Nucleotide triphosphatase/ helicase of hepatitis C virus as a target for antiviral therapy. Antiviral Res 2002; 55: 397-412.

[214] Urbani A, De Francesco R, Steinkuhler C. Proteases of Infectious Agents. San Diego, CA: Academic Press 1999; pp. 61-91.

[215] Kim JL, Morgenstern KA, Lin C, *et al.* Crystal structure of the hepatitis C virus NS3 protease domain complexed with a synthetic NS4A cofactor peptide. Cell 1996; 87: 343-55.

[216] Pileri P, Uematsu Y, Campagnoli S, *et al.* Binding of hepatitis C virus to CD81. Science 1998; 282: 938-41.

[217] Takeda K, Kaisho T, Akira S. Toll-like receptors. Annu Rev Immunol 2003; 21: 335-76.

[218] Iwasaki A, Medzhitov R. Toll-like receptor control of the adaptive immune responses. Nat Immunol 2004; 5: 987-95.

[219] (a) Elbashir SM, Harborth J, Lendeckel W, *et al.* Duplexes of 21-nucleotide RNAs mediate RNA interference in cultured mammalian cells. Nature 2001; 411: 494-8.; (b) Manoharan M. RNA interference and chemically modified small interfering RNAs. Curr Opin Chem Biol 2004; 8: 570-9.

[220] Vincent W-F, Tai DG, Daniel J, *et al.* Design and synthesis of spirocyclic compounds as HCV replication inhibitors by targeting viral NS4B protein. Bioorg Med Chem Lett 2014; 24: 2288-94.

[221] Cannalire R, Barreca ML, Manfroni G, Cecchetti AV. Journey around the Medicinal Chemistry of Hepatitis C Virus Inhibitors Targeting NS4B: From Target to Preclinical Drug Candidates. J Med Chem 2016; 59: 16-41.

[222] Rai R, Deval J. New opportunities in anti-hepatitis C virus drug discovery: Targeting NS4B. Antiviral Res 2011; 90: 93-101.

[223] Gosert R, Egger D, Lohmann V, *et al.* Identification of the hepatitis C virus RNA replication complex in Huh-7 cells harboring subgenomic replicons. J Virol 2003; 77: 5487-92.

[224] Zhang N, Zhang X, Zhu J, *et al.* Structure-Activity Relationship (SAR) Optimization of 6-(Indol-2-yl)pyridine-3-sulfonamides: Identification of Potent, Selective, and Orally Bioavailable Small Molecules Targeting Hepatitis C (HCV) NS4B. J Med Chem 2014; 57: 2121-35.

[225] Zhao C, Wang Y, Ma S. Recent advances on the synthesis of hepatitis C virus NS5B RNA-dependent RNA-polymerase inhibitors. Eur J Med Chem 2015; 102: 188-214.

[226] Priet S, Zlatev I, Barvik I Jr, *et al.* 3'-Deoxy Phosphoramidate Dinucleosides as Improved Inhibitors of Hepatitis C Virus Subgenomic Replicon and NS5B Polymerase Activity. J Med Chem 2010; 53: 6608-17.

[227] Schoenfeld RC, Bourdet DL, Brameld KA, *et al.* Discovery of a Novel Series of Potent Non-Nucleoside Inhibitors of Hepatitis C Virus NS5B. J Med Chem 2013; 56: 8163-82.

[228] Nichols DB, Fournet G, Gurukumar K, *et al.* Inhibition of hepatitis C virus NS5B polymerase by S-trityl-L-cysteine derivatives. Eur J Med Chem 2012; 49: 191-9.

[229] Ding M, He F, Poss MA, *et al.* The synthesis of novel heteroaryl-fused 7,8,9,10-tetrahydro--H-azepino[1,2-a]indoles,4-oxo-2,3-dihydro-1H-[1,4]diazepino[1,7a]indoles and 1,2,4,5- tetrahydro-[1,4]oxazepino[4,5-a]indoles. Effective inhibitors of HCV NS5B polymerase. Org Biomol Chem 2011; 9: 6654-62.

[230] Haudecoeur R, Ahmed-Belkacem A, Yi W, *et al.* Discovery of Naturally Occurring Aurones That Are Potent Allosteric Inhibitors of Hepatitis C Virus RNA-Dependent RNA Polymerase. J Med Chem 2011; 54: 5395-402.

[231] Manfroni G, Cannalire R, Barreca ML, *et al.* The Versatile Nature of the 6-Aminoquinolone Scaffold: Identification of Submicromolar Hepatitis C Virus NS5B Inhibitors. J Med Chem 2014; 57: 1952-63.

[232] Leivers M, Miller JF, Chan SA, *et al.* Imidazopyridazine Hepatitis C Virus Polymerase Inhibitors. Structure-Activity Relationship Studies and the Discovery of a Novel, Traceless Prodrug Mechanism. J Med Chem 2013; 57: 1964-75.

[233] Beaulieu PL, Tsantrizos YS. Inhibitors of the HCV NS5B polymerase: new hope for the treatment of hepatitis C infections. Curr Opin Investig Drugs 2004; 5: 838-50.

[234] Lesburg CA, Cable MB, Ferrari E, Hong Z, Mannarino AF, Weber PC. Crystal structure of the RNA-dependent RNA polymerase from hepatitis C virus reveals a fully encircled active site. Nat Struct Biol 1999; 6: 937-43.

[235] McCown MF, Rajyaguru S, Le Pogam S, *et al.* The hepatitis C virus replicon presents a higher barrier to resistance to nucleoside analogs than to nonnucleoside polymerase or protease inhibitors. Antimicrob Agents Chemother 2008; 52: 1604-12.

[236] Sofia MJ, Chang W, Furman PA, Mosley RT, Ross BS. Nucleoside, Nucleotide, and Non-Nucleoside Inhibitors of Hepatitis C Virus NS5B RNA-Dependent RNA-Polymerase. J Med Chem 2012; 55: 2481-531.

[237] Jiao P, Xue W, Shen Y, Jin N, Liu H. Understanding the drug resistance mechanism of hepatitis C virus NS5B to PF-00868554 due to mutations of the 423 site: a computational study. Mol Biosyst 2014; 10: 767-77.

[238] Beaulieu PL, Bousquet Y, Gauthier J, *et al.* Non-nucleoside benzimidazole-based allosteric inhibitors of the hepatitis C virus NS5B Polymerase: inhibition of subgenomic hepatitis C virus RNA replicons in Huh-7 cells. J Med Chem 2004; 47: 6884-92.

[239] LaPlante SR, Gillard JR, Jakalian A, *et al.* Importance of ligand bioactive conformation in the discovery of potent indole-diamide inhibitors of the hepatitis C virus NS5B. J Am Chem Soc 2010; 132: 15204-12.

[240] Stansfield I, Pompei M, Conte I, *et al.* Development of carboxylic acid replacements in indole-Nacetamide inhibitors of hepatitis C virus NS5B polymerase. Bioorg Med Chem Lett 2007; 17: 5143-9.

[241] Bourgeois S, Reesink HW, Leempoels J, *et al.* 1188 combination therapy of TMC647055 with simeprevir (TMC435) in chronic hepatitis C patients. J Hepatol 2013; 58: 483-3.

[242] Hernando JI, Ontoria JM, Malancona S, *et al.* Optimization of thienopyrrole-based finger-loop inhibitors of the hepatitis C virus NS5B polymerase. ChemMedChem 2009; 4: 1695-713.

[243] Wei Y, Li J, Qing J, *et al.* Discovery of Novel Hepatitis C Virus NS5B Polymerase Inhibitors by Combining Random Forest. Multiple e-Pharmacophore Modeling and Docking PLOS ONE 2016.

[244] Harper S, Avolio S, Pacini B, *et al.* Potent Inhibitors of Subgenomic Hepatitis C Virus RNA Replication through Optimization of Indole-*N*-Acetamide Allosteric Inhibitors of the Viral NS5B Polymerase. J Med Chem 2005; 48: 4547-57.

[245] Rehmana S, Ijazb B, Fatimac N, *et al.* Therapeutic potential of Taraxacum officinale against HCV NS5B polymerase: In-vitro and In silico study. Biomed Pharmacother 2016; 83: 881-91.

[246] Beaulieu PL, Gillard J, Jolicoeur E, *et al.* Poupart From benzimidazole to indole-5-carboxamide Thumb Pocket I inhibitors of HCV NS5B polymerase. Part 1: Indole C-2 SAR and discovery of diamide derivatives with nanomolar potency in cell-based subgenomic replicons. Bioorg Med Chem Lett 2011; 21: 3658-63.

[247] de Vicente J, Hendricks RT, Smith DB, *et al.* Non-nucleoside inhibitors of HCV polymerase NS5B. Part 2: Synthesis and structure-activity relationships of benzothiazine-substituted quinolinediones. Bioorg Med Chem Lett 2009; 19: 3642-6.

[248] Beaulieu PL, Bös M, Cordingley MG, *et al.* Discovery of the First Thumb Pocket 1 NS5B Polymerase Inhibitor (BILB 1941) with Demonstrated Antiviral Activity in Patients Chronically Infected with Genotype 1 Hepatitis C Virus (HCV). J Med Chem 2012; 55: 7650-66.

[249] Smith AA, Zuwala K, Kryger MB, *et al.* Macromolecular prodrugs of ribavirin: towards a treatment for co-infection with HIV and HCV. Chem Sci (Camb) 2015; 6: 264-9.

[250] Cho A, Zhang L, Xu J, *et al.* Discovery of the First C-Nucleoside HCV Polymerase Inhibitor (GS-6620) with Demonstrated Antiviral Response in HCV Infected Patients. J Med Chem 2014; 57: 1812-25.

[251] Zhao F, Liu N, Zhan P, Jiang X, Liu X. Discovery of HCV NS5B thumb site I inhibitors: Core-refining from benzimidazole to indole scaffold. Eur J Med Chem 2015; 94: 218-28.

[252] Manfroni G, Cannalire R, Barreca ML, *et al.* The Versatile Nature of the 6-Aminoquinolone Scaffold:Identification of Submicromolar Hepatitis C Virus NS5B Inhibitors. J Med Chem 2014; 57: 1952-63.

[253] Hassan MZ, Osman H, Ali MA, Ahsan MJ. Therapeutic potential of coumarins as antiviral agents. Eur J Med Chem 2016; 123: 236-55.

[254] Du J, Chun B-K, Mosley RT, *et al.* Use of 2'-Spirocyclic Ethers in HCV Nucleoside Design. J Med Chem 2014; 57: 1826-35.

[255] Hutchinson DK, Flentge CA, Donner PL, *et al.* Hepatitis C NS5B polymerase inhibitors: Functional equivalents for the benzothiadiazine moiety. Bioorg Med Chem Lett 2011; 21: 1876-9.

[256] Hirashima S, Suzuki T, Ishida T, *et al.* Benzimidazole Derivatives Bearing Substituted Biphenyls as Hepatitis C Virus NS5B RNA-Dependent RNA Polymerase Inhibitors: Structure-Activity Relationship Studies and Identification of a Potent and Highly Selective Inhibitor JTK-109. J Med Chem 2006; 49: 4721-36.

[257] Chen KX, Vibulbhan B, Yang W, *et al.* Structure-Activity Relationship (SAR) Development and Discovery of Potent Indole-Based Inhibitors of the Hepatitis C Virus (HCV) NS5B Polymerase. J Med Chem 2012; 55: 754-65.

[258] Chen KX, Lesburg CA, Vibulbhan B, *et al.* A Novel Class of Highly Potent Irreversible Hepatitis C Virus NS5B Polymerase Inhibitors. J Med Chem 2012; 55: 2089-101.

[259] Das D, Hong J, Chen S-H, *et al.* Recent advances in drug discovery of benzothiadiazine and related analogs as HCV NS5B polymerase inhibitors. Bioorg Med Chem 2011; 19: 4690-703.

[260] Manfroni G, Manvar D, Barreca ML, *et al.* New Pyrazolobenzothiazine Derivatives as Hepatitis C Virus NS5B Polymerase Palm Site I Inhibitors. J Med Chem 2014; 57: 3247-62.

[261] Biswal BK, Wand M, Cherney MM, *et al.* Non-nucleoside Inhibitors Binding to Hepatitis C Virus NS5B Polymerase Reveal a Novel Mechanism of Inhibition J. Mol Biol 2006; 361: 33.

[262] Canales E, Carlson JS, Appleby T, *et al.* Tri-substituted acylhydrazines as tertiary amide bioisosteres: HCV NS5B polymerase inhibitors. Bioorg Med Chem Lett 2012; 22: 4288-92.

[263] Camarasa M, de la Bellacasa R. Design, synthesis and biological evaluation of pyrido[2,3-d]pyrimidin-7-(8H)-ones as HCV inhibitors. Eur J Med Chem 2016; 115: 463-83.

[264] Barreca ML, Manfroni G, Leyssen P, *et al.* Structure-Based Discovery of Pyrazolobenzothiazine Derivatives As Inhibitors of Hepatitis C Virus Replication. J Med Chem 2013; 56: 2270-82.

[265] Gardelli C, Attenni B, Donghi M, *et al.* Phosphoramidate Prodrugs of 20-C-Methylcytidine for Therapy of Hepatitis C Virus Infection. J Med Chem 2009; 52: 5394-407.

[266] Beaulieu PL, Anderson PC, Bethell R, *et al.* Discovery of BI 207524, an Indole Diamide NS5B Thumb Pocket 1 Inhibitor with Improved Potency for the Potential Treatment of Chronic Hepatitis C Virus Infection. J Med Chem 2014; 57: 10130-43.

[267] Court JJ, Poisson C, Ardzinski A, *et al.* Discovery of Novel Thiophene-Based, Thumb Pocket 2 Allosteric Inhibitors of the Hepatitis C NS5B Polymerase with Improved Potency and Physicochemical Profiles. J Med Chem 2016; 59: 6293-302.

[268] Di Bisceglie AM, Sulkowski M, Gane E, *et al.* VX-222, a Non-Nucleoside NS5B Polymerase Inhibitor, in Telaprevir-Based Regimens for Genotype 1 Hepatitis C Virus Infection. Eur J Gastroenterol Hepatol 2014; 26(7): 761-73.

[269] Lazerwith SE, Lew W, Zhang J, *et al.* Discovery of GS-9669, a Thumb Site II Non-Nucleoside Inhibitor of NS5B for the Treatment of Genotype 1 Chronic Hepatitis C Infection. J Med Chem 2014; 57(5): 1893-901.

[270] Zhao Y, Podos S, Fabrycki JL, *et al.* ACH-3422, a novel HCV NS5B RNA polymerase nucleotide inhibitor, demonstrates improved potency over sofosvuvir against HCV gentoype 3 replicons *in vitro.*

Hepatology 2014; 60: 1163.

[271] Chen Z, Jochmans D, Ku T, *et al.* Bicyclic and Tricyclic "Expanded" Nucleobase Analogues of Sofosbuvir: New Scaffolds for Hepatitis C Therapies ACS. Infect Dis 2015; 1: 357-66.

[272] Chen KX, Venkatraman S, Anilkumar GN, *et al.* Discovery of SCH 900188: A Potent Hepatitis C Virus NS5B Polymerase Inhibitor Prodrug As a Development Candidate ACS Med. Chem Lett 2014; 5: 244-8.

[273] Hucke O, Coulombe R, Bonneau P, *et al.* Molecular Dynamics Simulations and Structure-Based Rational Design Lead to Allosteric HCV NS5B Polymerase Thumb Pocket 2 Inhibitor with Picomolar Cellular Replicon Potency J. Med Chem 2014; 57: 1932-43.

[274] Beaulieu PL, Dansereau N, Duan J, *et al.* Benzimidazole Thumb Pocket I finger-loop inhibitors of HCV NS5B polymerase: Improved drug-like properties through C-2 SAR in three sub-series Bioorg. &. Med Chem Lett 2010; 20: 1825-9.

[275] Narjes F, Crescenzi B, Ferrara M, *et al.* Discovery of (7R)-14-Cyclohexyl-7-{[2-(dimethyl-amino)ethyl](methyl) amino}-7,8-dihydro-6Hindolo [1,2-e] [1,5]benzoxazocine-11-carboxylic Acid (MK-3281), a Potent and Orally BioavailableFinger-Loop Inhibitor of the Hepatitis C Virus NS5B Polymerase. J Med Chem 2011; 54: 289-301.

[276] Jardim ACG, Igloi Z, Shimizu JF, Santos VAFFM. Natural compounds isolated from Brazilian plants are potent inhibitors of hepatitis C virus replication *in vitro*. Antiviral Res 2015; 115: 39-47.

[277] Rivero-Buceta E, Carrero P, DoyagA1/4ez EG, *et al.* Linear and branched alkyl-esters and amides of gallic acid and other (mono-, di- and tri-) hydroxy benzoyl derivatives as promising anti-HCV inhibitors. Eur J Med Chem 2015; 92: 656-71.

[278] Wittine K, Babic MS, Makuc D, *et al.* Novel 1,2,4-triazole and imidazole derivatives of L-ascorbic and imino-ascorbic acid: Synthesis, anti-HCV and antitumor activity evaluations Bioorg. &. Med Chem 2012; 20: 3675-85.

[279] Wang S-R, Min Y-Q, Wang J-Q, Liu C-X, Fu B-S, Wu F. A highly conserved G-rich consensus sequence in hepatitis C virus core gene represents a new anti-hepatitis C target Sci. Adv 2016; 2: e1501535.

[280] Kim S, Ryoo S-R, Na H-K, *et al.* Deoxyribozyme-loaded nano-graphene oxide for simultaneous sensing and silencing of the hepatitis C virus gene in liver cells. Chem Commun (Camb) 2013; 49: 8241-3.

[281] Pertusati F, McGuigan C. Diastereoselective synthesis of P-chirogenic phosphoramidate prodrugs of nucleoside analogues (ProTides) *via* copper catalysed reaction. Chem Commun (Camb) 2015; 51: 8070-3.

[282] Shimura S, Ishima M, Nakajima S, *et al.* Total Synthesis and Anti-Hepatitis C Virus Activity of MA026. J Am Chem Soc 2013; 135: 18949-56.

[283] Xiao S, Wang Q, Si L, *et al.* Synthesis and biological evaluation of novel pentacyclic triterpene a-cyclodextrin conjugates as HCV entry inhibitors. Eur J Med Chem 2016; 124: 1-9.

[284] Redwan E M, Almehdar H A. Potential antiviral activities of camel, bovine, and human lactoperoxidases against hepatitis C virus genotype 4 RSC Adv 2015; 5: 60441-52.

[285] Wagner CE, Mohler ML, Kang GS, *et al.* Synthesis of 1-Boraadamantaneamine Derivatives with Selective Astrocyte *vs* C6 Glioma Antiproliferative Activity. A Novel Class of Anti-Hepatitis C Agents with Potential to Bind CD81. J Med Chem 2003; 46: 2823-33.

[286] Reddy PG, Chun B-K, Zhang H-R, *et al.* Stereoselective Synthesis of PSI-352938: A β-D-2'-Deox--2'-α-fluoro-2'-β-C-methyl-3',5'-cyclic Phosphate Nucleotide Prodrug for the Treatment of HCV. J Org Chem 2011; 76: 3782-90.

[287] Wang H, Wang S, Cheng L, *et al.* Discovery of Imidazo[1,2-α][1,8]naphthyridine Derivatives as Potential HCV Entry Inhibitor. ACS Med Chem Lett 2015; 6: 977-81.

[288] Shaw J, Harris M, Fishwick CW. Identification of a lead like inhibitor of the hepatitis C virus non-structural NS2 autoprotease. Antiviral Res 2015; 124: 54-60.

[289] Ye N, Chen H, Wold EA, Shi P-Y, Zhou J. Therapeutic Potential of Spirooxindoles as Antiviral Agents ACS. Infect Dis 2016; 2: 382-92.

[290] Draffan AG, Frey B, Fraser BH, *et al.* Derivatives of imidazotriazine and pyrrolotriazine C-nucleosides as potential new anti-HCV agents Bioorg. &. Med Chem Lett 2014; 24: 4984-8.

[291] Magri A, Reilly R, Scalacci N, *et al.* Rethinking the old antiviral drug moroxydine: Discovery of novel analogues as anti-hepatitis C virus (HCV) agents. Bioorg Med Chem Lett 2015; 25: 5372-6.

[292] Luscombea CA, Huangb Z, Murrayb MG, *et al.* A novel Hepatitis C virus p7 ion channel inhibitor, BIT225, inhibits bovine viral diarrhea virus *in vitro* and shows synergism with recombinant interferon-α-2b and nucleoside analogues. Antiviral Res 2010; 86: 144-53.

[293] Morris WJ, Muppalla KK, Cowden C, Ball RG. Stereoselective Addition of 2-Phenyloxazol-4-yl Trifluoromethanesulfonate to N-Sulfinyl Imines: Application to the Synthesis of the HCV Protease Inhibitor Boceprevir. J Org Chem 2013; 78: 706-10.

[294] (a) Torssell S, Kienle M, Somfai P. 1,3-Dipolar Cycloadditions of Carbonyl Ylides to Aldimines: A Three-Component Approach to syn-a-Hydroxy-b-amino Esters. Angew Chem Int Ed 2005; 44: 3096.; (b) Aoyagi Y, Jain RP, Williams RM. Stereocontrolled Asymmetric Synthesis of R-Hydroxy-â-amino Acids. A Stereodivergent Approach. J Am Chem Soc 2001; 123: 3472.; (c) Sleebs BE, Hughes AB. Diastereoselective Synthesis of r-Methyl and r-Hydroxy-α-Amino Acids *via* 4-Substituted-1-3-Oxazinan-6-ones. J Org Chem 2007; 72: 3340.

[295] Zhou L, Zhang H, Tao S, *et al.* Synthesis and Evaluation of 2,6-Modified Purine 2'-C-Methyl Ribonucleosides as Inhibitors of HCV Replication. ACS Med Chem Lett 2016; 7: 17-22.

[296] He S, Xiao J, Dulcey AE, *et al.* Discovery, Optimization, and Characterization of Novel Chlorcyclizine Derivatives for the Treatment of Hepatitis C Virus Infection. J Med Chem 2016; 59: 841-53.

[297] Huang S, Qing J, Wang S, Wang H, Zhang L, Tang Y. Design and synthesis of imidazo[1,2-α][1,8]-naphthyridine derivatives as anti-HCV agents *via* direct C-H arylation. Org Biomol Chem 2014; 12: 2344-8.

[298] Peng H-K, Chen W-C, Lee J-C, *et al.* Novel anilinocoumarin derivatives as agents against hepatitis C virus by the induction of IFN-mediated antiviral responses. Org Biomol Chem 2013; 11: 1858-66.

[299] Maiti M, Maiti M, Rozenski J, Jonghea SD, Herdewijn P. Aspartic acid based nucleoside phosphoramidate prodrugs as potent inhibitors of hepatitis C virus replication. Org Biomol Chem 2015; 13: 5158-74.

[300] Liu R, Huang Z, Murray MG, Guo X, Liu G. Quinoxalin-2(1H)-One Derivatives As Inhibitors Against Hepatitis C Virus. J Med Chem 2011; 54: 5747-68.

[301] Kazmierski WM, Hamatake R, Duan M, *et al.* Discovery of Novel Urea-Based Hepatitis C Protease Inhibitors with High Potency against Protease-Inhibitor-Resistant Mutants. J Med Chem 2012; 55: 3021-6.

[302] McGuigan C, Madela K, Aljarah M, *et al.* Phosphorodiamidates as a Promising New Phosphate Prodrug Motif for Antiviral Drug Discovery: Application to Anti-HCV Agents. J Med Chem 2011; 54: 8632-45.

[303] Hwang D-R, Wu Y-S, Chang C-W, *et al.* Synthesis and anti-viral activity of a series of sesquiterpene lactones and analogues in the subgenomic HCV replicon system. Bioorg Med Chem 2006; 14: 83-91.

[304] Stachulski AV, Pidathala C, Row EC, *et al.* Thiazolides as Novel Antiviral Agents. 2. Inhibition of Hepatitis C Virus Replication. J Med Chem 2011; 54: 8670-80.

[305] aTakaya D, Yamashita A, Kamijo K, *et al.* A new method for induced fit docking (GENIUS) and its

application to virtual screening of novel HCV NS3-4A protease inhibitors. Bioorg Med Chem 2011; 19: 6892-905.; bGogineni V, Schinazi RF, Hamann MT. Role of Marine Natural Products in the Genesis of Antiviral Agents. Chem Rev 2015; 115: 9655-706.

[306] Li W, Xiao F, Zhou M, *et al.* 3D-QSAR study and design of 4-hydroxyamino a-pyranone carboxamide analogues as potential anti-HCV agents. Chem Phys Lett 2016; 661: 36-41.

[307] He S, Jain P, Lin B, *et al.* High-Throughput Screening, Discovery, and Optimization To Develop a Benzofuran Class of Hepatitis C Virus Inhibitors. ACS Comb Sci 2015; 17: 641-52.

[308] Massarotti A, Coluccia A, Sorba G, Silvestri R, Brancale A. De novo computer-aided design of novel antiviral agents. Drug Discov Today Technol 2012; 9(3): e213-8.

[309] Clercq ED. Antivirals: Past, present and future. Biochem Pharmacol 2013; 85: 727-44.

[310] Hung CC, Wu SM, Lin PH, *et al.* Increasing incidence of recent hepatitis D virus infection in HIV-infected patients in an area hyperendemic for hepatitis B virus infection. Clin Infect Dis 2014; 58: 1625-33.

[311] Taylor JM. Virology of hepatitis D virus. Semin Liver Dis 2012; 32: 195-200.

[312] Karatayli SC, Bozdayi M, Karatayli E, *et al.* Interleukin-28 gene polymorphisms may contribute to HBsAg persistence and the development of HBeAg-negative chronic hepatitis B. Liver Int 2015; 35: 846-53.

[313] Onali S, Figorilli F, Balestrieri C, *et al.* Can antiretroviral therapy modify the clinical course of HDV infection in HIV-positive patients? Antivir Ther 2015; 20: 671-9.

[314] Koh C, Canini L, Dahari H, *et al.* Oral prenylation inhibition with lonafarnib in chronic hepatitis D infection: a proof-of-concept randomised, double-blind, placebo-controlled phase 2A trial. Lancet Infect Dis 2015; 15: 1167-74.

[315] Pischke S, Wedemeyer H, Hepatitis E. Virus Infection: multiple faces of an underestimated problem. J Hepatol 2013; 58: 1045-6.

[316] Pischke S, Hardtke S, Bode U, *et al.* Ribavirin treatment of acute and chronic hepatitis E: a single center experience. Liver Int 2013; 33: 722-6.

[317] Honer zu. Chronic HEV infection beyond transplantation or HIV infection. Hepatology 2014; 60: 1112-3.

[318] Kamar N, Izopet J, Tripon S, *et al.* Ribavirin for chronic hepatitis E virus infection in transplant recipients. N Engl J Med 2014; 370: 1111-20.

[319] Payne AW, Glen RC. Molecular recognition using a binary genetic search algorithm. J Mol Graph 24(11): 74-91.2011;

CHAPTER 6

Antimicrobial Peptides against Microbial Biofilms: their Structures and Modes of Action

Sudhir K. Shukla[1,2], **Dugeshwar Karley**[1] and **T. Subba Rao**[1,2,*]

[1] *Biofouling & Thermal Ecology Section, Water & Steam Chemistry Division, BARC Facilities, Kalpakkam, 603 102, India*

[2] *Homi Bhabha National Institute, Mumbai 400094, India*

Abstract: The formation of biofilms contributes significantly to bacterial resistance to antibiotics, innate host defences and in persistent infections. In this era of multidrug-resistant bacterial infections, the discovery of novel antibacterial agents is required to treat infections that kill these organisms *via* novel mechanisms of action. Antimicrobial peptides, also known as host-defence peptides are short polypeptides (<40 amino acids) and are an integral part of the innate immune system that protects a host from bacterial infection. This chapter discusses the potential of anti-microbial peptides as an anti-infective agent, its advantages, disadvantages, their structures and mechanisms of action. A perception of the bacteriostatic and bactericidal mechanism of antimicrobial peptides is required to facilitate the rational design of novel antimicrobial agents. Thus a deeper understanding of the mechanism of natural AMPs will also aid in developing new antibacterial agents. Furthermore, the chapter also considers the possibility of the use of synthetic antimicrobial peptides containing both natural and unnatural amino acids as anti-infective agents. Apart from the antibacterial property, AMPs are also being used as drug delivery vectors to transport the cell impermeable drugs to the cell interior. The diversity and broad spectrum antimicrobial activity of AMPs along with its multidimensional properties could be exploited as a potential and promising drug candidate.

Keywords: Antimicrobial peptides, Human β-defensin, Indolicidin, Synthetic peptide, biofilms, host defences, host-defence peptides, unnatural amino acids, β-peptides.

BIOFILMS AND ANTIBIOTICS RESISTANCE

The breakthrough in antibiotics production is one of the paramount achievements in the history of medicine. Antibiotics are used in the treatment of small to life-threatening infections, in organ transplantation, in oncology to give higher doses

* **Corresponding author T. Subba Rao:** Biofouling & Thermal Ecology Section, BARC Facilities, Kalpakkam, 603102, India; Tel: 044 - 27480500 ext.: 22607; Fax: 044 – 27480097; Email. subbarao@igcar.gov.in

Atta-ur-Rahman & M. Iqbal Choudhary (Eds.)

of chemotherapy for cancer treatment. However, the emergence of antibiotic resistant bacteria is alarming, which are undoing all the earlier advances and forcing a return to the pre-antibiotic era [1]. In the recent years, antibiotic-resistant bacteria have emerged as a biggest challenge for the medical community. The major reason behind enhanced antibiotic resistance was the persistent biofilm formation, which was previously neglected during the development phase of new antibiotics. Bio-molecular matrix enclosed microbial biomasses that stick on to biological or non-biological surfaces are called biofilms. Microbial biofilms protect the bacterial communities present inside antagonistic environment [2]. The production of biofilms and enhanced antibiotic resistance are linked each other. Most of the antibiotics are tested against the bacterial community growing in planktonic growth. Microbial communities growing inside biofilms need 1000 times higher dose of antibiotics to kill them. This demonstrates the striking difference in nature of planktonic life and biofilm-associated bacteria [3]. Bacterial communities residing in biofilm matrix are highly complex to treat with conventional antibiotics [4]. In hospitals, major antibiotic-resistant bacteria develop due to poor practice of handling antimicrobial drugs and the emerging resistant bacteria [5]. The problem of antibiotic resistance can be minimized by preventing unnecessary usages of antibiotics, which is the major reason behind the development of antibiotic resistance among bacteria [6]. The phenomenon of "persistence "also affects antibiotics action against bacterial communities. Persister cells are a small sub-population of microbes that survive the lethal effects of a drug and after the effect of the drug is minimized, they start growing again. The phenomenon of survival of persistent cells against antibiotics is illustrated in Fig. (**1**). When the antibiotic treatment is applied it kills a majority of cells but fails to eradicate a small subset of the population known as persister cells. When the presence of antibiotic is removed, persister cells resume growth and cause the recurrent infection. The persister cells are slightly different from resistant cells. Antibiotic resistant cells can grow even in the presence of antibiotics, but persister cells cannot. The persister cells can survive and grow after the release of antibiotics pressure. Unlike resistance, persistence is not an inherited phenotype, which is shown by the fact that once the organisms resume normal growth they remain drug sensitive similar to the initial population. In this context, persistent *Mycobacterium* infection is well studied and the results showed that such infections need a longer course of treatment, which is comprised of various antibiotics combinations. Infections with these are real challenges in medical science [7]. In the present scenario, there is a need to find out a new alternative antimicrobial drug which can work equally against bacterial community residing inside and outside the biofilm matrix.

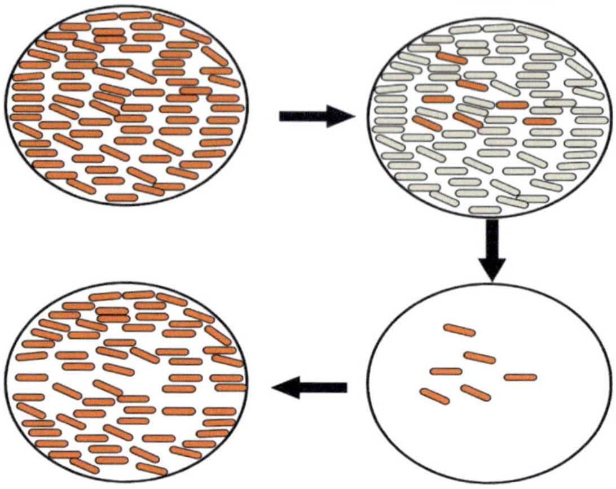

Fig. (1). Illustration showing the survival of persistent cells against antibiotics.

In the past 30 years, no new class of antibiotics had come in the market and a major reason is the increase in resistivity. In 1994, the WHO Scientific Group dealing with antibiotic resistance and surveillance stated that resistance to antibacterial agents is already a serious public health problem [8].Therefore, the current interest is antimicrobial peptides [9] which is mainly due to their ability to kill bacteria quickly by compromising the cell membrane integrity, hence they do not face the problem of resistance development against AMPs. AMPs are an intrinsic factor of the host's innate immune system in higher organisms [9]. AMPs are produced in response to various bacterial infections. AMPs are showing promising action to deal with antibiotic resistant bacteria in the present scenario [10]. AMPs which are distributed plentifully in nature can be a potential substitute to current anti-microbial drugs. The effectiveness of AMPs is broad-spectrum as they can act on a variety of bacteria, fungi, viruses, and parasites, and even cancerous cells [11]. Due to their ability to exert direct and/or indirect antimicrobial action, they are also termed as host-defence peptides [12].

BIOLOGICAL ROLES OF AMPS

Antimicrobial peptides belong to a diverse group with multi-dimensional properties and functional roles, that can't be denied. Apart from having antimicrobial activity, AMPs are also involved in the various intracellular processes such as angiogenesis, wound-healing, inflammatory response, and cell signalling. Different AMPs can perform differently as signalling molecules, mitogen, antitumor, immune modulators, and even as contraceptive agents (Table **1**). This unique characteristic makes AMPs among different types of antimicrobial compound, a perfect candidate for the profound study and development of novel drugs. Species-specific AMPs form species-specific bacterial relations [13]. For example, in the case of oral cavity infections, the role of defensins and cathelicidins as antimicrobial agents were identified by various researchers [14]. AMPs are not only effective in general bacterial infections, but can also be utilized as therapeutic agents against life-threatening bacterial or viral infections, for example; Retrocyclin-101 (RC101) and Protegrin-1 (PG1) are particularly used against HIV-1 or sexually transmitted infections [15].

Table 1. Different biological functions of antimicrobial peptides.

S. NO	Biological function	Peptide	Ref.
1	Direct chemotaxis of cell types such asneutrophils, monocytes, DCs, T cells and eosinophils	LL-37, PR-39, HNP-1,HNP-2, hBD-1 andhBD-2	[17 - 21]
2	Induction of chemokine expression	LL-37, hBD-2, hBD-3,IDR-1 and IDR-1002	[22 - 26]
3	Regulation of chemokine receptor expression,	LL-37	[26]
4	Suppression of neutrophil apoptosis	LL-37 and hBD-3	[27,28]
5	Induction of anti-inflammatory cytokines, *e.g.* IL-10 and IL-1RA	LL-37, IDR-1 and IDR-1002	[26, 29 - 31]
6	Suppression of pro-inflammatory mediators, *e.g.* IL-1, IL-6, TNF-α, and nitric oxide	LL-37, IDR-1 and IDR-1002	[26, 29, 31, 32]
7	Activation of ERK1/2 and p38 MAPK signalling pathways	LL-37 and hBD-2 61	[25, 33, 34]
8	Modification of DC differentiation, endocytic capacity, phagocytic receptor expression and cytokine secretion	LL-37 and HNP-1–3	[35 - 38]
9	Enhancement of phagocytosis HNP-1–3 Induction of autophagy	LL-37	[39]
10	Promotion of wound/vascular healing	LL-37, HNP-1, hBD-2 andhBD-3	[40,41]
11	Regulation of angiogenesis and arteriogenesis	LL-37 and PR-39	[42,43]
12	Activation and de-granulation of mast Cells	LL-37 and hBD-2–4	[44,45]
13	Regulation of T and B lymphocyte response	CRAMP	[46]

1. Antibacterial Activity (Direct)

Antimicrobial peptides can be used directly to overcome the problem of emerging antibiotic resistance due to their unique antimicrobial action. Among the various explained models of AMPs mechanism (discussed later in the chapter), membrane-disruption mode is primarily used as a major mechanism to exhibit its antimicrobial activity. The process of membrane disruption involves electrostatic binding of the negatively charged microbial surface to the positively charged AMPs. This results in significant perturbation in stability and negatively-charged phospholipid bilayer organization which leads to the disruption of microbial membrane integrity. Subsequent permeabilization of the membrane andosmolysis results in the death of a microbial cell [16].

2. Immune Modulation (Indirect Antibacterial Activity)

Direct antimicrobial activities of AMPs are considered to use AMPs as anti-infective drugs, however, in few cases, immuno-modulatory functions are a possible reason for antimicrobial property. AMPs have been found to be involved in many activities such as exhibiting immuno-modulatory actions, as well as anti-infective and selective anti-inflammatory properties *etc*. Around 2000 peptides have been reported in eukaryotes and in bacteria. The main function for these AMPs is direct antimicrobial action. Innate Defence Regulator (IDR) and Host Defence Peptides (HDPs) are important factors that are involved in immuno-modulatory function. The importance of the above two factors can be understood as illustrated in Fig. (**2**).

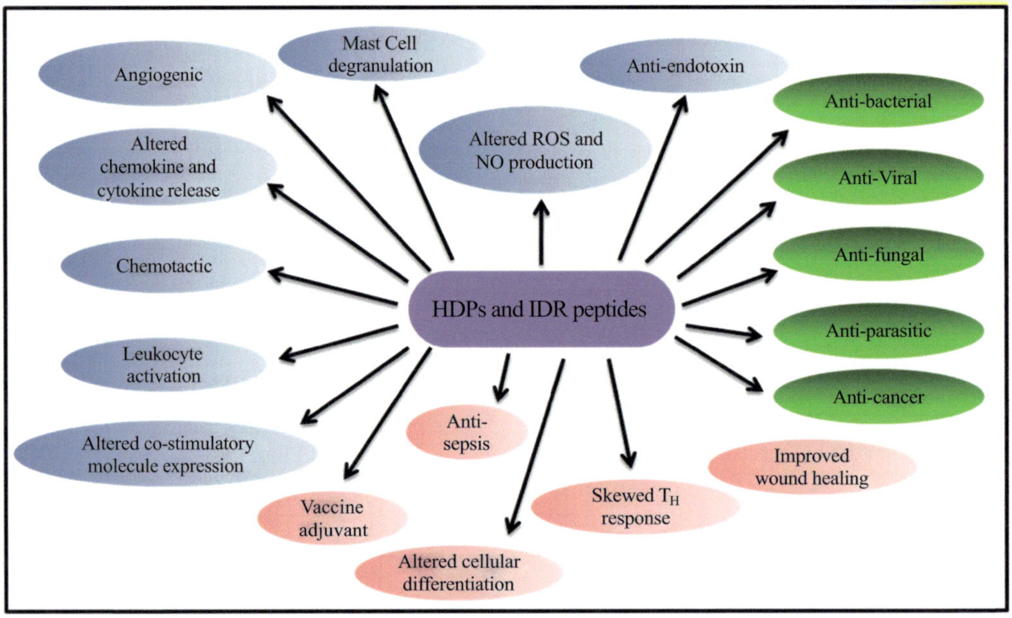

Fig. (2). Overview of the biological activities of HDP and IDR peptides: Direct cytotoxic activities are shown in green, direct immuno-modulatory peptides are shown in blue and indirect immuno-modulatory properties that are consequence of direct immuno-modulatory action.

DIFFICULTIES IN TESTING ANTIBIOFILM PROPERTIES

As bacteria are more resistant to a range of antimicrobial agents inside biofilms, so the focus now is on nontoxic antibiofilm agents, since it is believed that such molecules would not lead to drug resistance in future [47]. Biofilm-associated infections are more resilient to antibiotics and they act as a reservoir of drug resistant microorganisms, ultimately increasing the rate of failure of anti-infective healing. The identification as well as validation of newly invented antibiofilm agents is a crucial step. Testing these newly invented antibiofilm agents is not an easy process to experiment. There is a need for a wide range of procedural changes, and the criticism to be faced by microbiologists and infectious disease specialists will be large [48]. The exopolymeric substance (EPS) is also called "the house of biofilm cells". This surrounding substance shelters the biofilm microbial communities. EPS constitutes 90% of the total dry biomass, which provide high strength to the cells and cell-to-surface adhesion [49]. Many novel AMPs are being tested against mature and immature biofilms in recent years. Different AMPs are having distinct physical and physiochemical properties which make the process of testing their efficiency against biofilms tougher. As shown in many studies strain-to-strain variability is also one of the biggest problems to test AMPs as antibiofilm agents. To assess the antibiofilm activity of AMPs there were many studies with diverse methodologies which make the AMP assay non-universal [49]. The testing methods are different like in some cases the whole biomass has to be tested where viability of cell does not matter while in some techniques viability has to be tested. Furthermore, different components of biofilm play a specific role in the biofilm milieu. It should be noted that each kind of testing method as mentioned above does not give the same results. The diversity of testing method and its varied results make the testing process even more difficult [49]. *In-vitro* studies have shown that AMPs show better efficacy in combination with other antibiotics as compared to when used alone. The difference in efficacy of AMPs against biofilm and planktonic cells also demonstrates the difficulties of testing biofilms [50]. The variable range of biofilm architecture includes flat homogenous layers of cells or an organized cell cluster that makes the process of testing even more difficult. Other factors which play an important role, are higher frequency of mutation when compared to planktonic cells, the presence of low nutrient zones throughout biofilms, the oxidative stress development, the presence of polymers in biofilm matrix which obstruct their action and the presence of antibiotic-degrading enzymes that deactivate them [51]. Therefore, drug selection for biofilms needs a new test regime which can overcome these problems as discussed above. Activation of efflux pumps, acquisition of new enzymes and mutations of the drug targets have some impact on the presence of biofilms. Bacteria adopt a dormant mode of growth to overcome the toxic effects of the drugs. Selection of the best antibiotics to treat biofilm-associated incidents is a vital clinical confront [52].

ADVANTAGES OF AMPS OVER CONVENTIONAL ANTIBIOTICS

Antimicrobial peptides have captivated substantial attention as a new class of antimicrobial drugs for several reasons like their broad activity spectrum, selectivity towards a specific target, rapid action of mechanics and the lower rate of recurrence of resistant strains. AMPs have the ability to penetrate through cytoplasmic membranes by forming pores and thus have high potential against slow growing or even non-growing bacteria. This exceptional characteristic makes AMPs a future weapon against biofilms mode of infections [53]. AMPs have been isolated from most of the living organism as an innate machinery of their non-specific defences against infectious organisms. These isolates were taken as templates to design artificial AMPs in both chemical and biological mode. Few of these designed AMPs have been tested against specific pathogens are in use at present with mixed success. However, their assorted range of structures, activity band, biological roles, and modes of action, provide wide potential [54]. The effectiveness of AMPs to kill a number of pathogens such as bacteria, fungi, and viruses *via* a peculiar action mechanism makes it popular among the researchers. Moreover, as multi-drug/multi-antibiotics resistant pathogens can also be killed with AMPs, this property makes AMPs highly important. AMPs are able to disrupt the normal functioning of cellular membranes and sometimes directly interact with DNA to affect the expression of genes. AMPs are used for therapeutic application in two ways; either as single anti-infective agents or in combination with conventional antibiotics to increase their efficacy. Major advantages of AMPs over conventional antibiotics are that they illustrate broad-spectrum activity, quick onset of killing, cidal activity, potentially low levels of induced resistance and concomitant broad anti-inflammatory property [55]. AMPs illustrate broad immune modulatory effect when the pathogenic microbes or viruses infect host organism whereas antibiotics do not. They do not trigger adaptive immunity but fairly enhance the efficiency with the help of adjuvant activity (Table **2**). Highly diverse kind of AMPs are present, but they share few common properties like small size normally ~40 amino acids, binding to biological membranes, amphipathic secondary topology while they interact with membranes, a positive net charge under physiological circumstances and usually the ability to kill invading microorganisms within minutes [56]. The use of AMPs in the coating of medical implants has also been successfully tested. The AMPs coated over medical implants shown to be effective against bacterial and viral infections. Medical implants associated infections play a foremost hurdle in the use of medical devices in patients. Few studies have shown the efficiency of an AMP preventing implant-associated infections in an infectious keratitis model.

The results indicate that there is a promising future for AMPs as an antibiofilm drug [57].

Table 2. A comparison of conventional antibiotics with AMPs.

Property	Conventional Antibiotics	Antimicrobial Peptides
Spectrum of Activity	Bacterial infections (often selective)	Bacterial, fungal and viral infections; septicaemia; and inflammation
Uptake	Specific mechanisms	Relatively non-specific: based on charge. Self-promoted uptake
Targets	Usually one dominating target or class of targets (*e.g.* penicillin-binding proteins, topo-isomerases ribosomes)	Relatively less specific (possibly multiple targets in any given cell)
Resistance Rate and Mechanism	Resistance mechanisms involve degradation of antibiotics, reduced uptake or increased efflux, chemical modification or altered target Resistance, Resistance develops at frequencies of $10^{-7}$to 10^{-10}, or after a few passages at sub-MIC.	Resistance caused by mechanisms such as an impermeable outer membrane or specific proteases. Resistance development needs multiple passages on sub-MIC concentrations and can be overcome by amino acids alterations or replacement with D-amino acids)
Additional Activities	No	Boost innate immunity
Pharmacokinetics	Varies but once per week antimicrobials underdevelopment	Short systemic half-life due to proteolytic degradation
Toxicology	Safe	No known topical toxicities; systemic toxicity issues remain undefined
Manufacturing Costs	Production is quite cheap	Expensive ($40–400/gram)

Conventional antibiotics can be helped with the AMPs, the cumulative effect increased when they are used in combination. A brief comparison between conventional antibiotics and AMPs is given in Table **2** [58]. The AMPs as new kind of antibiotic offer a different approach against microbially related diseases. They offer many advantages for over conventional antibiotics for the commercial development, together with a broad range of action. The mode of action of AMPs against bacteria is normally through pore formation in the cell membrane, a very different way of action mechanism [59]. On the other hand, the emergence of AMP-resistant strains is very less. Along with plenty of advantages, AMPs are having some disadvantages too like instability, haemolytic activity, high cost of production and salt sensitivity [60].

STRUCTURES OF AMPS THAT INFLUENCE ANTIMICROBIAL ACTIVITY

Antimicrobial peptides structure plays an important role in determining its antimicrobial activity. Mode of action of AMPs is determined by the basic structure that required an improved structural categorization at the molecular level. Finding structural characteristics is a big challenge. While determining the anti-microbial activity of an AMP, many factors such as its secondary structure, orientation and tilt, topology of individual residues, *etc.*, all are taken into account [59]. AMPs are tremendously uneven in amino acid composition, size, and secondary structure, but they can acquire different membrane bound amphipathic conformation. A remarkable feature among AMPs as a group is that they have a conserved structure and charge across the diverse host environment.

Whether synthetically synthesized with and L- and D- amino acids, or from mRNA, AMPs acquire amphipathic structures and are mostly cationic at physiological conditions. Certain net charge (positive or negative) and amphipathicity are the conserved characteristics among almost all the AMPs. The charge affinity is probably one of the critical factors that confer selectivity to AMPs. In the context of these assumptions, the following key factors determine the molecular basis of antimicrobial activity as well as the selectivity of AMPs. Several aspects of AMPs structure that play role in antimicrobial activity and selective toxicity are described topically. As said earlier, structural parameters such as charge (Q), conformation (χ), amphi-pathicity (A), hydrophobic moment (MH), polar angle (θ), and hydrophobicity (H), determines the structure of AMPs (Fig. **3**) [60]. As these molecular determinants are interdependent, therefore, modification of any one of these parameters would lead to compensatory modulation in others. This holistic view of the peptide structure-activity relationship communicates to each of the key properties, thereby influencing the mechanisms of action of AMPs. Therefore, changes in the sequence, amino acid composition, and intra-molecular bonds have a significant effect on the structure-activity relationships of AMPs while interacting with membranes, or as they may undergo conformational phase transition to activated states. The optimal AMPs efficacy is derived from the coordination of these relationships as they relate to host cells *versus* pathogen target (Fig. **3**). When AMPs interact with specific pathogens in a specific physiologic micro-environment, these structural features become more critical factors for distinct peptides.

AMPs can acquire their antimicrobial activity by the modulation of different key cellular processes [61]. They compose a collection of various molecules that contribute to the innate immunity of numerous organisms. Biochemical characteristics play an important role in recognition and designing of new AMPs [62]. The structure may differ according to the source of production of AMPs (like bacteria, frogs, mammals, including humans *etc.*). Researchers have established a databases for AMPs, which helps to distinguish the structural difference between different AMPs [63]. There were also studies to identify some basic characteristics of human AMPs, which are over 100 such peptides, from different tissues and epithelial surfaces, including eyes, skin, oral cavities, ears, immune, gut, and excretory systems. Most of the natural AMPs are cationic in charge and a significant proportion (~60%) of peptide is comprised of hydrophobic residues. Whereas few AMPs, such as dermcidin, are anionic in charge, however, other biological actions appear to be more important for these peptides [64]. The size and amino acid composition of each AMPs are different [65]. The amino acid composition varies from 15 to 140 amino acids with a net charge varying from −3 and +20 and a hydrophobic content less than 60%, which allows human AMPs to adopt various structures [66]. Identifying and structural database formation for AMPs is very helpful to understand the mechanism of action and the possible role of the particular AMP.

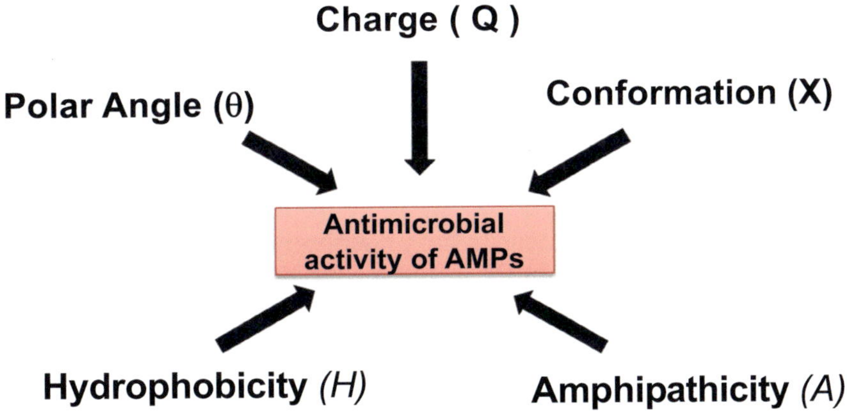

Fig. (3). Structural determinants of antimicrobial activity in antimicrobial peptides. The amino acid sequence as well as overall ccomposition influences not only the biochemical properties of the peptide but also govern their overall stereo geometry.

Primarily, a cationic charge and induced amphipathic conformations are vital for the antimicrobial activity. The membrane lipid composition specifically non-bilayer lipids is also an important element, apart from peptide conformation, in determining the peptide activity. Most of the studies have been concentrated mainly on the chemical and structural properties of these peptides. Membrane components may also play a crucial role in action and their proper study is need of the present day. The multiplicity of lipids between microorganisms may very well describe the differences in activity of a single peptide between these species. To understand the accurate mechanism a proper study of the relationship between peptides and lipids for a different organism is required [67]. The AMPs present in nature are generally from 12 to 50 amino acid chains, and most of them fit into four major structural groups, namely, α-helices, β-sheets, extended helices, and loops (Fig. **4**) [68].

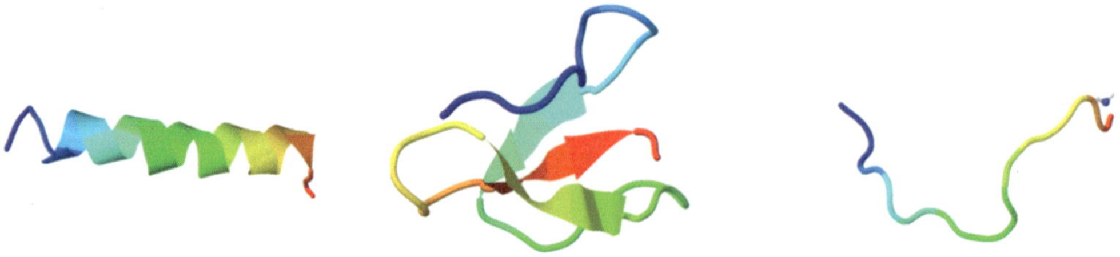

Fig. (4). Major structure classes of antimicrobial peptides. (a) α- helical peptides, example: Magainin-2 [PDB Id: 2MAG](b) β- sheet peptides, example: Human β-defensin-3 [PDB Id: 1KJ5](c) extended peptides, example- Indolicidin [PDB ID: 1G89].

1. α-Helical AMP

Peptides fold into as amphipathic α-helical are one of the prime groups among all peptides [69, 70]. The amphipathicity of the α-helix peptides is usually distributed along the axis in such way that one side of the helices is hydrophobic and the opposite side is charged. Thus, the peptide can lie parallel to the membrane plane during the initial lipid interactions *via* a hydrophobic interface, exposing the charged side facing outward towards the phospholipid head groups. Thus, overall biophysical properties of the α-helix influence the extent of membrane association with the membrane and, in turn, the antimicrobial activity [71]. Studies have shown that α- helices peptides with more continuous hydrophobic surface, can also become a contributing factor to cytotoxicity to the host (mammalian) cells [72, 73]. Activity modulation is majorly influenced by its structure, for example like its helicity. Indeed, few AMPs with low cytotoxicity but with substantial antimicrobial activity do need a membranous environment for proper folding. Such AMPs often have a proline- or glycine-induced link in the middle of the α-helix. Some studies showed that increase in the number of proline residues decreased the helicity, and is usually accepted as a helix breaker. Primary studies were focused towards improving the antimicrobial efficacy by proper amino acid substitution to increase peptide helicity [74]. Change in the peptide sequence can influence bacterial inner membrane permeability, insertion into liposomes, and hemolysis *etc.* [75]. Studies have shown that anα-helical peptide may turn into a toxin just by substituting of a single proline.

Antimicrobial peptide induced pore formation in the cell membrane is often associated with the temporary change in membrane thickness [76]. Most of the α-helices do have a length that is almost similar to the thickness of the cell membrane bilayers. Any misalignment between the hydrophobic cell membrane core and the hydrophobic portion of the helices strongly influence the orientation and lateral motion of AMPs within the membranes [77, 78]. An imperfect amphipathicity *i.e.* the presence of some charged or polar residues along the hydrophobic face of an AMP facilitates in the pulling of lipid head groups towards the membrane core, which aids in the pore formation. On the contrary, a perfect hydrophobic face on a peptide would bring the peptide in a parallel orientation with respect to the membrane surface. Imperfect amphipathicity is a key feature that explains the interfacial activity model [79] but also describes the disordered toroidal pore model up to some extent. The key difference between these two models is that in interfacial activity model AMP interaction with membrane causes the membrane disruption without the self-assembly of a peptide. In carpet model, AMPs act more like a detergent to dissociate the membrane lipids into micelle-like structures. This model is an extreme extension of the toroidal pore model which is described later in this chapter (Fig. **6**). Carpet model fits best wherein high concentrations of α-helical AMPs come into picture [80].

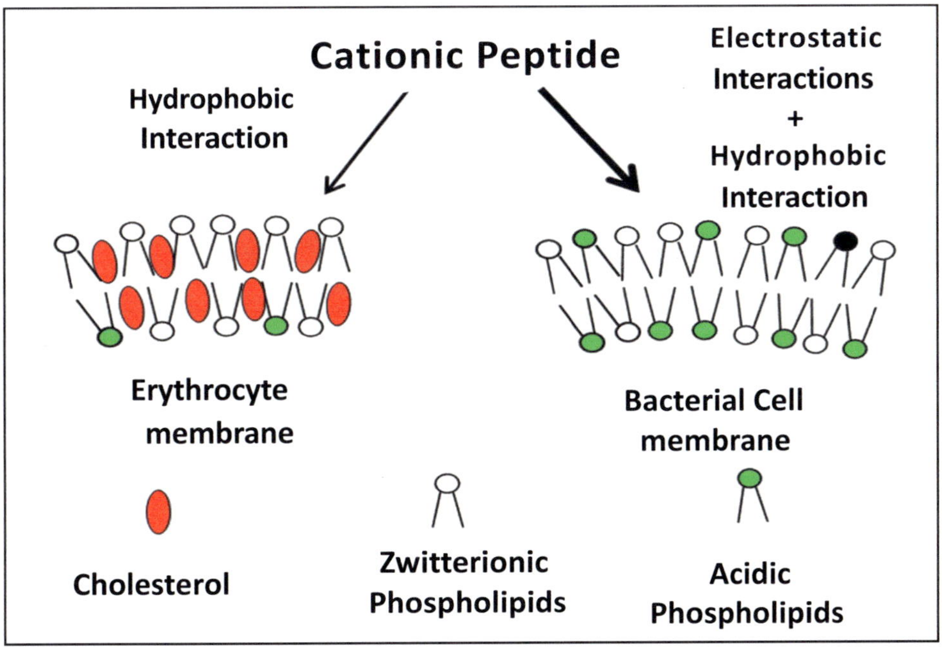

Fig. (5). Differential interaction of AMP molecules with eukaryotic membrane and bacterial cell membrane. Eukaryotic membrane surface is predominantly hydrophobic whereas bacterial cell membrane involves both electrostatic and hydrophobic interactions.

Few α-helical AMPs show pH-dependent mode of action. For instance, clavanin A which is a His-, Phe-, and Gly-rich peptide, permeabilizes membranes at neutral pH like regular α-helical AMPs which occurs *via* lipid interactions. However, at a slightly acidic pH, it manifests inhibitory interactions by interfering with proteins that are involved in maintaining the pH gradient across the membrane [81]. Buforin II, a peptide derivative from *Bufobufo gargarizans*, does not cause membrane disruption as most α-helical peptides do [82], however, the overall membrane lipid composition significantly affects its entry into the cell [83]. Once synthesized, buforin II exerts its antimicrobial activity by adapting an extended or polyproline II conformation to interact with DNA [84].

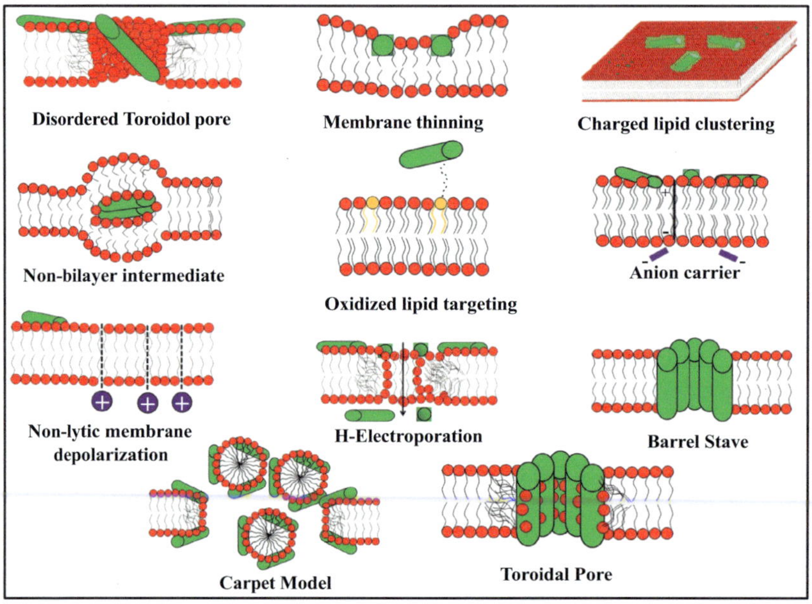

Fig. (6). Different models defining cell membranes disruptions. A- Disordered toroidol pore, B- Membrane thinning, C- Charged lipid clustering, D- Non-bilayer intermediate, E- Oxidized lipid targeting, F- Anion carrier, G- Non-lytic membrane depolarization, H-Electroporation, I- Barrel Stave, J- Carpet Model, K, Toroidal Pore, L- Bacterial Membrane, M- Peptides.

2. β-Sheet AMPs

β-sheet AMPs comprises the second most abundant group of AMPs that includes several β-hairpin peptides. These peptides disrupt bacterial membranes by forming toroidal pore structures in the membrane. These peptides form oligomeric transmembrane β-barrels in anionic membranes, but forms β-sheet aggregates on the surface of cholesterol containing membranes [61]. Certain β-sheet peptides also deploy non-lytic mechanisms. For instance, a membrane-active peptide, tachyplesin, is capable of binding to the minor groove of DNA and interferes with DNA–protein interactions [80]. The β-hairpin peptide bovine lactoferricin can affect the trans-membrane potential and proton motive force, resulting in inhibition of ATP-dependent multidrug efflux pumps [85]. Additionally, it can localize in the cytoplasm where it can inhibit protein synthesis as well as DNA, RNA synthesis. Due to these additional activities, such β-hairpin peptides can act synergistically if employed with other antimicrobial agents. Similarly, many peptide-mimetic analogs of AMPs often employ a new bactericidal mechanism involving a specific target but do not exhibit much membrane activity. For instance, few peptide-mimetic analogues of protegrin-I affect the outer membrane biosynthesis but do not have membrane activity [86]. In some studies, it was shown that the spectrum of peptide analogs was narrowed to *Pseudomonas aeruginosa* strains. On the other hand, human defensins, in which most are membrane active, few of them can bind to the peptidoglycan precursor lipid II to inhibit the cell wall synthesis in *Staphylococci* species [87].

The β-hairpin motif or β-sheet secondary structures of AMPs are often stabilized by disulphide covalent bonds between Cys residues. Studies have shown that linear derivatives of β-sheet tachyplesin and lactoferricin retained their antimicrobial activity, but lost the hemolytic activity which indicates that covalent bonds do not play a necessary role in antimicrobial activity [85]. A detailed study of tachyplesin and its two linear analogs, in which the four Cys residues were substituted by either Ala or Phe residues, showed that all three peptides are positioned at the membrane interface and adopt similar β-sheet conformations on anionic membranes. However, the Cys-to-Phe peptide was equally active as naïve tachyplesin, whereas the Cys-to-Ala peptide was found to be inactive [88]. Therefore, it is concluded that it is the peptide dynamics rather than their secondary structures which determine their functional activities. In human β-defensin-3, an α-helical turn followed by a three-stranded anti-parallel β-sheets are held together by three disulfide bonds in a definite pattern which distinguishes the β-defensins from the α-defensins. Rearrangement or reduction of these disulphide bond pattern in HBD-3 neither alters their antimicrobial activity, nor it abolishes the overall formation of the native secondary structure [61, 89]. However, their chemotactic activities are decreased for the analogs with non-native disulfide linkages.

3. Extended AMPs

Extended AMPs are short peptides which do not fold into regular secondary structures and often contain high proportions of certain amino acids, specifically Trp, Arg or Pro. Many of the extended peptides need not necessarily to be membrane active, they can exert their antimicrobial activity *via* other mechanisms. For instance, Proline rich AMPs drosocin, pyrrhocoricin, and apidaecin peptides penetrate through the membrane and do exert their antimicrobial activities by disruptive interactions with other essential intracellular metabolic proteins [80]. Sometimes extended AMPs can be fungicidal and anti-parasitic without having any bacteriostatic or bactericidal property; such as in the case of Histidine rich salivary histatin [90].

Two of the shortest known active peptides, RRWQWR and RAWVAWR, have been identified as the active antimicrobial fragments from bovine lactoferricin and human lysozyme, respectively. Trp and Arg residues are normally prominent in such short extended peptides [91]. Though, these peptides are not membrane active, but can fold into defined amphipathic molecules in the membranous environment and accumulate in the cytoplasm. On the other hand, 13-residue long Arg- and Trp-rich tritrpticin and indolicidin peptides can cause membrane leakage [91]. Both peptides comprise multiple Proline-induced turns that give them amphipathic boat-like conformations in a membranous environment (Fig. **5**). As these peptides are very small any residue substitutions do have a substantial effect on their overall structural and functional properties. For example, replacing the two Pro residues with Ala in tritrpticin transforms it into an α-helical peptide with slightly enhanced membrane and antimicrobial activity [92]. Indolicidin has been used as a template for the development of many analogous AMPs [93]. A number of factors contribute to the high efficacy of indolicidin, such as activation of phospholipase A2 secretion by human lacrimal fluid to hydrolyze anionic membranes [80] or acting as a small anion carrier across the membrane or a direct membrane action [94, 95]. It also has intracellular targets and can interfere with DNA-binding proteins [96]. It is unclear how the short and unique sequence of indolicidin can exhibit so many activities and which of the proposed mechanisms contributes to its activity *in vivo*.

Antimicrobial peptides display antibacterial activity against a broad-spectrum of microbes, including antibiotic resistant strains, and are less susceptible to resistance development [97]. In past one decade, many AMPs have been developed which includes β-peptides, arylamide oligomers, peptoids, and β-turn mimetic. Recently, a new class of AMPs has been recognised which are termed as "AA-peptides". AA-peptides are comprised of N-acylated-N-amino-ethyl amino acid units that are derived from chiral peptide nucleic acid backbones [98, 99]. They are highly resistant to proteolytic degradation and their amphipathic secondary structures mimicking the bactericidal mechanism of known AMPs. The two subclasses of these peptides termed as α-AA-peptides and γ-AA-peptides, have been designated depending on the position of the side chain which can bond with either α-C or γ-C (with respect to =CO group) [100]. The relationship between the structure and function of these peptides must be considered. Interestingly, AMPs may be designed by joining amphiphilic peptide building blocks. In this context, broad-spectrum antimicrobial activity of an AMP can be fine-tuned by changing the ratio of hydrophobic and charged by adding hydrophobic building blocks. This also suggests that the structural relationships in AMPs indicate the balance of forces required for bactericidal activity. To date, new synthetic AMPs are designed by cyclization of linear peptides or coupling with stable unnatural amino acids [101]. A dedicated library of linear γ-A-

-peptide sequences containing γ-1, γ-2, γ-3, and γ-4 has been prepared. It was found that γ-AA-peptides have had enhanced bactericidal activity against Gram-positive strains, indicating that γ-AA-peptides are very potent and can be developed as antimicrobial agents to treat Gram-positive bacterial infections [102]. However, they are quite toxic to blood cells as well as other mammalian cells. In fact, the antimicrobial activity of γ-AA-peptides are likely to be enhanced if the overall hydrophobicity increases, which at the same time also leads to increased hemolytic activity and cytotoxicity. Nevertheless, cationic residues can be introduced to minimize the hemolytic activity and cytotoxicity. Increasing hydrophobicity may increase antimicrobial activity, but can have low toxicity to mammalian cells [103].

MECHANISM OF ACTION OF AMPS

The relationship between AMPs structure and antibacterial activity has been described by many researchers but the molecular basis of noticeable dissimilarity in peptide activity and specificity has to be investigated (Table **3**). Membrane lipid composition is of significant importance for the action of AMPs. Bacteria with cytoplasmic membranes that have higher acidic phospholipids content were found to be more vulnerable to AMPs [80]. Cellular inactivation is a major consequence of the physical interaction of α-helical AMPs with membranes as defined in carpet model (Fig. **6**). Better understanding of the behaviour of natural α-helical AMPs and toxins would furnish a framework for the construction of the synthetic AMPs with optimized activity/selectivity profiles for possible biomedical applications [104]. Some AMPs present in human body help us to understand the structure and working mechanism. In human body AMPs are present in abundance and are widely distributed in human and animal tissues, they are mainly engaged in host defence. Models defined by different researchers explained that at the time of the natural attack by foreign molecules the defensins and other AMPs function as natural antibiotics in infected tissues [105].

All biological membranes are composed of proteins and lipids in a fluid mosaic arrangement. In some organisms, sterols and glycerides also contribute to the lipid surface array and the architecture of the cell membranes. Nevertheless, fundamental differences exist between microbial and host membranes that represent potential selective targets for AMPs. However, pharmacological application of AMPs relies on the degree to which they can differentiate, or engineered to differentiate between microbial targets and normal host cells.AMPs target the microbes by distinguishing the basic dissimilarity in the arrangement of the membrane components of the microbes and multi-cellular animals. For example, a bacterial membrane is covered by the outermost layer with negatively charged phospholipid head groups. On the other hand, the outermost layer in plant and animal cell membranes is made up of lipids with no charge [106]. The phenomena described can be clearly understood in Fig. (**5**). Zwitter ionic or acidic lipids are the crucial part of lipid bilayer membranes where they play an important role in living cells. AMPs carry a net positive charge and they bind to negatively charged outermost leaflet of the bacterial membrane with the help of hydrophobic and electrostatic relations. Typically AMPs fold into amphipathic secondary structures, α-helices and β-sheets. This action kills the bacteria *via* either physical, chemical, or biological processes [107].

The mode of action of AMPs in not known completely but proposed models portray dealings of peptides with microbial membrane and pore formation which leads to one or more of many processes that include micellization, membrane depolarization, cytoplasmic leakage, and internalization of biocidal peptides or break to intracellular macromolecule synthesis [108]. Three-dimensional arrangement and communication of AMPs with the microbial membrane *via* hydrophobic or electrostatic forces defines the mode of action [109]. More than 1700 natural AMPs have been identified and thousands of derivatives and analogues have been computationally designed, engineered or synthetically generated using natural AMPs as templates [109].

Earlier antimicrobial mechanism of AMPs was thought to be solely dependent on its ability to increase membrane permeability of microbes. However, various studies showed that this is not completely true. AMPs can exert its antimicrobial activity by restraining processes such as protein and cell wall synthesis, as well as enzyme activity, among the others [110]. The ability to damage cell membrane is a classical action of the mechanism but inhibition of cell wall synthesis, inhibition of nucleic acid and protein synthesis, induction of cell death are some actions of AMPs against different pathogens [110]. For almost three decades, AMPs have been investigated, but still, the mechanism of action is not fully understood. Some models (Fig. **6**) have been proposed that are helpful to explain its antimicrobial mechanism. Different models were described by various researchers like inter-facial activity model [79], Carpet like or detergent like [111 - 113], Membrane thinning [114 - 116], Aggregate type [117 - 119], Toroidal pore [80, 119], Barrelstave [122]. Each model defines its a specific plan of action. (Table **3**) describe specific action mechanisms of membrane-active AMPs.

Table 3. The action mechanisms of membrane-active AMPs.

Model	Mechanism
Carpet Like (Detergent-like)	First, peptide micelles come in the contact of membrane and mask a small area of the membrane. Then AMP molecules penetrate the lipid bilayer to let pore formation occur leaving holes behind.

(Table 3) contd.....

Model	Mechanism
Membrane Thinning	AMPs insert themselves into only one side of the lipid bilayer. It can form a gap between lipid molecules at the chain region. This gap creates a force and pulls the neighbouring lipid molecules to fill it.
Aggregate	AMPs stick to the membrane parallel to the surface. Then reorientation of AMPs occurs and they insert themselves into the membrane vertically to form sphere-like structures.
Toroidal Pore	AMPs align perpendicularly into the bilayer structure with their hydrophobic regions associated with the centre part of the lipid bilayer and their hydrophilic regions facing the pore
Barrel-stave	First, staves are formed parallel to the cell membrane followed by barrel formation. Then AMPs are inserted perpendicularly to the plane of the membrane bilayer.

Looking at all different models, one common theme in the mechanism of AMPs action appears to integrate the following factors: 1) initial interaction with target cells due to electrostatic and hydrophobic interactions. 2) biochemical and biophysical connections, conformational phase transition in the framework of the target membrane (*e.g.*, transition to α-helical conformational dynamics); 3) accumulation up to a threshold stoichiometry facilitating active peptide monomer or multimer nonspecific membrane disruption (*i.e.,* carpet mechanism), or self-association and ensuing pore or channel formation (*i.e.*, barrel-stave or toroid pore mechanisms); 4) transient or prolonged membrane disruption yielding permeability, depolarization, and related perturbations that may cause direct and indirect dysfunction and 5) peptide translocation across the membrane to access and inhibit intracellular targets (Fig. **7**).

The fluid mosaic model which defines the structure of functional cell membranes is composed of proteins and phospholipids. In some organisms, glycerides and sterols too take part the building of bio-membranes. Based on the basic differences in the membrane design the target for AMPs will be changed. Several AMPs are supposed to exist in comparatively amorphous or absolute shape prior to contact with target cells. Others are held in specific conformations by intramolecular bonds. Peptides may change their conformation into helical after binding to the pathogen cell membrane. AMPs structure determination is inter-related with different components, such as charge (Q), amphipathicity (A), hydrophobicity (H) and their three-dimensional configuration [*e.g.*, conformation (X), polar angle (θ), and overall stereo geometry (Fig. **3**). Therefore, best possible AMP efficiency slander in the applicable coordination of these relationships as they relate to microbial target *versus* host cells in a particular context of infection [60].

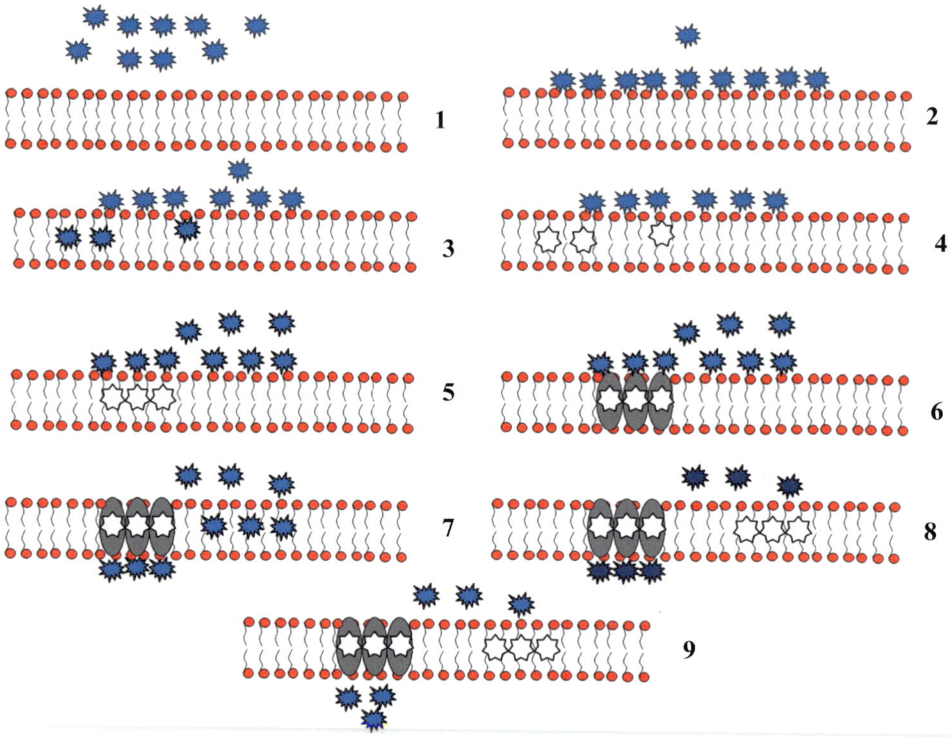

Fig. (7). Sequence of different steps in generalised theme of antibacterial activity of AMPs. Sequence of events associated with inhibition or killing of pathogen cells includes: 1) initial electrostatic and hydrogen bond interaction; 2) hydrophobic interactions when the AMPs come along the target surface; 3) accumulation and conformational modification of AMPs above the threshold concentration and subsequent early membrane deformation; 4) conformational phase transition aids AMP molecule insertion into the membrane core; 5) self-association and multimerization; 6) formation of quaternary peptide complexes with different configurations such as barrel-stave or toroid pore; 7) translocation of peptide to the inner facet of the cytoplasmic membrane; 8) ongoing peptide accumulation and interactions as described above; and 9) access and targeting of essential intracellular structures and functions. Native AMPs are indicated as coloured stars, whereas activated or conformation-transformed peptides are depicted as white stars.

RESISTANCE MECHANISM OF MICROBES TO AMPS

Microbial pathogens capable of surviving on exposure to AMPs generally employ two fundamentally distinct strategies: 1) constitutive resistance and 2) inducible resistance. A constitutive or passive mechanism of resistance refers to inherent properties of an organism that confer resistance and are normally expressed even in the absence of peptide exposure. On the other side, inducible (adaptive) resistance mechanisms include those triggered in response to the AMP or due to the target cell stresses. Anyway, these strategies exist as a coordinated response system that provides the pathogenic bacteria with the greater chance of survival in diverse environments.

A. Passive Resistance

A study has to be done to fully explain the inherent ability of certain microorganisms to resist killing by diverse types of AMPs. For example, in a variety of studies, *Serratia, Proteus,* and *Providencia* species showed to have refractoriness to inhibition or cell death by cationic AMPs [120]. *Pseudomonas* species also exhibit broad resistance to AMPs which was demonstrated by *in vitro* studies [121]. These studies illustrate that a few bacterial pathogens are inherently more resistant to AMPs due to their structural stability of membranes, functional properties and their unique pathogenic strategies. There are multiple factors which contribute to passive resistance to AMPs such as electrostatic shielding, altered membrane energetics, niche specific resistance *etc.*

1. Electrostatic Shielding/ Anionic Capsule Shielding

Most bacterial and fungal pathogens synthesize EPS as a means of adhering to biotic substratum or to escape opsonization and phagocytosis in the host. Thus, EPS production is an important virulence factor in those microorganisms, which infect the human bloodstream, respiratory tract, and gastrointestinal mucosa and is also a critical factor in biofilm stability. However, there is relatively little information available to assess the role of EPS expression in relation to resistance to AMPs. EPS compositions vary widely among different organisms. However, the capsular exopolymers of many pathogenic bacteria are often composed of an anionic complex of carbohydrates and phosphates. Therefore, it is rational to speculate that exopolymeric matrices such as those which sequester cationic AMPs, preventing them from accessing their intended targets. For instance, studies by Friedrich *et al.* [122] showed that purified alginate, which is a highly anionic capsular exo-polysaccharide produced by most of the virulent strains of *P. aeruginosa,* interferes with the antimicrobial activities of cationic AMPs *in vitro*. Thus, the AMPs, thereby confer the resistance against peptide-mediated killing. The complete molecular mechanism for peptide resistance is not yet clear. However, several captivating observations provide insights into the possible reasons. During the course of action of mechanism the, AMPs interact with the outermost surface, *i.e.* the cell membrane of the target pathogen. Thus, it can be conceived that such surfaces inherently lack electrostatic affinity and may even repel cationic AMPs (see Fig. **7**).

2. Reduced Negative Charge on Cell Membrane

Certain *Staphylococcus* species constitutively articulate cell membrane with reduced negative charge. *Staphylococcus aureus* strains that differ in susceptibility or resistance to AMPs showed constitutive alterations in cytoplasmic membrane structure. This could have been the key to inherent AMP resistance in *S. aureus* which subverts peptide-induced membrane dysfunction and cell death due to altered membrane energetics as they relate to peptides with specific mechanisms of action (see Fig. **6**). Experimental observations revealed that selective toxicity and potential antimicrobial spectra of such peptides is unique. Nonetheless, it is also speculated that some pathogenic bacteria employ regulation of energy status as a means of subverting the mechanisms of AMPs. Notable modifications in the outer membrane of some Gram-negative bacteria are also assumed to preserve membrane integrity in the presence of AMPs. Thus, intrinsic characteristics of microbial phospholipid membranes are likely related to constitutive AMPs resistance. Nahaie *et al.* [123] examined the constitutive phospholipids composition of a group of *Staphylococcus* species. These *Staphylococcus* species, displayed polar lipid profiles consisting predominantly of phosphatidyl-glyceroland di-phosphatidyl-glycerol. However, among the organisms tested, *S. aureus* was unique in having a lipid composition enriched in unsaturated menaquinones with eight isoprene units, and lysyl-phosphatidy-glycerol, a derivative of phosphatidyl-glycerol that is considerably less electronegative. In *Enterococcus* species resistance to AMPs has been associated with broad resistance to a group of cationic AMPs and heavy metal ions. However, the unusual susceptibility and resistance patterns to conventional antibiotics that target their cell membrane or cell wall do persist. Studies have shown that an inverse correlation exists between glycol-peptide susceptibility and resistance to cationic AMPs or oxidized heavy metal ions among clinical enteric bacteria. This finding suggested that mechanisms conferring inherent resistance to AMPs may prompt some bacterial pathogens to the inhibitory action. Phylogenetic scrutiny also supports the concept that distinct microorganisms possess constitutive structural features that confer AMP resistance.

3. Niche-specific Resistance

The perception of niche specific resistance to AMPs integrates many aspects of constitutive resistance as described above. However, this model is based on the assumption that some bacterial pathogens may resist AMPs to which they would otherwise be susceptible, simply by virtue of their affinity for or exploitation of certain anatomical or physiological niches of the host. For example, *P. aeruginosa* is an opportunistic pathogen that preferentially colonizes tissues having abnormal osmotic or ionic strength. Studies suggested that the protective role of AMPs may be diminished in relatively high ionic strength microenvironments, such as the kidney, when compared with cardiac or splenic tissues. Similarly, differences in other immune mechanisms in such tissues may also contribute to this phenomenon. Recorded observations, such as these accentuate the likelihood that some bacterial pathogens would exploit specific tissues or physiologic micro-environments to subvert the host defence contributions of AMPs.

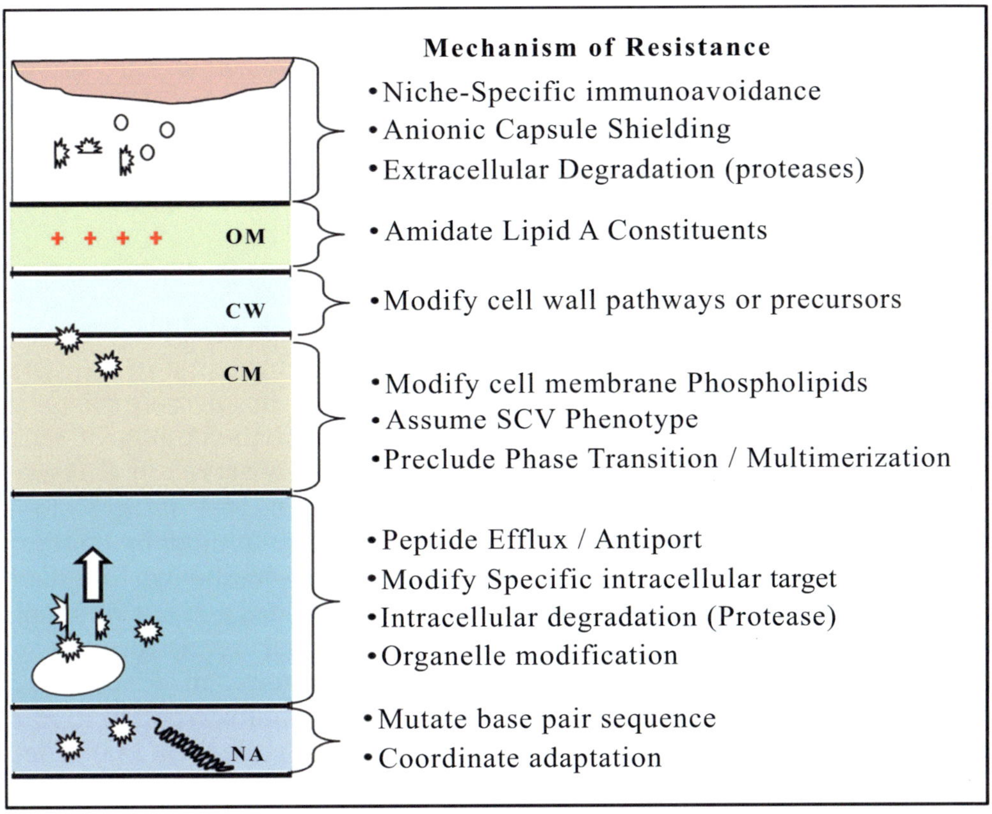

Fig. (8). A schematic showing the various mechanisms of microbial resistance against AMPs. Star and rectangle shape structures show inactive and active AMPs respectively. OM, Outer Membrane; CW, Cell Wall; CM, Cytoplasmic Membrane; CY, Cytoplasm; NA, Nucleic Acid.

B. Adaptive/Inducible Resistance

Microbial pathogens are exposed to several potentially lethal host defence mechanisms, one of which is AMPs (Fig. **8**). The organisms must negotiate many tolerant conditions at the host milieu in order to sustain its pathogenicity, survival, and proliferation. To counter such anti-microbial factors, many pathogenic bacteria have evolved an assortment of inducible countermeasures aimed to suppress the effects of the host defence mechanisms. Therefore, adaptive responses of pathogenic bacteria may range from quick activation of inducible virulence factors and the responses required for continued existence to elicit chronic strategies that eventually lead towards permanent cellular modifications to manifest its growth and proliferation. Moreover, most mechanisms of peptide resistance correspond to microbial responses that are completely opposed to mechanisms of peptide action. Constitutive and inducible mechanisms of resistance to AMPs are becoming clearer with the advent of genetically modified pathogens and the availability of native or synthetic AMPs. In a case of constitutive response, many of the mechanisms responsible for inducible resistance involve modifications of the pathogen's cell membrane and/or extracellular conformation of the cytoplasmic membrane, which directly offset the mechanism of peptide action. The following are the main action mechanisms to encounter AMPs toxicity by bacterial cells.

1. Activation of PhoP/PhoQ regulon in Microbial Response to AMP Stress

Exposure to AMPs results in a lethal stress condition, which would trigger a rapid activation of conserved response pathways in the cell. This surge in response is referred to as the starvation/stress or stringent response. In microorganisms, the inducible resistance to AMPs is largely controlled *via* a two-component sensor-transducer response system. This phenomenon was first observed in *Salmonella* sp, where the specific genetic locus of the pathogen was integral to the intracellular survival in macrophages as well as virulence in mice by conferring resistance to a defensin AMP [124]. Several two-component regulatory mechanisms have now been recognized and which activates a series of adaptive responses different pathogens. For example, sub-lethal levels of cecropins reported to induce hyper-osmotic stress response systems in *E. coli* [125]. Whereas, Hong *et al.* [126], showed that similar treatment of cecropinin in *E. coli* prompted a genomic response which was very distinguishable from that of lethal concentrations, and distinct from hyper-osmotic stress response.

PhoP-PhoQ is a two-component system that governs virulence, and regulates numerous cellular activities in several gram-negative species. It consists of the inner membrane sensor PhoQ and the cytoplasmic regulator PhoP [127]. The PhoP-PhoQ system is encoded by the *phoP* locus, which was first identified in *Salmonella enteric* serovar *Typhimurium* as controlling the expression of a nonspecific acid phosphatase [128]. It is now known that the PhoP/PhoQ system also activates the transcription of specific genes that encode inducible surface and secretory proteins, enzymes that modify lipopolysaccharide, lipid, and outer membrane protein constituents to mitigate the actions of AMPs. It also activates few specific extracellular proteases that are likely to degrade certain AMPs (see Fig. **9**). This whole systemic response is regulated by two sets of genes knows as 'phoP-activated genes (*pag*)', and 'phoP-repressed genes(*prg*)'. *Pag* clusters up-regulate the expression of pathways that actively defend against AMPs such as proteases, and enzymatic modification of surface structures and whereas *prg* gene cluster suppress the expression of structural or functional features vulnerable to AMPs action [129].

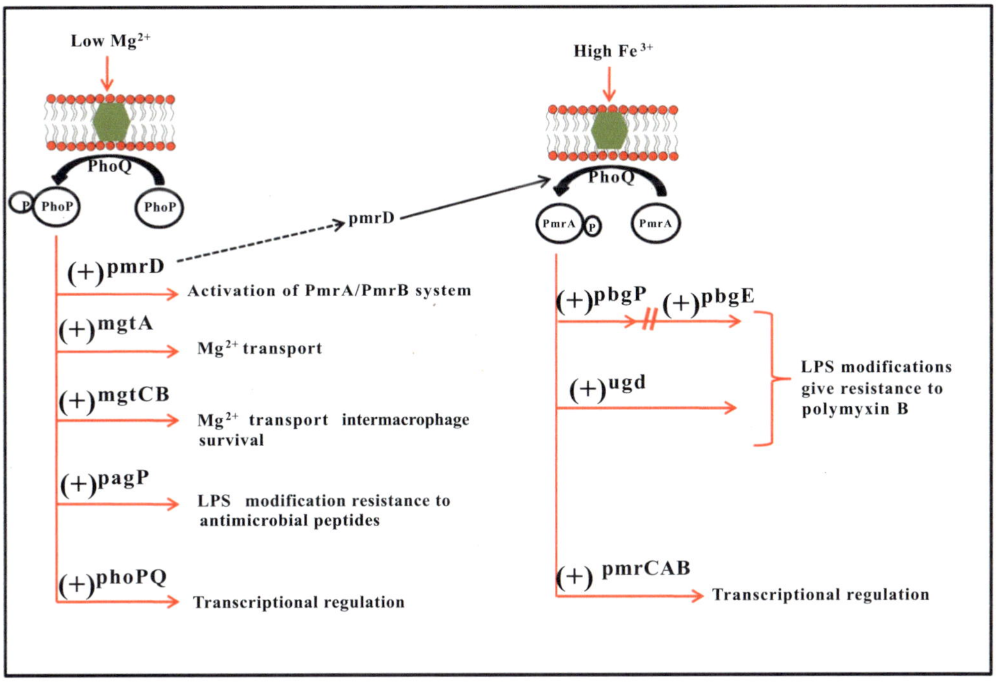

Fig. (9). Adaptive/Inducible Resistance: A coordinated microbial response to AMP stress *via* PhoP-PhoQ and PmrA/PmrB system activation.

Apart from PhoP/PhoQ, a distinct two-component regulatory system, PmrA/PmrB, also coordinates the expression of a different set of genes which appear to be necessary for synthesis and addition of amino-arabinose onto lipid A in the Gram-negative bacterial outer membrane [130], imparting more cationic charge to the membrane, thus enhancing the electrostatic shielding and in turn higher resistance towards cationic AMPs. PhoP/PhoQ and PmrAB regulatory systems also PagB, regulator of PhoP/PhoQ system, activates the two-component pmrA-pmrB regulon, which confers *Salmonella* resistance to numerous cationic AMPs, including polymyxin B, azurocidin, bactericidal activity, permeability increasing factor, protamine, and polylysine. PhoP/PhoQ also regulates pagP, encoding an acyl-transferase that catalyzes lipid Apalmitoylation in *Salmonella*. This outer membrane modification is believed to reduce AMP accessibility to the cytoplasmic membrane. Thus, the PhoP/PhoQ and PmrA/PmrBsystems act synergistically and the likelihood function will complement in AMPs degradation and confer peptide resistance through the surface and envelope modifications, respectively [129].

2. Proteases and Peptidases.

Protease-mediated resistance to AMPs was described from well-characterized studies examining the pathogenic Gram-negative bacteria. Many microbial systems regulate the countermeasures employed by bacteria to resist AMPs. Among them, the PgtE protein was recently demonstrated and found to be an outer membrane endo-peptidase in the case of *Salmonella* [131]. This protein molecule was identified as having structural features consistent with the outer membrane protease families [132]. These proteases specifically cleave peptides between paired basic amino acid residues and at the carboxy-terminal aspect of basic amino acid residues that precede a nonpolar residue. Thus, a variety of amphipathic and cationic AMPs are a probable substrate to PgtE protease [132]. It is intriguing to note that, in *Salmonella*, a *pgtE* deletion strain exhibited increased *in vitro* sensitivity to a number of α-helical peptides that contain predicted cleavage sites. However, PgtE protease did not confer any enhanced resistance to amphipathic β-sheet peptides (*e.g.,* defensins or protegrins). Therefore, the three-dimensional structures of the latter peptides will likely create steric hindrance that is protective against the activity of PgtE protease.

OmpT, a homolog of PgtE in *E. coli*, has shown to promote AMP resistance in *Salmonella*, as well as in *E. coli.* Studies showed that expression of OmpT increases the survival of *E. coli* in the presence of protamine, which is a DNA binding and cationic AMP [133]. Results also showed OmpT to be capable of degrading protamine in low or high Mg^{2+} concentrations, although degradation of the peptide was slower in conditions of higher ionic strength. These findings suggest that OmpT functions to degrade AMPs at the extracellular facet of the outer membrane of *E. coli*. OmpT provides *E. coli.* with an important survival advantage against host innate immunity, thus it has been implicated as a key virulence factor.

3. Extracellular Structural Modification

The initial target of AMPs was to interact with the external appendages of the cytoplasmic membrane. With exposure to AMPs, bacterial pathogens have developed mechanisms by which these targets can be modified to resist peptide targeting and circumvent the ensuing antimicrobial mechanism. Coordinate systems commonly regulate expression of countermeasures needed for pathogen survival in response to AMP exposure. Theoretically, this feedback mechanism should rapidly induce and trigger in part the peptide action itself. For example, major variations in Mg^{2+} or Ca^{2+} concentrations (intracellular or trans-cellular) induced by AMPs action can activate the *Salmonella* PhoP/PhoQ locus [127]. Cationic AMPs can likely displace or mobilize these ions or perturb their transmembrane gradient as part of their mechanism of action against organisms unable to respond defensively. Therefore, it is likely that one mechanism of action of these peptides involves the inactivation and/or deregulation of these or other resistance countermeasures.

4. Modification of Cytoplasmic Membrane

Microbial pathogens adaptively modify their cytoplasmic membrane to resist cationic AMP through a highly regulated mechanism involving cytoplasmic membrane modification in Gram-positive as well as in Gram-negative bacterial pathogens. In a study by Dorrer and Teuber [134], it was found that when *Pseudomonas fluorescens* culture was shifted from phosphate-rich to phosphate-limited medium, a dramatic decline in anionic phospholipids composition of cytoplasmic membrane occurred. Interestingly concomitant with these changes in anionic phospholipids, a cationic ornithine-amide constituent emerged in membranes. This increase in cationic ornithine-amide constituent was also correlated with increasing resistance to polymyxin B. Another observation that intact cells, in addition to isolated cytoplasmic or outer membranes of resistant organisms, have displayed significantly reduced binding capacities for polymyxin B. This has further substantiated the speculation that cationic polymyxin B exerts its antibiotic activity *via* high-affinity binding to electronegative bacterial membrane constituents.

THERAPEUTIC TARGETS OF ANTIMICROBIAL PEPTIDES

Recent studies have contributed significantly to enhance our current understanding of poorly understood action mechanisms AMPs and resistance against it. These advances have highlighted potentially vulnerable microbial structures and functions. A better understanding of AMP action against planktonic microbes and biofilms would facilitate the further development and design of novel anti-biofilm agents or treatment strategies. For example, new efforts are being made towards targeting sensitive microbial structures or functions, exploiting specific contexts or virulence factors characteristic of infection, and hampering pathogen adaptive response mechanisms. These approaches may take advantage of unique situations associated with pathogenesis or host response to govern and optimize AMPs targeting and selective toxicity. The following concepts are the emerging highlights in the area of AMPs:

A. Synergistic Effect on Conventional Antibiotics Efficacy

The prospective therapeutic applications of AMPs are related to their use to enhance the antibacterial efficiency of conventional antibiotics. For example, the tendency of AMPs to permeate microbial cell membranes may facilitate the conventional antibiotics by enhancing penetration/diffusion of antibiotics and to overcome the resistance mechanisms such as reduced uptake. On the other hand, AMPs that interact with intracellular processes or targets can be coaxed so that they noncompetitively boost the mechanisms of typical antibiotics. The potential for synergistic activities among AMPs in combination is recently being appreciated [135]. Although many credible examples of the favourable interactions were observed by *in vitro* studies, yet the challenge to understand and apply the mechanistic basis is not clear.

The configuration and functional attributes that are distinctive to AMPs interactions with bacterial pathogens present new insights for the development of novel anti-infective agents that are derived from host defence bio-molecules. Molecular determinants that are arising as likely targets for AMP strategies include; bacterial receptors, metabolic processes and essential pathways, virulence factors (adhesins and envelope proteins), as well as ribosomes, mitochondria, or nucleic acids which are intracellular targets. Besides, AMPs may be useful in potentiating microbial targets that are vulnerable to host cellular immune mechanisms.

B. Strategic Microbial Response Pathways

AMPs target constitutive and inducible assets of pathogenic bacteria as targets of their mechanisms of action. For example, adaptations to characteristic membrane energetics, surface moieties, or expression of virulence factors are exploited by AMPs in host defence. In addition, AMP-induced responses that certainly evoke global changes in pathogen status and virulence capability. Such as, responses necessary for survival upon exposure to AMPs may prompt microorganisms to considerably compromise virulence factor or surface feature expressions that are required for adhesion, colonization and to avoid the immune response. Similarly, the unregulated activation of signalling pathways on exposure to AMPs or their analogues such as synthetic peptides may lead to pathogen injury and cell death due to deregulation. Although nonlethal, the effects will render pathogens to greatly increase susceptibility to host defence mechanisms.

BIOLOGICAL PRODUCTION OF AMPS

During early stages of host response to pathogens, AMPs together with antimicrobial metabolites and stress related proteins act as components of non-specific basic defence mechanisms [136]. As stated earlier, AMPs are produced by all kinds of organisms, from bacteria to mammals. AMPs display lower cytotoxicity to mammalian cells and exhibit a unique mode of action. Active peptides can be synthesized by using different bacterial expression system. Most of the bacteriocins are produced as precursor peptides and then modified inside the cell exterior as the final product. Degradation of larger proteins can be used to produce small peptides [137]. The widely dispersed AMPs in the phylogenetically distant organisms ranging from bacteria and primitive invertebrates to humans shows that they are ancient evolutionary molecules [138]. AMPs can be isolated from plants too like from roots, seeds, flowers, stems, and leaves of a variety of species. Plants produce a lot of toxic molecules as a part of the resistance response which includes AMPs as well [139]. Plants can be used for AMPs production and will be an excellent alternative for expensive peptide production. Larger precursors like signal sequence changed or modified into AMPs in most of the cases. Post-translational modifications include proteolytic processing, glycosylation, and amino-acid isomerisation are some of the precursors [140]. These host-defense peptides can be categorized by the name of the target, against which it shows its cidal action. AMPs are most studied against bacteria, however, antifungal peptides, and anti-parasitic peptides also exist [141].

A. Over-expression of AMPs in Heterologous Host

Expression of AMPs in recombinant bacterial expression systems has been found in several cases. Expression of AMPs by using a recombinant system helps to make the process economically viable, which helps in mass production. Insect, baculo virus [142], yeast [143], and *Escherichia coli* [144 - 146] based systems have been used by researchers. Various systems have been developed for the expression of AMPs, which includes Translational Coupled Two-Cistron Expression System [147], a recombinant system in *E. coli, etc* [148]. Expressing AMPs directly in *E. coli* may also sometimes cause numerous difficulties such as AMP toxicity to the host cell, its vulnerability towards proteolytic degradation, *etc*. To overcome this problem, sometimes, it can be over expressed with a fusion partner that can be helpful in enhancing its stability and ease the product recovery, in tern, its productivity [149]. Fission by chemical or enzymatic cleavage helps the peptide to release [150]. Bacteria are not only in use for the AMPs production but also to bioengineer "bugs", which can be of use for both the production and characterization of AMPs. Most of the AMPs are produced in their host organisms but their recovery from their respective host species are neither reasonably nor realistically practicable and it might even result in environmental issues. Synthesis of amino acid sequence is economically viable if only when its size is short, however, with increase in the peptide length it becomes a highly expensive process [151]. As already described above, many microbial streams were used for the production and expression of numerous AMPs, *e.g.* dermicin [152], moricidin [153], defensins [154] and buforin [155].

B. New Synthetic Peptides and Their Function

For few decades new synthetic AMPs have been used to prevent or treat bacterial infections. For example, gramicidins, polymyxins, and bacitracin were found in many topical applications. For many years, lantibiotics *i.e.,* bacteria derived AMPs have been in use to preserve livestock feed. Many AMPs are under clinical trials to assess their efficacies as topical and systemic peptide drug, but yet to get federal approval for manufacturing and commercial use. Thus, the concept that AMPs may be utilized to prevent or treat disease is not very new. However, advances in understanding the structural and mechanistic aspects of AMPs may accelerate the development of improved, new and effective anti-infective agents. For example, how AMPs differentiate between pathogen and host cells provide the inputs to enable design new peptides with higher selectivity. In this context, efforts to identify and constrain peptides to antimicrobial conformations may allow the engineering of novel peptides with potent efficacy against even the most antibiotic resistant pathogens. Studies that guide the identification and formulation of the most selective peptide-antibiotic and peptide-peptide combinations with an equivalent *in vivo* demonstration are warranted. The possibility of the emergence of drug resistance bacteria against AMPs needs to be evaluated by detailed studies. Some research work should be focused on the development of AMPs against Gram-negative bacteria, which are more difficult to kill when compared to Gram-positive bacteria.

CONCLUSION

The early period of antibiotic discovery came as a boon in the field of bacteria related infections, however, the emergence of multi-antibiotic resistant bacteria have forced the scientific community to look for quick alternative drugs to treat such infections. Multi-drug resistance at present is an ever-growing universal public health risk that entails all major microbial pathogens and antimicrobial drugs [156]. Increasing understanding of AMPs structure and their mode of actions has shown promising future for the development of AMPs against medical biofilms as an alternative to antibiotics in the post-antibiotic era. To use AMPs for biofilm therapies, biofilm>related resistance to AMPs also needed to be addressed. In particular, AMP repulsion or sequestration by the biofilm matrix and proteolytic degradation by microbial proteases are known to limit AMPs efficacy, particularly against biofilm control. The synergistic effect with conventional antibiotics offered by peptides, further expand the promising use of AMPs. The composition of AMPs shows a potential substitute to therapeutic agents against a variety of pathogenic microbes. The isolation of these therapeutic agents is possible from a variety of organisms. In this context, synthetic biology using computational approaches may also provide valuable contributions in AMPs rational design. More engineered AMPs *via* molecular modelling method can clarify AMP mechanisms of action on the bacterial membrane or even on the biofilm matrix. Protein engineering by modifying one or two amino acids to generate more effective AMPs gives hope that more effective AMPs that are less toxic to host cells may be designed specifically against biofilms. However, while the AMPs are recognized as essential components of natural host innate immunity against microbial infections, their usefulness as a new class of antimicrobial drugs still has to be realized after looking into various concerns.

CONFLICT OF INTEREST

The authors declare no conflict of interest, financial or otherwise.

ACKNOWLEDGEMENTS

Declared none.

REFERENCES

[1] Watkins RR, Bonomo RA. Overview: Global and Local Impact of Antibiotic Resistance. Infect Dis Clin North Am 2016; 30(2): 313-22.
[http://dx.doi.org/10.1016/j.idc.2016.02.001] [PMID: 27208761]

[2] Morandi S, Cremonesi P, Capra E, *et al.* Molecular typing and differences in biofilm formation and antibiotic susceptibilities among *Prototheca* strains isolated in Italy and Brazil. J Dairy Sci 2016; 99(8): 6436-45.
[http://dx.doi.org/10.3168/jds.2016-10900] [PMID: 27236754]

[3] Dheilly A, Soum-Soutéra E, Klein GL, *et al.* Antibiofilm activity of the marine bacterium *Pseudoalteromonas sp. strain* 3J6. Appl Environ Microbiol 2010; 76(11): 3452-61.
[http://dx.doi.org/10.1128/AEM.02632-09] [PMID: 20363799]

[4] Nouraldin AA, Baddour MM, Harfoush RA, Essa SA. Bacteriophage-antibiotic synergism to control planktonic and biofilm producing clinical isolates of *Pseudomonas aeruginosa.* Alexandria Med J 2016; 52: 99-105.
[http://dx.doi.org/10.1016/j.ajme.2015.05.002]

[5] Ory J, Bricheux G, Togola A, *et al.* Ciprofloxacin residue and antibiotic-resistant biofilm bacteria in hospital effluent. Environ Pollut 2016; 214: 635-45.
[http://dx.doi.org/10.1016/j.envpol.2016.04.033] [PMID: 27131824]

[6] Centner TJ. Efforts to slacken antibiotic resistance: Labeling meat products from animals raised without antibiotics in the United States. Sci Total Environ 2016; 563-564: 1088-94.
[http://dx.doi.org/10.1016/j.scitotenv.2016.05.082] [PMID: 27236477]

[7] Cohen NR, Lobritz MA, Collins JJ. Microbial persistence and the road to drug resistance. Cell Host Microbe 2013; 13(6): 632-42.
[http://dx.doi.org/10.1016/j.chom.2013.05.009] [PMID: 23768488]

[8] Hancock RE. Peptide antibiotics. Lancet 1997; 349(9049): 418-22.
[http://dx.doi.org/10.1016/S0140-6736(97)80051-7] [PMID: 9033483]

[9] Sampson M, Phillips C, Blake R. Influence of the attachment of acidophilic bacteria during the oxidation of mineral sulfides. Miner Eng 2000; 13: 373-89.
[http://dx.doi.org/10.1016/S0892-6875(00)00020-0]

[10] Andersson DI, Hughes D, Kubicek-Sutherland JZ. Mechanisms and consequences of bacterial resistance to antimicrobial peptides. Drug Resist Updat 2016; 26: 43-57. [http://dx.doi.org/10.1016/j.drup.2016.04.002] [PMID: 27180309]

[11] Lakshmaiah Narayana J, Chen J-Y. Antimicrobial peptides: Possible anti-infective agents. Peptides 2015; 72: 88-94. [http://dx.doi.org/10.1016/j.peptides.2015.05.012] [PMID: 26048089]

[12] Bauer ME, Shafer WM. On the *in vivo* significance of bacterial resistance to antimicrobial peptides. BBA Biomembranes 2015; 1848: 3101-11.

[13] Franzenburg S, Walter J, Künzel S, *et al.* Distinct antimicrobial peptide expression determines host species-specific bacterial associations. Proc Natl Acad Sci USA 2013; 110(39): E3730-8. [http://dx.doi.org/10.1073/pnas.1304960110] [PMID: 24003149]

[14] Tao R, Jurevic RJ, Coulton KK, *et al.* Salivary antimicrobial peptide expression and dental caries experience in children. Antimicrob Agents Chemother 2005; 49(9): 3883-8. [http://dx.doi.org/10.1128/AAC.49.9.3883-3888.2005] [PMID: 16127066]

[15] Lee SB, Li B, Jin S, Daniell H. Expression and characterization of antimicrobial peptides Retrocyclin-101 and Protegrin-1 in chloroplasts to control viral and bacterial infections. Plant Biotechnol J 2011; 9(1): 100-15. [http://dx.doi.org/10.1111/j.1467-7652.2010.00538.x] [PMID: 20553419]

[16] Augustyniak D, Nowak J, Lundy FT. Direct and indirect antimicrobial activities of neuropeptides and their therapeutic potential. Curr Protein Pept Sci 2012; 13(8): 723-38. [http://dx.doi.org/10.2174/138920312804871139] [PMID: 23305360]

[17] Tjabringa GS, Ninaber DK, Drijfhout JW, Rabe KF, Hiemstra PS. Human cathelicidin LL-37 is a chemoattractant for eosinophils and neutrophils that acts *via* formyl-peptide receptors. Int Arch Allergy Immunol 2006; 140(2): 103-12. [http://dx.doi.org/10.1159/000092305] [PMID: 16557028]

[18] Soehnlein O, Zernecke A, Eriksson EE, *et al.* Neutrophil secretion products pave the way for inflammatory monocytes. Blood 2008; 112(4): 1461-71. [http://dx.doi.org/10.1182/blood-2008-02-139634] [PMID: 18490516]

[19] Yang D, Chen Q, Chertov O, Oppenheim JJ. Human neutrophil defensins selectively chemoattract naive T and immature dendritic cells. J Leukoc Biol 2000; 68(1): 9-14. [PMID: 10914484]

[20] Territo MC, Ganz T, Selsted ME, Lehrer R. Monocyte-chemotactic activity of defensins from human neutrophils. J Clin Invest 1989; 84(6): 2017-20. [http://dx.doi.org/10.1172/JCI114394] [PMID: 2592571]

[21] Huang HJ, Ross CR, Blecha F. Chemoattractant properties of PR-39, a neutrophil antibacterial peptide. J Leukoc Biol 1997; 61(5): 624-9. [PMID: 9129212]

[22] Ghosh SK, Gupta S, Jiang B, Weinberg A. Fusobacterium nucleatum and human beta-defensins modulate the release of antimicrobial chemokine CCL20/macrophage inflammatory protein 3α. Infect Immun 2011; 79(11): 4578-87. [http://dx.doi.org/10.1128/IAI.05586-11] [PMID: 21911466]

[23] Montreekachon P, Chotjumlong P, Bolscher JG, Nazmi K, Reutrakul V, Krisanaprakornkit S. Involvement of P2X(7) purinergic receptor and MEK1/2 in interleukin-8 up-regulation by LL-37 in human gingival fibroblasts. J Periodontal Res 2011; 46(3): 327-37. [http://dx.doi.org/10.1111/j.1600-0765.2011.01346.x] [PMID: 21338358]

[24] Nijnik A, Madera L, Ma S, *et al.* Synthetic cationic peptide IDR-1002 provides protection against bacterial infections through chemokine induction and enhanced leukocyte recruitment. J Immunol 2010; 184(5): 2539-50.

[http://dx.doi.org/10.4049/jimmunol.0901813] [PMID: 20107187]

[25] Mookherjee N, Lippert DN, Hamill P, *et al.* Intracellular receptor for human host defense peptide LL-37 in monocytes. J Immunol 2009; 183(4): 2688-96. [http://dx.doi.org/10.4049/jimmunol.0802586] [PMID: 19605696]

[26] Scott MG, Davidson DJ, Gold MR, Bowdish D, Hancock RE. The human antimicrobial peptide LL-37 is a multifunctional modulator of innate immune responses. J Immunol 2002; 169(7): 3883-91. [http://dx.doi.org/10.4049/jimmunol.169.7.3883] [PMID: 12244186]

[27] Nagaoka I, Niyonsaba F, Tsutsumi-Ishii Y, Tamura H, Hirata M. Evaluation of the effect of human β-defensins on neutrophil apoptosis. Int Immunol 2008; 20(4): 543-53. [http://dx.doi.org/10.1093/intimm/dxn012] [PMID: 18308714]

[28] Nagaoka I, Tamura H, Hirata M. An antimicrobial cathelicidin peptide, human CAP18/LL-37, suppresses neutrophil apoptosis *via* the activation of formyl-peptide receptor-like 1 and P2X7. J Immunol 2006; 176(5): 3044-52. [http://dx.doi.org/10.4049/jimmunol.176.5.3044] [PMID: 16493063]

[29] Turner-Brannen E, Choi K-Y, Lippert DN, *et al.* Modulation of interleukin-1β-induced inflammatory responses by a synthetic cationic innate defence regulator peptide, IDR-1002, in synovial fibroblasts. Arthritis Res Ther 2011; 13(4): R129. [http://dx.doi.org/10.1186/ar3440] [PMID: 21835002]

[30] Mookherjee N, Hamill P, Gardy J, *et al.* Systems biology evaluation of immune responses induced by human host defence peptide LL-37 in mononuclear cells. Mol Biosyst 2009; 5(5): 483-96. [http://dx.doi.org/10.1039/b813787k] [PMID: 19381363]

[31] Scott MG, Dullaghan E, Mookherjee N, *et al.* An anti-infective peptide that selectively modulates the innate immune response. Nat Biotechnol 2007; 25(4): 465-72. [http://dx.doi.org/10.1038/nbt1288] [PMID: 17384586]

[32] Mookherjee N, Brown KL, Bowdish DM, *et al.* Modulation of the TLR-mediated inflammatory response by the endogenous human host defense peptide LL-37. J Immunol 2006; 176(4): 2455-64. [http://dx.doi.org/10.4049/jimmunol.176.4.2455] [PMID: 16456005]

[33] Bowdish DM, Davidson DJ, Speert DP, Hancock RE. The human cationic peptide LL-37 induces activation of the extracellular signal-regulated kinase and p38 kinase pathways in primary human monocytes. J Immunol 2004; 172(6): 3758-65. [http://dx.doi.org/10.4049/jimmunol.172.6.3758] [PMID: 15004180]

[34] Tjabringa GS, Aarbiou J, Ninaber DK, *et al.* The antimicrobial peptide LL-37 activates innate immunity at the airway epithelial surface by transactivation of the epidermal growth factor receptor. J Immunol 2003; 171(12): 6690-6. [http://dx.doi.org/10.4049/jimmunol.171.12.6690] [PMID: 14662872]

[35] Rodríguez-García M, Oliva H, Climent N, *et al.* Impact of α-defensins1-3 on the maturation and differentiation of human monocyte-derived DCs. Concentration-dependent opposite dual effects. Clin Immunol 2009; 131(3): 374-84. [http://dx.doi.org/10.1016/j.clim.2009.01.012] [PMID: 19237318]

[36] Funderburg N, Lederman MM, Feng Z, *et al.* Human -defensin-3 activates professional antigen-presenting cells via Toll-like receptors 1 and 2. Proc Natl Acad Sci USA 2007; 104(47): 18631-5. [http://dx.doi.org/10.1073/pnas.0702130104] [PMID: 18006661]

[37] Bandholtz L, Ekman GJ, Vilhelmsson M, *et al.* Antimicrobial peptide LL-37 internalized by immature human dendritic cells alters their phenotype. Scand J Immunol 2006; 63(6): 410-9. [http://dx.doi.org/10.1111/j.1365-3083.2006.001752.x] [PMID: 16764694]

[38] Davidson DJ, Currie AJ, Reid GS, *et al.* The cationic antimicrobial peptide LL-37 modulates dendritic cell differentiation and dendritic cell-induced T cell polarization. J Immunol 2004; 172(2): 1146-56. [http://dx.doi.org/10.4049/jimmunol.172.2.1146] [PMID: 14707090]

[39] Jo E-K. Innate immunity to mycobacteria: vitamin D and autophagy. Cell Microbiol 2010; 12(8): 1026-35. [http://dx.doi.org/10.1111/j.1462-5822.2010.01491.x] [PMID: 20557314]

[40] Soehnlein O, Wantha S, Simsekyilmaz S, *et al.* Neutrophil-Derived Cathelicidin Protects from Neointimal Hyperplasia. Sci Transl Med 2011; 3(3): 103-98. [http://dx.doi.org/10.1126/scitranslmed.3002531]

[41] Steinstraesser L, Koehler T, Jacobsen F, *et al.* Host defense peptides in wound healing. Mol Med 2008; 14(7-8): 528-37. [http://dx.doi.org/10.2119/2008-00002.Steinstraesser] [PMID: 18385817]

[42] Koczulla R, von Degenfeld G, Kupatt C, *et al.* An angiogenic role for the human peptide antibiotic LL-37/hCAP-18. J Clin Invest 2003; 111(11): 1665-72. [http://dx.doi.org/10.1172/JCI17545] [PMID: 12782669]

[43] Li J, Post M, Volk R, *et al.* PR39, a peptide regulator of angiogenesis. Nat Med 2000; 6(1): 49-55. [http://dx.doi.org/10.1038/71527] [PMID: 10613823]

[44] Niyonsaba F, Ushio H, Hara M, *et al.* Antimicrobial peptides human β-defensins and cathelicidin LL-37 induce the secretion of a pruritogenic cytokine IL-31 by human mast cells. J Immunol 2010; 184(7): 3526-34. [http://dx.doi.org/10.4049/jimmunol.0900712] [PMID: 20190140]

[45] Niyonsaba F, Someya A, Hirata M, Ogawa H, Nagaoka I. Evaluation of the effects of peptide antibiotics human β-defensins-1/-2 and LL-37 on histamine release and prostaglandin D(2) production from mast cells. Eur J Immunol 2001; 31(4): 1066-75. [http://dx.doi.org/10.1002/1521-4141(200104)31:4<1066::AID-IMMU1066>3.0.CO;2-#] [PMID: 11298331]

[46] Kin NW, Chen Y, Stefanov EK, Gallo RL, Kearney JF. Cathelin-related antimicrobial peptide differentially regulates T- and B-cell function. Eur J Immunol 2011; 41(10): 3006-16. [http://dx.doi.org/10.1002/eji.201141606] [PMID: 21773974]

[47] Rabin N, Zheng Y, Opoku-Temeng C, Du Y, Bonsu E, Sintim HO. Agents that inhibit bacterial biofilm formation. Future Med Chem 2015; 7(5): 647-71. [http://dx.doi.org/10.4155/fmc.15.7] [PMID: 25921403]

[48] Costerton W, Veeh R, Shirtliff M, Pasmore M, Post C, Ehrlich G. The application of biofilm science to the study and control of chronic bacterial infections. J Clin Invest 2003; 112(10): 1466-77. [http://dx.doi.org/10.1172/JCI200320365] [PMID: 14617746]

[49] Batoni G, Maisetta G, Esin S. Antimicrobial peptides and their interaction with biofilms of medically relevant bacteria. BBA Biomembrane 2016; 1858: 1044-60.

[50] Mataraci E, Dosler S. *In vitro* activities of antibiotics and antimicrobial cationic peptides alone and in combination against methicillin-resistant *Staphylococcus aureus* biofilms. Antimicrob Agents Chemother 2012; 56(12): 6366-71. [http://dx.doi.org/10.1128/AAC.01180-12] [PMID: 23070152]

[51] Jorge P, Lourenço A, Pereira MO. New trends in peptide-based anti-biofilm strategies: a review of recent achievements and bioinformatic approaches. Biofouling 2012; 28(10): 1033-61. [http://dx.doi.org/10.1080/08927014.2012.728210] [PMID: 23016989]

[52] Chen L, Wen YM. The role of bacterial biofilm in persistent infections and control strategies. Int J Oral Sci 2011; 3(2): 66-73. [http://dx.doi.org/10.4248/IJOS11022] [PMID: 21485310]

[53] Batoni G, Maisetta G, Brancatisano FL, Esin S, Campa M. Use of antimicrobial peptides against microbial biofilms: advantages and limits. Curr Med Chem 2011; 18(2): 256-79. [http://dx.doi.org/10.2174/092986711794088399] [PMID: 21110801]

[54] Hancock RE, Patrzykat A. Clinical development of cationic antimicrobial peptides: from natural to novel antibiotics. Curr Drug Targets Infect Disord 2002; 2(1): 79-83. [http://dx.doi.org/10.2174/1568005024605855] [PMID: 12462155]

[55] Gordon YJ, Romanowski EG, McDermott AM. A review of antimicrobial peptides and their therapeutic potential as anti-infective drugs. Curr Eye Res 2005; 30(7): 505-15. [http://dx.doi.org/10.1080/02713680590968637] [PMID: 16020284]

[56] Park S-C, Park Y, Hahm K-S. The role of antimicrobial peptides in preventing multidrug-resistant bacterial infections and biofilm formation. Int J Mol Sci 2011; 12(9): 5971-92. [http://dx.doi.org/10.3390/ijms12095971] [PMID: 22016639]

[57] Tan XW, Goh TW, Saraswathi P, *et al.* Effectiveness of antimicrobial peptide immobilization for preventing perioperative cornea implant-associated bacterial infection. Antimicrob Agents Chemother 2014; 58(9): 5229-38. [http://dx.doi.org/10.1128/AAC.02859-14] [PMID: 24957820]

[58] Marr AK, Gooderham WJ, Hancock RE. Antibacterial peptides for therapeutic use: obstacles and realistic outlook. Curr Opin Pharmacol 2006; 6(5): 468-72. [http://dx.doi.org/10.1016/j.coph.2006.04.006] [PMID: 16890021]

[59] Salditt T, Li C, Spaar A. Structure of antimicrobial peptides and lipid membranes probed by interface-sensitive X-ray scattering. BBA Biomembranes 2006; 1758: 1483-98.

[60] Yeaman MR, Yount NY. Mechanisms of antimicrobial peptide action and resistance. Pharmacol Rev 2003; 55(1): 27-55. [http://dx.doi.org/10.1124/pr.55.1.2] [PMID: 12615953]

[61] Nguyen LT, Haney EF, Vogel HJ. The expanding scope of antimicrobial peptide structures and their modes of action. Trends Biotechnol 2011; 29(9): 464-72. [http://dx.doi.org/10.1016/j.tibtech.2011.05.001] [PMID: 21680034]

[62] Ruiz J, Calderon J, Rondón-Villarreal P, Torres R. Analysis of Structure and Hemolytic Activity Relationships of Antimicrobial Peptides (AMPs). In: Castillo FL, Cristancho M, Isaza G, Pinzón A, Rodríguez CJM, Eds. Proceedings of the 2nd Colombian Congress on Computational Biology and Bioinformatics (CCBCOL). 253-8. [http://dx.doi.org/10.1007/978-3-319-01568-2_36]

[63] Wang Z, Wang G. APD: the Antimicrobial Peptide Database. Nucleic Acids Res 2004; 32(Database issue): D590-2. [http://dx.doi.org/10.1093/nar/gkh025] [PMID: 14681488]

[64] Harris F, Dennison SR, Phoenix DA. Anionic antimicrobial peptides from eukaryotic organisms. Curr Protein Pept Sci 2009; 10(6): 585-606. [http://dx.doi.org/10.2174/138920309789630589] [PMID: 19751192]

[65] Kaushal A, Gupta K, Shah R, van Hoek ML. Antimicrobial activity of mosquito cecropin peptides against Francisella. Dev Comp Immunol 2016; 63: 171-80. [http://dx.doi.org/10.1016/j.dci.2016.05.018] [PMID: 27235883]

[66] Wang G. Human antimicrobial peptides and proteins. Pharmaceuticals (Basel) 2014; 7(5): 545-94. [http://dx.doi.org/10.3390/ph7050545] [PMID: 24828484]

[67] Powers J-P, Hancock RE. The relationship between peptide structure and antibacterial activity. Peptides 2003; 24(11): 1681-91. [http://dx.doi.org/10.1016/j.peptides.2003.08.023] [PMID: 15019199]

[68] Bhattacharjya S, Ramamoorthy A. Multifunctional host defense peptides: functional and mechanistic insights from NMR structures of potent antimicrobial peptides. FEBS J 2009; 276(22): 6465-73. [http://dx.doi.org/10.1111/j.1742-4658.2009.07357.x] [PMID: 19817858]

[69] Zasloff M. Antimicrobial peptides of multicellular organisms. Nature 2002; 415: 389-95.

[70] Haney EF, Hunter HN, Matsuzaki K, Vogel HJ. Solution NMR studies of amphibian antimicrobial peptides: linking structure to function? BBA Biomembranes 2009; 1788: 1639-55.

[71] Haney EF, Nazmi K, Lau F, Bolscher JG, Vogel HJ. Novel lactoferrampin antimicrobial peptides derived from human lactoferrin. Biochimie 2009; 91(1): 141-54. [http://dx.doi.org/10.1016/j.biochi.2008.04.013] [PMID: 18534196]

[72] Takahashi D, Shukla SK, Prakash O, Zhang G. Structural determinants of host defense peptides for antimicrobial activity and target cell selectivity. Biochimie 2010; 92(9): 1236-41. [http://dx.doi.org/10.1016/j.biochi.2010.02.023] [PMID: 20188791]

[73] Zelezetsky I, Tossi A. Alpha-helical antimicrobial peptides-using a sequence template to guide structure–activity relationship studies. BBA Biomembranes 2006; 1758: 1436-49.

[74] Dathe M, Wieprecht T. Structural features of helical antimicrobial peptides: their potential to modulate activity on model membranes and biological cells. Biochim Biophys Acta 1999; 1462(1-2): 71-87. [http://dx.doi.org/10.1016/S0005-2736(99)00201-1] [PMID: 10590303]

[75] Zhang L, Benz R, Hancock RE. Influence of proline residues on the antibacterial and synergistic activities of α-helical peptides. Biochemistry 1999; 38(25): 8102-11. [http://dx.doi.org/10.1021/bi9904104] [PMID: 10387056]

[76] Lohner K. New strategies for novel antibiotics: peptides targeting bacterial cell membranes. Gen Physiol Biophys 2009; 28(2): 105-16. [http://dx.doi.org/10.4149/gpb_2009_02_105] [PMID: 19592707]

[77] Holt A, Killian JA. Orientation and dynamics of transmembrane peptides: the power of simple models. Eur Biophys J 2010; 39(4): 609-21. [http://dx.doi.org/10.1007/s00249-009-0567-1] [PMID: 20020122]

[78] Ramadurai S, Holt A, Schäfer LV, *et al.* Influence of hydrophobic mismatch and amino acid composition on the lateral diffusion of transmembrane peptides. Biophys J 2010; 99(5): 1447-54. [http://dx.doi.org/10.1016/j.bpj.2010.05.042] [PMID: 20816056]

[79] Wimley WC. Describing the mechanism of antimicrobial peptide action with the interfacial activity model. ACS Chem Biol 2010; 5(10): 905-17. [http://dx.doi.org/10.1021/cb1001558] [PMID: 20698568]

[80] Brogden KA. Antimicrobial peptides: pore formers or metabolic inhibitors in bacteria? Nat Rev Microbiol 2005; 3(3): 238-50. [http://dx.doi.org/10.1038/nrmicro1098] [PMID: 15703760]

[81] van Kan EJ, Demel RA, Breukink E, van der Bent A, de Kruijff B. Clavanin permeabilizes target membranes *via* two distinctly different pH-dependent mechanisms. Biochemistry 2002; 41(24): 7529-39. [http://dx.doi.org/10.1021/bi012162t] [PMID: 12056883]

[82] Nicolas P. Multifunctional host defense peptides: intracellular-targeting antimicrobial peptides. FEBS J 2009; 276(22): 6483-96. [http://dx.doi.org/10.1111/j.1742-4658.2009.07359.x] [PMID: 19817856]

[83] Fleming E, Maharaj NP, Chen JL, Nelson RB, Elmore DE. Effect of lipid composition on buforin II structure and membrane entry. Proteins 2008; 73(2): 480-91. [http://dx.doi.org/10.1002/prot.22074] [PMID: 18452210]

[84] Lan Y, Ye Y, Kozlowska J, Lam JK, Drake AF, Mason AJ. Structural contributions to the intracellular targeting strategies of antimicrobial peptides. BBA Biomembranes 2010; 1798: 1934-43.

[85] Gifford JL, Hunter HN, Vogel HJ. Lactoferricin: a lactoferrin-derived peptide with antimicrobial, antiviral, antitumor and immunological properties. Cell Mol Life Sci 2005; 62(22): 2588-98. [http://dx.doi.org/10.1007/s00018-005-5373-z] [PMID: 16261252]

[86] Srinivas N, Jetter P, Ueberbacher BJ, *et al.* Peptidomimetic antibiotics target outer-membrane

biogenesis in *Pseudomonas aeruginosa.* Science 2010; 327(5968): 1010-3. [http://dx.doi.org/10.1126/science.1182749] [PMID: 20167788]

[87] Sass V, Schneider T, Wilmes M, *et al.* Human β-defensin 3 inhibits cell wall biosynthesis in *Staphylococci.* Infect Immun 2010; 78(6): 2793-800. [http://dx.doi.org/10.1128/IAI.00688-09] [PMID: 20385753]

[88] Doherty T, Waring AJ, Hong M. Dynamic structure of disulfide-removed linear analogs of tachyplesin-I in the lipid bilayer from solid-state NMR. Biochemistry 2008; 47(4): 1105-16. [http://dx.doi.org/10.1021/bi701390t] [PMID: 18163648]

[89] Wu Z, Hoover DM, Yang D, *et al.* Engineering disulfide bridges to dissect antimicrobial and chemotactic activities of human β-defensin 3. Proc Natl Acad Sci USA 2003; 100(15): 8880-5. [http://dx.doi.org/10.1073/pnas.1533186100] [PMID: 12840147]

[90] Luque-Ortega JR, van't Hof W, Veerman EC, Saugar JM, Rivas L. Human antimicrobial peptide histatin 5 is a cell-penetrating peptide targeting mitochondrial ATP synthesis in Leishmania. FASEB J 2008; 22(6): 1817-28. [http://dx.doi.org/10.1096/fj.07-096081] [PMID: 18230684]

[91] Chan DI, Prenner EJ, Vogel HJ. Tryptophan-and arginine-rich antimicrobial peptides: structures and mechanisms of action. BBA Biomembranes 2006; 1758: 1184-202.

[92] Schibli DJ, Nguyen LT, Kernaghan SD, Rekdal Ø, Vogel HJ. Structure-function analysis of tritrpticin analogs: potential relationships between antimicrobial activities, model membrane interactions, and their micelle-bound NMR structures. Biophys J 2006; 91(12): 4413-26. [http://dx.doi.org/10.1529/biophysj.106.085837] [PMID: 16997878]

[93] Melo MN, Dugourd D, Castanho MA. Omiganan pentahydrochloride in the front line of clinical applications of antimicrobial peptides. Recent Pat Antiinfect Drug Discov 2006; 1(2): 201-7. [http://dx.doi.org/10.2174/157489106777452638] [PMID: 18221145]

[94] Rokitskaya TI, Kolodkin NI, Kotova EA, Antonenko YN. Indolicidin action on membrane permeability: carrier mechanism versus pore formation. BBA Biomembranes 2011; 1808: 91-7.

[95] Mattila J-P, Sabatini K, Kinnunen PK. Oxidized phospholipids as potential molecular targets for antimicrobial peptides. BBA Biomembranes 2008; 1778: 2041-50.

[96] Marchand C, Krajewski K, Lee H-F, *et al.* Covalent binding of the natural antimicrobial peptide indolicidin to DNA abasic sites. Nucleic Acids Res 2006; 34(18): 5157-65. [http://dx.doi.org/10.1093/nar/gkl667] [PMID: 16998183]

[97] Pletzer D, Hancock RE. Anti-biofilm peptides: Potential as broad-spectrum agents. J Bacteriol 2016; 00017-6.

[98] Hu Y, Li X, Sebti SM, Chen J, Cai J. Design and synthesis of AApeptides: a new class of peptide mimics. Bioorg Med Chem Lett 2011; 21(5): 1469-71. [http://dx.doi.org/10.1016/j.bmcl.2011.01.005] [PMID: 21292484]

[99] Niu Y, Wu H, Li Y, *et al.* AApeptides as a new class of antimicrobial agents. Org Biomol Chem 2013; 11(26): 4283-90. [http://dx.doi.org/10.1039/c3ob40444g] [PMID: 23722277]

[100] Méndez-Samperio P. Peptidomimetics as a new generation of antimicrobial agents: current progress. Infect Drug Resist 2014; 7: 229-37. [http://dx.doi.org/10.2147/IDR.S49229] [PMID: 25210467]

[101] Niu Y, Hu Y, Wu H, Cai J. Synthesis of AApeptides. Peptide Modifications to Increase Metabolic Stability and Activity. 2013; 1081: pp. 35-46. [http://dx.doi.org/10.1007/978-1-62703-652-8_3]

[102] Niu Y, Padhee S, Wu H, *et al.* Identification of γ-AApeptides with potent and broad-spectrum antimicrobial activity. Chem Commun (Camb) 2011; 47(44): 12197-9.

[http://dx.doi.org/10.1039/c1cc14476f] [PMID: 21963627]

[103] Barbu EM, Shirazi F, McGrath DM, *et al.* An antimicrobial peptidomimetic induces Mucorales cell death through mitochondria-mediated apoptosis. PLoS One 2013; 8(10): e76981. [http://dx.doi.org/10.1371/journal.pone.0076981] [PMID: 24098573]

[104] Zelezetsky I, Tossi A. Alpha-helical antimicrobial peptides-Using a sequence template to guide structure–activity relationship studies. BBA Biomembranes 2006; 1758: 1436-49.

[105] Ganz T. Defensins: antimicrobial peptides of innate immunity. Nat Rev Immunol 2003; 3(9): 710-20. [http://dx.doi.org/10.1038/nri1180] [PMID: 12949495]

[106] Matsuzaki K. Why and how are peptide-lipid interactions utilized for self-defense? Magainins and tachyplesins as archetypes. Biochim Biophys Acta 1999; 1462(1-2): 1-10. [http://dx.doi.org/10.1016/S0005-2736(99)00197-2] [PMID: 10590299]

[107] Chen L, Gao L, Fang W, Golubovic L. How the Antimicrobial Peptides Kill Bacteria: Computational Physics Insights. Commun Comput Phys 2012; 11: 709-25. [http://dx.doi.org/10.4208/cicp.071210.240511a]

[108] Melo MN, Ferre R, Castanho MA. Antimicrobial peptides: linking partition, activity and high membrane-bound concentrations. Nat Rev Microbiol 2009; 7(3): 245-50. [http://dx.doi.org/10.1038/nrmicro2095] [PMID: 19219054]

[109] Holaskova E, Galuszka P, Frebort I, Oz MT. Antimicrobial peptide production and plant-based expression systems for medical and agricultural biotechnology. Biotechnol Adv 2015; 33(6 Pt 2): 1005-23. [http://dx.doi.org/10.1016/j.biotechadv.2015.03.007] [PMID: 25784148]

[110] Guilhelmelli F, Vilela N, Albuquerque P, Derengowski LdaS, Silva-Pereira I, Kyaw CM. Antibiotic development challenges: the various mechanisms of action of antimicrobial peptides and of bacterial resistance. Front Microbiol 2013; 4: 353. [http://dx.doi.org/10.3389/fmicb.2013.00353] [PMID: 24367355]

[111] Bechinger B. Detergent-like properties of magainin antibiotic peptides: a 31P solid-state NMR spectroscopy study. Biochim Biophys Acta 2005; 1712: 101-8.

[112] Bolintineanu DS, Kaznessis YN. Computational studies of protegrin antimicrobial peptides: a review. Peptides 2011; 32(1): 188-201. [http://dx.doi.org/10.1016/j.peptides.2010.10.006] [PMID: 20946928]

[113] Pouny Y, Rapaport D, Mor A, Nicolas P, Shai Y. Interaction of antimicrobial dermaseptin and its fluorescently labeled analogues with phospholipid membranes. Biochemistry 1992; 31(49): 12416-23. [http://dx.doi.org/10.1021/bi00164a017] [PMID: 1463728]

[114] Chen F-Y, Lee M-T, Huang HW. Evidence for membrane thinning effect as the mechanism for peptide-induced pore formation. Biophys J 2003; 84(6): 3751-8. [http://dx.doi.org/10.1016/S0006-3495(03)75103-0] [PMID: 12770881]

[115] Ludtke S, He K, Huang H. Membrane thinning caused by magainin 2. Biochemistry 1995; 34(51): 16764-9. [http://dx.doi.org/10.1021/bi00051a026] [PMID: 8527451]

[116] Mecke A, Lee DK, Ramamoorthy A, Orr BG, Banaszak Holl MM. Membrane thinning due to antimicrobial peptide binding: an atomic force microscopy study of MSI-78 in lipid bilayers. Biophys J 2005; 89(6): 4043-50. [http://dx.doi.org/10.1529/biophysj.105.062596] [PMID: 16183881]

[117] Matsuzaki K. Magainins as paradigm for the mode of action of pore forming polypeptides. Biochim Biophys Acta 1998; 1376(3): 391-400. [http://dx.doi.org/10.1016/S0304-4157(98)00014-8] [PMID: 9804997]

[118] Matsuzaki K, Murase O, Fujii N, Miyajima K. An antimicrobial peptide, magainin 2, induced rapid

flip-flop of phospholipids coupled with pore formation and peptide translocation. Biochemistry 1996; 35(35): 11361-8.
[http://dx.doi.org/10.1021/bi960016v] [PMID: 8784191]

[119] Wu M, Maier E, Benz R, Hancock RE. Mechanism of interaction of different classes of cationic antimicrobial peptides with planar bilayers and with the cytoplasmic membrane of *Escherichia coli.* Biochemistry 1999; 38(22): 7235-42.
[http://dx.doi.org/10.1021/bi9826299] [PMID: 10353835]

[120] Viljanen P, Vaara M. Susceptibility of gram-negative bacteria to polymyxin B nonapeptide. Antimicrob Agents Chemother 1984; 25(6): 701-5.
[http://dx.doi.org/10.1128/AAC.25.6.701] [PMID: 6331296]

[121] Manniello JM, Heymann H, Adair FW. Resistance of spheroplasts and whole cells of *Pseudomonas cepacia* to polymyxin B. Antimicrob Agents Chemother 1978; 14(3): 500-4.
[http://dx.doi.org/10.1128/AAC.14.3.500] [PMID: 213017]

[122] Friedrich C, Scott MG, Karunaratne N, Yan H, Hancock RE. Salt-resistant alpha-helical cationic antimicrobial peptides. Antimicrob Agents Chemother 1999; 43(7): 1542-8.
[PMID: 10390200]

[123] Nahaie MR, Goodfellow M, Minnikin DE, Hájek V. Polar lipid and isoprenoid quinone composition in the classification of *Staphylococcus*. J Gen Microbiol 1984; 130(9): 2427-37.
[PMID: 6502136]

[124] Fields PI, Groisman EA, Heffron F. A Salmonella locus that controls resistance to microbicidal proteins from phagocytic cells. Science 1989; 243(4894 Pt 1): 1059-62.
[http://dx.doi.org/10.1126/science.2646710] [PMID: 2646710]

[125] Oh J-T, Cajal Y, Dhurjati PS, Van Dyk TK, Jain MK. Cecropins induce the hyperosmotic stress response in *Escherichia coli.* Biochim Biophys Acta 1998; 1415(1): 235-45.
[http://dx.doi.org/10.1016/S0005-2736(98)00195-3] [PMID: 9858741]

[126] Hong RW, Shchepetov M, Weiser JN, Axelsen PH. Transcriptional profile of the *Escherichia coli* response to the antimicrobial insect peptide cecropin A. Antimicrob Agents Chemother 2003; 47(1): 1-6.
[http://dx.doi.org/10.1128/AAC.47.1.1-6.2003] [PMID: 12499161]

[127] Groisman EA. The pleiotropic two-component regulatory system PhoP-PhoQ. J Bacteriol 2001; 183(6): 1835-42.
[http://dx.doi.org/10.1128/JB.183.6.1835-1842.2001] [PMID: 11222580]

[128] Kier LD, Weppelman RM, Ames BN. Regulation of nonspecific acid phosphatase in *Salmonella*: phoN and phoP genes. J Bacteriol 1979; 138(1): 155-61.
[PMID: 374361]

[129] Gunn JS, Miller SI. PhoP-PhoQ activates transcription of pmrAB, encoding a two-component regulatory system involved in *Salmonella typhimurium* antimicrobial peptide resistance. J Bacteriol 1996; 178(23): 6857-64.
[http://dx.doi.org/10.1128/jb.178.23.6857-6864.1996] [PMID: 8955307]

[130] Gunn JS, Lim KB, Krueger J, *et al.* PmrA-PmrB-regulated genes necessary for 4-aminoarabinose lipid A modification and polymyxin resistance. Mol Microbiol 1998; 27(6): 1171-82.
[http://dx.doi.org/10.1046/j.1365-2958.1998.00757.x] [PMID: 9570402]

[131] Guina T, Yi EC, Wang H, Hackett M, Miller SI. A PhoP-regulated outer membrane protease of Salmonella enterica serovar typhimurium promotes resistance to alpha-helical antimicrobial peptides. J Bacteriol 2000; 182(14): 4077-86.
[http://dx.doi.org/10.1128/JB.182.14.4077-4086.2000] [PMID: 10869088]

[132] Sugimura K, Nishihara T. Purification, characterization, and primary structure of *Escherichia coli* protease VII with specificity for paired basic residues: identity of protease VII and OmpT. J Bacteriol

1988; 170(12): 5625-32.
[http://dx.doi.org/10.1128/jb.170.12.5625-5632.1988] [PMID: 3056908]

[133] Stumpe S, Bakker EP. Requirement of a large K+-uptake capacity and of extracytoplasmic protease activity for protamine resistance of *Escherichia coli.* Arch Microbiol 1997; 167: 126-36.
[http://dx.doi.org/10.1007/s002030050425]

[134] Dorrer E, Teuber M. Induction of polymyxin resistance in *Pseudomonas fluorescens* by phosphate limitation. Arch Microbiol 1977; 114(1): 87-9.
[http://dx.doi.org/10.1007/BF00429636] [PMID: 199125]

[135] Tang Y-Q, Yeaman MR, Selsted ME. Antimicrobial peptides from human platelets. Infect Immun 2002; 70(12): 6524-33.
[http://dx.doi.org/10.1128/IAI.70.12.6524-6533.2002] [PMID: 12438321]

[136] Bent AF, Mackey D. Elicitors, effectors, and R genes: the new paradigm and a lifetime supply of questions. Annu Rev Phytopathol 2007; 45: 399-436.
[http://dx.doi.org/10.1146/annurev.phyto.45.062806.094427] [PMID: 17506648]

[137] Faye T, Brede DA, Langsrud T, Nes IF, Holo H. An antimicrobial peptide is produced by extracellular processing of a protein from *Propionibacterium jensenii.* J Bacteriol 2002; 184(13): 3649-56.
[http://dx.doi.org/10.1128/JB.184.13.3649-3656.2002] [PMID: 12057960]

[138] Yevtushenko DP, Misra S. Transgenic Expression of Antimicrobial Peptides in Plants: Strategies for Enhanced Disease Resistance, Improved Productivity, and Production of Therapeutics. Small Wonders: Peptides for Disease Control: Am Chem Soc. 2012; pp. 445-58.

[139] Nawrot R, Barylski J, Nowicki G, Broniarczyk J, Buchwald W, Goździcka-Józefiak A. Plant antimicrobial peptides. Folia Microbiol (Praha) 2014; 59(3): 181-96.
[http://dx.doi.org/10.1007/s12223-013-0280-4] [PMID: 24092498]

[140] Simmaco M, Mignogna G, Barra D. Antimicrobial peptides from amphibian skin: what do they tell us? Biopolymers 1998; 47(6): 435-50.
[http://dx.doi.org/10.1002/(SICI)1097-0282(1998)47:6<435::AID-BIP3>3.0.CO;2-8] [PMID: 10333736]

[141] Bahar AA, Ren D. Antimicrobial peptides. Pharmaceuticals (Basel) 2013; 6(12): 1543-75.
[http://dx.doi.org/10.3390/ph6121543] [PMID: 24287494]

[142] Andersons D, Engström A, Josephson S, Hansson L, Steiner H. Biologically active and amidated cecropin produced in a baculovirus expression system from a fusion construct containing the antibody-binding part of protein A. Biochem J 1991; 280(Pt 1): 219-24.
[http://dx.doi.org/10.1042/bj2800219] [PMID: 1720614]

[143] Reichhart J-M, Petit I, Legrain M, *et al.* Expression and secretion in yeast of active insect defensin, an inducible antibacterial peptide from the fleshfly Phormia terranovae. Invertebr Reprod Dev 1992; 21: 15-24.
[http://dx.doi.org/10.1080/07924259.1992.9672215]

[144] Cipáková I, Hostinová E, Gasperík J, Velebný V. High-level expression and purification of a recombinant hBD-1 fused to LMM protein in *Escherichia coli.* Protein Expr Purif 2004; 37(1): 207-12.
[http://dx.doi.org/10.1016/j.pep.2004.04.024] [PMID: 15294300]

[145] Hwang SW, Lee JH, Park HB, *et al.* A simple method for the purification of an antimicrobial peptide in recombinant *Escherichia coli.* Mol Biotechnol 2001; 18(3): 193-8.
[http://dx.doi.org/10.1385/MB:18:3:193] [PMID: 11503514]

[146] Zhang L, Falla T, Wu M, *et al.* Determinants of recombinant production of antimicrobial cationic peptides and creation of peptide variants in bacteria. Biochem Biophys Res Commun 1998; 247(3): 674-80.
[http://dx.doi.org/10.1006/bbrc.1998.8848] [PMID: 9647752]

[147] Jang SA, Sung BH, Cho JH, Kim SC. Direct expression of antimicrobial peptides in an intact form by a translationally coupled two-cistron expression system. Appl Environ Microbiol 2009; 75(12): 3980-6.
[http://dx.doi.org/10.1128/AEM.02753-08] [PMID: 19363064]

[148] Ingham AB, Moore RJ. Recombinant production of antimicrobial peptides in heterologous microbial systems. Biotechnol Appl Biochem 2007; 47(Pt 1): 1-9.
[http://dx.doi.org/10.1042/BA20060207] [PMID: 17432953]

[149] Kim JM, Jang SA, Yu BJ, Sung BH, Cho JH, Kim SC. High-level expression of an antimicrobial peptide histonin as a natural form by multimerization and furin-mediated cleavage. Appl Microbiol Biotechnol 2008; 78(1): 123-30.
[http://dx.doi.org/10.1007/s00253-007-1273-5] [PMID: 18094965]

[150] Zorko M, Japelj B, Hafner-Bratkovič I, Jerala R. Expression, purification and structural studies of a short antimicrobial peptide. BBA Biomembranes 2009; 1788: 314-23.

[151] Li C, Blencke H-M, Paulsen V, Haug T, Stensvåg K. Powerful workhorses for antimicrobial peptide expression and characterization. Bioeng Bugs 2010; 1(3): 217-20.
[http://dx.doi.org/10.4161/bbug.1.3.11721] [PMID: 21326929]

[152] Cipáková I, Gasperík J, Hostinová E. Expression and purification of human antimicrobial peptide, dermcidin, in *Escherichia coli.* Protein Expr Purif 2006; 45(2): 269-74.
[http://dx.doi.org/10.1016/j.pep.2005.07.002] [PMID: 16125410]

[153] Hara S, Yamakawa M. Production in *Escherichia* of moricin, a novel type antibacterial peptide from the silkworm, Bombyx mori. Biochem Biophys Res Commun 1996; 220(3): 664-9.
[http://dx.doi.org/10.1006/bbrc.1996.0461] [PMID: 8607822]

[154] Xu Z, Peng L, Zhong Z, Fang X, Cen P. High-level expression of a soluble functional antimicrobial peptide, human beta-defensin 2, in *Escherichia coli.* Biotechnol Prog 2006; 22(2): 382-6.
[http://dx.doi.org/10.1021/bp0502680] [PMID: 16599550]

[155] Lee JH, Minn I, Park CB, Kim SC. Acidic peptide-mediated expression of the antimicrobial peptide buforin II as tandem repeats in *Escherichia coli.* Protein Expr Purif 1998; 12(1): 53-60.
[http://dx.doi.org/10.1006/prep.1997.0814] [PMID: 9473457]

[156] Levy SB, Marshall B. Antibacterial resistance worldwide: causes, challenges and responses. Nat Med 2004; 10(12) (Suppl.): S122-9.
[http://dx.doi.org/10.1038/nm1145] [PMID: 15577930]

SUBJECT INDEX

A

B

C

D

E

F

G

H

I

P

Q

R

S

Made in the USA
Las Vegas, NV
03 November 2026

57425096R00326